Community-Based Nursing

Community-Based Nursing

AN INTRODUCTION

Melanie McEwen, RN, PhD, CS
Baylor University
School of Nursing
Dallas, Texas

W.B. Saunders Company
A Division of Harcourt Brace & Company
Philadelphia London Toronto Montreal Sydney Tokyo

W.B. SAUNDERS COMPANY
A Division of Harcourt Brace & Company

The Curtis Center
Independence Square West
Philadelphia, Pennsylvania 19106

Library of Congress Cataloging-in-Publication Data

McEwen, Melanie.
Community-based nursing: an introduction/Melanie McEwen.—1st ed.

p. cm.

ISBN 0–7216–6109–2

1. Community health nursing.
[DNLM: 1. Community Health Nursing. WY 106 M478c 1998]

RT98.M3 1998 610.73′43—dc21

DNLM/DLC 97-41326

COMMUNITY-BASED NURSING: AN INTRODUCTION ISBN 0–7216–6109–2

Printed in the United States of America.

Last digit is the print number: 9 8 7 6 5 4 3 2 1

Preface

No one disputes that the health care delivery system in the United States has changed rapidly. Cost containment measures, technology, and political decisions have altered *how* health care is provided, *who* is responsible for care delivery, *what* care is provided, and *when* clients are seen. One of the most significant changes, however, has been *where* care is given.

No longer is the hospital the central site for health care. Health care today is being provided in community-based settings such as homes, schools, clinics, offices, churches, and work sites, and even over the telephone. Correspondingly, there is a need for nurses prepared to practice in those settings. Therefore, nursing education must include course content and clinical experiences.

Community-Based Nursing: An Introduction is written to be both a core and a supplemental textbook for nursing students who have an opportunity to deliver nursing care to clients in community-based settings. It can be the first text a student studies, or it can be used throughout a program to bring other texts up to date in concept. The purpose of this book is to introduce community-based practice to nursing students in 2-, 3-, and 4-year programs.

Organization

Community-Based Nursing: An Introduction brings together the essential information for nurses practicing in community settings. It includes content "hidden" in the major nursing textbooks that cover related material, information that may not be included in other resources, and content found in other books but presented from a different perspective.

For example, Chapter 2 discusses roles and interventions emphasized in community-based nursing care and how they differ from roles and interventions in acute care settings. Chapter 3 gives an overview of the health care delivery system designed to help the reader understand *why* health care is becoming increasingly community based. Chapter 6 explores cultural influences on health and health care–seeking behaviors.

Likewise, Chapter 12 discusses care of infants, children, and teenagers. Here, focus is on health promotion and illness prevention. Information for community-based nursing care includes nutrition needs, growth and development guidelines, immunization schedules, and suggested screenings. This chapter also discusses care of children with minor acute episodic illnesses usually managed at home, such as gastroenteritis, chicken pox, strep throat, or pediculosis (head lice). In pediatric nursing textbooks, these topics are discussed from an acute care perspective, and the information may be difficult to apply in community settings. This book presents the material in a format that emphasizes teaching and care by the family.

The textbook is divided into five units and subdivided into two to four chapters per unit. Unit I outlines changes in settings for provision of health care and corresponding opportunities for nurses to practice within the changing system. It also includes information on roles and interventions used by nurses working in community settings and how they might differ from those of nursing in hospitals.

Unit II presents information on factors that influence health and health care. Chapter topics are the health care delivery system, how epidemiology affects nursing practice, environmental health issues, and cultural influences.

Unit III describes "traditional" settings for community-based nursing care. Because of the increasing importance of home health nursing in the delivery of care, three chapters are devoted to it. Chapter 7 provides an overview of home health nursing, Chapter 8 walks the reader through the *process* of home health nursing, and Chapter 9 covers a number of areas of specialization in home health care, including intravenous therapy, enterostomal care, and caring for clients with special needs (e.g., high-risk perinatal care, postpartum care, and caring for individuals with mental illnesses) in their homes.

Nursing in a variety of ambulatory settings is described in Chapter 10. This chapter covers such topics as public health nursing; parish nursing; school nursing; and working in clinics, physicians' offices, and outpatient surgery centers.

Unit IV provides detailed information on health promotion; care of clients with acute conditions; and care of clients with chronic conditions, including children, adults, and older adults, in community-based settings. Issues in women's health care are also described.

Unit V details special needs encountered in community practice, including prevention and management of communicable disease in general, which is described in Chapter 15. Chapter 16 focuses on community-based strategies for prevention of human immunodeficiency virus infection and community-based care of persons who have been infected. Finally, Chapter 17 describes strategies for promotion of mental health and identification and management of threats to mental health and management of mental illness.

This book includes material that will help direct nursing students in community-based practice, whatever the setting and whoever the population being served. For example, if the student is working with a home health care nurse providing skilled nursing services for older adults in their home, helpful content would be found in Chapters 7, 8, and 14. If the student is working in an elementary school, the section in Chapter 10 describing school nursing, as well as information in Chapter 13, will be beneficial. Or, if the student is working in a women's clinic, appropriate information is found in Chapter 12 and possibly in Chapters 15 and 16 (sexually transmitted diseases and human immunodeficiency virus and acquired immunodeficiency syndrome, respectively).

Much of the content of this book focuses on material that should be part of client education (e.g., smoking cessation guidelines, how to bathe a newborn, fall prevention measures for elders); guidelines for health promotion and illness prevention for all age groups (e.g., immunizations, screenings, risk identification); how to identify, intervene in, and refer for a variety of health problems and health threats in a variety of settings; and description, elaboration, and simplification of content the student needs to become community focused (e.g., cultural issues, the health care delivery system, and epidemiology). Because of the breadth of the content and practical method of its presentation, this book will be useful from the first day of nursing school through the first years of transition practice—no matter what the setting.

Acknowledgments

I would like to thank Ilze Rader (formerly a Senior Editor for W.B. Saunders Company) for her vision, understanding, and patience throughout the process of writing this book. In addition, thanks to Rachel Hubbs for her persistence and focus in its development.

I would like to acknowledge the following reviewers for their help in developing this text: Alyce Smithson Ashcraft, RN, MSN, Blinn College, Bryan, Texas; Frances M. Hammerly, RNCS, MSN, Stark State College of Technology, Canton, Ohio; Charlotte H. Mackey, RN, MSN, Eastern College, Elyria, Ohio; and Betty L. Whigham, RN, MEd, ARNP, Hillsborough Community College, Tampa, Florida.

I also want to thank the staff and faculty at Baylor University School of Nursing for their support and encouragement. In particular, thanks to those working in the LRC for allowing me to keep books and other resources for months at a time and for helping me acquire obscure reference materials (you guys are amazing).

Finally, much appreciation, gratitude, respect, and love go to my husband, Scott, for his many hours of help; for keeping me supplied with the latest computer gadgetry; for responding immediately whenever the computer would crash or "eat" my work; and for putting up with the horrible mess I made of his office. Scott, I *truly* could not have done it without you.

Melanie McEwen

Contents

NOTICE

Community Health Nursing is an ever-changing field. Standard safety precautions must be followed, but as new research and clinical experience broaden our knowledge, changes in treatment and drug therapy become necessary or appropriate. Readers are advised to check the product information currently provided by the manufacturer of each drug to be administered to verify the recommended dose, the method and duration of administration, and contraindications. It is the responsibility of the treating physician relying on experience and knowledge of the patient to determine dosages and the best treatment for the patient. Neither the publisher nor the editor assumes any responsibility for any injury and/or damage to persons or property.

THE PUBLISHER

UNIT

I

Introduction to Community-Based Nursing Practice

1

Opportunities in Community-Based Nursing Practice

Case Study

Martha McDonald will complete her nursing program and take the National Council Licensure Examination (NCLEX) in 3 months. Although she has enjoyed nursing school, Martha can't wait to graduate and begin her new career. Anticipating graduation, she has begun the process of looking for employment and has been somewhat surprised and concerned by her findings.

For the past year, Martha has worked three or four evenings each week as a "student nurse tech" on a general medical floor of a large, nonprofit hospital. Through conversations at work and at school, she is aware that nursing positions in area hospitals are becoming increasingly scarce, and there are rumors that jobs will be difficult to find for her graduating class. Indeed, the hospital where she works closed a floor 6 months ago, and although no nurses were laid off at the time, there were changes in scheduling and a dramatic reduction in overtime for all nursing personnel. Martha has since learned that reduction in numbers of hospital beds and "downsizing" have become a national trend.

Martha began her job search by reviewing the employment classified advertisements in the local Sunday paper. Surprisingly, many of the ads for Registered Nurses (RNs) were in the areas of home health nursing, case management, and managed care groups, such as health maintenance organizations (HMOs). In addition, there were opportunities for RNs to work in nursing homes and a variety of outpatient settings, such as day surgery centers and minor emergency or primary care clinics.

Martha then discussed employment opportunities with the job placement office and several of her nursing instructors. She was encouraged to discover that although nursing jobs in acute care institutions were not as commonplace as during the last decade, there were many other avenues to explore. After a month of interviews and weighing options, Martha chose a position as a staff nurse in a geriatric clinic affiliated with one of the large nonprofit health care organizations in her city.

Regardless of what happens in Congress at the federal level, health care reform has already begun. Cost-consciousness among insurers at all levels has mandated massive alterations in health care delivery. This has resulted in the phenomenal decrease in average length of hospital stays for virtually all illnesses and procedures. No one argues that patients are being discharged "sicker and quicker" now than in the past. Additionally, there is (finally and thankfully) increasing emphasis on health promotion and illness prevention throughout society, with recognition of the impact of lifestyle choices and behavior on individual and aggregate health. There is little doubt that health care delivery is moving from an acute care focus, and hospital-based delivery of care, to illness prevention and management and community-based delivery of care. As a result, hospitals are reducing capacity and downsizing, becoming specialized or closing altogether. This, in turn, has resulted in loss of employment for many nurses in acute care settings.

That is the "bad news"; now for the "good news." For jobs lost in the hospital, jobs are created in community-based settings, whether in home care, HMOs, clinics, or "other." Nurses, therefore, must be equipped to make the transition.

In a position statement on the future of nursing education, the National League for Nursing (NLN) (1993) focused on the importance of moving much of the content and clinical focus in nursing education from acute care settings into community settings. Nursing educators, including both associate and baccalaureate degree holders, have recognized the trends in health care and understand the need to incorporate community-based nursing concepts and clinical experiences into curricula. In baccalaureate programs, this often means expansion or integration of community content and clinical experiences throughout programs rather than confining them to the study of "community health nursing" near the end of the program, where they have been traditionally.

Associate degree nursing programs have also recently acknowledged the need to include community-based experiences and related content. In October 1994, the NLN Council of Associate Degree Programs (NLN/CADP) held a national video conference to discuss the "examination of opportunities for clinical learning available in community-based settings and the potential role of the associate degree nurse in these settings" (p. 1). The discussions from this conference underscored the need to promote community-based clinical opportunities and offered a number of suggestions for settings and learning experiences for students pursuing an Associate Degree of Nursing (ADN). Tagliareni and Murray (1995) agreed, stating that the "next step in curricular reform". . . is to include . . . "community-based experiences in the AD curriculum" (p. 366).

Community-Based Health Care and Nursing Practice

Nursing's Agenda for Health Care Reform (known as *Nursing's Agenda*) (1991) was composed in response to the expansive debate on health care reform, health care delivery, health care financing, and increasing emphasis on health promotion and illness prevention. *Nursing's Agenda* was the result of a combined effort of the American Nurses' Association (ANA) and the NLN to improve access to health care for all individuals. Following its publication in late 1991, *Nursing's Agenda* was quickly endorsed by more than 60 nursing and health care organizations (Meierhoffer, 1992). Table 1–1 summarizes this document.

As described in *Nursing's Agenda*, the "cornerstone of nursing's plan for reform is the delivery of primary health care services to households and individuals in convenient, familiar places" (ANA, 1991, p. 9). Homes, work sites, schools, churches, and neighborhood clinics are among the settings suggested to serve as "convenient familiar places" to enhance the delivery of preventive, systematic, and comprehensive health care. The emphasis on health care delivery in community-based settings has moved beyond *primary* health care (prevention activities, such as well child check-ups, routine physical examinations, prenatal care and diagnosis, and treatment of common acute or episodic illnesses), however, and now encompasses secondary and tertiary care.

Secondary health care typically refers to relatively serious or complicated care that has histori-

TABLE 1–1 Components of *Nursing's Agenda for Health Care Reform*

- Restructured health care system, including enhanced access to services delivering primary care in community-based settings, promotion of consumer responsibility for personal health and informed decision-making, and focus on utilizing the most cost-effective providers and therapeutic options
- Federally defined and financed standard package of essential health services available to all United States citizens and residents, including "essential services" coverage for children, pregnant women, and "vulnerable" populations
- Planned change in anticipation of health service needs to correlate with demographics
- Steps to reduce costs, including encouragement of managed care, controlled growth of the health care system through planning and resource allocation, incentives for consumers and providers to be cost-efficient, development of health care policies based on outcomes research, assurance of direct access to a full range of qualified providers, and elimination of bureaucratic controls and administrative procedures
- Case management for persons with continuing health needs
- Provision for long-term care
- Insurance reform to ensure improved access to coverage
- Establishment of public and private sector review to determine resource allocation, allowable insurance premiums, and consistent reimbursement for all levels of providers

Data from American Nurses' Association. (1991). *Nursing's Agenda for Health Care Reform.* Washington, D. C., American Nurses' Association.

cally been provided to patients in hospitals. However, recent changes in techniques, procedures, and medical practice have moved much of secondary health care into community settings. Examples of community-based secondary health care include

- Outpatient surgery for several serious conditions that would have required hospitalization just a few years ago (e.g., cholecystectomy, hysterectomy, appendectomy, herniorrhaphy)
- Treatment of serious illnesses (e.g., chemotherapy, radiotherapy)
- A wide variety of diagnostic testing procedures (e.g., computed tomography, magnetic resonance imaging, angiography)

Similarly, *tertiary* care (management of chronic, complicated, long-term health problems) is now frequently delivered in community settings. Rehabilitation centers for clients with neurologic conditions (e.g., spinal cord injuries, multiple sclerosis, amyotropic lateral sclerosis), centers for cardiac rehabilitation, home health care for bed-bound older people, home care for respirator-dependent infants, and hospice care for the terminally ill are examples of tertiary health care that is commonly provided in nonhospital settings.

Nursing care is an essential component in each of these settings and for each level of care described. Nursing practice in community settings is similar to nursing practice in acute care facilities as nurses perform assessments, administer procedures, teach clients and their caregivers, counsel, and work to ensure that clients receive needed care and services. Nursing practice in community settings, however, may differ markedly from nursing practice in the hospital. In the community setting, there is often less structure, less formality, and more independence. There is much less reliance on technology and a "controlled" environment, and there is enhanced recognition of the importance of knowing and understanding the patient's unique situation and individual needs. Thus, the application of the nursing process (assessment, analysis, planning, intervention, and evaluation) must take into account information beyond the immediate physical and psychosocial needs that are addressed in the formal and controlled hospital setting. In community-based practice, environmental threats, availability of resources, financial burdens, family concerns, lifestyle choices, and a variety of management issues for clients and their caregivers are often of primary concern.

Employment Opportunities in Community Settings

DIFFERENTIATED PRACTICE ISSUES

The movement of nursing out of traditional, structured roles found in acute care settings has given new direction to the debate on "differentiated practice," sparking questions on whether Associate Degree or diploma-prepared nurses are educationally equipped to practice in less structured, community-based settings. Although the ANA's published 1965 and 1984 position statements outlining two entry levels for nursing practice (the "technical" nurse and the "professional" nurse) were widely debated, there has been little action toward an official distinction in levels of practice. In 1995, only two states—North Dakota and Maine—required a baccalaureate degree for a professional nurse's license (Kovner, 1995).

Discussion of the merits of differentiated practice is beyond the scope of this book. When appropriate, however, specific educational requirements and recommendations for nurses using advanced knowledge, working with designated populations, or in specialized settings, are included.

CURRENT TRENDS IN NURSING EMPLOYMENT

In the case study mentioned earlier, what Martha discovered when she began her job search is not unusual. As a result of cost-containment measures and medical practice modifications, nursing employment in acute care settings has changed during the past several years. The Public Health Service's Division of Nursing has chronicled this change in practice settings through periodic surveys of RNs. The 1993 National Sample Survey of Registered Nurses (U. S. Department of Health and Human Services [USDHHS], 1993) discovered that:

- The rate for RNs who work outside of hospitals is 33.5%.
- Although the *number* of RNs working in hospitals increased, the *proportion* of nurses working in hospitals declined between 1988 and 1992.
- Increases in hospital employment between 1988 and 1992 were greatest in outpatient departments.
- Nurses in community/public health nursing showed a 38% increase between 1988 and 1992 that was largely the result of an increase in nurses working in home health care.
- The number of nurses in nursing homes and other extended care facilities increased almost 20% between 1988 and 1992.

Reforms in health care delivery appear to dictate that these trends will continue well into the 21st century. Table 1–2 presents data detailing employment settings for RNs practicing in the United States.

Another finding of the National Nursing Survey (USDHHS, 1993) was that the Registered Nurses supply, like that of other health providers, has a problem with geographic maldistribution. States in the south-central regions have approximately half the number of nurses per 100,000 people as the New England and Midwest states. For example, Mississippi, Texas, and Oklahoma have 510 to 530 RNs per 100,000 people in contrast to Massachusetts, Rhode Island, and North Dakota, which have 960 to 1,060 per 100,000 people. It is interesting that the District of Columbia has the greatest per capita concentration, with 1,927 RNs per 100,000 people. Rural areas, in particular, are understaffed with RNs because 83% of all nurses work in urban areas.

EMPLOYMENT OPPORTUNITIES

The movement from an illness-oriented, "cure," perspective in acute care, hospital-based health settings, to a focus on health promotion and primary health care in community-based settings, combined with changing demographics (an aging population) cost-consciousness, and changes in medical technology and treatments, all have dramatically changed employment opportunities for today's RNs. This shift of emphasis to primary care and outpatient treatment and management of both acute and chronic health conditions will continue. As a result, employment growth in a variety of ambulatory care settings, home health care, nursing homes, occupational health, school health, and parish care programs can be expected. Table 1–3 lists current and future employment options for RNs in non–acute care settings.

As shown in the table, nursing opportunities in

TABLE 1–2 **Summary of Employment Settings for All Registered Nurses**

Setting	Estimated Total	Estimated Percent
Hospitals	1,233,000	66.5
Nursing home/extended care facilities	129,000	7.0
Nursing education	36,500	2.0
Community/public health settings (includes Visiting Nurse Association and other home health agencies)	180,000	9.7
School health services	50,600	2.7
Occupational health	19,200	1.0
Ambulatory care settings	144,100	7.8
Other	56,200	3.0

From U. S. Department of Health and Human Services (USDHHS), Division of Nursing, Bureau of Health Professions, Public Health Service. (1993). *The Registered Nurse Population: Findings for the National Sample Survey of Registered Nurses, March 1992.* Washington, D.C., Government Printing Office.

community settings are extensive and varied. New graduates as well as experienced nurses should have a number of alternatives to explore to meet individual professional interests. For instance:

- If pediatrics is the nurse's primary area of interest, employment choices include working in a pediatrician's office, a pediatric hospital-based clinic, a school health program, and a well-child clinic.
- If the nurse enjoys working with older people, there are many options, including adult day care, geriatric clinics, home health, and nursing homes.
- If surgery is an interest, the nurse should realize that about half of all surgical procedures are now performed on an outpatient basis (Mezey and Lawrence, 1995).

As a result, employment opportunities in both freestanding and hospital-based day surgery centers have increased and include not only operating room nursing but also postanesthesia care, intake/admissions, and patient education positions. In addition, post–day surgery home care is becoming increasingly popular.

CHARACTERISTICS OF COMMUNITY-BASED NURSING

Although opportunities for employment in community-based settings are impressive, a baccalaureate degree may be required for some positions. Many school health programs and most public health departments, for example, will hire only nurses with a Bachelor of Science in Nursing (BSN) degree. Furthermore, experience may be necessary for many nursing positions in nonhospital settings. Home health agencies, for example, have preferred 1 to 2 years of recent, acute care experience when hiring RNs.

There are many advantages to practicing in community settings. Many nurses prefer the emphasis on health promotion and illness prevention that is a major focus of primary health care. The opportunity to get to know clients and their families by seeing them in their own homes, workplaces, schools, or communities, and to provide more holistic care, has also been cited as an advantage of nursing in the community setting. Another advantage has been the customary Monday-to-Friday, daytime work schedule. Although a hospital must be staffed around the clock, 7 days per week, few non–acute care facilities have required staffing for night shifts, weekends, and holidays. As more services are provided in the community, however, hours may expand.

Wages and salaries, on the other hand, have tended to be somewhat lower for RNs in community-based practice. This is, in part, reflective of the lack of evening, night, and weekend differential payment. As a result, nurses who work in community settings may occasionally supplement

TABLE 1–3 **Community-Based Employment Opportunities for Registered Nurses**

Ambulatory Care

- Physician's offices (solo, partnership, or private group practice)
- Managed health care organizations/insurers
  - Health maintenance organizations (HMOs)
  - Utilization review
  - Case management
- Hospital-based ambulatory services
  - Hospital clinics
  - Day surgery
- Freestanding ambulatory surgery centers
- Freestanding Emergi-centers
- Categorical clinics and services (may be hospital-based or freestanding)
  - Intravenous therapy and chemotherapy clinics
  - Dialysis units
  - Adult day care centers
  - Day care centers for ill children
  - Mental health clinics
  - Family planning clinics
  - Cardiac rehabilitation programs
  - Neuro rehabilitation programs (spinal cord injuries, multiple sclerosis, amyotrophic lateral sclerosis)
  - Geriatric clinics
  - Migrant health clinics
  - AIDS clinics
  - Diabetes management and education services
  - Pulmonary clinics (asthma, chronic obstructive pulmonary disease, cystic fibrosis)
  - Genetic screening and counseling services
  - Bloodmobiles
- Freestanding diagnostic centers
  - Diagnostic imaging centers
  - Mobile mammography centers

Health Department Services

- Maternal/child health clinics
- Family planning clinics
- Communicable disease control programs
  - HIV/AIDS (testing, counseling, and treatment)
  - Tuberculosis (testing, treatment, and surveillance)
  - Sexually transmitted diseases (testing, counseling, and treatment)
  - Immunization clinics
- Neighborhood clinics serving disenfranchised populations
- Mobile clinics serving disenfranchised populations
- Substance abuse programs
- Jails and prisons
- Indian health services

Home Health Care Services

- Skilled nursing care
- Intravenous therapy
- High-risk pregnancy/neonate care
- Maternal/child newborn care
- Private duty (hourly care)
- Respite care
- Hospice care

Long-Term Care

- Skilled nursing facilities
  - Hospital-based facilities
  - Freestanding/nursing home-based facilities
  - Hospice facilities
- Nursing Homes
  - Skilled nursing care
  - Assisted living

Other Community Health Settings

- School health programs
- Occupational health programs
- Parish nursing programs
- Summer camp programs
- Childbirth education programs

AIDS = acquired immunodeficiency syndrome; HIV = human immunodeficiency virus.

their income by working two to three shifts per month in hospitals. Some nurses report concern over the relative lack of a controlled environment and lack of immediate access to support from other nurses when providing nursing care in some community-based settings. This lack of support, or structure, may be a difficult adjustment for some nurses.

NATIONAL GOALS

In 1990, the USDHHS published *Healthy People 2000: National Health Promotion and Disease Prevention Objectives*. This document was written to commit the United States to the attainment of three broad goals:

- Increasing the span of healthy life for United States residents
- Reducing health disparities among this population
- Achieving access to preventive services for all residents

These goals are to be accomplished through implementation of a number of activities (1) to meet specified objectives identified, (2) to prevent premature death and disability, (3) to preserve a physical environment that supports human life, to cultivate family and community support, and (4) to enhance individual abilities to achieve and maintain a maximum level of functioning.

The goals of *Healthy People 2000* are divided into the four broad categories:

- Health promotion
- Health protection
- Preventive services
- Surveillance and data systems

These are further divided into 22 priority areas, which are then separated into a set of objectives for each. Table 1–4 depicts the category divisions and the priority areas. In 1996, *Healthy People 2000: Midcourse Review and 1995 Revisions* was published; this document addressed the progress being made toward meeting goals.

Implementation of activities and interventions to achieve most of the goals for *Healthy People 2000* rests on health care providers in community-based practice. Furthermore, meeting these objectives requires changing the focus of practice from illness and cure to health promotion and illness prevention. Throughout this book, related objectives from *Healthy People 2000* are presented, and practical methods to achieve them are discussed.

TABLE 1–4 ***Healthy People 2000:* Priority Areas**

Health Promotion

1. Physical activity and fitness
2. Nutrition
3. Tobacco
4. Alcohol and other drugs
5. Family planning
6. Mental health and mental disorders
7. Violent and abusive behavior
8. Educational and community-based programs

Health Protection

9. Unintentional injuries
10. Occupational safety and health
11. Environmental health
12. Food and drug safety
13. Oral health

Preventive Services

14. Maternal and infant health
15. Heart disease and stroke
16. Cancer
17. Diabetes and chronic disabling conditions
18. Human immunodeficiency virus (HIV) infection
19. Sexually transmitted diseases
20. Immunization and infectious diseases
21. Clinical preventive services

Surveillance and Data Systems

22. Surveillance and data systems

Age-Related Objectives

Children
Adolescents and young adults
Adults
Older adults

From U. S. Department of Health and Human Services (USDHHS). (1990). *Healthy People 2000: National Health Promotion and Disease Prevention Objectives.* Washington, D. C., Government Printing Office.

SUMMARY

Health care at all levels is becoming increasingly community-based. In response, nurses must be educationally and experientially prepared to provide care in very diverse settings. This chapter has introduced the recognition of, and rationale for, enhancing educational opportunities for all nurses in community-based settings. Related information is presented in Chapter 2, which discusses differences and similarities between nursing roles and interventions in acute care settings and community settings.

Key Points

- The *health care delivery system* is changing; care is becoming more focused on *health promotion* and *illness prevention* and moving from acute care and hospital-based delivery to prevention and management in *community-based settings.*
- Nurses have recognized the need to adapt *delivery of care* and *nursing education* to meet the needs of the population and the changing health care system as described in *Nursing's Agenda for Health Care Reform.*
- Like *primary* health care (preventive services and diagnosis and treatment of common acute episodic illnesses), *secondary* health care (relatively serious or complicated care traditionally provided in hospitals) and *tertiary* health care (management of chronic, complicated, long-term health problems) are increasingly being delivered in community-based settings.
- Although most nurses still work in hospitals, the *proportion* is changing with nurses increasingly being employed in community-based settings. This trend is expected to continue.
- There are *numerous* and *diverse* opportunities for nurses to work in community-based settings.
- The document *Healthy People 2000: National Health Promotion and Disease Prevention Objectives* was developed to (1) increase the span of healthy life for United States residents, (2) reduce health disparities among this population, and (3) achieve access to preventive services for all residents. *Comunity-based* health care providers are responsible for implementation of *activities* and *interventions* to achieve most of the goals.

Learning Activities and Application to Practice

- Obtain a copy of *Nursing's Agenda for Health Care Reform* (ANA, 1991). Discuss sections of the document relevant to movement of health care delivery from acute care settings to community-based settings. Which components have been implemented and which have not? What factors have hindered implementation? How can nurses join together to help make these changes?
- Obtain a copy of *The Registered Nurse Population: Findings from the National Sample Survey of Registered Nurses* (USDHHS, 1993). Review changes in the geographic region in which students practice. Compare local statistics with those of other regions of the United States.

- Obtain a copy of *Healthy People 2000* (USDHHS, 1990). Encourage students to discuss the document and the implications for nursing practice.
- Assign a group of students to research local employment opportunities for Registered Nurses in both hospital and community-based settings. Where are there more opportunities? Are there differences in Salaries? Hours? Experience requirements?

REFERENCES

American Nurses' Association. (1991). *Nursing's Agenda for Health Care Reform*. Washington, D. C., American Nurses' Association.

American Nurses' Association. (1965). *Educational Preparation for Nurse Practitioners and Assistants to Nurses: A Position Paper.* Kansas City, MO, American Nurses' Association.

Kovner, C. (1995). Nursing. In A. R. Kovner (Ed). *Jonas's Health Care Delivery in the United States*. New York: Springer Publishing Co.

Meierhoffer, L. L. (1992). State associations support nursing's agenda. *American Journal of Nursing, 24*(3), 6–7.

Mezey, A. P. and Lawrence, R. S. (1995). Ambulatory care. In A. R. Kovner (Ed). *Jonas's Health Care Delivery in the United States*. New York: Springer Publishing Co.

National League for Nursing (NLN). (1993). *A Vision for Nursing Education*. New York, National League for Nursing.

National League for Nursing/Council of Associate Degree Programs (NLN/CADP) (1994). *Web of Inclusion: Faculty Helping Faculty—Evaluation Summary.* National Video Conference, October 14, 1994.

Tagliareni, M. E. and Murray, J. P. (1995). Community-focused experiences in the AND curriculum. *Journal of Nursing Education, 34*(8), 366–371.

U. S. Department of Health and Human Services (USDHHS), Division of Nursing, Bureau of Health Professions, Public Health Service. (1993). *The Registered Nurse Population: Findings for the National Sample Survey of Registered Nurses, March 1992.* Washington, D. C., Government Printing Office.

U. S. Department of Health and Human Services (USDHHS). (1990). *Healthy People 2000: National Health Promotion and Disease Prevention Objectives*. Washington, D. C., Government Printing Office.

U. S. Department of Health and Human Services (USDHHS). (1996). *Healthy People 2000: Midcourse Review and 1995 Revisions*. Washington, D. C., Government Printing Office.

2

Roles and Interventions in Community-Based Nursing Practice

Case Study

Sally Smith is a home health nurse for a hospital-based agency in a small city. Last Tuesday, Sally saw five clients: Mrs. Black, to perform a fasting blood glucose tolerance test and to teach about insulin-dependent diabetes mellitus (IDDM); Mr. Johnson, for twice-a-day dressing changes following an amputation of his left great toe; Mrs. Garcia, to teach about anticoagulant therapy and to draw blood to monitor clotting times; Mrs. Gray, who has a diagnosis of Alzheimer's disease, and her family, who are considering placing her in a nursing home because they can no longer care for her at home; and Mr. Jones, who was recently discharged from the hospital following an episode of congestive heart failure, and who needs to be evaluated for fluid retention, hypertension, and heart and lung function.

Sally performs a number of roles and interventions in her practice as a home health care nurse. In preparation, Sally must schedule the day's visits on the basis of several factors. For example, she needs to see Mrs. Black before breakfast in order to obtain an accurate fasting glucose value and allow her to maintain her normal insulin and breakfast schedule. Mr. Johnson must be seen fairly early too, as his dressing changes are scheduled for early to mid-morning and early evening. To ensure accuracy, Mrs. Garcia's blood sample must be taken to the laboratory within 30 minutes and the results should to be reported to her physician by 3:00 pm. Finally, the visit to Mrs. Gray and her family is to be coordinated with one of the agency's medical social workers. Sally must consider each of these factors, calculate the distance that must be covered between the residences of the clients, ensure that all supplies are available (dressing materials, laboratory supplies), and schedule with other providers when planning the day's visits. Thus, management, including management of self, time, patient's care needs and schedules, and resources, is a key component of Sally's workday.

In addition to her management roles, Sally performs numerous skilled nursing interventions, such as physical assessment, wound care, blood glucose monitoring, and venipuncture. She is continually teaching her clients about their health and health care management. She collaborates closely with clients, their caregivers, the social worker, physicians, other home health care nurses, and a variety of other providers (e.g., aides, therapists, laboratory technicians), and she routinely acts as a counselor, advocate, and role model for her clients, their families, and other caregivers.

Nursing Roles and Interventions in Community-Based Practice

Nursing practice in community settings differs considerably from practice in the hospital. And, just as nursing practice in acute care institutions varies greatly from one area to another (operating room differs from intensive care unit, which differs from post partum, which differs from acute psychiatric care), it can be very different between community settings. Home health nursing is very different from school nursing, which, in turn, is very different from working in a health maintenance organization (HMO) or clinic. But, just as there are similarities in nursing practice in acute care settings (following physician orders, medication administration, and taking vital signs), there are similarities throughout community settings (emphasis on health promotion, teaching, counseling, advocacy, and ensuring continuity of care).

Nursing Roles in Community Settings

Shortened hospital stays, proliferation of day surgery, emphasis on health promotion, recognition of the unique health care needs of older clients and the underserved, and the desire to decrease costs have changed the health care system and the practice of nursing (see Chapter 1). Although performing traditional nursing skills (e.g., injections, vital signs, dressing changes) in the role of "care provider" is still an integral part of nursing practice, the importance of other roles is increasing. Although the variety of roles that make up nursing practice are the same, no matter what the setting is, the emphasis varies greatly. This chapter describes some of the roles common to nursing practice, how the roles differ in community-based practice compared with hospital-based practice, and how they might differ between community settings.

CARE PROVIDER

The care provider role involves the direct delivery of care. Performing tasks or skills for which the nurse has been trained and that are typically associated with nursing practice (e.g., client assessment, taking vital signs, administering injections, changing dressings, and inserting catheters) is the essence of the role of care provider.

This role constitutes much of nursing practice in acute care settings, where patients are typically hospitalized after surgery or for treatment of serious or complex medical conditions. For example, most of an ICU nurse's time (~70–80%) is spent in direct care provision. A nurse working on a "general medicine" floor devotes about 50% of the time in direct delivery of care; in contrast, the amount of time spent in direct care delivery for a nurse working in a postpartum unit is 40–50%, and for the nurse working in an inpatient psychiatric unit, it is 20–30%.

Even though direct care provision is an important part of community-based nursing practice, this task tends to occupy less time than in acute care settings. In community settings, direct care provision might be most time-intensive for the nurse in home health (35–40%); it is less significant in occupational health or school health (10–15%); and it might be minimal at an HMO practice. As a result, many nursing students and Registered Nurses (RNs) who are new to community-based practice often discount the nurse's importance in health care delivery in these settings because the nurses are not seen doing tasks (i.e., giving medication, performing hygiene procedures, managing intravenous lines). It is imperative, therefore, that nurses recognize the difference in emphasis on roles and that they be educationally and experientially equipped to identify, and intervene to meet, the needs of their patients.

EDUCATOR

Regardless of the setting, health education is an essential component of quality nursing care. Education in hospitals typically focuses on client instructions for post-hospital discharge and is often severely restricted because of time limitations, as hospital stays have become shortened. The limited amount of time for teaching, coupled with the acuity level of the client and stress on the family, often means that health teaching is marginally effective. Incorporation of written discharge instructions with verbal explanations as well as other techniques, including post-discharge telephone calls, has helped improve the assimilation of information by clients and caregivers in acute care settings.

Although health education is an important role for nursing in acute care settings, it is often the most significant role of the nurse working in community settings. Teaching individuals, families, and groups about maintenance of health, threats to health, and relevant lifestyle choices that affect health is integral in all community settings. The information presented should allow clients to make informed decisions on health matters and to direct self-care to follow treatment regimens.

The educator role makes up much of community-based nursing practice.

- School nurses often spend 30–40% of their time providing health education in areas such as prevention of sexually transmitted diseases (STDs), basic hygiene, and dental care.
- Occupational health nurses instruct clients on issues such as accident prevention, ergonomics, smoking cessation strategies, and the importance of physical fitness.
- Home health nurses spend much of their time teaching clients and families self-care strategies (e.g., dressing changes, diabetes management, colostomy care).
- Nurses in ambulatory clinic settings teach infant nutrition to new parents, signs and symptoms of infection to clients with acquired immunodeficiency syndrome (AIDS), principles of a low-fat diet to clients with coronary artery disease, and medication management to clients with congestive heart failure (CHF).

Health education goes beyond simple dissemination of information. Whether the information is instruction concerning the schedule and potential side effects of a prescribed medication, nutritional principles to reduce blood lipids, or breastfeeding, it must be presented appropriately for the individual client. As health educators, nurses should consider such factors as the client's developmental stage, learning readiness, language, educational level, and perceived learning needs. Additionally, the nurse must evaluate the learner's level of understanding accurately and must reinforce it accordingly.

All RNs should be familiar with basics of client teaching. Theories, models, and principles of teaching as well as experience in applying principles needs to be part of every introductory or nursing fundamentals course. A variety of tools (e.g., written materials, visual aids, models) and techniques (e.g., demonstration, observation, repetition) should be incorporated into the teaching plan. Use of appropriate, familiar terminology (i.e., avoidance of medical jargon), consideration of cultural variables, and encouraging or enabling the client to ask questions are essential. Evaluation of the client's level of understanding is accomplished through questioning, the use of return demonstration, or both.

COUNSELOR

Counseling involves listening to clients and their families, encouraging them to explore issues and options, and enabling them to manage their personal situations. Assistance with identification of problems and possible solutions and guidance through the problem-solving process are functions of nurses in most community-based settings. Indeed, counseling represents a significant component of quality, community-based nursing care. For example, a clinic nurse may discuss contraception options with a young mother; a school nurse might talk with a high school student perceived to be "at risk" for using drugs or alcohol; or a hospice nurse might discuss the importance of respite care and caring for the caregiver with the family of a terminally ill client.

In contrast, nurses in acute care settings typically spend considerably less time counseling clients. Because much of the care in hospitals is directed by hospital procedure or physician orders, there tends to be less emphasis on this role. Exceptions may include nursing care in psychiatric settings, where counseling might constitute the greatest percentage of the nurse's time, and nursing care for families of very seriously ill clients, where the family must weigh options for treatment and long-term care.

ADVOCATE

A nurse advocate is one who acts on behalf of, or intercedes for, the client. Frequently, clients, particularly children, elderly people, and the disadvantaged, are unable to obtain needed care and services within today's health care system. Advocates ensure that clients receive necessary care and services.

Nurses act as client advocates in all settings. In hospitals, nurses work as advocates through creative interventions, such as

- Ensuring that clients are as pain-free as possible by phoning a physician at 1:00 am to change a medication
- Participating with administrators to plan visiting hours to accommodate individual and family needs
- Helping parents to stay with small children
- Protecting a client's desires regarding advanced directives

In community settings, the nurse's role as an advocate is vital. Because they often work with vulnerable populations, nurses in community settings serve as client advocates constantly. For example, it is often the school nurse who identifies a source of funding to pay for eyeglasses for the child whose parents cannot afford them or identifies and reports suspected child abuse or neglect. The occupational health nurse's responsibility is to ensure that Occupational Safety and Health Administration (OSHA) guidelines for employee safety are carried out. The home health nurse may be the one who finds a way to provide insulin for an older client who cannot afford to pay for medications and the nurse in the homeless shelter clinic ensures that clients receive blankets and coats in the winter.

MANAGER

The role of the nurse as manager in a community-based practice is possibly most similar to the role of the nurse in an acute care setting. Nursing care in both hospital and community settings involves management of the nurse's time, limited resources, other personnel, and program organization and coordination as well as the management of the client's care. The management role includes planning, organizing, coordinating, marketing, controlling, and evaluating care and care delivery.

In community settings, school nurses

- Manage clinics
- Ensure that student records are complete
- Perform and document legally mandated services, such as vision and hearing screenings
- Direct clinic volunteers

As described in the case study earlier, home health nurses

- Coordinate scheduled visits based on client needs (i.e., fasting blood glucose or three times daily intravenous administration), estimating distances between client's homes and services to be provided
- Ensure that other professional services (part-time or overtime) are delivered when necessary
- Monitor or oversee the practice of a home health aide

- Use each client's resources to develop a plan of care

Nurses in clinics or physician offices perform *triage* so that clients in need of immediate help are treated first, ensure that supplies and equipment are available, and assist in ensuring that clients are seen on a timely basis.

OTHER ROLES IN COMMUNITY-BASED NURSING

Care provider, educator, manager, counselor, and advocate are the roles performed by most nurses most often. Additional roles that *all* nurses should perform routinely or occasionally include

- Collaborator
- Role model
- Researcher
- Leader

Each role is described briefly, and examples for application of each role to community-based nursing practice are presented.

Collaborator

Changes in health care delivery have included a move from the reliance on an individual physician as the sole director of care, and thereby responsible for all aspects of care, to a more comprehensive, interdisciplinary approach wherein several health care team members are responsible for various facets of care. *Collaboration* refers to the process of making decisions regarding health care management where individuals from various professions work with the client and the family or caregivers to jointly determine the course of care. Through interactions, discussion, and coordination, goals are set and a plan of care is formed to meet those goals. For clients with a complex or chronic health problem, such as coronary artery disease, Alzheimer's disease, or renal failure, the nurse must work with other health providers to deliver the most comprehensive, effective, cost-conscious care possible. Caring for a stroke victim, for example, may involve collaboration between physicians, nurses, physical therapists, occupational therapists, speech therapists, and possibly, others in both community and hospital settings.

Similarly, health promotion interventions need to be collaborative. For example, a team of professionals in a senior health clinic might work with an elderly client with diabetes to teach principles of nutrition, medication management, and foot care. The nurse in this setting might collaborate with a dietitian, pharmacist, diabetes educator, and others to seek the best management of client care.

Role Model

A role model is a person who demonstrates an action or behavior that is learned by others. *Role modeling* is both conscious and unconscious, and nurses in all settings, whether "on the job" or at home, demonstrate to others both positive and negative actions and attitudes related to health and health care. In community-based practice, nurses serve as role models to clients, their caregivers, and other health professionals. For example, a student receiving helpful, therapeutic, understanding care from the school nurse might be motivated to become a nurse; the caregiver of an elderly woman watching the professional, matter-of-fact changing of a sterile dressing may be convinced that he or she, too, may be able to learn to perform this task; or a nurse working with immigrant families in a community clinic can demonstrate care, empathy, and appreciation for cultural differences of clients to new employees and nursing students working in the clinic.

Researcher

Nurses, whatever their practice setting or primary population served, must remain informed of developments that are relative to their individual practice. Nurses should be careful, discriminating consumers of research. They should critically review research findings for merit and applicability to practice and should determine care accordingly. Nurses in obstetric clinics, for example, should be aware of the latest recommendations regarding dietary guidelines during pregnancy and the rationale behind these recommendations. Similarly, nurses working with new families should share the most recent findings about sleeping positions for newborns; and nurses who work with adults should be aware of new guidelines and rationale for prostate and breast screenings as well as exercise and diet recommendations. Very often, the client is unaware of recent discoveries and innovations related to health, and it is the nurse's responsibility to share them when relevant.

Occasionally, a nurse in community-based practice may be a part of a research study. Identifying problems or questions for investigation, participating in approved research studies, and disseminating research findings to clients and other professionals are appropriate actions for all nurses.

Leader

Leadership refers to the ability to influence the behavior of others. In community settings, the nurse may assume the role of a leader with clients and their families, other health care providers, public officials, local leaders, or employers. As a leader, the nurse might work with others to identify and assess threats to health and to intervene to remove or lessen these threats. For example, a nurse employed in a manufacturing setting might direct a group in establishing a health promotion program; a school nurse might lead a coalition of concerned parents to improve the nutritional value of hot lunches; and a nurse working in a clinic for low-income families might undertake the establishment of evening hours to meet the scheduling needs of the working poor.

Comparison of Nursing Roles in Hospitals and Community Settings

Although each of the many roles should be part of quality, comprehensive nursing care in any setting, role emphasis varies according to each client's needs and from setting to setting. Figure 2–1 visually depicts *estimates* of time spent by nurses in various roles in selected community and acute care settings. The time spent in any role varies according to each client's specific needs. Remember, these are estimates and are *not* meant to be examples of ideal amounts of time spent in each role; furthermore, they are not necessarily accurate for each nurse in each setting. Instead, the purpose of the diagrams is to illustrate the various nursing roles in different settings.

Nursing Interventions in Community Settings

Nursing interventions have been defined as "any treatment, based upon clinical judgment and knowledge, that a nurse performs to enhance patient/client outcomes," and they include both direct and indirect care that may be nurse-initiated, physician-initiated, or other provider-initiated treatments (McCloskey and Bulechek, 1996, p. xvii). Because nursing roles vary, often dramatically, between acute care and community settings and between different community settings, nursing interventions also vary.

The Nursing Interventions Classification (NIC) system (Iowa Intervention Project) (McCloskey and Bulechek, 1996) is the most comprehensively developed taxonomy of nursing interventions. The NIC system has more than 400 nursing interventions that have been defined and developed to include examples of appropriate nursing activities (behaviors or actions that implement the intervention) for each. The identified nursing interventions are divided into six "domains":

1. *Physiological: basic*—care that supports physical functioning
2. *Physiological: complex*—care that supports homeostatic regulation
3. *Behavioral*—care that supports psychosocial functioning and facilitates lifestyle changes
4. *Safety*—care that supports protection against harm
5. *Family*—care that supports the family unit

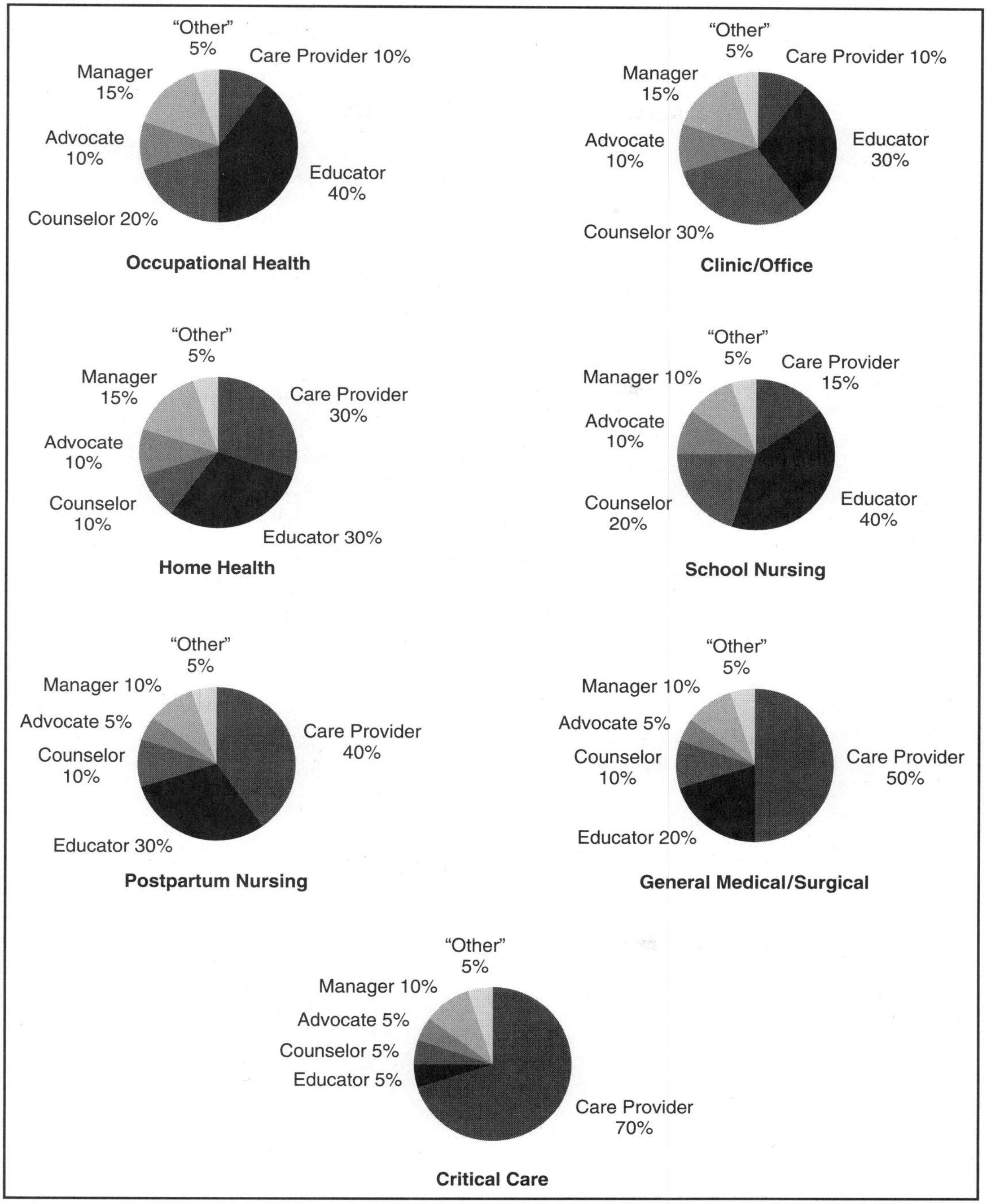

FIGURE 2–1 Comparison of nursing roles in selected settings.

6. *Health system*—care that supports effective use of the health care delivery system

Each domain is further divided into "classes" into which individual interventions are grouped. Some interventions fall into more than one class or domain. The remainder of the chapter describes some of the similarities and differences in nursing interventions in community and in acute care settings.

"UNIVERSAL" NURSING INTERVENTIONS

Certain nursing interventions are required of virtually all nurses in almost all settings (McCloskey and Bulechek, 1996). Examples of universal nursing interventions are as follows:

- *Documentation*—recording of pertinent patient data in a clinical record
- *Environmental management: safety*—monitoring and manipulation of the physical environment to promote safety
- *Anticipatory guidance*—preparation of patient for an anticipated developmental and/or situational crisis
- *Infection control*—minimizing the acquisition and transmission of infectious agents
- *Laboratory data interpretation*—critical analysis of patient laboratory data in order to assist with clinical decision-making
- *Learning facilitation*—promoting the ability to process and comprehend information
- *Patient rights protection*—protection of health care rights of a patient, especially a minor, or an incapacitated or incompetent patient unable to make decisions
- *Physician support*—collaborating with physicians to provide quality patient care
- *Vital signs monitoring*—collection and analysis of cardiovascular, respiratory, and body temperature data to determine and prevent complications

NURSING INTERVENTIONS IN ACUTE CARE

Some nursing interventions are very specialized, and nurses would provide those related activities only when delivering care in certain settings. For example, in critical care settings, nurses frequently perform many of the nursing interventions, termed "physiological complex" (i.e., acid-base management, cerebral edema management, circulatory care: mechanical assist device) but rarely perform many from the "behavioral" domain (i.e., behavior modification, learning readiness enhancement, health education).

Alternatively, many of the interventions in the "family" domain are directed specifically to the practice of perinatal nursing, including

- Cesarean section care
- Electronic fetal monitoring: intrapartum care
- High-risk pregnancy care

A number of nursing interventions are performed only rarely outside the acute care setting. Some of these include

- Anesthesia administration
- Autotransfusion
- Artificial airway management
- Cardiac care: acute
- Cerebral edema management
- Circulatory care
- Electronic fetal monitoring
- Endotracheal extubation
- Gastrointestional intubation
- Hemorrhage control
- Intrapartal care: high-risk delivery
- Mechanical ventilation
- Traction and immobilization care
- Tube care: chest

NURSING INTERVENTIONS FREQUENTLY USED IN COMMUNITY PRACTICE

A number of nursing interventions are commonly used throughout all community settings and more often than in acute care settings. For example, *abuse protection* (identification of high-risk, dependent relationships and actions to prevent further infliction of physical or emotional harm) is appropriate for home health nurses who see caregivers of seriously ill or infirm clients who need respite care. Similarly, school nurses and nurses in geriatric or pediatric clinics and similar settings should monitor for signs of neglect or unexplained illness or injury and should seek to identify parents or caregivers who might be at risk of being abusers (alcoholics or substance abusers or those abused as children).

Other nursing interventions identified by McCloskey and Bulechek (1996) commonly found throughout community-based practice are as follows:

Health education—developing and providing instruction and learning experiences to facilitate voluntary adaptation of behavior conductive to health in individual, families, groups, or communities

Health screening—detecting health risks or problems by means of history, examining, and other procedures

Health system guidance—facilitating a patient's location and use of appropriate health services

Medication administration—preparing, giving, and evaluating the effectiveness of prescription and nonprescription drugs

Teaching: prescribed medication—preparing a patient to safely take prescribed medications and monitoring for their effects

Nutritional counseling—using an interactive helping process, with focus on the need for diet modification

Referral—arranging for services by another care provider or agency

Risk identification—analyzing potential risk factors, determining health risks, and prioritizing risk reduction strategies for an individual or group

Teaching: individual—planning, implementing, and evaluating a teaching program designed to address a patient's particular needs

Telephone consultation—exchanging information, providing health education and advice, managing symptoms, or performing triage over the telephone

Although not all of these interventions are implemented by all nurses working in community settings, they are performed by most nurses.

Table 2–1 compares typical nursing interventions for several settings, both hospital-based and community-based. As with the comparison of nursing roles in various settings, these are examples only and the lists are by no means comprehensive or exclusive. Nursing in each area involves many more interventions than are presented here, and there may be significant overlap and exceptions in all areas.

SUMMARY

A number of nursing roles and nursing interventions are required to deliver comprehensive, competent, appropriate, and effective client care in any setting. This chapter has described some of the most important nursing roles and has shown how they are distinctive in both acute care and community settings. Likewise, nursing interventions are numerous and diverse, and their implementation may vary significantly from setting to setting. Similarities and differences have been discussed to encourage nurses to recognize and appreciate some of the unique characteristics of nursing care in a wide variety of settings.

Key Points

- Nursing practice in community-based settings differs considerably from practice in the hospital, and nursing practice also differs across various community settings.
- Nursing roles in community-based practice that are most frequently used are educator, counselor, manager, advocate, and care provider. The amount of time spent in each role varies from setting to setting, patient to patient, and day to day.

TABLE 2–1 **Commonly Used Nursing Interventions in Selected Settings**

Physiologic	Behavioral	Safety	Family	Health System
Home Health				
Teaching prescribed medications Wound care Cardiac care: rehabilitative Phlebotomy: venous blood sample *IV teams* IV therapy Medication administration Chemotherapy management	Anxiety reduction Teaching: disease process Teaching: preoperative Teaching: prescribed medication Teaching: prescribed activity/exercise Teaching: prescribed diet	Risk identification Prevention of falls	Caregiver support Home maintenance assistance Normalization promotion Family involvement Respite care	Culture brokerage Discharge planning Health system guidance Insurance authorization Supply management Multidisciplinary care conference Referral Telephone consultation
School Nursing				
Oral health promotion Medication administration: oral Heat/cold application Exercise promotion	Substance use prevention Behavior management: overactivity/inattention Teaching: group Teaching: sexuality Distraction	First aid Abuse protection: child Health screening Immunization/vaccination administration Risk identification	Developmental enhancement Family involvement Family integrity promotion Parent education: childrearing family Parent education: adolescent	Health policy monitoring Supply management Multidisciplinary care conference Referral
Ambulatory Care Nursing (Clinic or Physician's Office)				
Phlebotomy: venous blood sample Exercise promotion Weight management Weight reduction assistance Medication administration	Self-responsibility facilitation Smoking cessation assistance Substance use prevention Substance use treatment Communication enhancement: hearing deficit Coping enhancement Decision-making support Teaching: disease process Teaching: preoperative Teaching: prescribed diet Teaching: safe sex	First aid Triage Abuse protection: child Abuse protection: elder Health screening Immunization/vaccination administration Risk identification	Caregiver support Family mobilization Developmental enhancement Family involvement Family integrity promotion Parent education: childrearing family	Referral Telephone consultation Insurance authorization Health system guidance Controlled substance checking Supply management Health care information exchange

Occupational Health Nursing				
Weight management Exercise promotion Weight reduction assistance Stress management	Health education Self-responsibility facilitation Smoking cessation assistance Substance use prevention Coping enhancement Decision-making support Teaching: safe sex Support group Teaching: group	Environmental management: worker safety First aid Emergency care Health screening Risk identification Surveillance: safety	Role enhancement Family integrity promotion Parent education: childrearing family Family support	Referral Telephone consultation Insurance authorization Health system guidance Controlled substance checking Supply management Health policy monitoring
Critical Care Nursing				
Acid-base management Airway suctioning Artificial airway management Bowel management Cardiac care: acute Cerebral edema management Circulatory care Electrolyte management Phlebotomy: arterial blood sample Tube care: chest IV therapy Embolus precautions Pain management	Dying care Emotional support Presence	Code management Area restriction	Family involvement Family process maintenance Family mobilization	Delegation Emergency cart checking Order transcription Shift report Visitation facilitation Bedside laboratory testing Technology management
General Medical/Surgical Nursing				
Exercise therapy: ambulation Self care assistance Cough enhancement IV therapy Incision site care Venous access device maintenance Self-care assistance	Anxiety reduction Teaching: disease process Teaching: preoperative Teaching: prescribed medication Teaching: prescribed activity/exercise Teaching: prescribed diet	Code management	Family involvement Family process maintenance Family mobilization Normalization promotion	Admission care Discharge planning Bedside laboratory testing Delegation Emergency cart checking Order transcription Shift report

TABLE 2–1 **Commonly Used Nursing Interventions in Selected Settings** *Continued*

Physiologic	Behavioral	Safety	Family	Health System
		Postpartum Nursing		
Perineal care	Grief work facilitation: perinatal death	Code management	Postpartal care	Admission care
Constipation management	Support system enhancement	Area restriction	Attachment promotion	Discharge planning
Pelvic floor exercise	Family planning: contraception		Breastfeeding assistance	Bedside laboratory testing
Self-care assistance	Parent education: childbearing family		Environmental management: attachment process	Delegation
Pain management	Teaching: infant care		Infant care	Emergency cart checking
Bleeding reduction: postpartum uterus			Newborn monitoring	Order transcription
			Caregiver support	Shift report
			Family integrity promotion	

Data from McCloskey, J. C. and Bulechek, G. M. (1996). *Nursing Interventions Classifications (NIC)* (2nd ed). St. Louis: Mosby.
IV = intravenous.

- Nursing interventions vary, often dramatically, between acute care and community-based settings and between different community settings.

Learning Activities and Application to Practice

In Class

- Have students discuss or debate how the various roles of the nurse differ from setting to setting. What role or roles do the students see as most important in each setting? Why?
- Obtain a copy of *Nursing Interventions Classifications* (McCloskey and Bulechek, 1996). Outline examples of nursing interventions that would be appropriate in a number of settings in both hospital and community settings. Discuss similarities and differences.

In Clinical

- Encourage students to estimate the amount of time they spend during the clinical day in each of the nursing roles described. Keep track of these estimates in a log or diary. Do nursing roles change between settings? How and why? Encourage comparison with students in other settings.
- Have students list nursing interventions performed in each clinical setting in a log or diary. How are interventions different in each setting? Do students feel some interventions are more "important" or "necessary" than others? Why or why not?

REFERENCE

McCloskey, J. C. and Bulechek, G. M. (1996). *Nursing Interventions Classifications (NIC).* (2nd ed). St. Louis, Mosby-Year Book.

UNIT II

Factors That Influence Health and Health Care

3

Overview of the Health Care Delivery System

Case Study

Carol Clark is employed as a head nurse for the evening shift in the emergency department of a large, nonprofit hospital in an urban area. Carol has been a nurse for 20 years, and during that time she has witnessed dramatic changes in health care provision and in the health care delivery system. Carol knows that reimbursement issues are extremely important to the hospital, but she finds it confusing and even unfair that a patient's care is often affected by his or her health care insurance coverage or lack of coverage. It concerns her that one of the first questions she must ask clients as they come into the emergency department is "Do you have health insurance?"

One recent Monday, Carol saw Melissa Mills, a 34-year-old woman, for lower abdominal pain; George Green, a 76-year-old man with chest pain; Beth Bell, a 12-year-old girl who had sprained her ankle; Nancy Nelson, a 19-year-old prima gravida in active labor; and Andy Adams, a 46-year-old man experiencing an acute asthma attack. During the evening, Carol wondered whether the care given each of these clients was influenced by insurance coverage and insurer requirements. Following the shift, Carol reviewed the disposition of each case from a financial standpoint and this is what she learned:

Ms. Mills—insured through a large health maintenance organization (HMO). It was determined that her pain was caused by ovulation, and she was sent home with pain medication. Because she was not referred to the emergency department by her primary care provider (gatekeeper), it is unlikely that the HMO will pay for the visit.

Mr. Green—insured by Medicare parts A and B. Admitted into the coronary care unit for observation. Hospital coverage is fairly comprehensive and based on the prospective payment system. Medical coverage is at 80% following a deductible.

Beth B.—health care financed by "traditional" insurance through her father's employer. Hospital and medical coverage will be 80 to 100% after a predetermined deductible.

Ms. Nelson—has no health insurance. As it was determined that delivery was not imminent, she was sent to the local county hospital, which provides care for indigent clients. She is eligible for Medicaid but has not applied.

Mr. Adams—has no health insurance. Because his asthma attack was severe and he was in danger of respiratory arrest, Mr. Adams was kept for treatment and observation. Although Mr. Adams has no insurance, he is responsible for the costs of his health care and will be billed. Because he is only sporadically employed, Mr. Adams will be unable to pay most of the bill, which totals several thousand dollars, and the hospital will incur the cost of his care as bad debt. (Bad debt is covered by increasing charges to paying patients.)

Carol, like many other health care providers, is struggling to understand the health care delivery system and to be informed about financing of health care and differing health plans and reimbursement methods. She, along with other providers, must learn to practice within the context of constant change and to work with multiple insurance plans and providers.

To better understand the context in which they practice, it is essential that all nurses—particularly nurses working in primary care or community-based settings, including emergency departments—acquire a working knowledge of the health care delivery system (HCDS). This chapter presents basic concepts, information, illustrations, and tables to reinforce the nurse's understanding of the HCDS, including the structure of the system, health care settings and organizations, provider roles, and health care financing. Understanding these concepts will assist the nurse to deliver the highest-quality, most cost-effective care possible.

Structure of the Health Care Delivery System

Organizationally, the HCDS can be divided into "public sector" and "private sector" components. The public sector of the HCDS can be subdivided into federal, state, and local level divisions and is typically concerned with the health of populations and the provision of a healthy environment. The private sector includes nonprofit and proprietary organizations (e.g., hospitals, clinics, home health agencies, voluntary groups) and providers (e.g., physicians, dentists, therapists) whose primary focus is health care for individuals and families.

PUBLIC SECTOR

The U. S. Department of Health and Human Services (USDHHS) is the federal cabinet department that directly or indirectly oversees most components of the HCDS. Most USDHHS agencies have regional, state, or local offices that may be contacted for specific needs or questions. For example, regional or local offices of the Social Security Administration, the Administration on Aging, and Aid to Families with Dependent Children should be accessed to obtain information on services, eligibility, and other issues.

The organizational structure for the USDHHS is depicted in Figure 3–1. The U. S. Public Health Service, one of the major components of the USDHHS, is concerned with direct monitoring and care delivery to improve the health of U. S. residents. As illustrated in Figure 3–1, the agencies that compose the Public Health Service include the Centers for Disease Control and Prevention, the Food and Drug Administration, and the National Institutes of Health. Each of these agencies and organizations is responsible for oversight or regulation of differing issues related to health and health care delivery. The National Institutes of Health, for example, finances a significant amount of research related to health; the Food and Drug Administration is responsible for monitoring and regulating the safety of pharmaceuticals, food additives, and other consumer goods, as well as health care products and equipment; and the Centers for Disease Contol monitors infectious diseases and directs programs to control and prevent

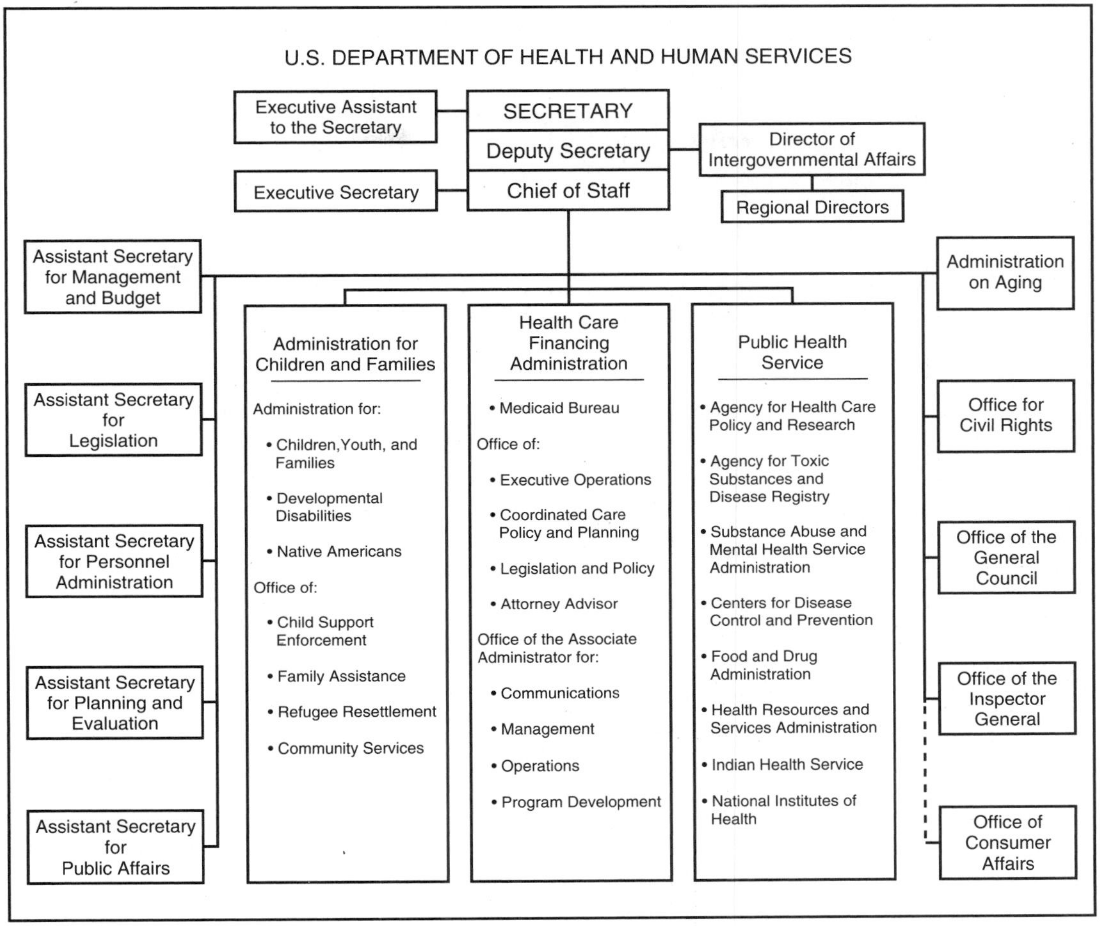

FIGURE 3–1 Organizational structure of the U. S. Department of Health and Human Services.

diseases. The impact of these agencies and other components of the USDHHS on health and the health care system cannot be overstated, and all nurses should be familiar with the various components of the USDHHS. Thus, listings and functions of most of the offices and agencies within the USDHHS are presented in Table 3–1.

Each state maintains a state health department, usually located in the state capitol. Most state health departments are headed by a health officer or commissioner and are funded through state taxes and federal monies (e.g., grants, matching funds). Local health departments may reside within a city, county, municipality, or district. State legislatures generally define the responsibilities and roles of the local health agency. Funding for local activities comes from a combination of local and state taxes and federal grants. Although roles, functions, and services vary, state and local health departments are typically responsible for the activities listed in Table 3–2.

PRIVATE SECTOR

The private sector of the health care delivery system is composed of a variety of providers (e.g.,

TABLE 3–1 U. S. Department of Health and Human Services—Selected Agencies and Units

The USDHHS is divided into three agencies, which are subdivided into units. The addresses and telephone numbers of some of the agencies and selected units are listed here.

Agency or Organization	Function
Department of Health and Human Services (202) 619-0257	Oversees, manages, and finances most of the products, organizations, and interests related to health
Public Health Service 5600 Fisher's Lane Rockville, MD 20857 (301) 443-2403	Coordinates federal health programs
Centers for Disease Control and Prevention 1600 Clifton Road, NE Atlanta, GA 30333 (404) 639-3311	Monitors and supports programs to prevent and control infectious diseases
Food and Drug Administration 5600 Fisher's Lane Rockville, MD 20857 (301) 443-2410	Provides surveillance for the safety of pharmaceuticals and other consumer goods
Health Resources and Services Administration 5600 Fisher's Lane Rockville, MD 20857 (301) 443-2216	Provides health care to Native Americans, federal prisoners, and underserved populations
National Institutes of Health 9000 Rockville Pike Bethesda, MD 20892 (301) 496-4000	Conducts and funds health-related research
Substance Abuse and Mental Health Services Administration 5600 Fisher's Lane Rockville, MD 20857 (301) 443-4513	Supports research and programs related to substance abuse and mental health
Agency for Toxic Substances Disease Registry 200 Independence Avenue, SW Washington, D.C. 20201	Prevents or mitigates environmental exposure to hazardous substances
Agency for Health Care Policy and Research 2101 East Jefferson Street Rockville, MD 20852 (301) 594-6662	Coordinates health care research to determine what practices work best and at what cost
Office of Disease Prevention and Health (202) 205-5968	Carries out the goals of *Healthy People 2000*
Health Care Financing Administration 200 Independence Avenue, SW Washington, D.C. 20201 (202) 245-6726	Funds federal health programs
Social Security Administration 6401 Security Building Baltimore, MD 21235 (410) 965-8882 (800) 772-1213	Administers Social Security

TABLE 3–1 **U. S. Department of Health and Human Services—Selected Agencies and Units** *Continued*

The USDHHS is divided into three agencies, which are subdivided into units. The addresses and telephone numbers of some of the agencies and selected units are listed here.

Agency or Organization	Function
Administration for Children and Families 901 D Street SW, Suite 600 Washington, D.C. 20447 (202) 401-9215	Coordinates efforts for children and families, including Head Start, Job Opportunities and Basic Skills Training (JOBS), and AFDC
Office of Family Assistance (202) 401-9275	Oversees AFDC and JOBS programs
Administration for Children, Youth and Families 330 C Street SW Washington, D.C. 20201 (202) 205-8347	Operates Head Start and other programs on child care, foster care, adoption, child abuse, and runaways
Administration for Native Americans (202) 690-7776	Promotes the well-being and economic self-sufficiency of Native Americans
Administration on Developmental Disabilities (202) 690-5504	Promotes self-sufficiency and protects the rights of U. S. residents with developmental disabilities
Office of Child Support (202) 401-9370	Seeks to ensure that children receive adequate support from absent parents
Office of Community Services (202) 401-9333	Administers grants to states and community-based organizations for a variety of human services
Administration on Aging (202) 619-1006	Represents the concerns of older U. S. residents
Office of Civil Rights (202) 619-1587	Enforces federal laws prohibiting discrimination by health care providers
Office of Consumer Affairs (202) 634-4310	Ensures that the consumer's voice is heard in the federal government
Office of the Inspector General (202) 619-1142	Investigates fraud, waste, and abuse in health and welfare programs

physicians, nurses, dentists, pharmacists), organizations (e.g., American Red Cross, American Heart Association, American Cancer Society), institutions (e.g., hospitals, clinics), industries and corporations (e.g., pharmaceutical companies, hospital equipment manufacturers), and insurers (e.g., Blue Cross/Blue Shield, CIGNA). Although most components of the private sector of the HCDS are income producing or "for profit," others are designated "nonprofit" and thus tax exempt. Nonprofit, private sector organizations include "voluntary" agencies, such as the Red Cross and the American Cancer Society, and direct care providers, including the Visiting Nurses Associations and many hospitals and community clinics.

The individuals and organizations that compose the private sector of the HCDS work more or less independently to produce goods and services to promote the health of U. S. residents, as well as treat and manage health threats, diseases, and related conditions. However, the public component of the HCDS maintains a degree of control over the private sector through a variety of means, as described previously. Licensure of most direct

TABLE 3–2 **Functions and Services of State and Local Health Departments**

State Health Departments	
Administer Medicaid	
Operate state mental hospitals	
Provide licensure and regulation of	
Health practitioners	
Health facilities	
Regulate insurance companies	
Communicable disease control and monitoring	
Enforcing and overseeing environmental programs	
Health planning and development	
Maintenance of vital records for the state	
Local Health Departments	
Provision of direct health services, such as family planning and WIC	
Recording of local vital statistical data and reporting them to the state	
Local communicable disease control and prevention	
Direct environmental services, such as monitoring water quality, inspection of food services, and vector control	

providers (e.g., physicians, nurses, dentists) is required by all states; federal approval is needed for all new medications and devices used in medical treatment before marketing; and recommendations and federal and state requirements for communicable disease prevention, management, and reporting are examples of how the public sector of the HCDS directly affects the private sector in health care delivery. The following sections provide more examples and details about various organizations and providers.

Health Care Provider Organizations

The U. S. HCDS is composed of a multitude of providers and organizations serving the population at many levels and for a vast array of needs. Chapter 1 included a discussion of "primary," "secondary," and "tertiary" heath care. You will recall that *primary health care* refers to basic care for preventive services or treatment of common acute illnesses and conditions (e.g., sore throat, otitis media, pregnancy) or routine chronic conditions (e.g., diabetes, hypertension, arthritis) in ambulatory settings. *Secondary health care* refers to more intensive or complicated care, usually provided in acute care settings (usually a hospital [e.g., open-heart surgery, treatment of complications of diabetes]). Finally, *tertiary health care* is long-term care for complex, chronic, and complicated health problems. Facilities, organizations, and providers for each of these levels are described here.

AMBULATORY HEALTH CARE

Primary health care is provided to "ambulatory" clients in community-based settings. Ambulatory care is commonly thought of as health care provided to an individual who is not a bed patient in a health care institution (Mezey and Lawrence, 1995).

The numbers and types of ambulatory care settings and providers are rapidly growing. There are two basic types of ambulatory care: (1) care provided by private physicians in solo, partnership, or group practice on a fee-for-service basis or preferred provider organization (PPO)–type arrangement and (2) care provided in organized settings that "have an identity independent from that of the individual physicians practicing in it" (Mezey and Lawrence, 1995, p. 123). These include HMOs, hospital-based ambulatory services, hospital-sponsored group practices, surgicenters, "urgicenters" or emergicenters, neighborhood health centers, organized home care, and school and workplace health services. Providers of care in ambulatory settings include physicians, dentists, nurses, social workers, therapists, pharmacists, optometrists, and chiropractors. Specific information regarding some of the many health care providers is presented later in this chapter.

According to a survey performed in 1992, U. S. residents averaged six physician contacts each year, and 78% of U. S. residents reported that they had seen a physician in the previous year (USDHHS, 1994). The number of yearly physician contacts varied greatly based on age (approximately 7 contacts per year for infants and small children; 4.5 contacts per year for young and middle-aged adults; and 10–12 contacts per year for those older than 65 years), sex (males had five contacts per year; females, seven contacts per year), and income (surprisingly, those with annual incomes under $10,000 averaged eight contacts per year, and those with incomes greater than $35,000 per year averaged six contacts per year). Other factors, such as race and geographical region, however, had very little influence on the number of physician contacts. Williams (1993) reported that the 10 most common principal diagnoses for office visits in 1990 were

1. Essential hypertension
2. Normal pregnancy
3. Otitis media
4. General medical examination
5. Acute upper respiratory infection
6. Health supervision of infant or child
7. Diabetes mellitus
8. Allergic rhinitis
9. Bronchitis
10. Acute pharyngitis

U. S. residents average about two visits each year for dental care. In contrast to physician care, dental visits are fewest for small children (less than one visit per year) and greatest between the ages of 5 and 14 and 45 and 64 (average, 2.3 visits per year). Although there is very little variation in the number of yearly dental visits between men and women, there is marked difference between races (whites, 2.1 visits per year; black, 1.3 visits per year) and with family income (those with annual incomes less than $10,000, 1.3 visits per year; those with annual incomes greater than $35,000, 2.7 per year) (Aday, 1993). Most dental visits are for preventive care (e.g., cleaning and fluoride treatment) and to obtain fillings.

Innovations in anesthesiology and surgical techniques have led to rapid growth in the number of "outpatient" surgery and "day surgery" procedures. Begun in the early 1970s as a cost-cutting measure, ambulatory surgery is now very common. Indeed, it is estimated that about half of all surgical procedures are performed on an outpatient basis.

Likewise, the growth of freestanding emergicenters is attributed to attempts to lower costs by decreasing the use of expensive hospital emergency rooms for nonurgent primary care. Emergicenters offer convenient locations, flexible hours, and short waiting periods at significantly lower costs for services. As emergicenters have increased in number and in acceptance by clients, they have evolved to offer a combination of walk-in and appointment services. They provide a wide range of primary care, including preventive care (e.g., physical examinations), in addition to diagnosis and treatment of acute, episodic illnesses (e.g., bronchitis, influenza), and injuries (e.g., minor lacerations, sprains, and strains).

HOSPITALS

Acute care hospitals are the principal settings for provision of secondary health care. "Hospitals differ from one another based on size, mission, ownership, complexity, competitive environment, population served, endowment and financial situation, physical facilities and costs per day of care or cost by patient diagnostic category" (Kovner, 1995, p. 166). Hospitals may range in size from less than 30 beds to more than 500 beds, may serve special populations (e.g., children, elders, disabled), may care for clients with specific diagnoses (e.g., acquired immunodeficiency syndrome, tuberculosis, cancer), and/or may support a defined mission of service (e.g., hospice, rehabilitation). Hospitals in which the average stay is less than 30 days are called short-term hospitals.

Collectively, hospitals are among the largest industries in the United States in terms of the number of employees and revenue. About three fourths (or 75%) of health care personnel work in hospitals, and about 38% of health care expenditures are to hospitals (Haglund and Dowling, 1993).

Hospitals may be publicly or privately funded. Those that are privately funded may be nonprofit or proprietary. Examples of each are found in Table 3–3. The distinction between public and privately funded institutions is not absolute, as

TABLE 3–3 **Types of Hospitals**

Public			Private	
Federal	***State***	***Local***	***Nonprofit***	***Proprietary***
Veterans Administration hospitals Federal prison hospitals Military hospitals "Special" hospitals (e.g., Native Americans, Hansen's disease)	State mental facilities Tuberculosis hospitals Teaching hospitals associated with state universities (also local)	City/county general or "charity" hospitals	Religious based (e.g., Catholic, Christian, or Jewish) Foundation, charity, or voluntary (e.g., many children's hospitals, Masonic hospitals)	Corporately owned (e.g., Humana, Columbia/HCA, National Medical Enterprises) Group owned (typically physician groups)

virtually all public facilities accept private-pay clients, and many private hospitals will take uninsured clients and/or may be reimbursed by public monies.

It is important to note that the number of hospitals decreased rather significantly during the past decade. Cost containment strategies, the increasing use of outpatient care, and many other factors have resulted in hospital closures throughout the nation. These same factors have prompted a reduction in hospital beds in many other hospitals. Table 3–3 lists the various types of hospitals, and Table 3–4 illustrates the trend in reduction in the number of hospitals over the past decade.

LONG-TERM CARE FACILITIES

Tertiary, or long-term, care includes institutional health services, mental health services, and residential services provided to temporarily or chronically disabled persons over an extended period. The goal of long-term care is to provide services that enhance the "functional ability" of these individuals.

Functional ability refers to a person's capacity to perform basic self-care activities such as eating, dressing, and personal care (e.g., bathing, showering, oral care, and maintenance of bowel and bladder control). These activities are generally termed activities of daily living (ADL). Long-term care may also assist the client in performance of instrumental activities of daily living; e.g., shopping, housekeeping, meal preparation, and managing of monetary affairs (Evashwick, 1993).

The need for long-term care may be temporary (e.g., an older person's recovery from joint replacement surgery or rehabilitative care for a client with a spinal cord injury) or permanent (e.g., institutional care for an individual who is profoundly mentally retarded or for a bed-bound, frail older person). Functional disability, particularly in the elderly, often results from chronic conditions such as arthritis, hearing impairment, vision impairment, diabetes, and respiratory or cardiac disease. The need for more and higher-quality long-term care facilities and providers is evident with the increase in the number of elderly and chronically ill (Bodenheimer and Estes, 1994; Rice, 1991; Richardson, 1995). Examples of long-term care facilities, and some of the services they provide, are listed in Table 3–5.

In general, long-term care is financed through governmental programs, including Medicaid, Medicare, and state funding for care of the mentally ill, as well as out-of-pocket payment. Nursing home care of the elderly, for example, is largely financed through a combination of Medicaid and out-of-pocket payment. It is important to note that approximately 40% of Medicaid expenditures are

TABLE 3–4 **Hospital Facts—1981 and 1991**

Type or Size of Hospitals	Hospitals—1981 (n)	Hospitals—1991 (n)
Public		
Federal	348	334
State psychiatric	549	800
State respiratory (tuberculosis)	11	4
Long-term general	146	126
State and local government	1,744	1,429
Private		
Nonprofit	3,340	3,175
Proprietary	729	738
6–24 beds	244	222
25–49 beds	977	922
50–99 beds	1,449	1,244
100–199 beds	1,402	1,311
200–299 beds	717	741
300–399 beds	427	398
400–499 beds	276	223
500+ beds	330	281

Data from American Hospital Association. (1993–1994). *Hospital Statistics*. Chicago, American Hospital Association.

for long-term care for older people (Birchfield, 1996). Detailed information on financing of health care services is discussed later in this chapter.

Health Care Professionals

Kovner (1995) states that health care in the United States is "provided by doctors and nurses and by more than 200 different occupational groups, ranging from physical therapists to lab technicians" (p. 7). Although most consumers have a general understanding of the roles and functions of providers, there remains much room for misunderstanding. For example, what are the educational requirements for a "nurse?" What is the difference between a psychologist, a psychiatrist, and a psychotherapist or an M. D. and a D. O.? Does a specific client need to see an audiologist or a speech therapist?

Because of the importance of collaboration and coordination in their practice, nurses working in community settings need to understand the practice parameters, roles, education, and credentialing requirements of the many health care providers. Knowledge of the different disciplines can assist the nurse in planning and implementation of health care and is an essential component of case management. Information on education, practice, and licensure for many health care providers is described here.

PHYSICIANS, PHYSICIAN ASSISTANTS, AND DENTISTS

Doctor of Medicine

Allopathic Doctors of Medicine (M. D.s) prevent, diagnose, and treat disease and injury. They prescribe medications, perform surgery, and direct many other health services (e.g., laboratory services, hospital use) and providers. Education requirements are 3 to 4 years of college (most have a bachelor's degree) and 4 years of medical school, followed by a 1-year internship. M. D.s who stop training at this point are nonspecialists, or "general practitioners." However, most M. D.s (80–90%) specialize. Specialization requires 3 to 4 years of additional, "residency" training. Medical specialties include internal medicine, general surgery, obstetrics, pediatrics, and radiology. Subspecialties include hematology, oncology, cardiology, orthopedic surgery, and thoracic surgery.

All states require physicians to be licensed. Requirements for licensure include graduation from an accredited professional school, passage of a licensing examination administered by the National Board of Medical Examiners (except Texas and Louisiana, which have their own examination), and successful completion of an accredited graduate medical education program (internship or residency).

TABLE 3–5 **Examples of Long-Term Care Facilities and Services**

Nursing homes—generic term that includes a wide spectrum of facilities such as retirement centers, convalescent homes, and skilled nursing facilities. Nursing homes are utilized by individuals who are not able to remain at home due to physical health problems, mental health problems, or functional disabilities.

Skilled nursing facilities—long-term care establishments that are designed to provide a higher level of care than custodial care facilities but at a level less intensive than care provided in short-term, acute care hospitals. Skilled nursing facilities must have a licensed nurse available at all times and are eligible for Medicare reimbursement.

Home health care—consists of a variety of nursing, therapy, and social support services provided to individuals and their families at their place of residence. Home health care can include skilled nursing care, nurse's aide services, physical therapy, occupational therapy, and speech therapy. Home health care must include a plan of care prescribed by a physician for Medicare reimbursement.

Adult day care—refers to a variety of health and social services for the elderly during the day and out of the home. Adult day care provides respite care to delay or prevent institutionalization, particularly for elders in families in which the caregivers work or when the elder lives alone.

Respite care—provides a temporary "respite," or break for the caregivers of frail elderly or disabled chronically ill. Respite care may be provided in or out of the client's home and may include homemaker services and/or assistance with ADL. Medicaid and Medicare will pay for respite care in some circumstances.

Hospice—refers to the provision of care for the terminally ill. Hospice care may be delivered at home or in an institutional setting and is directed toward symptom management; pain control; and psychological, social, and spiritual care for the client and the family.

Assisted living arrangements—refers to "any group or residential setting (licensed or unlicensed) providing personal care and meeting unscheduled needs for older, disabled persons" (Richardson, 1995, p. 211). Assisted living facilities vary greatly with regard to size, funding sources, target populations, services, and staffing. There are several models, including

Congregate living arrangements—group-living and supportive service facilities, typically multiunit apartment complexes, where residents can live and eat independently

Board-and-care homes—provide rooms, meals, assistance with ADL, and some protective oversight and may be licensed or unlicensed

Continuing care communities—comprehensive service settings providing three levels of living: independent, assisted, and nursing home care; a resident can join a continuing care community as an "independent" resident and progress through the services if physical or mental disabilities dictate

Data from Richardson, H. (1995). Long-term care. In A. R. Kovner (Ed.). *Jonas' Health Care Delivery in the United States* (5th ed.). New York, Springer Publishing Co., pp. 194–231; Evashwick, C. J. (1993). The continuum of long-term care. In S. J. Williams and P. R. Torrens (Eds.). *Introduction to Health Services* (4th ed.). Albany, NY, Delmar Publishers, pp. 177–218.

Doctor of Osteopathy

Like M. D.s, Doctors of Osteopathy (D. O.s) prevent, diagnose, and treat diseases. Osteopathy, however, emphasizes that the body can make its own remedies given normal structural relationship, environmental conditions, and nutrition. Education requirements and specialties are similar to those for an M. D. and include instruction in body mechanics and manipulative methods in diagnosis and treatment, as well as medicinal and surgical treatments.

Physician Assistant

The role of the physician assistant (PA) developed in the 1960s in response to a shortage of primary care physicians in certain areas. PAs practice medicine under the supervision of a licensed physician, and their practice includes physical examination, ordering and interpretation of laboratory tests, and making tentative diagnoses and prescribing treatments under protocol and direct and/or indirect supervision of physicians. Education requirements are 3 to 4 years of college (a bachelor's degree is usually required) and 2 years of PA school. PA programs are located in medical schools, universities, or schools of allied health. Most offer a bachelor's degree as the basic degree, although some offer a master's degree. A few PA programs award a certificate.

All states except Mississippi require licensure to practice as a PA. Graduation from an accredited professional school is necessary for licensure. Specialization is possible, and specialty areas include surgery, emergency medicine, and orthopedics.

Doctor of Dental Surgery and Doctor of Dental Medicine

Dentists may obtain one of two degrees: Doctor of Dental Surgery (DDS) and DDM (Doctor of Dental Medicine). Dentists prevent, diagnose, and treat problems of the teeth and tissues of the mouth. Education requirements are similar to those for an M. D., with an additional four academic years in dental school. Most dentists (85%) are generalists. Specialization requires 2 years or more of additional training and includes endodontics (treatment of the roots of teeth), orthodontics (straightening of teeth), periodontics (treatment of the gums and bone supporting the teeth), and pedodontics (children's dentistry).

All states require dentists to be licensed. Licensure requires graduation from an accredited dental school and successful completion of a licensing examination, including written and practical components.

NURSES

Nurses use the nursing process in the promotion and maintenance of health; management of illness, injury, or infirmity; restoration of optimum function; or achievement of a dignified death. Nursing practice varies depending on education, licensure, and credentialing.

Licensed Practical Nurse or Licensed Vocational Nurse

Education programs for licensed practical nurses (LPNs) or licensed vocational nurses (LVNs) are 12 to 18 months and are available in trade, technical, and vocational schools and community colleges. All states require LPNs/LVNs to be licensed, and requirements include graduation from a state-approved program in practical nursing or vocational nursing and successful completion of a licensing examination.

Registered Nurses

Education for a Registered Nurse (RN) may be in associate degree (2 years of community college), diploma (2–3 year hospital-based), or baccalaureate (4–5 years in colleges or universities) programs. All states require RNs to be licensed. Requirements include graduation from a state-approved nursing program and successful completion of the National Council Licensure Examination (NCLEX), a written examination administered by each state.

Advanced Practice Nurses

Advanced practice nurses (APNs) may be nurse practitioners, clinical nurse specialists, certified nurse-midwives, or certified registered nurse-anesthetists. They conduct assessments and diagnose and treat clients, usually following a predefined protocol. Most APNs are in specialty practices such as anesthesia, pediatrics, geriatrics, gynecology, and obstetrics. Education requirements generally include a basic undergraduate degree in nursing, with additional graduate education. Most APN programs award master's degrees. Licensure requirements vary between states but typically include graduation from an accredited APN program, completion of a certification examination conducted by a nationally recognized organization, and completion of a requisite number of hours in advanced practice. Scope of practice parameters for APNs in such areas as prescriptive authority and third party reimbursement also vary between states and are detailed in each state's Nurse Practice Act.

THERAPISTS

A number of different types of therapists practice in the U. S. HCDS. Some of those more commonly encountered in community-based practice are described here.

Physical Therapists

Physical therapists (PTs) plan, organize, and administer treatments to restore functional mobility, relieve pain, and prevent or limit permanent disability. In addition, some PTs perform diagnostic testing to determine joint measurement, functional activity, and voluntary muscle power. Although education requirements vary somewhat, the minimum educational requirement for practice is a bachelor' degree. Some programs will confer a certificate (for those who hold a degree in another field), and others confer a master's degree. All states require PTs to be licensed, and requirements include graduation from an accredited professional school and successful completion of a licensing examination. Specialization requires additional educational preparation, 2 years or more of practice experience, and successful completion of a certification examination. Specialization areas include pediatrics, sports therapy, geriatrics, and orthopedics. Physical therapy technicians usually have a 2-year associate degree education.

Occupational Therapists

Occupational therapists (OTs) employ a number of techniques to help clients who are mentally, physically, developmentally, or emotionally disabled maintain daily living skills and cope with physical and emotional effects of disability. OTs assist clients in learning or relearning ADL and help them establish as independent, productive, and satisfying a lifestyle as possible. Educational preparation requires a bachelor's degree. Some programs confer a master's degree if the student is postbaccalaureate. Most states regulate OTs through licensure. Requirements include degree or certificate from an accredited program and successful completion of the OT National Certification Examination.

Speech Therapists and Audiologists

Speech therapists (STs), or language pathologists, diagnose and treat persons experiencing speech or language problems resulting from conditions such as hearing loss, brain injury (cerebrovascular accident), cleft palate, and voice pathology. *Audiologists* assess, diagnose, treat, and work to prevent hearing problems. Educational preparation for STs and audiologists is generally at the graduate level. Specialty areas include pediatrics, geriatrics, and linguistics. Most states mandate licensure for STs and audiologists, and requirements include graduation from an accredited master's degree program, completion of a licensing examination, and supervised clinical experience.

OTHER HEALTH CARE PROVIDERS

There are a number of other health care providers with whom nurses in community-based practice may work. These include optometrists, pharmacists, psychologists, dietitians, and social workers.

Optometrists

Optometrists are primary eye care providers who diagnose and treat common vision problems and prescribe eye glasses, contact lenses, and vision therapy. Most optometrist programs require 2 to 3 years of undergraduate study (most optometrists have a bachelor's degree) followed by completion of a 4-year program to obtain a Doctor of Optometry degree. All states require optometrists to be licensed.

Psychologists

Psychologists study the behavior of individuals to understand and identify fundamental processes of behavior; develop, administer, and score a variety of psychological tests; provide counseling and therapy to persons suffering emotional or adjustment problems; conduct research to improve diagnosis and treatment of mental and emotional disorders; and study human and animal behavior.

A psychologist's education is 7 years or more. Typically, a psychologist has an undergraduate degree in psychology and 3 to 5 years of graduate study. A master's degree (Master of Arts, Master of Science, or Master of Education) allows for provision of supervised psychological services, whereas a doctoral degree (Doctor of Philosophy [PhD], Doctor of Psychiatry, or Doctor of Education) is the standard entry-level degree required for independent practice. A *psychiatrist* is a physician who has completed a 3-year residency in psychiatry and can diagnose and treat mental illness using a variety of therapies, including pharmacotherapeutics. All states require licensure or certification of psychologists, although requirements vary.

Pharmacists

Pharmacists dispense medicines prescribed by physicians, podiatrists, and dentists and advise health professionals on medication selection and use. A bachelor's degree is the standard entry-level requirement for the practice of pharmacy. Graduate preparation confers a master's degree, Doctor of Pharmacy (PharmD), or a PhD and is necessary for educators, researchers, and specialists. All states require pharmacists to be licensed. Requirements include graduation from an accredited program, successful completion of a licensing examination, supervised clinical experience or internship, and that the pharmacist be over 21 years of age. Pharmacology technicians generally have an associate degree and work under the supervision of a pharmacist.

Dietitians

Dietitians teach individuals and health professionals about the science of food and nutrition. The entry level for practice as a dietitian is the bachelor's degree. A 6- to 12-month supervised internship is required if the graduate desires licensure.

Social Workers

Social workers work with individuals and families to address a wide variety of social problems and issues. Medical social workers refer clients to community resources, assist clients in attaining needed social and health care services, and help plan for institutional community placement (e.g., nursing home or extended-care facility). Identification of community resources, financial assistance, and referral for additional services are part of the practice of many social workers. The bachelor's degree is the minimum entry level for practice as a social worker. Master's and advanced master's degrees (e.g., doctoral level training) are necessary for licensure in some states and for the provision of some interventions such as counseling. Licensure for practicing social workers is required by all states, and most states recognize more than one category of social worker based on education and work experience.

Health Care Financing

Financing of health care is becoming increasingly complex and confusing. Over the past 50 years, the HCDS has evolved from being a simple, fee-for-service enterprise to a very complex entity in which a variety of individuals, groups, corporations, and/or insurers contract with providers and organizations to deliver care to individuals, families, and groups. Because of their important role in coordination and management of care, all nurses should be aware of the payment structure for health care. Understanding of eligibility requirements, copayments, deductibles, and the variety of third party reimbursement strategies can assist nurses in planning and implementing appropriate, cost-effective, and reimbursable care. Table 3–6 provides definitions of terms frequently used in describing the financial structure of the HCDS to assist nurses working in community settings.

THE HIGH COST OF HEALTH CARE

Knickman and Thorpe (1995) report that current health care expenditures represent an estimated

TABLE 3–6 Terms Used in Health Care Financing

Capitation—in managed care, capitation describes a negotiated, prepaid fixed fee for each covered individual or family. For the capitation fee, the managed care organization agrees to provide the services for which the contract calls, for a specified time period.

Coinsurance—coinsurance is a predetermined amount or percentage of the cost of covered services that the beneficiary will pay. The coinsurance may be an agreed-on percentage of the fee (20–30% is typical) or the balance of the total for fixed price services. For example, if the insurer contracts to pay $2,000 to an obstetrician for a vaginal delivery and the obstetrician charges $2,500, the client is responsible for the difference.

Copayment—a copayment is a specified flat fee per unit of service or time that the individual pays, while the insurer pays the remaining costs (example $10 per visit or $100 per day).

Deductible—a deductible is a sum that must be paid each calendar year before the insurance policy becomes active. Deductible amounts vary greatly, from almost nothing to several thousand dollars.

Diagnosis-related group (DRG)—DRGs represent a classification system that groups patients into categories based on the coding system of the International Classification of Disease, Ninth Revision-Clinical Modification (ICD-9-CM). DRGs are used to establish health care payments under Medicare.

Gatekeeper—The primary care physician within managed care plans is frequently referred to as the "gatekeeper." Usually the gatekeeper is a family practitioner, internist, pediatrician, or gynecologist who is responsible for all primary care for the enrolled patient. To avoid duplication of services and overuse of specialists, the gatekeeper coordinates all care and determines when to refer the client to a specialist.

Health maintenance organization (HMO)—An HMO is a managed care organization that contracts with an individual, group, or organization to provide health care for enrollees. The HMO agrees to provide a set of services for a set fee (typically a capitated fee). HMOs attempt to provide services to clients at a cost lower than the fee paid and thereby profit by delivering less costly care and less total services and by minimizing referrals to other providers. HMOs provide care to clients with no or minimal deductibles and copayments. There are two basic types of HMOs—the "staff" model or group practice HMO and the independent practice association:

- **Group or staff model HMO**—The "traditional" type of HMO is the group or staff model, in which the fiscal agent, or insurer, employs salaried physicians who generally spend all their time delivering services to the HMO's enrollees.
- **Independent practice association (IPA)**—IPAs are affiliations of independent practitioners who, in addition to their fee-for-service patients, contract to provide care for prepaid enrolled individuals. The IPA pays participating physicians on either a capitated or fee-for-service basis.

Managed care—*managed care* is the "umbrella," or generic, term that describes a variety of prepaid and managed fee-for-service health care plans. Managed care plans are designed to encourage greater control over the use and cost of health care services through 1) providing incentives to contain costs, 2) providing barriers to inappropriate use of specialists, 3) administrative management of the use of services, and 4) facilitating the paperwork required on the part of consumers.

Managed competition—*managed competition* is a term coined in the health care reform debates and plan posed by President and Mrs. Clinton. In theory, managed competition would reform the health care system by dividing physicians and hospitals into competing economic units that would contract with insurance-purchasing groups or organizations to provide standardized packages of health care benefits for fixed per capita rates. It is believed that this use of competition and market-based principles would create cost savings and improve access.

Medicaid—Medicaid is a national and state-sponsored public assistance (welfare) health program. Enacted by Title XIX of the Social Security Act of 1965, Medicaid is financed jointly by the states and federal government, with the federal contributions matching 50 to 77% of state contributions.

Medicare—Medicare is a national health insurance plan begun in 1965 under Title XVIII of the Social Security Act. Those eligible for Medicare are 1) persons 65 years of age and older; 2) disabled individuals who are entitled to Social Security benefits, and 3) end-stage renal disease patients. Medicare uses indirect financing and service delivery administered by the HCFA branch of the USDHHS, which contracts with independent providers.

TABLE 3–6 **Terms Used in Health Care Financing** *Continued*

Preferred provider organizations (PPOs)—PPOs are business arrangements or contracts between a panel of health care providers, usually hospitals and physicians, and purchasers of health care services (e.g., self-insured employers or health insurance companies). The providers agree to supply services to a defined group of patients on a discounted fee-for-service basis. In PPOs, the organization, usually a health insurer, contracts to provide health services for a set fee using selected physicians. The physician agrees to the fee structure of the PPO in return for the PPO providing patients. The fees are typically lower than those that the physicians charge non-PPO clients.

Third party reimbursement—within health care, third party reimbursement refers to fiscal payment by an intermediary or "third party" such as an insurance company (e.g., Blue Cross, Aetna), Medicare, or Medicaid. This third party insures beneficiaries against health expenses. The individual pays a premium for coverage, and the insurer then pays health care bills on his or her behalf.

Utilization review—utilization review is a process of monitoring and evaluating the quality of health care, including necessity, appropriateness, and efficiency. The goal of utilization review is to monitor and provide incentives to influence the use of health care services through examination of hospitalization rates, admissions, length of stay, frequency of diagnostic and therapeutic procedures, and appropriateness and efficacy of practice patterns.

Worker's compensation—begun in the early 1900s as a "social insurance" system operated by each state, worker's compensation provides covered workers with protection against the costs of medical care and loss of income resulting from work-related injury or illness. Worker's compensation laws vary greatly between the states.

Data from Williams, S. J. and Torrens, P. R. (1993). Managed care: Restructuring the system. In S. J. Williams and P. R. Torrens (Eds.). *Introduction to Health Services* (4th ed.). Albany, NY, Delmar Publishers; Inglehart, J. K. (1994). Managed competition. In P. R. Lee and C. L. Estes (Eds.). *The Nation's Health* (4th ed.). Boston, Jones and Bartlett; Knickman, J. R. and Thorpe, K. E. (1995). Financing for health care. In A. R. Kovner (Ed.). *Jonas's Health Care Delivery in the United States* (5th ed.). NY, Springer Publishing Co.; Koch, A. L. (1993). Financing health services. In S. J. Williams and P. R. Torrens (Eds.). *Introduction to Health Services* (4th ed.). Albany, NY, Delmar Publishers.

15.6% of the U. S. gross national product (up from 12.2% in 1990, 9.4% in 1980, and 7.3% in 1970), or about $4,000 per capita. This per capita expenditure is by far the highest in the world. By comparison, Sweden, France, Germany, and Canada spent 8.5 to 9.0% of their gross national products on health care during 1990, and Japan and Great Britain spent about 6.5 to 6.8% (Koch, 1993).

Reasons for the expenditures and the phenomenal growth of the cost of health care are numerous and interrelated. The growth in private insurance and third party payment for services and general economic inflation are two of the most often cited reasons for increasing health care costs. In addition, the rapid increase in the income of health care providers, most notably physicians, has profoundly affected the health care expenditures. During the 1980s, physician income grew faster than that of any other profession, and according to a report by the American Medical Association in 1993, mean physician *net* income ranges from $111,500 (general/family practice) to $233,800 (surgery) (Salsberg and Kovner, 1995). This represents an almost 100% increase in income since 1982 using constant dollars. During the same time period, the average income of year-round, full-time workers increased from about $25,000 to $30,000 (or about 20%).

Another factor that affects the costs of health care is the changes in population demography. As Americans age, more expensive and intensive health care is required. Lifestyle choices, including smoking, alcohol consumption, high-fat diets, obesity, lack of exercise, use of legal (e.g., alcohol) and illegal (e.g., cocaine) substances, and indiscriminate sexual practices have contributed to chronic diseases such as lung cancer, heart disease, diabetes, and acquired immunodeficiency syndrome. Growth in the numbers of uninsured individuals has contributed indirectly to the increase in health care costs, as health care providers raise charges and fees for those able to pay to offset bad debt.

Dependence on technology by health care providers and insistence on high-tech care by consumers contributes to misuse and abuse of technology. Overuse of expensive care and procedures (e.g., cesarean section, hysterectomy, cataract surgery, prostatectomy), medications (e.g., use of a very expensive antibiotic when penicillin would produce the same result), and failure to encourage preventative interventions such as immunizations and health promotion activities (e.g., stopping smoking, lowering cholesterol, exercising regularly) have also contributed to inefficiency, waste, and overuse of care. The increase in costs of health care also include the costs incurred in research and development; manufacture and marketing; and profits made on new medications, equipment, and techniques. Finally, malpractice insurance premiums and alterations in practice to address potential litigation and forestall malpractice claims ("defensive medicine") have been cited as contributing factors to rapid increase in health care costs.

The current system of health care financing is composed of a combination of fee-for-service, public sector payment, and third party (e.g., health insurance) reimbursement. Financing sources and distribution of health care expenditures are presented in Figure 3–2. As indicated in this illustration, payment for health care services comes from a combination of governmental sources (e.g., Medicare, Medicaid, Veteran's Administration, military service) and private sources (e.g., private health insurance, direct payment). Additionally, the greatest percentage of payment went to hospital care (38%), followed by "personal care" (e.g., medications, outpatient laboratory services, dental care, eyeglasses) and physicians' services.

PUBLIC FINANCING

As discussed, local, state, and federal governments combine to finance about 42% of health care. As Medicare and Medicaid are very important sources of health care financing, it is imperative that nurses be aware of specific components of these programs, including eligibility parameters, reimbursement requirements, and which services are or are not covered.

Medicare

"Medicare is a federal health insurance program for people 65 and older and certain disabled people" (USDHHS/Health Care Financing Administration [HCFA], 1995 p. 1), which was established by Title XVIII of the Social Security Act in 1965. Medicare is financed through tax wages, administered by the Social Security Administration, which is responsible for application and determining eligibility, and funded through the HCFA.

Medicare is divided into Part A and Part B. Medicare Part A insures qualified individuals for hospital and skilled nursing facility care, as well as for home health and hospice care. Part A has deductibles and coinsurance, but most people do not have to pay premiums for coverage. Medicare Part B insures qualified individuals for physician services, outpatient hospital services, durable medical equipment, and other medical services and supplies not covered by Part A. Part B requires monthly premiums for all subscribers, as well as deductibles and coinsurance for which the individual is responsible.

Most U. S. residents (about 98%) are eligible for premium-free Medicare Part A benefits when they reach age 65, based on their own or their spouse's employment. Medicare Part A benefits are also available for individuals who rely on dialysis for permanent kidney failure or who have had a kidney transplant and for those who are disabled and eligible for Social Security benefits. Table 3–7 provides detailed, specific information on Medicare Parts A and B, including services, benefits, premiums, coinsurance, and deductibles.

Prior to 1983, Medicare paid physicians and other providers on a fee-for-service basis and hospitals on a cost-based retrospective basis (Koch, 1993). In an attempt to better manage costs and to stop the rapid increase in expenditures, Congress enacted the Social Security Amendment of 1983 (Public Law 98–21). This act ended the cost-

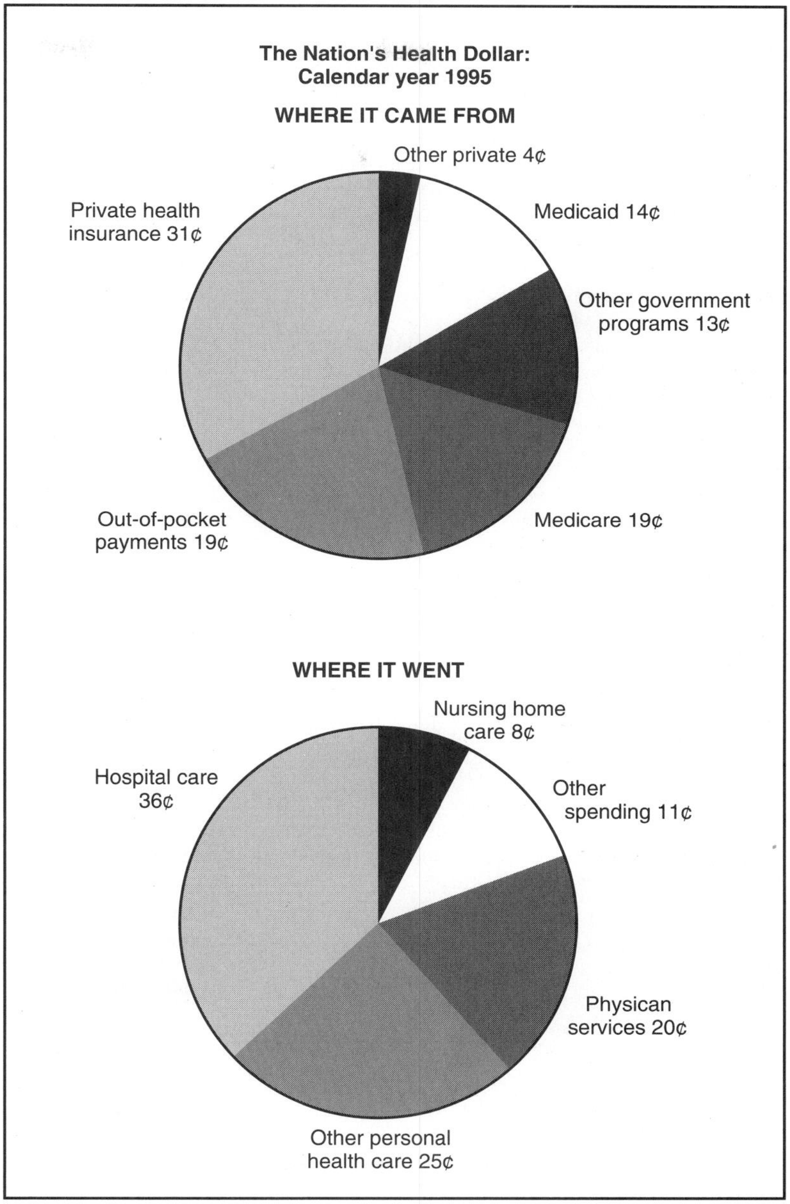

FIGURE 3–2 Health care funding sources and expenditures. (From Letsch, S. W., Lazenby, H. C., Levit, K. R., and Cowan, C. A. (1994). National health expenditures, 1991. In P. R. Lee and C. L. Estes (Eds.). *The Nation's Health* (4th ed.). Boston, Jones and Bartlett, p. 253.)

TABLE 3–7 **Medicare-Covered Services and Fees**

Medicare Part A: 1996

Services	*Benefits*	*Medicare Pays*	*You Pay**
Hospitalization—semiprivate room and board, general nursing, and other hospital services and supplies (Medicare payments based on benefit periods; see p. 7)	First 60 days 61st to 90th day 91st to 150th day† Beyond 150 days	All but $736 All but $184 a day All but $368 a day Nothing	$736 $184 a day $368 a day All costs
Skilled nursing facility care—semiprivate room and board, skilled nursing, and rehabilitative services and other services and supplies (Medicare payments based on benefit periods; see p. 7)	First 20 days Additional 80 days Beyond 100 days	100% of approved amount All but $92 a day Nothing	Nothing Up to $92 a day All costs
Home health care—part-time or intermittent skilled care, home health aide services, durable medical equipment and supplies, and other services	Unlimited as long as you meet Medicare conditions	100% of approved amount; 80% of approved amount for durable medical equipment	Nothing for services; 20% of approved amount for durable medical equipment
Hospice care—pain relief, symptom management, and support services for the terminally ill	For as long as doctor certifies need	All but limited costs for outpatient drugs and inpatient respite care	Limited costs for outpatient drugs and inpatient respite care
Blood—when furnished by a hospital or skilled nursing facility during a covered stay	Unlimited if medically necessary	All but first three pints per calendar year	For first three pints‡

1996 Part A monthly premium: $289 with fewer than 30 quarters of Medicare-covered employment; $188 with more than 30 quarters but fewer than 40 quarters of covered employment. Most beneficiaries do not have to pay a premium for Part A.

plus, fee-for-service system and introduced the prospective payment system for hospital coverage. The prospective payment system uses 468 diagnosis-related groups to classify cases for payment, and reimbursement is based on a fixed price per case. The prospective payment system requires that all providers bill Medicare directly for reimbursement for services. Medicare claims are paid indirectly by the HCFA through the use of "fiscal intermediaries." These intermediaries are typically insurance companies who contract with Medicare to review, process, and pay all claims.

Medicaid

The Medicaid program was initiated in 1965 by Title XIX of the Social Security Act. Medicaid is a public assistance welfare program that provides financial assistance to pay for health care for the poor, blind, and disabled, and families with dependent children. Medicaid is funded jointly by the federal government and each state. Eligibility, coverage, and payment for services vary greatly from state to state.

Although covered services vary, federal require-

TABLE 3–7 **Medicare-Covered Services and Fees** *Continued*

Medicare Part B: 1996

Services	***Benefits***	***Medicare Pays***	***You Pay****
Medical expenses—Doctors' services, inpatient and outpatient medical and surgical services and supplies, physical and speech therapy, diagnostic tests, durable medical equipment and other services	Unlimited if medically necessary	80% of approved amount (after $100 deductible) Reduced to 50% for most outpatient mental health services	$100 deductible plus 20% of approved amount and limited charges above approved amount
Clinical laboratory services—Blood tests, urinalyses, and more	Unlimited if medically necessary	Generally 100% of approved amount	Nothing for services
Home health care—Part-time or intermittent skilled care, home health aide services, durable medical equipment, and supplies and other services	Unlimited as long as you meet Medicare conditions	100% of approved amount; 80% of approved amount for durable medical equipment	Nothing for services; 20% of approved amount for durable medical equipment
Outpatient hospital treatment—Services for the diagnosis or treatment of illness or injury	Unlimited if medically necessary	Medicare payment to hospital based on hospital cost	20% of whatever the hospital charges (after $100 deductible)
Blood	Unlimited if medically necessary	80% of approved amount (after $100 deductible and starting with fourth pint)	First three pints plus 20% of approved amount for additional pints (after $100 deductible)‖
Ambulatory surgical services	Unlimited if medically necessary	80% of predetermined amount (after $100 deductible)	$100 deductible plus 20% of predetermined amount

1996 Part B monthly premium: $42.50 (premium may be higher if you enroll late).

From USDHHS/HCFA. (1996). *Your Medicare Handbook, 1996.* Publication No. HCFA-10050. Baltimore, Government Printing Office.

*Either you or your insurance company are responsible for paying the amounts listed in the "You Pay" column.

†This 60-reserve-days benefit may be used only once in a lifetime (see p. 7).

‡Blood paid for or replaced under Part B of Medicare during the calendar year does not have to be paid for or replaced under Part A.

‖Blood paid for or replaced under Part A of Medicare during the calendar year does not have to be paid for or replaced under Part B.

ments dictate that Medicaid cover certain services in all states. These include inpatient and outpatient hospital care; skilled nursing care; physician services; family planning services; home health care; and early and periodic screening, diagnosis, and treatment services for eligible children. Additional services that may be covered in some states include dental care, eye care, and medications. Table 3–8 provides detailed information on Medicaid beneficiaries and services. A comparison of Medicare and Medicaid appears in Table 3–9.

It is important to note that both the legislative and executive branches of the federal government are exploring ways to decrease health care costs. Several states, including Arizona, Massachusetts, Hawaii, and Oregon, are experimenting with plans to reduce costs through a variety of changes (Stanhope, 1996). Reduction of coverage for certain services, prioritizing care based on specified criteria such as effectiveness and benefit, refusal to pay for certain procedures or services, encouraging participants to use managed care, and other efforts have been proposed and are being tested. All health providers, as well as consumers, are advised to closely monitor the ongoing debates and support legislative efforts that control costs and maintain quality.

TABLE 3–8 **Medicaid Beneficiaries and Services**

Medicaid Recipients	Major Benefits under Medicaid
Federally Dictated Recipients	***State-Determined Optional Services***
• All persons in federal aide programs, including Supplemental Security Income (SSI) and Aid to Families with Dependent Children (AFDC) • Pregnant women and children up to 6 years of age with a family income below 133% of the poverty level • Children 18 years of age and younger, born after September 30, 1983, with a family income below the poverty level • Medicare beneficiaries with income below the poverty level (but only for payment of Medicare premiums and cost sharing)	• Drug therapy • Dental care • Physical therapy • Eyeglasses • Podiatry • Optometry • Clinical services • Transportation • Residential intermediate care facilities for the mentally retarded (ICF-MR) • Nursing facility services for people under 21 years of age • Prescription drugs • Prosthetic devices
Optional Recipients	***Federally Required Services***
• Medically needy families with incomes above AFDC limits with sick children • Medically needy older persons not qualified for income assistance (welfare)	• Inpatient and outpatient hospital care • Physician services • Diagnostic services (e.g., laboratory tests, radiographs) • Skilled nursing home care • Home health care • Family planning • Nurse-midwife services • Certified family or pediatric nurse practitioner services • Ambulatory services provided in federally qualified health centers • Early and periodic screening, diagnosis, and treatment (EPSDT) for people under 21 years of age

From National Heritage Insurance Company. (1992). *Medicaid Provider Procedures Manual: Texas Department of Human Services.* Austin, TX: National Heritage Insurance Company.

Note: Covered services are provided to those groups with federally required coverage. Mandated services to optional groups are less comprehensive.

From Congressional Budget Office Staff Memorandum, May 1992.

TABLE 3–9 **Comparison of Medicare and Medicaid**

Medicare	Medicaid
• A federal health *insurance* program for persons 65 years and older, disabled persons, and persons with end-stage renal disease	• A welfare *assistance* program for the poor; those eligible for Medicaid include families receiving Aid to Families with Dependent Children, individuals receiving benefits for the Supplemental Security Income Program due to age or disability, and the "medically needy" whose incomes fall below a certain percentage of the poverty level; each state determines eligibility requirements, payment for services, and type of services provided (with some federal restrictions)
• Financed through Social Security taxes and monthly premiums	• Jointly funded by the states and the federal government
• Administered by the HCFA within the USDHHS • HCFA contracts with insurance companies to process and pay claims submitted by beneficiaries	• Administered by a designated state agency and the HCFA
• Medicare Part A covers inpatient hospital care, home health care, hospice care and skilled nursing care • Medicare Part B covers physicians' services; covered services provided by other health professions, including RNs, nurse practitioners, chiropractors, psychologists, and social workers; outpatient hospital services, ambulance services, ambulatory surgery, outpatient physical, occupational and speech therapy, radiation therapy, durable medical equipment, surgical dressing, screening examinations are also covered	• Medicaid benefits include inpatient and outpatient hospital services; prenatal care; outpatient diagnostic and laboratory services; home health care; physicians' services; screening, diagnosis, and treatment of children; family planning services. States may add additional benefits, including prescription medications, dental services, ambulance services, psychiatric care, medical supplies, optometrists' services, and eyeglasses
• Medicare enrollees in Part B pay a monthly premium of $42.50 per month for coverage	• There is no cost to those eligible for Medicaid
• Payment may be fee-for-service or option of enrolling in an HMO or comprehensive medical plan	• Payment to providers is a combination of fee-for-service based on "reasonable charges" and a state-defined "Medicaid fee schedule"
• Payment to hospitals is based on diagnosis-related groups (DRGs) or audited costs	• Payment to hospitals is based on DRGs, with some exceptions

From National Heritage Insurance Company. (1995). *Medicaid Provider Procedures Manual: Texas Department of Human Services.* Austin, TX, National Heritage Insurance Company; USDHHS/HCFA. (1996). *Your Medicare Handbook.*

PRIVATE FINANCING

The greatest percentage of health care is financed by private health insurance (see Fig. 4–3). At present, the structure of the private sector health insurance system is very complex. In the United States, health care insurance is frequently provided by employers and has become an expected benefit of employment. Typically, employer-provided health insurance covers both the employee and his or her family, and both the employer and the employee contribute to the cost of premiums.

As insurance premium costs have increased dramatically over the past two decades, alterations in the structure and coverage parameters of this system have altered and continue to do so. The result has been an increase in managed care plans; changes in premiums, coinsurance and deductibles; limits to coverage; and refusal to pay for "preexisting conditions." Health care insurance programs and options include a variety of financial arrangements, such as traditional, indemnity health insurance coverage; PPOs, and HMOs. Each is described briefly.

Traditional Health Insurance

In the United States, health insurance began when teachers in Dallas, Texas devised a way to finance and share the costs of health care. In 1929, Dallas public school teachers contracted with Baylor Hospital to provide specified health care services for a predetermined cost. By 1939, this insurance plan had grown to include many other groups and became Blue Cross-Blue Shield (Clemen-Stone et al., 1995). The idea of health insurance grew very rapidly, and currently about 73% of United States residents are covered by private health insurance.

Health insurance organizations may be nonprofit (e.g., Blue Cross-Blue Shield) or commercial, for profit (e.g., Aetna, CIGNA). Under traditional contracts, the insurance company finances care for enrollees. Premiums, deductibles, and copayments or coinsurance are required by indemnity policies. Premiums have increased dramatically since the 1980s, prompting cost-containment strategies by most employers. These strategies include encouraging the use of managed care, reducing reliance on traditional insurers through increasing self-funding of health benefits, and increasing the share of health care expenses paid by the employees. Many insurers now provide options for enrollees whereby they may choose traditional coverage or care through an HMO or PPO.

Preferred Provider Organizations

Preferred provider organizations are business arrangements, or contracts, between a group of health care providers (e.g., hospitals or physicians) and a purchaser of health care services (e.g., employers or insurance companies). PPOs began during the mid-1980s to decrease the costs of health care insurance. In these arrangements, the providers agree to supply services to a defined group of patients (e.g., employees of company "X") at a discounted fee-for-service basis. According to Koch (1993), PPOs have five elements: a limited number of physicians and hospitals, negotiated fee schedules, utilization review or utilization management, consumer choice of providers with incentives to use participating providers, and expedient settlement of claims. As of 1992, about 13% of private insurance was through PPOs (Knickman and Thorpe, 1995), and the percentage is growing.

Health Maintenance Organizations

An HMO is an organized health care system that provides health services to enrolled individuals for a fixed, prepaid (i.e., capitated) fee. HMOs typically possess an organized system to provide health care in a particular geographical area, an agreed-on set of services for health maintenance and treatment, voluntarily enrolled membership, and rates similar to those of providers in the community (Clark, 1995). HMOs provide fairly comprehensive coverage in return for the prepaid fee, usually without deductibles and with minimal copayments ($10–$20 per visit is common). HMOs are intended to reduce hospitalizations and health care costs by encouraging illness prevention and health maintenance and reducing "inappropriate care." There is evidence of success in these goals, as Knickman and Thorpe (1995) report that HMOs have resulted in a 40% reduction in hospital use for enrollees.

In the United States, the concept of the HMO began in 1929 at a private health clinic in Los Angeles, which expanded in 1930 as the Kaiser company provided coverage for workers building the Grand Coulee Dam (Koch, 1993). The number of prepaid insurance plans, however, grew very slowly until the 1970s. The cost of health care had already become a concern, and, in response, the HMO Act of 1973 (Public Law 93–222) was passed. Subsequent amendments have encouraged rapid growth through the 1980s through use of incentives to employers and providers. Estimates indicate that members enrolled in HMO plans have climbed dramatically, growing from 9.1 million (1980), to 18.9 million (1985), to 36.5 million (1990), to 41.4 million (1992) (Knickman and Thorpe, 1995).

There are several basic HMO models including

the "staff" model, the "group" model, and the "independent practice association," with some variations in each. In the traditional, or "staff" model, HMO, the HMO is an organization that employs physicians and other providers to deliver services to the HMO's enrollees. In the "group" model HMO, a group or association of physicians contracts with the fiscal agent to provide services to enrollees. Finally, in the independent practice association model, the fiscal agent contracts with a range of physicians who are not associated with each other and work in independent practices to provide services on a capitated basis.

Because of capitated payments, physicians working in HMOs usually have incentives to use resources efficiently. Reportedly, some HMOs offer bonuses to physicians if services, such as specialists and expensive procedures, are not significantly utilized, and HMOs might reprimand providers for overuse of services and specialists.

Health maintenance organizations usually require that enrollees designate one primary care provider as a "gatekeeper." The gatekeeper may be a family practitioner, internist, pediatrician, or, in some cases, an obstetrician/gynecologist. This primary care physician determines when referral to a specialist is needed and provides oversight for all of the patient's health care needs. Other cost-containment strategies employed by HMOs, as well as other health care insurers, include second surgical opinions, preauthorization for most hospital admissions, case management, and utilization review (Stanhope, 1996; Williams and Torrens, 1993). The preauthorization requirement and second surgical opinions were developed to correct the practice of unnecessary surgeries and unneeded hospitalizations.

Table 3–10 presents a simplified comparison of HMOs, PPOs, and "traditional" health insurance. An understanding of the requirements of each increases the nurse's awareness of the similarities and differences in the programs to encourage care planning that is sensitive to the financial needs and resources of the client.

CARING FOR THE UNINSURED

In the United States, an estimated 31 to 43 million individuals have no health insurance on any given day, and an additional 30 million (12%) are considered "underinsured" (Friedman, 1991; Stanhope, 1996). Thus, at any given time in the United States, as many as 25% of Americans have no or inadequate health care coverage. The typical uninsured individual is a member of a family in which the adults are unemployed or underemployed and thereby ineligible for employee-paid health insurance coverage. Children, young adults, and members of minorities are disproportionately represented among uninsured persons (Friedman, 1991).

The lack of insurance affects health and well-being in many ways. Lack of access to timely and affordable health care discourages the use of preventive services and early treatment for acute, episodic illnesses. Failure to seek preventive care (for example, prenatal care) contributes to an increase in complications of pregnancy, such as low–birth-weight infants. Likewise, failure to adequately immunize infants and small children puts them at risk for a variety of illnesses. People who have no health care coverage often wait to seek care until the illness has progressed to a stage requiring more extensive, and therefore more costly, treatment. Emergency departments are more accessible to the uninsured and are often their only source of health care.

The lack of accessible health care services for those who are uninsured or underinsured has, by default, created health care rationing, in which only those who can afford treatment receive it. Uncompensated care continues to drain many regional and public hospitals and also affects private health providers and society at large. Public hospitals must incur a very large share of uncompensated care, which results in increased taxes and higher insurance costs for everyone. Recognition of these problems has resulted in efforts to reform the HCDS, and many proposals have been made to address these issues and institute some form of universal coverage. Nurses are encouraged to stay informed of legislative efforts at all levels and to support efforts to provide care to all.

SUMMARY

It is incumbent on all health care providers, including nurses, to have a basic understanding of the

TABLE 3–10 **Comparison of Private Insurance Plans**

Traditional Indemnity	Preferred Provider Organization	Health Maintenance Organization: Staff Model	Health Maintenance Organization: Individual Practice Association, and Group Models
Free choice of providers without any restrictions	Free choice of providers; lower costs if providers are within "network" of preferred providers	Choice of providers limited to physicians and other providers employed by the HMO	Choice of providers limited to physicians under contract with the HMO
No referral necessary for specialty care	No referral necessary for specialty care; use of specialists within PPO encouraged through financial incentives	Designated primary care provider (gatekeeper) must approve treatment and determines when referrals are made to specialists; specialists within the HMO are used whenever possible	Designated primary care provider (gatekeeper) must approve treatment and determines when referrals are made to specialists; Individual Practice Association specialists are used whenever possible
Providers use their own office; referrals for specialized care may not be conveniently located	Providers use their own offices	Centralized facility allows for convenience and coordination of care	Providers use their own offices
Costs of premiums highest of all insurance plans; deductibles required; copayments 20–30% of total medical care	Premiums and deductible are lower than traditional insurance; copayment or coinsurance is usually required; costs to the insured if providers are outside of the PPO	Premiums and copayments are lower than traditional indemnity and PPOs	Premiums and copayments are lower than traditional indemnity and PPOs
No coordination of care; each provider works independently	Limited coordination of care	Care coordinated through primary care provider; case management may be utilized	Care coordinated through primary care provider; case management may be utilized
Provider or insured must file claim forms for reimbursement; processing time may be lengthy	May require additional paperwork or approval for some services	No paperwork required for basic services	No paperwork required for basic services
Preventive care may or may not be covered	Preventive care may or may not be covered	Preventive care encouraged	Preventive care encouraged

HCDS. Financial and reimbursement considerations, current and anticipated need for health care, practice parameters for providers, and a variety of other factors influence how health care is delivered in the United States. These issues have been discussed in this chapter, and the reference list that follows provides several sources that include more detailed information on these and related topics.

Key Points

- The health care delivery system is divided into "public sector" and "private sector" components.
- The public sector is subdivided into federal, state, and local levels and is typically concerned with the health of populations and maintaining a healthy environment. At the federal level, the USDHHS oversees many of the issues related to health. Each state maintains a state health department and defines what services will be offered at the state level and at the local level.
- The private sector system is composed of a variety of providers, institutions, industries, corporations, and insurers. It can be further divided into "nonprofit" or "proprietary" components.
- The health care delivery system contains a multitude of organizations that serve the population at many levels and for many needs. These include ambulatory health care settings, hospitals, and long-term care facilities (e.g., nursing homes, skilled nursing units, hospice care).
- A number of different health care professionals provide care to members of the population. These include physicians, physician assistants, dentists, nurses, nurse practitioners, therapists, optometrists, psychologists and counselors, pharmacists, social workers, and many others.
- In the United States, health care is very expensive, representing about 15.6% of the gross national product. Reasons for the high cost of health care include growth in insurance and third party payment for services, general economic inflation, increases in the income of health care providers, changes in population demography (e.g., aging of U. S. residents), lifestyle choices that are detrimental to health (e.g., smoking, drug abuse, poor diet, indiscriminate sexual practices), and dependence on technology.
- Financing of health care is very complex and consists of a combination of fee-for-service, public sector payment, and third party reimbursement. Payment for health care comes from a combination of governmental sources (e.g., Medicare, Medicaid, Veteran's Administration) and private sources (e.g., private health insurance, direct payment).
- Medicare is the federal health insurance program for people 65 years of age and older and persons with certain disabilities. It is divided into parts A and B. Medicare Part A insures individuals for hospital and skilled nursing facility care, home health, and hospice care. Part A has deductibles and coinsurance, but most people do not pay premiums for coverage. Medicare Part B insures individuals for physician services, outpatient hospital services, medical equipment, and other medical services and supplies not covered by Part A. A monthly premium is required.

- Medicaid is a public assistance welfare program that pays for health care for the poor, blind, and disabled and families with dependent children. Medicaid is funded jointly by the federal government and each state. Eligibility, coverage, and payment for services are set by each state and vary greatly. Medicaid covers inpatient and outpatient hospital care; skilled nursing care; physician services; family planning services; home health care; and early periodic screening, diagnosis, and treatment services for eligible children. Other services that may be covered in some states include dental care, eye care, and medications.
- The greatest percentage of health care is financed by private health insurance. The health insurance system is very complex and is typically provided by an individual's employer, and both the employer and the employee contribute to the cost of premiums. Health care insurance programs include a variety of financial arrangements, including indemnity health insurance, PPOs, and HMOs.
- Approximately 25% of U. S. residents have no or inadequate health care coverage. Children, young adults, and members of minorities are disproportionately represented among the uninsured and underinsured.

Learning Activities and Application to Practice

In Class

- Obtain a copy of the current *Medicare Handbook* (USDHHS/HCFA, 1996). Discuss Medicare coverage and related fees. Discuss the importance of Medicare requirements, guidelines, and reimbursement parameters in directing health care payment for services (e.g., DRGs).
- With the students, create a list of local health care organizations (e.g., ambulatory care agencies, hospitals, voluntary organizations) according to source of payment (public or private) and whether they are nonprofit or for profit. Identify actual or perceived differences in services provided and mission.
- Encourage students to discuss their personal source of health care insurance. Compare coverage, costs, deductibles, and copayments. Have them share personal experiences with the costs of health care (e.g., recent pregnancy, chronic illness, having a check-up, medications). What are some student experiences with managed care?
- Have students debate the prospect of a national health insurance program sponsored by the federal government. What might be advantages? What would be disadvantages?

In Clinical

- In each setting to which they are assigned, have students gather information on the sources of, and procedure for, reimbursement. What is covered by insurance, Medicare, or Medicaid and what is not? How can services be provided efficiently and cost-effectively?

- Assign each student to briefly interview a health care professional from another discipline (e.g., physical therapist, medical technologist, pharmacist) they encounter during clinical. Encourage students to question the professional on issues such as education and licensure or certification requirements, practice, salary range, and related information. If possible, allow the student to spend a few hours observing this individual in practice and share observations with the other students.

REFERENCES

Aday, L. A. (1993). Indicators and predictors of health services utilization. In S. J. Williams and P. R. Torrens (Eds.). *Introduction to Health Services* (4th ed.). Albany, NY, Delmar Publishers, pp. 46–70.

American Hospital Association. (1993–1994). *Hospital Statistics*. Chicago, American Hospital Association.

Birchfield, P. C. (1996). Elder health. In M. Stanhope and J. Lancaster (Eds.). *Community Health Nursing: Promoting Health of Aggregates, Families and Individuals* (4th ed.). St. Louis, MO, Mosby-Year Book, pp. 581–600.

Bodenheimer, T. and Estes, C. L. (1994). Long term care: Requiem for commercial private insurance. In P. R. Lee and C. L. Estes (Eds.). *The Nation's Health* (4th ed.). Boston, Jones and Bartlett, pp. 350–358.

Clark, M. J. (1995). *Nursing in the Community* (2nd ed.). Norwalk, CT, Appleton & Lange.

Clemen-Stone, S., Eigsti, D. G., and McGuire, S. L. (1995). *Comprehensive Community Health Nursing* (4th ed.), St. Louis, MO, Mosby–Year Book.

Evashwick, C. J. (1993). The continuum of long-term care. In S. J. Williams and P. R. Torrens (Eds.). *Introduction to Health Services* (4th ed). Albany, NY, Delmar Publishers, pp. 177–218.

Friedman, E. (1991). The uninsured: From dilemma to crisis. *Journal of the American Medical Association, 265* (19), 2491–2495.

Haglund, C. L. and Dowling, W. L. (1993). The hospital. In S. J. Williams and P. R. Torrens (Eds.). *Introduction to Health Services* (4th ed). Albany, NY, Delmar Publishers, pp. 134–176.

Inglehart, J. K. (1994). Managed competition. In P. R. Lee and C. L. Estes (Eds.). *The Nation's Health* (4th ed.). Boston, Jones and Bartlett, pp. 224–237.

Knickman, J. R. and Thorpe, K. E. (1995). Financing for health care. In A. R. Kovner (Ed.). *Jonas's Health Care Delivery in the United States* (5th ed.). New York, Springer Publishing Co., pp. 267–293.

Koch, A. L. (1993). Financing health services. In S. J. Williams and P. R. Torrens (Eds.). *Introduction to Health Services* (4th ed). Albany, NY, Delmar Publishers, pp. 299–359.

Kovner, A. R. (1995). Introduction to Jonas's Health Care Delivery in the United States. In A. R. Kovner (Ed.). *Jonas's Health Care Delivery in the United States* (5th ed.). New York, Springer Publishing Co., pp. 3–9.

Lee, P. R., Soffel, D., and Luft, H. S. (1995). Costs and coverage: Pressures toward health care reform. In P. R. Lee and C. L. Estes (Eds.). *The Nation's Health* (4th ed.). Boston, Jones and Bartlett, pp. 204–213.

Letsch, S. W., Lazenby, H. C., Levit, K. R., and Cowan, C. A. (1993). National Health Expenditures, 1991. Report from the Office of National Health Statistics, Office of the Actuary, Health Care Financing Administration. In P. R. Lee and C. L. Estes (Eds.). *The Nation's Health* (4th ed.). Boston, Jones and Bartlett, pp. 252–263.

Mezey, A. P. and Lawrence, R. S. (1995). Ambulatory care. In A. R. Kovner (Ed.). *Jonas's Health Care Delivery in the United States* (5th ed.). New York, Springer Publishing Co., pp. 122–161.

National Heritage Insurance Company. (1992). *Medicaid Provider Procedures Manual: Texas Department of Human Services*. Austin, TX, National Heritage Insurance Company.

Rice, D. P. (1991). Health status and national health priorities. *Western Journal of Medicine, 154* (3), 294–302.

Richardson, H. (1995). Long-term care. In A. R. Kovner (Ed.). *Jonas's Health Care Delivery in the United States* (5th ed.). New York, Springer Publishing Co., pp. 194–231.

Salsberg, E. S. and Kovner, C. (1995). The health care workforce. In A. R. Kovner (Ed.). *Jonas's Health Care Delivery in the United States* (5th ed.). New York, Springer Publishing Co., pp. 55–100.

Stanfield, P. S. (1990). *Introduction to the Health Professions*. Boston, Jones and Bartlett Publishers.

Stanhope, M. (1996). Economics of health care delivery. In M. Stanhope and J. Lancaster (Eds.). *Community Health Nursing: Promoting Health of Aggregates, Families and Individuals* (4th ed.). St. Louis, MO, Mosby-Year Book, pp. 65–92.

U. S. Department of Health and Human Services. (1994). *Vital and Health Statistics: Current Estimates for the National Health Interview Survey, 1992.* DHHS Publication No. (Public Health Service) 94–1517. Hyattsville, MD, U. S. Department of Health and Human Services.

U. S. Department of Health and Human Services/Health Care Financing Administration (1996). *Your Medicare Handbook, 1995.* HCFA Publication No. 10050.

Williams, S. J. (1993). Ambulatory health care services. In S. J. Williams and P. R. Torrens (Eds.). *Introduction to Health Services* (4th ed.). Albany, NY, Delmar Publishers, pp. 108–133.

Williams, S. J. and Torrens, P. R. (1993). Managed care: Restructuring the system. In S. J. Williams and P. R. Torrens (Eds.). *Introduction to Health Services* (4th ed.). Albany, NY, Delmar Publishers, pp. 361–374.

4

Epidemiology

Case Study

Meg Henderson is a school nurse who cares for children of elementary school age in a small city. One of her primary responsibilities is prevention of communicable diseases. In addition to monitoring each child's immunization status, this includes identifying children with communicable diseases, excluding them from school, and then reinstating them, according to school district policy.

One recent Monday, Meg saw Elizabeth Ellis, a third grader, whose teacher sent her to the clinic because she was seen scratching her head repeatedly. Using applicators, Meg carefully examined Elizabeth's hair and saw evidence of head lice. When questioned, Elizabeth replied that her head had been itching "about 2 or 3 days." Meg learned that Elizabeth lives with her parents and older brother and younger sister, who are also students at the school. Following district guidelines, Meg examined both of Elizabeth's siblings and determined that they were also infected. She called Mrs. Ellis and informed her that she must come to school to get her children and treat the entire family for lice.

When Mrs. Ellis arrived to pick up her children, she was obviously embarrassed. Meg carefully explained that lice are a very contagious parasite, easily passed between children through sharing of brushes, combs, hats, or other items, and not *an indicator of poor hygiene. She also stated that head lice are easily treatable and gave Mrs. Ellis an information packet that she keeps in the clinic describing the transmission, identification, and treatment of head lice. She reviewed the information with Mrs. Ellis, informed her that the children can return to school after they have all been treated, and pointed out that they should be treated again in 2 weeks.*

After the Ellis family left, Meg examined all of the students from each of the Ellis children's classes for head lice. From the three classes, she identified seven more children with lice and then called their parents. These children had siblings in three more classes, and the children in each of these classes were also examined. At the end of the day, a total of 15 children had been excluded from school.

The following week, Meg reexamined all of the children in each class with an infected student. Two weeks after the incident, she examined all of the excluded children and determined that they had been successfully treated. No more cases of lice were identified that semester.

Much of nursing practice, particularly in community settings, involves prevention, early identification, and prompt treatment of health problems, as well as monitoring for emerging threats and unidentified patterns that might signify health problems. For example, a nurse working in an inner-city women's clinic might note that the diagnosis of cervical dysplasia among teenagers and women in their early 20s has increased over a period of time, associated with increases in human papillomavirus infection. In addition to assisting with treatment of the clients involved, she would inform officials from the county health department's sexually transmitted disease program or a regional medical school for further investigation.

Another example would be a nurse working in a manufacturing plant who notes an unusual increase in complaints of back strain. After assisting the workers with reducing their back pain, the nurse should collect data on cases of back strain during the past 6 months and look for trends. Further, he should inform the plant management and work with them to take appropriate steps to identify the cause of the problems and develop plant policy to minimize risks. Recording problems, keeping track of patterns, and thus identifying causes are all part of the science and practice of epidemiology.

Epidemiology is the basic science of public health and refers to "the study of the distribution and determinants of health-related states or events in a specified population, and the application of this study to the control of health problems" (Centers for Disease Control, 1992, p. 430). The science of epidemiology is based on the idea that disease, illness, and ill health are not randomly distributed in a population but rather that "each of us has certain characteristics that predispose us to, or protect us against, a variety of different diseases" (Gordis, 1996, p. 3). Identifying these characteristics and removing or minimizing them if they are harmful, or enhancing them or transferring them if helpful, are basic goals in epidemiology.

Nurses who work with clients in community settings are frequently in a position to assist in identification, management, treatment, and prevention of health problems, and, as a result, need a general understanding of the basic principles, theories, and concepts of epidemiology. In addition, a nurse needs to be able to read and interpret data about trends in diseases to carry out responsibilities in client teaching. Valanis (1992) outlines seven uses of epidemiology, which are depicted in Table 4–1.

Healthy People 2000 (U.S. Department of Health and Human Services, 1990), which was introduced in Chapter 1, was written based on epidemiological principles. This document presents health statistics and data; describes health threats; discusses interventions and plans; and set goals and objectives directed toward prevention, management, minimization, or elimination of the identified health threats. Table 4–2 presents examples of *Healthy People 2000*'s goals demonstrating epidemiological concepts that are described in this chapter (e.g., primary prevention, rates). In addition, selected goals from the "priority area" termed "Surveillance and Data Systems" (Objective 22) are listed.

This chapter presents basic concepts of epidemiology and describes how understanding the course or progression of a disease or health condition is important for nurses who practice in community settings. The use of epidemiological concepts and principles to identify risks and to assist in the prevention and management of disease also is discussed. As a starting point, Table 4–3 contains definitions of some important terms and concepts fundamental to epidemiology.

TABLE 4–1 **Uses of Epidemiology**

- Investigation of disease etiology and determination of the natural history of disease
- Identification of risks
- Identification of syndromes and classification of disease
- Differential diagnoses and planning clinical treatment
- Surveillance of the health status of population
- Community diagnosis and planning of health services
- Evaluation of health services and public health interventions

Data from Valanis, B. (1992). *Epidemiology in Nursing and Health Care.* Norwalk, CT, Appleton & Lange.

TABLE 4–2 ***Healthy People 2000*—Objectives Related to Epidemiology**

Objective	
1.1	Reduce coronary heart disease deaths to no more than 100 per 100,000 people (age-adjusted baseline: 135 per 100,000 in 1987)
4.1	Reduce death caused by alcohol-related motor vehicle crashes to no more than 8.5 per 100,000 people (baseline: 9.7 per 100,000 in 1987)
5.1	Reduce pregnancies among girls 17 years of age and younger to no more than 50 per 1,000 adolescents (baseline: 71.1 pregnancies per 1,000 girls 15 through 17 years of age in 1985)
8.1	Increase years of healthy life to at least 65 (baseline: an estimated 62 years in 1980)
9.5	Reduce drowning deaths to no more than 1.3 per 100,000 people (age-adjusted baseline: 2.1 per 100,000 people in 1987)
14.1	Reduce the infant mortality rate to no more than 7 per 1,000 live births (baseline: 10.1 per 1,000 live births in 1987)
16.3	Reduce breast cancer deaths to no more than 20.6 per 100,000 women (age-adjusted baseline: 22.9 per 100,000 in 1987)
18.2	Confine the prevalence of HIV infection to no more than 800 per 100,000 people (baseline: an estimated 400 per 100,000 in 1987)
20.4	Reduce tuberculosis to an incidence of no more than 3.5 per 100,000 people (baseline: 9.1 per 100,000 in 1988)
22.1	Develop a set of health status indicators appropriate for federal, state, and local health agencies and establish use of the set in at least 40 states
22.4	Develop and implement a national process to identify significant gaps in the nation's disease prevention and health promotion data, including data for racial and ethnic minorities, people with low incomes, and people with disabilities, and establish mechanisms to meet these needs

From U. S. Department of Health and Human Services. (1990). *Healthy People 2000: National Health Promotion and Disease Prevention Objectives.* Washington, D. C., Government Printing Office.

TABLE 4–3 **Epidemiological Terms and Concepts**

Epidemiology is derived from three Greek words: *epi* (upon), *demas* (the people), and *logos* (science). Traditionally, epidemiology is defined as "The study of the distribution and determinant of diseases and injuries in human populations" (Mausner and Kramer, 1985, p. 1).

More recently, epidemiology has been termed "The study of the distribution and determinants of health-related states or events in a specified population, and the application of this study to the control of health problems" (CDC, 1992, p. 430). The following terms are related to epidemiology:

- Agent—a factor, such as microorganism, chemical substance, or form of radiation, whose presence, excessive presence, or (in deficiency diseases) relative absence is essential for the occurrence of a disease.
- Carrier—a person or animal without apparent disease who harbors a specific infectious agent and is capable of transmitting the agent to others.
- Case definition—a set of standard criteria for deciding whether a person has a particular disease or health-related condition by specifying clinical criteria and limitations on time, place, and person.
- Cohort—a well-defined group of people who have had a common experience or exposure, who are then followed up for the incidence of new diseases or events, as in a cohort or prospective study.
- Common source outbreak (point source)—an outbreak that results from a group of persons being exposed to a common noxious influence, such as an infectious agent or toxin. If the group is exposed over a relatively brief time, so that all cases occur within one incubation period, then the common source outbreak is further classified as a point source outbreak.

Table continued on following page

TABLE 4–3 **Epidemiological Terms and Concepts** *Continued*

- Crude mortality rate—the mortality rate from all causes of death for a population.
- Direct transmission—the immediate transfer of an agent from a reservoir to a susceptible host by direct contact of droplet spread.
- Distribution—the frequency and pattern of health-related characteristics and events in a population.
- Endemic disease—the constant presence of a disease or infectious agent within a given geographical area or population group; it may also refer to the usual prevalence of a given disease within such an area or a group.
- Epidemic—the occurrence of more cases of disease than expected in a given area or among a specific group of people over a particular period.
- Herd immunity—the resistance of a group to invasion and spread of an infectious agent, based on the resistance to infection of a high proportion of individual members of the group. The resistance is a product of the number susceptible and the probability that those who are susceptible will come into contact with an infected person.
- High-risk group—a group in the community with an elevated risk of disease.
- Host—a person or other living organism that can be infected by an infectious agent under natural conditions.
- Incidence (incidence rate)—a measure of the frequency with which an event, such as a new case of illness, occurs in a population over a period. The denominator is the population at risk; the numerator is the number of *new* cases occurring during a given time.
- Indirect transmission—the transmission of an agent carried from a reservoir to a susceptible host by suspended air particles or by animate (vector) or inanimate (vehicle) intermediaries.
- Infectivitiy—the proportion of persons exposed to a causative agent who become infected by an infectious disease.
- Mortality rate—a measure of the frequency of occurrence of death in a defined population during a specified time interval.
- Natural history of disease—the temporal course of disease from onset (inception) to resolution.
- Outbreak—synonymous with *epidemic.* Sometimes the preferred word because it may escape sensationalism associated with the word *epidemic.* Alternatively, a localized as opposed to generalized epidemic.
- Pandemic—an epidemic occurring over a very wide area (several countries or continents) and usually affecting a large proportion of the population.
- Prevalence (prevalence rate)—The proportion of persons in a population who have a particular disease or attribute at a specified point in time or over a specified period of time.
- Propagated outbreak—an outbreak that does not have a common source but instead spreads from person to person.
- Risk—the probability that an event will occur; e.g., that an individual will become ill or die within a stated period of time or age.
- Risk factor—an aspect of personal behavior or lifestyle, an environmental exposure, or an inborn or inherited characteristic that is associated with an increased occurrence of disease or other health-related event or condition.
- Universal precautions—recommendations issued by the CDC to minimize the risk of transmission of bloodborne pathogens, particularly HIV and hepatitis B virus, by health care and public safety workers. Barrier precautions are to be used to prevent exposure to blood and certain body fluids of all patients.
- Vector—an animate intermediary in the indirect transmission of an agent that carries the agent from a reservoir to a susceptible host.
- Vehicle—an inanimate intermediary in the indirect transmission of an agent that carries the agent from a reservoir to a susceptible host.
- Years of potential life lost—a measure of the impact of premature mortality on a population, calculated as the sum of the differences between some predetermined minimum or desired life span and the age of death for individuals who died earlier than that predetermined age.
- Zoonoses—an infectious disease that is transmissible under normal conditions from animals to humans.

From Centers for Disease Control (1992). *Principles of Epidemiology* (2nd ed.). Atlanta, GA, Centers for Disease Control.

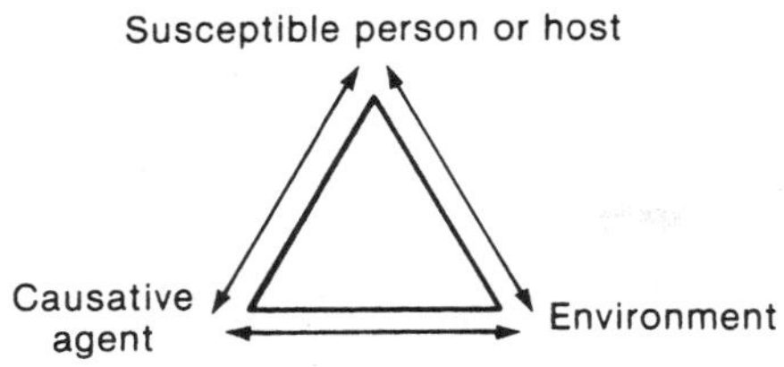

FIGURE 4–1 The epidemiological triangle. (From Smith, C. M. and Mauer, F. A. [1995]. *Community Health Nursing: Theory and Practice.* Philadelphia. W. B. Saunders, p. 274.)

Models of Disease Causation

A number of theories and models describe disease causation and the properties that relate to disease processes and prevention. Several of the most frequently encountered models are briefly discussed here.

THE EPIDEMIOLOGICAL TRIANGLE

The classic epidemiological model, particularly useful in the depiction of communicable disease, is the epidemiological triangle (Fig. 4–1). This model is often used to illustrate the interrelationships among the three essential components of *host, agent,* and *environment* with regard to disease causation. A change in any of the three components can result in the disease process. For example, exposure (environment) of a child who has not been immunized (host) to the measles virus (agent) will probably result in a case of measles. Another example would be respiratory difficulties resulting after an adult with chronic bronchitis (host) drives to work during rush hour (environment) on a day with excessive atmospheric ozone (agent).

Within the epidemiological triangle, prevention of the disease lies in preventing exposure to the agent, enhancing the physical attributes of the host to resist the disease, and minimizing any environmental factors that might contribute to disease development. Table 4–4 outlines host, agent, and environmental factors that affect health and could influence progression of the disease process.

THE WEB OF CAUSATION

The causes of most diseases are more complex. To explain disease and disability caused by multiple

TABLE 4–4 **Some Host, Agent, and Environmental Factors that Affect Health**

Host Factors

Demographic data: Age, gender, ethnic background, race, marital status, religion, education, economic status
Level of health: Genetic risk factors, physiological states, anatomical factors, response to stress, previous disease, nutrition, fitness
Body defenses: Autoimmune system, lymphatic system
State of immunity: Susceptibility versus active or passive immunity
Human behavior: Diet, exercise, hygiene, substance abuse, occupation, personal and sexual contact, use of health resources, food handling

Agent Factors (Presence or Absence)

Biological: Viruses, bacteria, fungi, and their mode of transmission, life cycle, virulence
Physical: Radiation, temperature, noise
Chemical: Gas, liquids, poisons, allergens

Environmental Factors

Physical properties: Water, air, climate, season, weather, geology, geography, pollution
Biological entities: Animals, plants, insects, food, drugs, food source
Social and economic consideration: Family, community, political organization, public policy, institutions, occupation, economic status, technology, mobility, housing, population density, attitudes, customs, culture, health practices, health services

From Smith, C. M. and Maurer, F. A. (1995). *Community Health Nursing: Theory and Practice.* Philadelphia, W. B. Saunders.

factors, MacMahon and Pugh (1970) developed the concept of "chain of causation," later termed the "web of causation." Chronic diseases such as coronary artery disease and most types of cancer are not attributable to one or two factors alone. Rather, the interaction of multiple factors is necessary to develop the disease. An example of the application of the web of causation to the development of coronary heart disease is presented in Figure 4–2.

The web of causation can also be applied to many health-related threats and conditions. The problem of teenage pregnancy, for example, is attributable to a complex interaction between a number of causative and contributing factors, including lack of knowledge about sexuality and pregnancy prevention, lack of easily accessible contraception, peer pressure to engage in sex, low self-esteem, social patterns that encourage early motherhood, and use of alcohol or other drugs. Patterns of family violence, cocaine use, and gang membership are examples of other threats to health and well-being that can be more accurately explained through a multiple-causation model.

Recognition that many health problems have multiple causes leads to the recognition that simple solutions to these health problems rarely exist. When trying to manage teenage pregnancy, for example, the solution is not as simple as addressing a "knowledge deficit about sexuality and contraception." Many (if not most) teens are well informed about contraception and the mechanics of how one gets pregnant and still fail to take preventative measures.

To prevent heart disease in an individual at risk, interventions include health education addressing

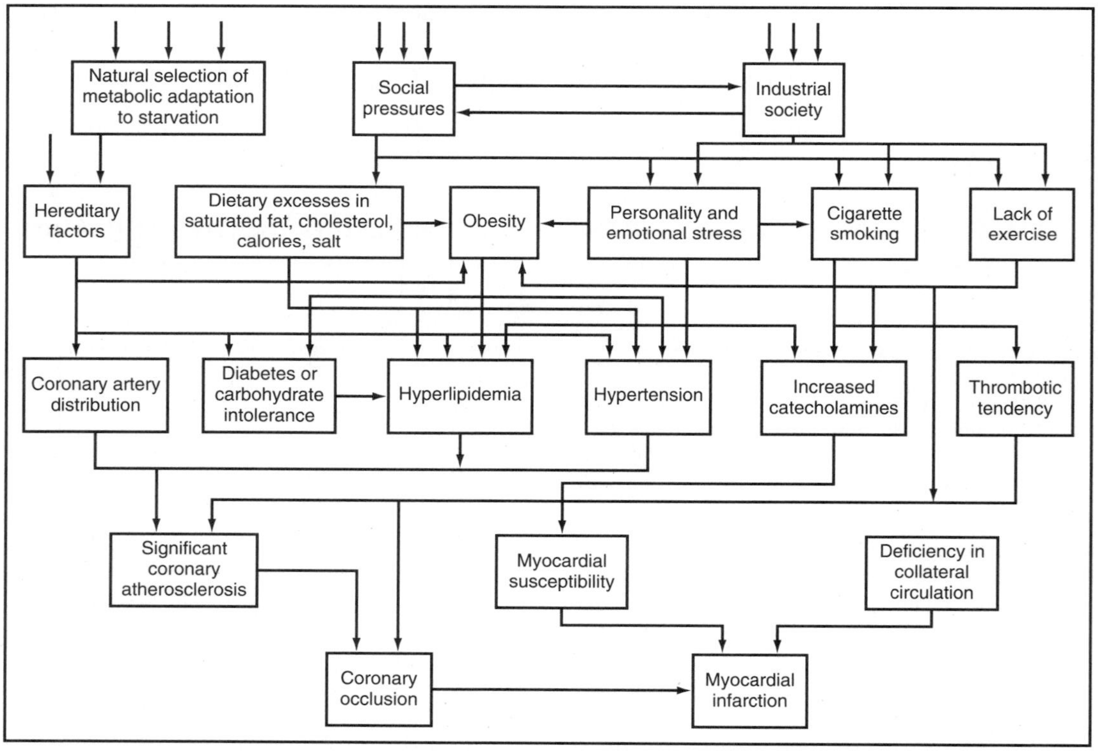

FIGURE 4–2 The web of causation for myocardial infarction. (From Frideman, G. D. [1987]. *Primer of Epidemiology.* New York, McGraw-Hill.)

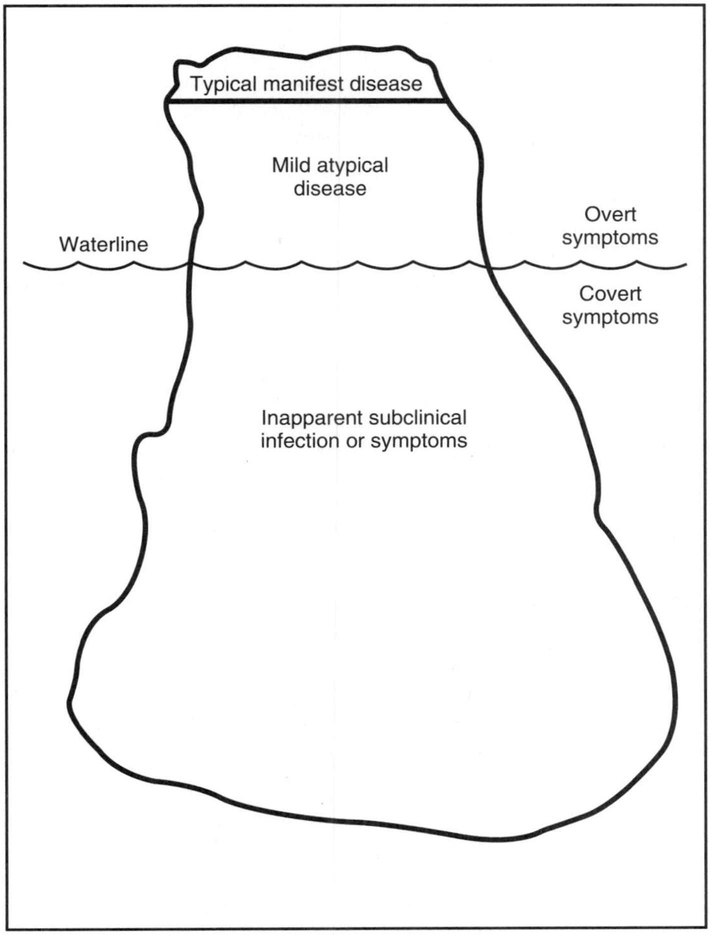

FIGURE 4–3 The iceberg model. (From Clemen-Stone, S., Eigsti, D. G. and McGuire, S. L. [1995]. *Comprehensive Community Health Nursing* [4th ed.]. St. Louis, Mosby-Year Book.)

a number of areas, including smoking cessation, reduction of blood pressure, weight loss, cholesterol reduction, and exercise. Interventions might also need to address lifestyle, stress management, social support, and personality traits, among others. Likewise, to prevent teenage pregnancy, interventions should include health teaching on improving self-esteem; role-playing exercises on how to say "no"; encouraging future orientation; enhancing parental supervision; and providing recreational alternatives (sports and other after-school activities), as well as information on sexuality, the mechanics of reproduction, and methods of contraception.

THE ICEBERG MODEL

The "iceberg model" or "iceberg principle" (Fig. 4–3) describes the phenomenon that at any given time there are a small number of "known" cases of a disease or condition at the early and advanced stages. These "known" cases are those that are "visible." However, like the iceberg, the greatest threat comes from the greater amount of unknown cases; i.e., those that are not identified.

Infection with human immunodeficiency virus (HIV) is an excellent illustration of this principle. The clinically diagnosed cases of acquired immunodeficiency syndrome (AIDS) (manifest disease) represent only a small fraction of all cases of those infected. Those known to have HIV infection (mild, atypical disease) make up a more significant part of the whole, but the greatest concern, and possibly the greatest threat, comes from those individuals who have not been diagnosed and may be transmitting HIV unknowingly.

NATURAL HISTORY OF DISEASE

The natural history of a disease refers to the progress of a disease process in an individual over time. Two periods in the natural history of disease, prepathogenesis and pathogenesis, were described by Leavell and Clark (1965) in what is now a classic model. In this model, the *prepathogenesis* stage occurs prior to interaction of the disease agent and human host, when the individual is susceptible. For example, an adult man may smoke, a teenage girl might consider becoming sexually active, or a preschooler attends a party also attended by a sick child. After exposure or interaction, the period of pathogenesis proceeds to early pathogenesis (e.g., alterations in lung tissue, pregnancy, or chicken pox) and on through the disease course to resolution—either death, disability, or recovery (e.g., lung cancer, teenage motherhood, immunity to chicken pox).

LEVELS OF PREVENTION

In addition to the description of the natural history of disease progression, Leavell and Clark (1965) also outlined three "levels of prevention"—primary prevention, secondary prevention, and tertiary prevention—that correlate with the stages of disease progression. These three levels are described as

- *Primary prevention*, which consists of activities that are directed at preventing a problem before it occurs. Altering susceptibility or reducing exposure for susceptible individuals in the period of prepathogenesis is primary prevention. Primary prevention consists of two categories—*general health promotion* (e.g., good nutrition, adequate shelter, rest, exercise) and *specific protection* (e.g., immunization, water purification).
- *Secondary prevention*, which refers to the early detection and prompt intervention in a disease or health threat during the period of early pathogenesis. Screening for disease and prompt referral and treatment are secondary prevention. Mammography, blood pressure screening, scoliosis screening, and Papanicolaou smears are examples of secondary prevention.
- *Tertiary prevention*, which consists of limitation of disability and rehabilitation during the period of advanced disease and convalescence, in which the disease has occurred and resulted in a degree of damage. Teaching how to perform insulin injections and teaching disease management to a diabetic, referral for occupational therapy and physical therapy for a head injury victim, and leading a support group for grieving parents are examples of tertiary prevention.

Much of nursing practice in community settings is intended to *prevent the progression of disease* at the earliest period or phase using the appropriate level or levels of prevention. Thus, when applying "levels of prevention" to AIDS, a nurse would

1. Educate clients on the practice of sexual abstinence or "safer sex" (primary prevention in the period of prepathogenesis)
2. Encourage testing and counseling for clients with known exposure or who are in high-risk groups; provide referrals for follow-up for clients who test positive for HIV (secondary prevention in the period of early pathogenesis for early diagnosis and prompt treatment)
3. Provide education on management of HIV infection, advocacy, case management and other interventions (tertiary prevention to limit disability through the periods of advanced disease)

Figure 4–4 illustrates the relationship between the levels of prevention and the natural history of disease, as described by Leavell and Clark (1965).

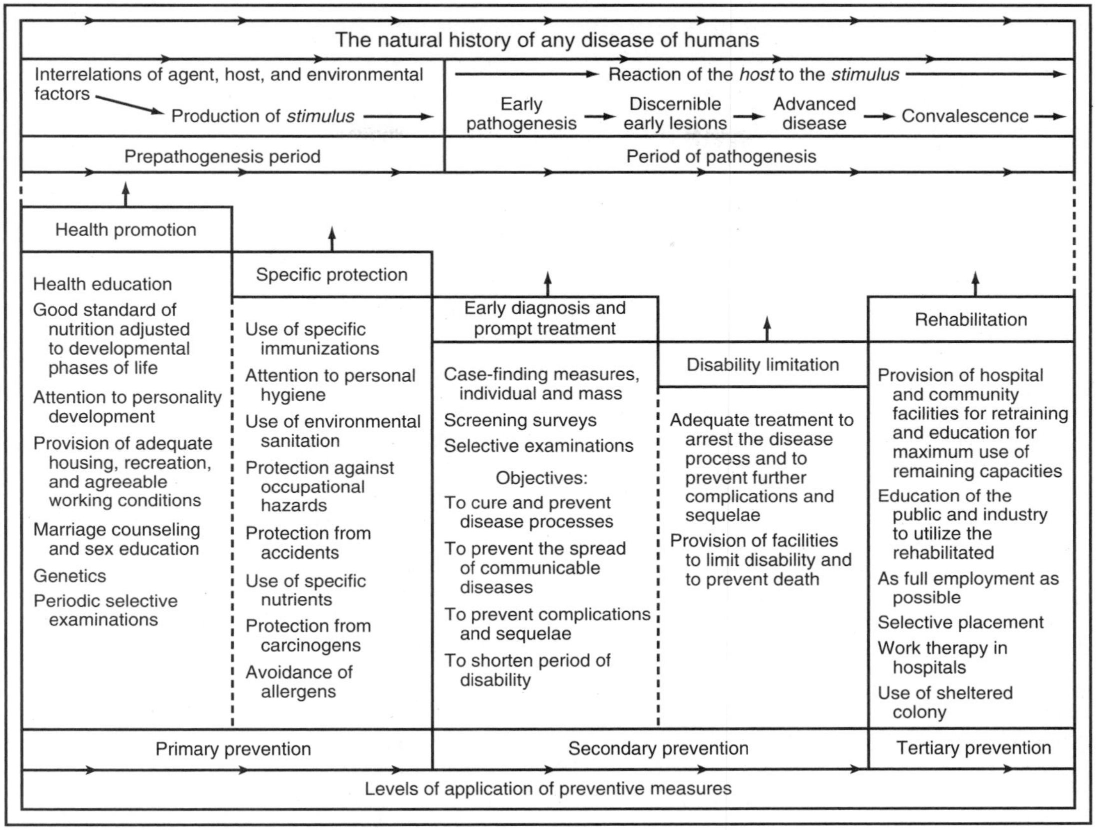

FIGURE 4–4 Levels of prevention in the natural history of disease. (From Leavell, H. R. and Clark, E. G. [1965]. *Preventive Medicine for the Doctor in His Community: An Epidemiologic Approach.* New York, McGraw-Hill.)

Epidemiological Tools in Community Health Practice

THE EPIDEMIOLOGICAL PROCESS

Closely related to the nursing process, the epidemiological process is a step-by-step method to assess, analyze, plan, and evaluate the study of disease. Table 4–5 outlines a comparison of the nursing process and the epidemiological process. The epidemiological process is particularly useful for nurses in community settings, as it defines or identifies assessment data that should be addressed or collected for planning interventions. Data should include distribution patterns (person, place, time) and frequency patterns (rates or statistical measures), as well as information on the host, agent, and environment. These components and related concepts are described further.

RATES—DESCRIPTION, CALCULATION, AND INTERPRETATION

In epidemiology, rates are used to make comparisons among groups or populations or to compare a subgroup of the population with the total population. Rates are essential tools in identifying

TABLE 4–5 **Comparison of the Nursing Process and the Epidemiological Process**

Nursing Process	Epidemiological Process
Assessing (data collection to determine nature of client problems)	I. Determine the nature, extent, and scope of the problem A. Natural life history of condition B. Determinants influencing condition 1. Primary data (essential agent) a. Parasite, bacterium, or virus b. Nutritional c. Psychosocial 2. Contributory data a. Agent b. Host c. Environment C. Distribution patterns 1. Person 2. Place 3. Time D. Condition frequencies 1. Prevalence 2. Incidence 3. Other biostatistical measures
Analyzing (formulation of nursing diagnosis or hypothesis)	II. Formulate tentative hypothesis(es) III. Collect and analyze further data to test hypothesis(es)
Planning	IV. Plan for control
Implementing	V. Implement control plan
Evaluating	VI. Evaluate control plan
Revising or terminating	VII. Make appropriate report
Research	VIII. Conduct research

From Clemen-Stone, S., Eigsti, D. G., and McGuire, S. L. (1995). *Comprehensive Community Health Nursing* (4th ed.). St. Louis, Mosby-Year Book.

actual and potential problems in a given community or population. Rates from a given aggregate or community can be compared with international, national, state, local, or regional rates; age-specific rates; gender-specific rates; or race-specific rates. Just as a nurse working in a hospital compares a complete blood count with a given norm or standard, nurses who work in community settings use rates to compare information on morbidity and mortality in their practice setting or aggregate with "norms," "standards," or "goals."

The use of rates allows the nurse working in any setting to recognize when a health threat or disease encountered is "normal" or typical, or if a problem or concern that warrants further investigation or intervention exists. For example, an elementary school nurse found that five children in her school of 500 have chicken pox (a rate of 10 children per 1,000). Should school be closed to prevent further infection? The nurse called the local health department and discovered that the current state incidence rate was 25 per 1,000 children and the county incidence rate was 20 per 1,000. Thus, she determined that the rate of chicken pox in her school was actually much lower than rates in comparison groups, so there was no reason to be concerned.

In calculating a rate, the numerator is the number of events, and the denominator is the total population at risk. The rate is usually converted to a standard base denominator (1,000; 10,000; or 100,000) to permit comparisons between various groups.

Measures of Morbidity. Measurement of morbidity and mortality is an integral part of public health. Table 4–6 lists measures of morbidity frequently used (or misused). The terms *incidence* and *prevalence* are used to measure and describe morbidity. Incidence refers to the number of *new* cases of an illness or injury that occur within a specified time. Prevalence refers to *all of the existing* cases of an illness at a given point of time. Incidence rates are most helpful in detecting and describing fluctuations in acute diseases, and prevalence rates are important in measuring chronic illness. Examples of the use of incidence rates are depicted in Figures 4–5 and 4–6, and prevalence rates, in Figures 4–7 and 4–8.

Figure 4–5 shows pockets of disease—in this case, diphtheria—in the former Soviet Union. As this figure charts the *incidence* of diphtheria, it is referring to the number of newly diagnosed cases of that illness during 1994. The use of a *rate* (number of cases per 100,000 population) allows for comparison between countries regardless of total population. Therefore, to interpret this figure, the incidence of diphtheria in the Russian Federation is *26 times greater* than that in Armenia or Lithuania, and that in Latvia is about *20 times greater* than that in neighboring Estonia. Based on this information, public health efforts to arrest this epidemic should be intensified in the countries with the highest incidence.

Figure 4–6 shows alarming concentrations of AIDS in Washington, D. C. (273 per 100,000), New York (84.8 per 100,000), and California (46.2 per 100,000). Montana (3.6 per 100,000), Iowa (3.5 per 100,000), and Idaho (5.2 per 100,000), on the other hand, have relatively few cases. Among other things, this information is useful for tracking the progression of the disease geographically, as well as in developing resources to manage AIDS where they are needed most.

To examine the extent of a particular health problem in a population, prevalence rates are extremely helpful. Figure 4–7, for example, delineates changes, as well as the extent of the chronic conditions, related to age. According to this chart, very few individuals younger than 45 years (about 50 per 1,000) have been diagnosed with arthritis, compared with more than half (550 per 1,000) of those older than 75. Likewise, the prevalence of hearing impairments and high blood pressure increases dramatically with age. Figure 4–8 breaks

Text continued on page 72

TABLE 4–6 **Frequently Used Measures of Morbidity**

Measure	Numerator (x)	Denominator (y)	Expressed per Number at Risk (10^n)
Incidence rate	Number of new cases of a specified disease reported during a given time interval	Average population during time interval	Varies: 10^n, where n = 2,3,4,5,6
Attack rate	Number of new cases of a specified disease reported during an epidemic period	Population at start of the epidemic period	Varies: 10^n, where n = 2,3,4,5,6
Secondary attack rate	Number of new cases of a specified disease among contacts of known cases	Size of contact population at risk	Varies: 10^n, where n = 2,3,4,5,6
Point prevalence	Number of current cases, new and old, of a specified disease at a given point in time	Estimated population at the same point in time	Varies: 10^n, where n = 2,3,4,5,6
Period prevalence	Number of current cases, new and old, of a specified disease identified over a given time interval	Estimated population at mid-interval	Varies: 10^n, where n = 2,3,4,5,6

From Centers for Disease Control. (1992). *Principles of Epidemiology* (2nd ed.). Atlanta, GA, Centers for Disease Control.

Reported incidence rate* of diphtheria—New Independent States of the former Soviet Union, 1994

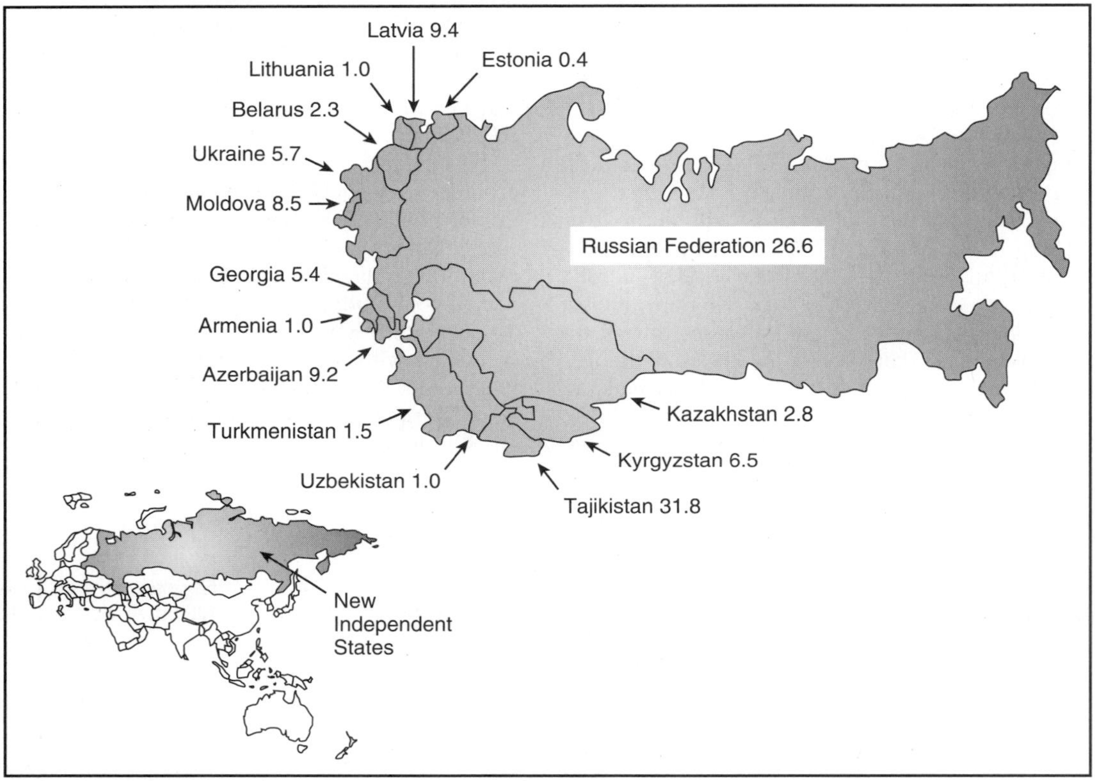

*Per 100,000 population.

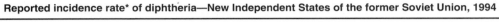

FIGURE 4–5 Morbidity rate examples—incidence. (From Centers for Disease Control and Prevention. [1995]. Diphtheria epidemic—new independent states of the former Soviet Union, 1990–1994. *Morbidity and Mortality Weekly Report, 44*[10], 177–179.)

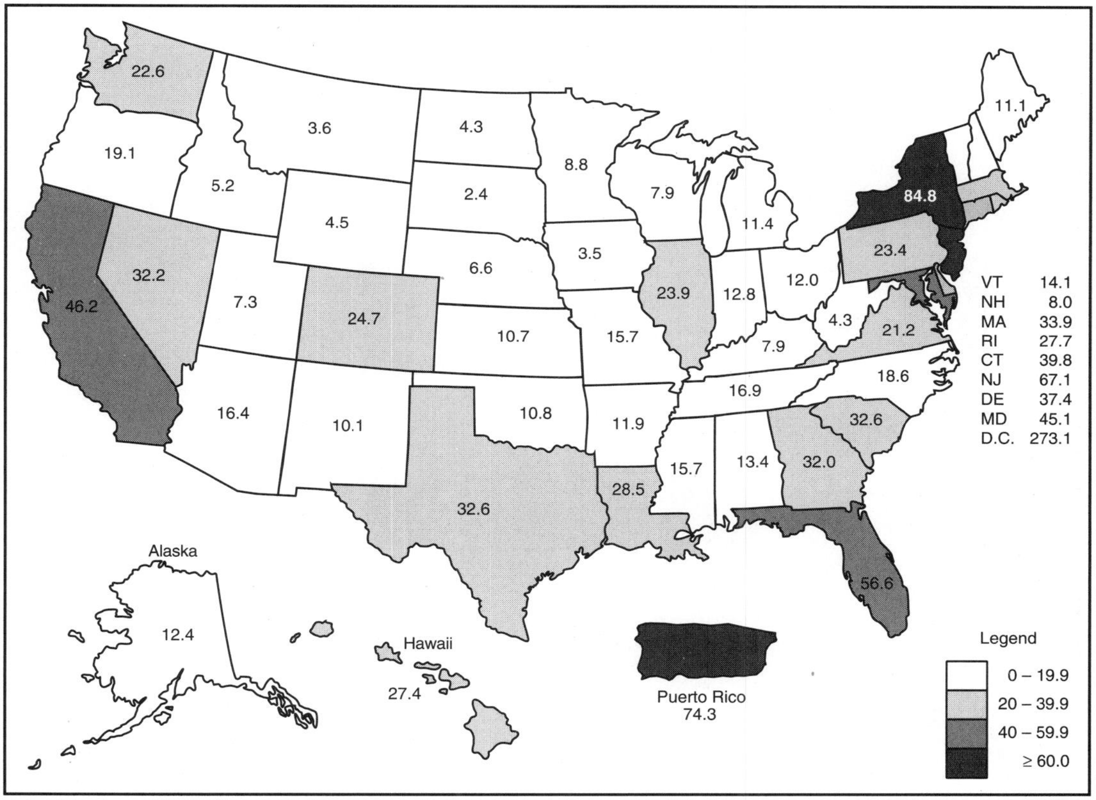

FIGURE 4–6 Morbidity rate examples—incidence. (From Centers for Disease Control and Prevention. [1994]. AIDS map. *Morbidity and Mortality Weekly Report, 43*[42], 776.)

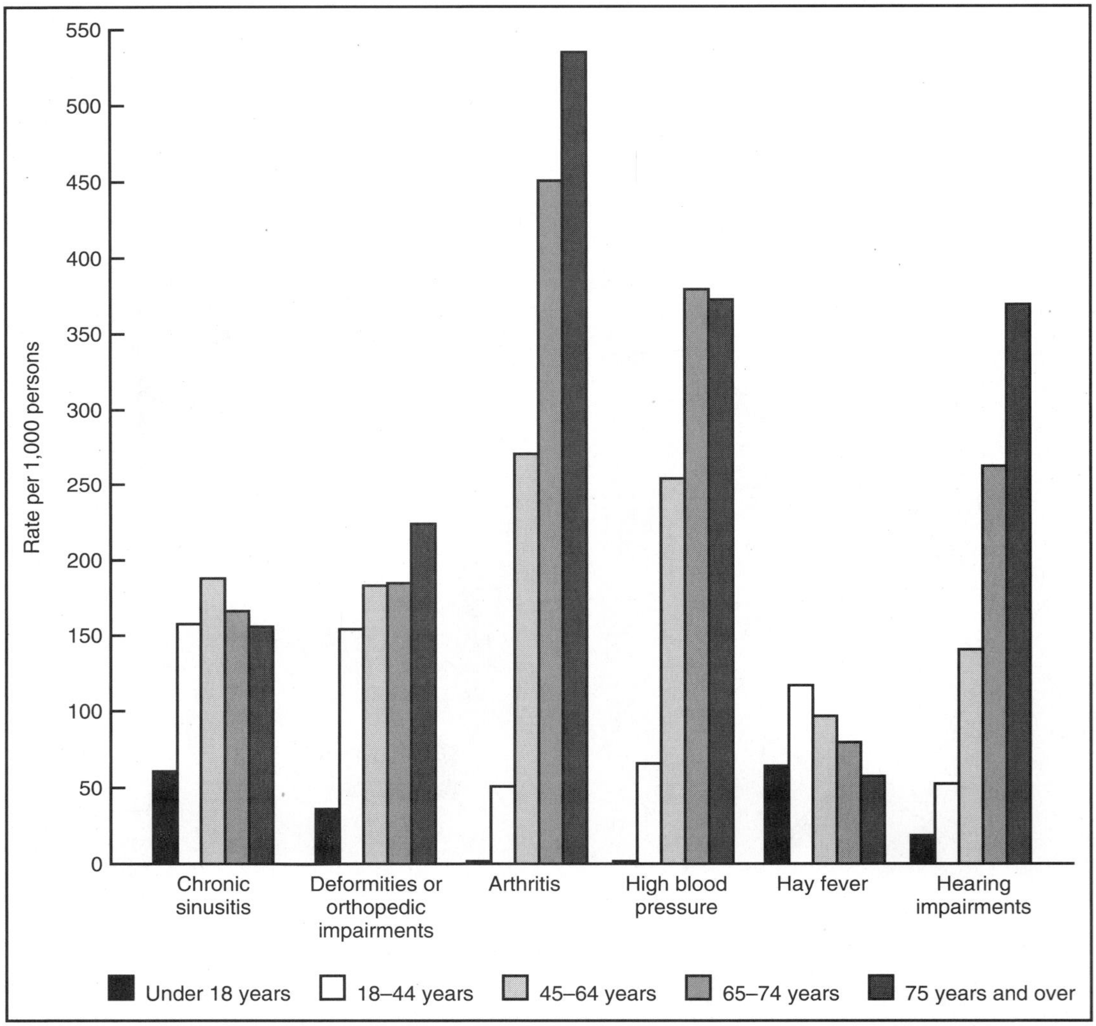

FIGURE 4–7 Morbidity rate examples—prevalence. (From National Center for Health Statistics. [1993]. *Prevalence of Selected Chronic Conditions: United States, 1986–88.* Series 10: Data from the National Health Survey, No. 192. DHHS Publication No. [PHS] 93–1510. Hyattsville, MD, Government Printing Office.)

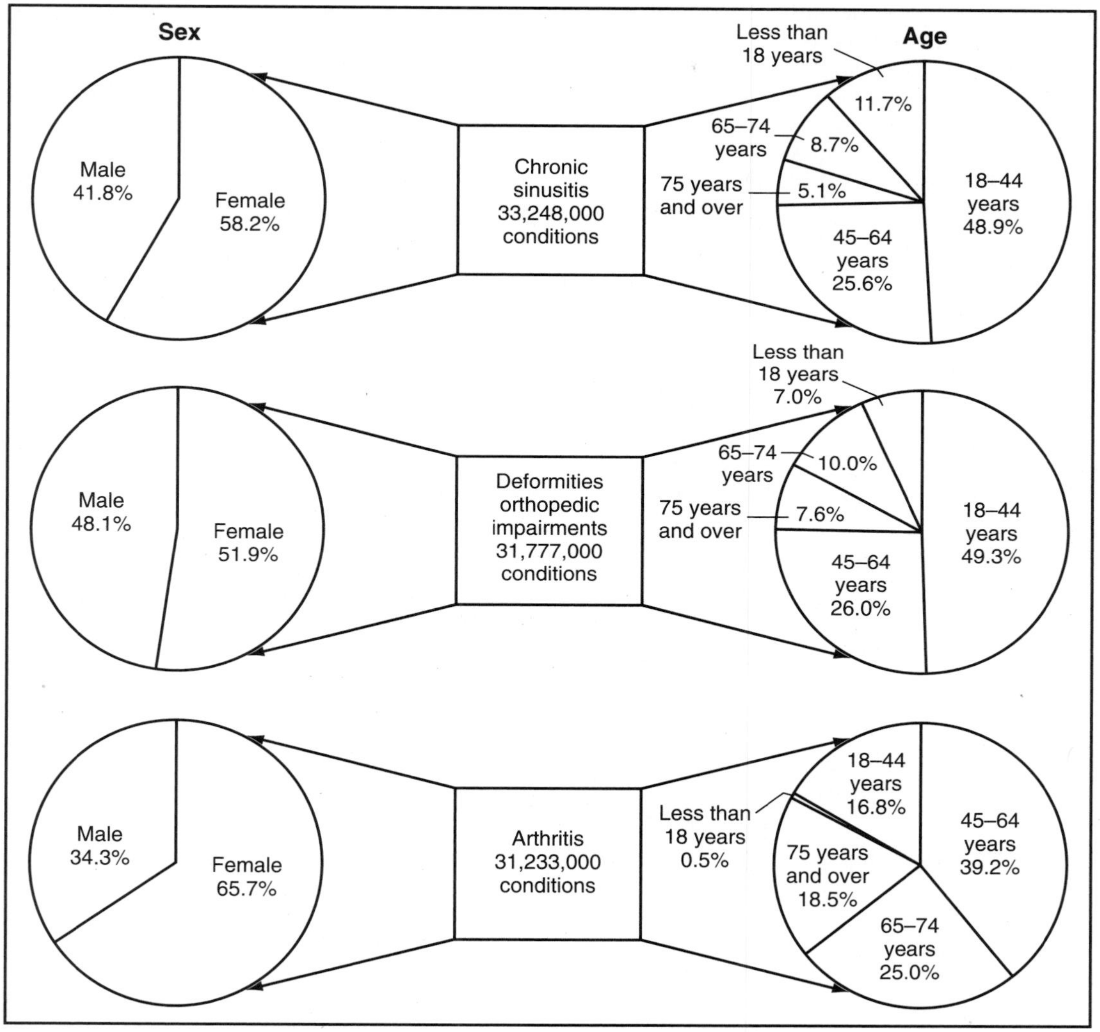

FIGURE 4–8 Morbidity rate examples—prevalence. (From National Center for Health Statistics. [1993]. *Prevalence of Selected Chronic Conditions: United States, 1986–88*. Series 10: Data from the National Health Survey, No. 182. DHHS Publication No. [PHS] 93–1510. Hyattsville, MD, Government Printing Office.)

down these data further into gender distribution as well as age categories. Information of this type is helpful in recognizing risk factors associated with certain conditions and in directing planning of interventions to meet identified and anticipated needs in specific populations.

The ability to read and interpret data of this type can be very important for nurses who work in community settings. Occasionally, nurses need to calculate rates to determine if rates for clients within their practice are above or below "expected" or referenced rates. To provide practice, Figure 4–9 presents exercises in calculating incidence and prevalence. Answers are at the end of this chapter.

Measures of Mortality. Just as different types of morbidity rates are used to measure and monitor illnesses, a number of different rates are used to measure attributes regarding death. Measures of mortality frequently used in public health are listed in Table 4–7. Of particular interest to nurses working in community settings are the infant mortality rate, crude death rate and the cause-specific death rated (e.g., how many individuals have died from AIDS or automobile accidents). Tables 4–8 and 4–9 show examples of mortality data.

Collection of Data: The Census, Vital Statistics, and Health Statistics

Sources of population-focused data for nurses in community-based practice include the census and local, state, and national vital statistics and health statistics. Each of these is discussed briefly. Much of the relevant information for nurses is available at local or state health departments as well as the local library. Sources of data on health issues from federal sources are listed in Table 4–10.

The Census. The Bureau of the Census is responsible for collection of data on the U. S. population. A census of the population to assess its

$$\text{Incidence rate} = \frac{\text{Number of NEW cases during a specified period}}{\text{Population at risk during the same period}} \times k$$

$$\text{Prevalence rate} = \frac{\text{Number of EXISTING cases at a specified time}}{\text{Population at risk at the same specified time}} \times k$$

$$\text{Crude death rate} = \frac{\text{Number of deaths in a population during a specified time}}{\text{Population estimate during the specific time}} \times k$$

$$\text{Crude birth rate} = \frac{\text{Number of live births in a population during a specified time}}{\text{Population estimate during the specified time}} \times k$$

$$\text{Cause-specific death rate} = \frac{\text{Number of deaths from a specific cause during a specified time}}{\text{Population estimate during the specified time}} \times k$$

$$\text{Age-specific death rate} = \frac{\text{Number of deaths for a specific age group during a specified time}}{\text{Population estimate for the age group during the specified time}} \times k$$

During 1994, 215 NEW cases of AIDS were reported in Acme, a city of 500,000. This brought the total of active cases of AIDS to 2,280. During that time, 105 deaths were attributable to the disease.

1. What is the incidence rate per 100,000 for AIDS during 1994?
2. What was the prevalence rate of AIDS per 100,000?
3. What is the cause-specific death rate for AIDS per 100,000?

Sun City is a small city with a mid-1994 population of 120,000. During 1994, 342 live births and 515 deaths occurred in Sun City. Sun City has a large elderly population, with approximately 24,000 of the population being older than 65 years. Of the 515 deaths during 1994, 425 were in individuals older than 65.

4. What is the crude birth rate for Sun City for 1994 per 1,000?
5. What is the crude death rate for Sun City for 1994 per 1,000?
6. What is the age-specific death rate for individuals older than 65 for Sun City for 1994 per 1,000?

FIGURE 4–9 *See legend on opposite page*

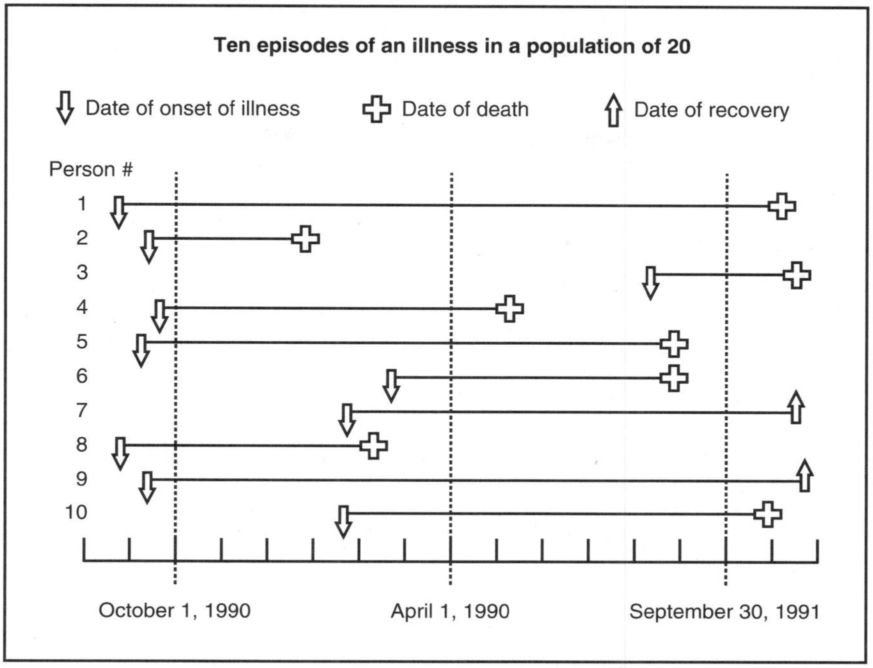

FIGURE 4–9 Calculation exercise—incidence and prevalence rate. (Answers are at the end of the chapter.) (Questions 7 & 8 from Centers for Disease Control. [1992]. *Principles of Epidemiology* [2nd ed.]. Washington, D. C., U. S. Department of Health and Human Services.)

For the hypothetical illness above, calculate the

7. Prevalence rate for October 1, 1990
8. Incidence rate for October 1, 1990 to September 30, 1991

characteristics has been conducted every 10 years since 1790 as mandated by the Constitution of the United States (Robey, 1989). Among other reasons, the census was undertaken to establish each state's representation in the House of Representatives.

The methodology of census taking has evolved over the decades. To make the task more manageable and the data more meaningful, census tracts were developed. Census tracts are relatively small, usually homogenous geographic areas that allow for analysis of small units within communities. Maps outlining boundaries for census tracts can be obtained from a local public library.

Census tract information can be extremely valuable for nurses and others involved in health program planning. Information elicited from the census questionnaire includes

- Name, sex, race, age, ethnicity, and marital status of everyone living in the household (including housemates, foster children, boarders, and live-in employees)
- Housing characteristics, including the type of dwelling (e.g., mobile home, single-family detached, duplex, apartment); age of the dwelling; number of rooms; number of bedrooms; presence of plumbing facilities; kitchen facilities; source of fuel; source of water; sewage system; yearly costs for electricity, gas, water
- Information on the ownership of the home (e.g., owned by the resident, rented, mortgaged), estimated value, monthly rent, length of time in residence, property taxes

TABLE 4–7 **Frequently Used Measures of Mortality**

Measure	Numerator (x)	Denominator (y)	Expressed per Number at Risk (10^n)
Crude death rate	Total number of deaths reported during a given time interval	Estimated mid-interval population	1,000 or 100,000
Cause-specific death rate	Number of deaths assigned to a specific cause during a given time interval	Estimated mid-interval population	100,000
Proportional mortality	Number of deaths assigned to a specific cause during a given time interval	Total number of deaths from all causes during the same interval	100 or 1,000
Death-to-case ratio	Number of deaths assigned to a specific disease during a given time interval	Number of new cases of that disease reported during the same time interval	100
Neonatal mortality rate	Number of deaths under 28 days of age during a given time interval	Number of live births during the same time interval	1,000
Postneonatal mortality rate	Number of deaths from 28 days to, but not including, 1 year of age, during a given time interval	Number of live births during the same time interval	1,000
Infant mortality rate	Number of deaths under 1 year of age during a given time interval	Number of live births reported during the same time interval	1,000
Maternal mortality rate	Number of deaths assigned to pregnancy-related causes during a given time interval	Number of live births during the same time interval	100,000

From Centers for Disease Control. (1992). *Principles of Epidemiology* (2nd ed.). Atlanta, GA, Centers for Disease Control.

TABLE 4–8 **Mortality Rate Examples: Number and Percentage of Pregnancy-Related Deaths,* by Cause of Death and Surveillance Method—Georgia, 1990–1992**

	Death Certificate Review Only		Death Certificate Review and Record Linkage	
Cause of Death	***Number***	***Percentage***	***Number***	***Percentage***
Hemorrhage	16	(28.6)	17	(23.3)
Embolism	12	(21.4)	16	(21.9)
Infection	6	(10.7)	8	(11.0)
Pregnancy-induced hypertension	4	(7.1)	4	(5.5)
Pulmonary problems	4	(7.1)	6	(8.2)
Anesthesia complications	3	(5.4)	3	(4.1)
Cardiovascular problems	2	(3.6)	3	(12.3)
Cardiomyopathy	2	(3.6)	6	(8.2)
Other causes	7	(12.5)	10	(13.7)
Total	**56**	**(100.0)**	**73**	**(100.0)**

*Defined by the American College of Obstetricians and Gynecologists and the Centers for Disease Control as the immediate result of complications of pregnancy, events initiated by the pregnancy, or an exacerbation of an unrelated condition by the physiological or pharmacological effects of the pregnancy.

From Centers for Disease Control. (1995). Pregnancy-related mortality—Georgia, 1990–1992. *Morbidity and Mortality Weekly Report, 44* (5), 95.

- Education attainment of all in the household
- Language spoken in the home
- Information related to occupation and work, including location of work, transportation to work (e.g., car, bus, subway, ferry, motorcycle), estimated time to get to work and home, employment information, type of work (e.g., manufacturing, wholesale trade, retail trade, agriculture, construction, service, government), retirement benefits, and income

This information is gathered during April of each new decade (i.e., 1980, 1990, 2000) for all individuals residing in the United States. Information on numerous divisions (e.g., U. S. geographical areas) and subdivisions (e.g., states, metropolitan areas, census tract) of the census can be obtained at a regional public library and from the Bureau of Census (see Table 4–9).

Vital Statistics. The term *vital statistics* refers to data collected about the significant events that occur within a population over a period. These data are systematically gathered by agencies at local, state, national, and international levels. Vital statistics data include the "data collected from ongoing recording, or registration, of all 'vital events'—births and adoptions; deaths and fetal deaths; marriages, divorces, legal separations, and annulments" (Mausner and Kramer, 1985, p. 70). Data on vital events are collected locally and reported to area and state office through channels dictated by each state. Figure 4–10 depicts the vital statistics registration system in the United States. Local vital statistics data can typically be obtained from the county or district records office and are often available at public libraries. State vital statistic information can be gathered from state records departments, and national information, from the National Center for Health Statistics (see Table 4–10).

Health Statistics. The Centers for Disease Control and Prevention (CDC), the National Institutes of Health (NIH), and the National Center for

TABLE 4–9 **Mortality Rate Example: Estimated Deaths, Death Rates, and Percent of Total Deaths for the 15 Leading Causes of Death: United States, 1992***

Rank	Cause of Death (ICD-9)	Number	Death Rate	Total Deaths (%)
	All causes	2,177,000	853.3	100.0
1	Diseases of heart	720,480	282.5	33.1
2	Malignant neoplasms, including neoplasms of lymphatic and hematopoietic tissues	520,090	204.3	23.9
3	Cerebrovascular diseases	143,640	56.3	6.6
4	Chronic obstructive pulmonary diseases and allied conditions	91,440	35.8	4.2
5	Accidents and adverse effects	86,310	33.8	4.0
	Motor vehicle accidents	41,710	16.4	1.9
	All other accidents and adverse effects	44,600	17.5	2.0
6	Pneumonia and influenza	76,120	29.8	3.5
7	Diabetes mellitus	50,180	19.7	2.3
8	Human immunodeficiency virus infection	33,590	13.2	1.5
9	Suicide	29,760	11.7	1.4
10	Homicide and legal intervention	26,570	10.4	1.2
11	Chronic liver disease and cirrhosis	24,830	9.7	1.1
12	Nephritis, nephrotic syndrome, and nephrosis	22,400	8.8	1.0
13	Septicemia	19,910	7.8	0.9
14	Atherosclerosis	16,100	6.3	0.7
15	Certain conditions originating in the perinatal period	15,790	6.2	0.7
	All other causes	298,430	117.0	13.7

*Data are provisional, estimated from a 10% sample of deaths. Rates per 100,000 population. Figures may differ from those previously published. Due to rounding, figures may not add to totals.

ICD-9 = Ninth revision, International Classification of Diseases, 1975.

From Centers for Disease Control. (1993). Annual summary of births, marriages, divorces, and deaths: United States, 1992. *Monthly Vital Statistics Report.* (CDC/NCHS-PHS. *Vol. 40,* No. 13). Washington, D. C., U.S. Government Printing Office.

Health Statistics (NCHS) (see Table 4–10) are the primary sources for morbidity and mortality data in the United States. Each of these organizations is a component of the Department of Health and Human Services, as discussed in Chapter 2.

The CDC, as has been discussed, has primary responsibility for monitoring communicable diseases and other actual and potential health threats. The CDC publishes information for health providers in the *Morbidity and Mortality Weekly Report* (*MMWR*). Included in this periodical are weekly updates on selected reportable diseases, brief articles on a variety of topics, periodic recommendations for prevention, detection, and treatment of diseases, and field reports detailing current and completed investigations into disease outbreaks. The *MMWR* can be found in most medical libraries, in public libraries with significant public document collections, and at local health departments.

The NIH is essentially concerned with research into numerous areas related to health. Information from the NIH primarily covers federally funded research projects. Information generated from the various studies is typically published in a variety of professional journals. In addition, selected major studies, reports, guidelines, and recommendations are published and available from the Government Printing Office.

TABLE 4–10 **Sources of Population Data**

Centers for Disease Control and Prevention	
1600 Clifton Rd	
Atlanta, GA 30333	
(404) 639-3311	
(404) 639-3534 (public inquiry)	
National Center for Health Statistics	
6526 Belcrest Road	
Hyattsville, MD 20782	
(301) 436-8500	
U. S. Department of Commerce	
Bureau of the Census	
Washington, D. C. 20233	
(301) 457-4608	
(301) 457-4784 (fax)	
National Institutes of Health	
9000 Rockville Pike	
Bethesda, MD 20892	
(301) 496-4000	
Government Printing Office	
Superintendent of Documents	
P. O. Box 371954	
Pittsburgh, PA 15250	
(202) 512-1800	

In addition to maintaining information on vital statistics (e.g., births, deaths) discussed here, the NCHS also monitors and publishes causes of morbidity and mortality.

Descriptive and Analytical Epidemiology

There are two basic types of epidemiology. *Descriptive* epidemiology examines the amount and distribution of a disease in terms of "person," "place," and "time" to distinguish characteristics of individuals who have a specific disease from those who do not. *Analytical* epidemiology investigates the etiology of disease. In analytical epidemiology, observational and experimental studies are used to establish a causal relationship between identified threats and development of disease or disability.

DESCRIPTIVE EPIDEMIOLOGY

Descriptive epidemiology considers the "amount" and "distribution" of disease within a population by person, place, and time. Table 4–11 details characteristics or descriptors frequently used in the study of the amount and distribution of disease.

As shown in these figures, epidemiological data is often presented in a manner that allows for interpretation and application to other populations. For example, Table 4–12 details characteristics of persons diagnosed with Hantavirus during 1993. According to this figure, the profile of individuals with this diagnosis are predominately Native American, most often male and young (younger than 40 years). Table 4–13 describes the incidence of vaccine-preventable diseases during 1993 and

TABLE 4–11 **Characteristics Assessed in Descriptive Epidemiology: Person, Place, and Time**

Person	Age
	Sex
	Ethnic group and race
	Social class
	Occupation
	Marital status
	Family variables (e.g., family size, birth order, maternal age, parental deprivation)
	Personal variables (e.g., blood type, environmental exposure, personality traits)
Place	Natural boundaries
	Political subdivisions
	Environmental factors
	Urban-rural differences
	International comparisons
Time	Secular trends
	Cyclic changes
	Clusters in time and place

Data from Mausner, J. S. and Kramer, S. (1985). *Epidemiology—An Introductory Text.* Philadelphia, W. B. Saunders.

RESPONSIBLE PERSON OR AGENCY	BIRTH CERTIFICATE	DEATH CERTIFICATE	FETAL DEATH REPORT (STILLBIRTH)
Hospital authority	1. Completes entire certificate in consultation with parent(s). 2. Files certificate with local office or state office, per state law	When death occurs in hospital, may initiate preparation of certificate: Completes name, date of death, and place of death information; obtains certification of cause of death from physician; and gives certificate to funeral director.	1. Completes entire report in consultation with parent(s). 2. Obtains cause of death from physician 3. Obtains authorization for disposition of fetus. 4. Files report with local office or state office, per state law.
Funeral director	↓	1. Obtains personal facts about decedent and completes certificates. 2. Obtains certification of cause of death from physician or medical examiner or coroner. 3. Obtains authorization for disposition, per state law. 4. Files certificate with local office or state office, per state law.	1. If fetus is to be buried, the funeral director is responsible for obtaining the authorization for disposition. NOTE: In some states, the funeral director, or person acting as such, is responsible for all duties shown above under hospital authority.
Physician or other professional attendant	Verifies accuracy of medical information and signs certificate.	Completes certification of cause of death and signs certificate.	Provides cause of fetal death information
Local office* (may be local registrar or city or county health department)	1. Verifies completeness and accuracy of certificate and queries incomplete or inconsistent certification. 2. If authorized, makes copy or index for local use. 3. Sends certificates to state registrar.	1. Verifies completeness and accuracy of certificate and queries incomplete or inconsistent certificates. 2. If authorized, makes copy or index for local use. 3. If authorized by state law, issues authorization for disposition upon receipt of completed certificate. 4. Sends certificates to state registrar.	If state law requires routing of fetal death reports through local office, the local office will perform the same functions as shown for the death certificate.

FIGURE 4–10 The vital statistics registration system. *Asterisk* indicates that some states do not have local vital registration offices. In these states, the certificates or reports are transmitted directly to the state office of vital statistics. (From Centers for Disease Control. [1992]. *Principles of Epidemiology* [2nd ed.]. Washington, D.C., U. S. Department of Health and Human Services.)

City and county health departments use data derived from these records in allocating medical and nursing services, follow-ups on infectious diseases, planning programs, measuring effectiveness of services, and conducting research studies.	
State Registrar, Office of Vital Statistics	1. Queries incomplete or inconsistent information. 2. Maintains files for permanent reference and as the source of certified copies. 3. Develops vital statistics for use in planning, evaluating, and administering state and local health activities and for research studies. 4. Compiles health-related statistics for state and civil divisions of state for use of the health department and other agencies and groups interested in the fields of medical science, public health, demography, and social welfare. 5. Sends copies of records or data derived from records to the National Center for Health Statistics.
Public Health Service–National Center for Health Statistics	1. Prepares and publishes national statistics of births, deaths, and fetal deaths and constructs the official U. S. life tables and related actuarial tables. 2. Conducts health and social research studies based on visual records and on sampling surveys linked to records. 3. Conducts research and methodological studies in vital statistics methods, including the technical, administrative, and legal aspects of vital records registration and administration. 4. Maintains a continuing technical assistance program to improve the quality and usefulness of vital statistics.

FIGURE 10 *Continued*

1994 and designates the number of cases in children younger than 5 from total cases. On review, it appears that of the two most common vaccine-preventable diseases, hepatitis B and pertussis, hepatitis B in children represents only about 1% of all cases. Pertussis in small children, on the other hand, accounts for about half of all cases. Examination of data with respect to person (e.g., age, gender), place, and time can therefore be very important in determining where problems and potential problems exist and where none exist. For example, studying age-related data on hepatitis B can raise the question of why we immunize all infants against this disease.

ANALYTICAL EPIDEMIOLOGY

Analytical epidemiology focuses study on the *determinants* of disease in a given population. The search for causes and effects, or to "quantify the association between exposures and outcomes and to test hypotheses about causal relationships," (CDC, 1992, p. 32) is the purpose of analytical epidemiology.

The process of identification of the etiology of a disease occurs following comparison of groups through epidemiological studies. Epidemiological studies are typically experimental or observational. Types and examples of each are listed in Figure 4–11.

SUMMARY

This chapter has sought to present and clarify some of the basic elements of epidemiology. Recognition of the causes and course of a disease or health problem and identification of methods to prevent progression of the disease is a very important component of nursing practice in any setting and essential when practicing in the community. Many of the concepts included here are carried throughout the remainder of this book. Each of the chapters on health promotion (Chapters 11, 12, 13 and 14), for example, includes a number of primary, secondary, and tertiary prevention interventions. Additionally, Chapters 15 and 16 take a closer look at disease transmission and epidemiology when discussing communicable disease and HIV and AIDS, respectively.

TABLE 4–12 Reported Example of "Descriptive Epidemiology": Characteristics of 53 Persons Reported with Hantavirus Pulmonary Syndrome, by Outcome—United States, May–December, 1993

Characteristic	Total	Deaths		Relative Risk	95% CI*
		Number	*Percentage*		
Age (years)					
<20	7	4	57	Referent	
20–29	14	7	50	0.9	0.4–2.0
30–39	18	14	78	1.4	0.8–2.7
≥40	14	7	50	0.9	0.4–2.0
Sex					
Female	23	13	57	Referent	
Male	30	19	63	1.1	0.7–1.8
Race					
Native American	26	15	58	Referent	
Other†	27	17	63	1.1	0.7–1.7

*Confidence interval.
†Non-Hispanic white, Hispanic, and non-Hispanic black.
From Centers for Disease Control. (1994). Characteristics of 53 persons reported with Hantavirus pulmonary syndrome, by outcome—United States, May–December, 1993. *Morbidity and Mortality Weekly Report, 43* (3), 45–48.

TABLE 4–13 Reported Example of "Descriptive Epidemiology": Number of Reported Cases of Diseases Preventable by Routine Childhood Vaccination—United States, December 1994 and 1993–1994

Disease	Cases, December 1994 (n)	Total Cases, January–December		Cases Among Children Younger than 5 Years, January–December (n)	
		1993	*1994*	*1993*	*1994*
Congenital rubella syndrome (CRS)	1	5	8	4	7
Diphtheria	0	0	1	0	1
Haemophilus influenzae	125	1,419	1,161	435	313
Hepatitis B	1,090	13,361	11,534	141	114
Measles	21	312	902	119	226
Mumps	172	1,692	1,455	284	232
Pertussis	616	6,586	3,832	3,924	2,046
Poliomyelitis, paralytic	0	3	1	1	1
Rubella	7	192	218	32	27
Tetanus	5	48	38	0	0

From Centers for Disease Control and Prevention. (1995). Monthly Immunization Table. *Morbidity and Mortality Weekly Report, 44* (5), 99.

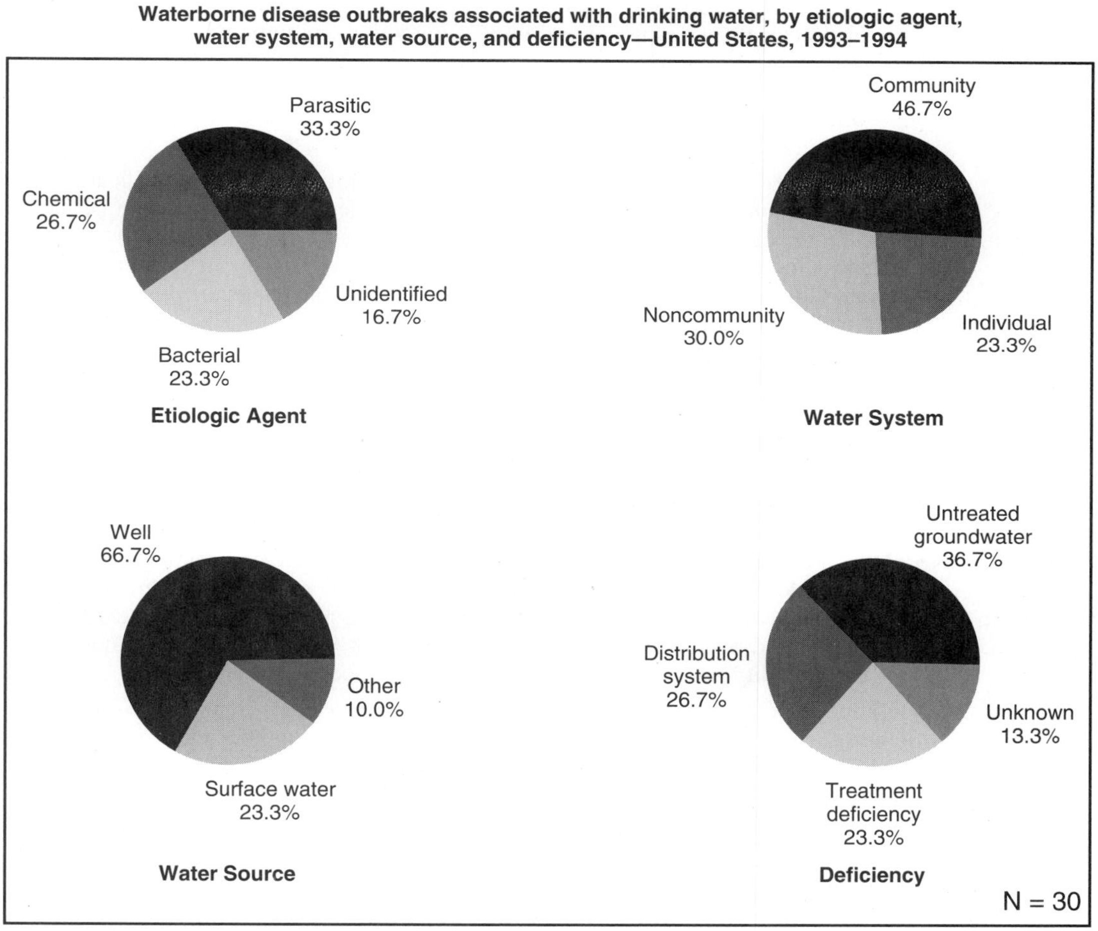

FIGURE 4–11 Examples of analytic epidemiology. (From Centers for Disease Control and Prevention. [1996]. Surveillance of Waterborne-disease outbreaks—United States, 1993–1994. *Morbidity and Mortality Weekly Report, 45*[SS-1], 1–40.)

Key Points

- Epidemiology is defined as the study of the distribution and determinants of disease in humans and the related application of this information to control health problems. Identification of characteristics or "risk factors" that predispose persons to, or protect them against, disease and removing or minimizing them if harmful or enhancing them if helpful, are basic goals in epidemiology. The use of epidemiological concepts and principles to identify risks and assist in the prevention and management of disease is important for nurses working in community-based practice.
- A basic understanding disease causation is important to assist in identification of risk factors and development of prevention strategies. Models of disease causation include the epidemiological triangle (host, agent, and environment triad), the web of causation (explains diseases of multiple causation), and the natural history of disease (demonstrates how a disease progresses through stages of prepathogenesis and pathogenesis).
- Much of nursing practice in community settings is intended to prevent the progression of disease at the earliest period or phase using the appropriate level of prevention. Nursing interventions can be delivered at three different levels of prevention—primary prevention (activities that prevent a problem before it occurs), secondary prevention (early detection and prompt intervention during the period of early pathogenesis), and tertiary prevention (efforts to limit disability and promote rehabilitation during the period of advanced disease and convalescence).
- Rates are statistical tools used to make comparisons between groups or populations or compare a subgroup of a population with the total population. Rates that measure the amount of morbidity associated with a particular illness include incidence and prevalence rates. Commonly used measures of mortality include the infant mortality rate, crude death rate, and cause-specific death rates.
- Sources of data on health-related issues include the census (population characteristics such as sex, race or ethnicity, age, housing characteristics, education levels, occupation information), vital statistics (e.g., registration of births, deaths), and health statistics (maintained by state health departments and the CDC).
- Descriptive epidemiology refers to the amount and distribution of a disease in terms of "person," "place," and "time." Analytical epidemiology investigates the etiology of disease through observational and experimental studies to identify causal relationships between identified threats and development of subsequent disease or disability.

Learning Activities and Application to Practice

In Class

- Select one or two "timely" illnesses or syndromes (e.g., breast cancer, Gulf War syndrome, AIDS, skin cancer). Examine the illness using the models of disease causation described. Which model best fits each illness? Are the models useful for determining appropriate interventions?

- For the illnesses or health conditions discussed in the previous exercise or other similar conditions, discuss primary-, secondary-, and tertiary-level interventions that nurses might be expected to deliver in community-based settings. During discussion, encourage students to come up with examples of each level of prevention.
- Obtain a copy of a recent *Morbidity and Mortality Weekly Report.* Discuss information presented in the report related to the chapter. For example, are there any graphs, maps, or tables of incidence or prevalence rates or other morbidity or mortality statistics? Are there examples of descriptive or analytical epidemiology?
- Complete the calculation exercises in Figure 4–9.

In Clinical

- Divide students into groups of three or four and assign each group to obtain selected census and vital statistics data on a local community or group. Have the students determine what data are pertinent to the health of members of the community or to management of health care resources (e.g., presence or absence of running water, number of persons in the household, number of small children, number of elders, number of deaths, number of live births). Have students share findings with other groups and compare.
- Have students observe for "clusters" of health problems that might indicate the need for comparison with other groups. For example, if the students are in schools and observe that many children seem to be having breathing difficulties or are being diagnosed with asthma, a comparison should be done with another school to see if one has higher rates of asthma than the other.

ANSWERS TO CALCULATIONS FOR FIGURE 4–9

1. 215/500,000 × 100,000 = 43 cases per 100,000
2. 2280/500,000 × 100,000 = 456 cases per 100,000
3. 105/500,000 × 100,000 = 21 deaths per 100,000
4. 342/120,00 × 1,000 = 2.85 births per 1,000
5. 515/120,000 × 1,000 = 4.29 deaths per 1,000
6. 425/24,000 × 1,000 = 17.71 deaths over age 65 per 1,000
7. 6/20 × 100 = 30 per 100
8. 4/18 (population at midpoint—20 − 2 = 18) × 100 = 22 per 100

REFERENCES

Centers for Disease Control. (1993). Annual summary of births marriages, divorces and deaths: United States, 1992. *Monthly Vital Statistics Report, 40* (13), 1–28.

Centers for Disease Control. (1992). *Principles of Epidemiology* (2nd ed.). Atlanta, GA, Centers for Disease Control.

Centers for Disease Control and Prevention. (1994). AIDS map. *Morbidity and Mortality Weekly Report, 43* (42), 776.

Centers for Disease Control and Prevention. (1995). Diphtheria epidemic—New Independent States of the Former Soviet Union, 1990–1994. *Morbidity and Mortality Weekly Report, 44* (10), 177–179.

Centers for Disease Control and Prevention. (1995). Pregnancy-related mortality—Georgia, 1990–1992. *Morbidity and Mortality Weekly Report, 44* (5), 93–96.

Clemen-Stone, S., Eigsti, D. G., and McGuire, S. L. (1995). *Comprehensive Community Health Nursing* (4th ed.). St. Louis, Mosby-Year Book.
Friedman, G. D. (1987). *Primer of Epidemiology.* New York, McGraw-Hill.
Gordis, L. (1996). *Epidemiology.* Philadelphia, W. B. Saunders.
Leavell, H. R. and Clark, E. G. (1965). *Preventive Medicine for the Doctor in His Community: An Epidemiologic Approach.* (2nd ed.). New York, McGraw-Hill.
MacMahon, B. and Pugh, T. F. (1970). *Epidemiologic Principles and Methods.* Boston, Little, Brown & Co.
Mausner, J. S. and Kramer, S. (1985). *Epidemiology: An Introductory Text.* Philadelphia, W. B. Saunders.
National Center for Health Statistics. (1993). *Prevalence of Selected Chronic Conditions: United States, 1986–1988.* Series 10: Data from the National Health Survey. DHHS Publication No. (PHS) 93–1510. Hyattsville, MD, Government Printing Office.
Robey, B. (1989). *Two Hundred Years and Counting: The 1990 Census.* Washington, D. C., Population Reference Bureau.
Smith, C. M. and Maurer, F. A. (1995). *Community Health Nursing: Theory and Practice.* Philadelphia, W. B. Saunders.
U. S. Department of Health and Human Services. (1990). *Healthy People 2000: National Health Promotion and Disease Prevention Objectives.* Washington, D. C., Government Printing Office.
Valanis, B. (1992). *Epidemiology in Nursing and Health Care.* Norwalk, CT, Appleton & Lange.

5

Environmental Health Issues

Case Study

Susan Baldwin is a Registered Nurse working in a pediatric, primary care clinic in an inner city. On Tuesday of this week, Susan assisted the Pediatric Nurse Practitioner with a routine well-child examination on Billy Benson, a 2-year-old boy who lives with his mother and three siblings in an area housing project. The health care professionals at the clinic follow the American Academy of Pediatrics recommendations for preventative care. In addition to overall physical assessment, the health professionals in the clinic perform various screenings, such as height and weight and vision and hearing testing, on the children, based on these recommendations.

One of the screening examinations recommended by the American Academy of Pediatrics is to test the level of lead in each child's blood. These recommendations have been established because an estimated 10% of inner-city children have serum lead levels above those recommended, and lead has been cited as the most common cause of mental impairment and mental retardation in children.

Susan understands the importance of lead screening and explained the problem of lead exposure and the rationale for testing to Billy's mother. She provided Mrs. Benson with pamphlets kept at the clinic explaining the basics of lead poisoning and prevention measures. While discussing the written materials with Mrs. Benson, Susan reviewed some of the main sources of lead contamination. These include paint in homes built before 1960, lead smelters, battery recycling plants, and hobbies that expose individuals to lead (e.g., ceramics, furniture refinishing, and stained glass work). Susan questioned Mrs. Benson and discovered that their residence was built in the late 1970s, which is not a problem, but learned that Billy regularly visits his grandmother, whose home was built in the 1940s. Mrs. Benson stated that she does not participate in any of the mentioned hobbies and knows of no area lead smelters or battery recycling plants.

Following guidelines set by the state health department, Susan drew a small tube of blood from a prick in Billy's finger, carefully labeled it, and completed the required forms. The specimen and accompanying paperwork were sent to the state laboratory for analysis. Susan explained to Mrs. Benson that the state health department has outlined a course of action for children with elevated lead levels based on Centers for

Disease Control and Prevention (CDC) recommendations, and if Billy's serum lead levels are elevated, further testing may be necessary.

Environmental factors play an important role in the processes of human development, health, and disease. Historically, public health efforts have addressed measures to improve or ensure adequate and safe supplies of food and water, manage waste disposal and sewage, and control or eliminate vectorborne illnesses (U. S. Department of Health and Human Services [USDHHS], 1990). Nationally, these efforts have been phenomenally successful and are largely responsible for the increase in life expectancy witnessed during the 20th century (McKeown, 1995).

According to the environmental health report presented in *Healthy People 2000*, contemporary challenges for environmental health come from "what is not known about the toxic and ecological effects of the use of fossil fuels and synthetic chemicals in modern society" (USDHHS, 1990, p. 314). Population growth, urbanization, technology, industrialization, and modern agricultural methods have demonstrated unprecedented progress in many areas but have concurrently created a number of hazards to human health. Risks from synthetic chemicals, naturally occurring radiation, and electromagnetic fields, as well as biological contamination of food and water supplies, remain potential threats to the health of United States citizens. In response to these potential threats to health, one priority area of *Healthy People 2000* is "Environmental Health," and consequently, a series of related objectives have been published. Table 5–1 presents selected goals from *Healthy People 2000* related to issues of environmental health.

Environmental threats to the health of individuals may come from a variety of different sources. Stevens and Hall (1993) categorize environmental health issues and concerns into nine "areas." These "Areas of Environmental Health" and corresponding definitions are listed in Table 5–2. Assessment and intervention strategies, along with general information for health education for each of these areas, with the exception of "violence risks," are discussed briefly. Violence risks and related nursing interventions are discussed in Chapters 12 and 13. In addition, concerns regarding housing and living patterns are addressed here.

Housing and Living Patterns

Numerous actual and potential threats to health related to housing and living patterns exist. Some common concerns include overcrowding, household chemical exposure, and violence. Table 5–3 describes sources of home pollution. Several related issues (e.g., radon gas, exposure to various chemicals, biological contaminants) are listed elsewhere in this chapter. This section discusses potential problems in housing and living conditions related to indoor air quality, lead exposure, and electromagnetic fields.

INDOOR AIR QUALITY

Indoor air quality in the home may significantly affect health. Concerns center on combustion pollutants (e.g., carbon monoxide, "secondhand smoke"), particles (e.g., asbestos, animal dander, pollen), and living organisms (e.g., dust mites, molds, bacteria). Several of these concerns (i.e., secondhand smoke, asbestos, and carbon monoxide poisoning) are addressed in detail.

Secondhand smoke refers to the combination of smoke given off by the burning of a cigarette, pipe, or cigar and the smoke exhaled from the lungs of smokers. Secondhand smoke has been classified by the Environmental Protection Agency (EPA) as a known carcinogen and is estimated to cause approximately 3,000 lung cancer deaths in nonsmokers each year (EPA, 1993c). Health threats to infants and children caused by secondhand smoke include increased risk of respiratory tract infection (e.g., pneumonia and bronchitis),

TABLE 5–1 *Healthy People 2000*—Selected Objectives for Environmental Health, Food Safety, and Occupational Health and Safety

Objective 11.3—Reduce outbreaks of waterborne disease for infectious agents and chemical poisoning to no more than 11 per year (baseline: average of 31 outbreaks per year during 1981–1988)

Objective 11.6—Increase to at least 40% the proportion of homes in which homeowners/occupants have tested for radon concentrations and that have either been found to pose minimal risk or have been modified to reduce risk to health (baseline: less than 5% of homes had been tested in 1989)

Objective 11.8—Reduce human exposure to solid waste–related water, air, and soil contamination, as measured by a reduction in average pounds of municipal solid waste produced per person each day to no more than 3.6 pounds (baseline: 4.0 pounds per person each day in 1988)

Objective 11.9—Increase to at least 85% the proportion of people who receive a supply of drinking water that meets the safe drinking water standards established by the EPA (baseline: 74% of 58,099 community water systems servicing approximately 80% of the population in 1988)

Objective 11.11—Perform testing for lead-based paint in at least 50% of homes built before 1950 (baseline data not available)

Objective 11.16—Establish and monitor in at least 35 state plans to define and track sentinel environmental diseases* (baseline: 0 states in 1990)

Food and Drug Safety

Objective 12.1—Reduce infections caused by key foodborne pathogens to indices of not more than the following:

Disease (per 100,000)	*1987 Baseline*	*2000 Target*
Salmonella species	18	16
Campylobacter jejuni	50	25
Escherichia coli	8	4
Listeria monocytogenes	0.7	0.5

Objective 12.3—Increase to at least 75% the proportion of households in which principal food preparers routinely refrain from leaving perishable food out of the refrigerator for over 2 hours and wash cutting boards and utensils with soap after contact with raw meat and poultry (baseline: for refrigeration of perishable foods, 70%; for washing cutting boards with soap, 66%; and for washing utensils with soap, 55% in 1988)

Occupational Health and Safety

Objective 1.10—Increase the proportion of worksites offering employer-sponsored physical activity and fitness programs as follows:

Work Site Size	*1985 Baseline (%)*	*2000 Target (%)*
50–99 employees	14	20
100–249 employees	23	35
250–749 employees	32	50
> 750 employees	54	80

Objective 3.11—Increase to at least 75% the proportion of work sites with a formal smoking policy that prohibits or severely restricts smoking at the workplace (baseline: 27% of work sites with 50 or more employees in 1985; 54% of medium and large companies in 1987)

Objective 10.1—Reduce deaths from work-related injuries to no more than 4 per 100,000 full-time workers (baseline: average of 6 per 100,000 during 1983–1987)

Objective 10.5—Reduce hepatitis B infections among occupationally exposed workers to an incidence of no more than 1,250 cases (baseline: an estimated 6,200 cases in 1987)

Objective 10.7—Reduce to no more than 15% the proportion of workers exposed to average daily noise levels that exceed 85 dBA (baseline data not available)

Objective 10.10—Implement occupational safety and health plans in 50 states for the identification, management, and prevention of leading work-related diseases and injuries within the state (baseline: 10 states in 1989)

*Note: Sentinel environmental diseases include lead poisoning, other heavy metal poisoning (e.g., cadmium, arsenic, and mercury), pesticide poisoning, carbon monoxide poisoning, heatstroke, hypothermia, acute chemical poisoning, methemoglobinemia, and respiratory diseases triggered by environmental factors (e.g., asthma).

From U. S. Department of Health and Human Services. (1990). *Healthy People 2000: National Health Promotion and Disease Prevention Objectives.* Washington, D. C., Government Printing Office.

TABLE 5–2 **Areas of Environmental Health**

Area	Definition
Living patterns	The relationships among persons, communities, and their surrounding environments that depend on habits, interpersonal ties, cultural values, and customs
Work risks	The quality of the employment environment, as well as the potential for injury or illness posed by working conditions
Atmospheric quality	The protectiveness of the atmospheric layers, the risks of severe weather, and the purity of the air available for breathing purposes
Water quality	The availability and volume of the water supply, as well as the mineral content levels, pollution by toxic chemicals, and the presence of pathogenic microorganisms; consists of the balance between water contaminants and existing capabilities to purify water for human use and plant and wildlife sustenance
Housing	As an environmental health concern, refers to the availability, safety, structural, strength, cleanliness, and location of shelter, including public facilities and individual or family dwellings
Food quality	The availability and relative costs of foods, their variety and safety, and the health of animal and plant food sources
Waste control	The management of waste materials resulting from industrial and municipal processes and human consumption, as well as efforts to minimize waste production
Radiation risks	Health dangers posed by the various forms of ionizing radiation relative to barriers preventing exposure of humans and other life forms
Violence risks	The potential for victimization through the violence of particular individuals, as well as the general level of aggression in psychosocial climates

From Stevens, P. E. and Hall, J. M. (1993). Environmental health. In J. M. Swanson and M. Albrecht (Eds.). *Community Health Nursing: Promoting the Health of Aggregates.* Philadelphia, W. B. Saunders.

decreased lung function and symptoms of chronic respiratory irritation, middle ear infections, and development and exacerbation of asthma. In adults, secondhand smoke causes eye, nose, and throat irritation and lung irritation and may affect the cardiovascular system. Table 5–4 lists the EPA's recommendations to reduce the health risks of passive smoking.

In 1971, the EPA identified asbestos as a hazardous air pollutant and in 1973 issued regulations to control asbestos emissions (EPA, 1989a). In the past, asbestos was commonly used in construction for insulation, fire-proofing, pipe insulation, roofing, and flooring. Asbestos-related health threats occur because of its tendency to break down into a dust of tiny fibers that remain suspended in the air for a long time and can be inhaled. These fibers can stay in the body for years and may cause long-term problems that develop 20 to 40 years after exposure. Lung cancer and mesothelioma are the most frequently seen asbestos-related diseases.

Nurses who practice in community settings should be familiar with measures and regulations taken to reduce asbestos exposure. Since the mid-1970s, the abatement of emissions from demolition and renovation of commercial and industrial buildings has been undertaken to protect citizens from asbestos exposure. Recent legislation includes the Asbestos School Hazard Abatement Act (1984) (which provides aid to schools to abate severe asbestos problems); the Asbestos Hazard Emergency Response Act (1986) (which required all primary and secondary schools in the United States to inspect for asbestos and take appropriate corrective actions); and the Asbestos Information Act (1988) (which requires manufacturers of asbestos or asbestos-containing materials to submit information about their products to the EPA for publication).

TABLE 5–3 **Sources of Home Pollution**

Pollutant	Description and Suggestions	Source and Examples of Substance in Home
Radon	Colorless, odorless, radioactive gas from the natural breakdown (radioactive decay) of uranium; it is estimated that radon causes up to 20,000 lung cancer deaths per year	Soil or rock under the home; well water; building materials
Asbestos	Mineral fiber used extensively in building materials for insulation and as a fire retardant; asbestos should be removed by a professional if it has deteriorated; exposure to asbestos fibers can cause irreversible and often fatal lung diseases, including cancer	Sprayed-on acoustical ceilings or textured paint; pipe and furnace insulation materials; floor tiles; automobile brakes and clutches
Biological contaminants	Include bacteria, mold and mildew, viruses, animal dander and saliva, dust mites, and pollen; these contaminants can provide infectious diseases or allergic reactions; moisture and dust levels in the home should be kept as low as possible	Mold and mildew; standing water or water-damaged materials; humidifiers; house plants; household pets; ventilation systems; household dust
Indoor combustion	Produces harmful gases (i.e., carbon monoxide, nitrogen dioxide), particles, and organic compounds (e.g., benzene); health effects range from irritation to the eyes, nose, and throat, to lung cancer; ventilation of gas appliances to the outdoors will minimize risks	Tobacco smoke; unvented kerosene or gas space heaters; unvented kitchen gas stoves; wood stoves or fireplaces; leaking exhaust flues from gas furnaces and clothes dryers; car exhaust from an attached garage
Household products	Can contain potentially harmful organic compounds; health effects vary greatly; the elimination of household chemicals through the use of nontoxic alternatives or by using only in well-ventilated rooms or outside minimizes risks	Cleaning products; paint supplies; stored fuels; hobby products; personal care products; mothballs; air fresheners; dry-cleaned clothes
Formaldehyde	Widely used chemical that is released to the air as a colorless gas; it can cause eye, nose, throat, and respiratory system irritation, headaches, nausea, and fatigue; may be a central nervous system depressant and has been shown to cause cancer in laboratory animals; remove sources of formaldehyde from the home if health effects occur	Particleboard, plywood, and fiberboard in cabinets, furniture, subflooring, and paneling; carpeting, durable-press drapes, other textiles; urea-formaldehyde insulation; glues and adhesives
Pesticides	Including insecticides, termiticides, rodenticides, and fungicides—all contain organic compounds; exposure to high levels of pesticides may cause damage to the liver and the central nervous system and increase cancer risks; when possible, nonchemical methods of pest control should be used: if the use of pesticides is unavoidable, they should be used strictly according to the manufacturer's directions	Contaminated soil or dust that is tracked in from outside; stored pesticide containers
Lead	A long-recognized harmful environmental pollutant; fetuses, infants, and children are more vulnerable to toxic effects; if the community health nurse suspects that a home has lead paint, it should be tested	Lead-based paint that is peeling, sanded, or burned; automobile exhaust; lead in drinking water; food contaminated by lead from lead-based ceramic cookware or pottery; lead-related hobbies or occupations

From Primomo, J. and Salazar, M. K. (1995). Environmental illness: At home, at work and in the community. In C. M. Smith and F. A. Maurer (Eds.). *Community Health Nursing: Theory and Practice.* Philadelphia, W. B. Saunders.

TABLE 5–4 **Reducing the Health Risks of Secondhand Smoking**

- Do not smoke in the home and do not permit others to do so
- If a family member insists on smoking indoors, increase ventilation in the area
- Do not smoke if children, particularly infants and toddlers, are present
- Do not smoke in an automobile with the windows closed if passengers are present
- Find out about the smoking policies of day care centers, schools, and other caregivers of children and take measures to ensure that children are not exposed
- Teach others about the risks associated with secondhand smoke
- Encourage and support policies that enact and maintain smoke-free workplaces
- Prohibit smoking indoors or limit smoking to rooms that have been specially designed to prevent smoke from escaping to other areas of the work site
- Encourage employer-supported smoking cessation programs
- Locate designated outdoor smoking areas away from building entrances or building ventilation system air intakes
- Know the local and state laws regarding smoking in public buildings
- Support stringent smoking control ordinances in the community

From the Environmental Protection Agency. (1993). *Secondhand Smoke.* EPA Publication: 402-F-93-004. Washington, D. C., Government Printing Office.

Pollution from indoor combustion comes from appliances such as space heaters, gas ranges and ovens, furnaces, gas water heaters, and wood- or coal-burning stoves and fireplaces. Potential problems from indoor combustion typically relate to ineffective or improper venting of the appliances, cracked heat exchangers, burning green or treated wood, or using the wrong fuel.

Carbon monoxide exposure is of particular importance, as more than 200 deaths each year are caused by accidental carbon monoxide poisoning. To reduce exposure to combustion pollutants, it is essential that combustion appliances undergo proper selection, installation, inspection, and maintenance. Suggestions to reduce or eliminate exposure to carbon monoxide and other combustion gases are discussed in Table 5–5.

LEAD EXPOSURE

According to *Healthy People 2000*, "high blood lead levels are among the most prevalent child-

TABLE 5–5 **Reducing Exposure to Carbon Monoxide and Other Indoor Combustion Pollutants**

- Choose vented appliances when possible
- Buy combustion appliances that have been tested and certified to meet safety standards
- Consider buying gas appliances that have electronic ignitions rather than pilot lights
- Buy appliances that are the correct size for the area to be heated
- Have appliances professionally installed
- If using an unvented gas space heater or kerosene heater, crack open a window and keep doors open to the rest of the house
- Use a hood fan if using a gas range
- Make sure vented appliances have the vent connected and nothing is blocking it
- Do not vent gas clothes dryers or water heaters into the house for heating
- Read and follow instructions for all appliances
- Always use the correct fuel for the appliance
- Never use a range, oven, or dryer to heat the home
- Never use an unvented combustion heater overnight or in a bedroom while sleeping
- Never ignore a safety device when it shuts off an appliance
- Never ignore the smell of fuel
- Have combustion appliances regularly inspected and maintained
- Have chimneys and vents inspected when installing or changing vented heating appliances
- Consider purchasing a carbon monoxide detector (available at hardware stores)

From U. S. Consumer Product Safety Commission/Environmental Protection Agency and American Lung Association. (1993). *What You Should Know About Combustion Appliances and Indoor Air Pollution.* United States: U. S. Consumer Product Safety Commission/Environmental Protection Agency and American Lung Association, Washington, D. C.

hood conditions and the most prevalent environmental threat to the health of children in the United States" (1990, p. 319). Therefore, reduction of blood lead levels is a national priority. Recent measures to reduce lead exposure through decreasing lead in gasoline, air, food, and industrial sources have worked to lower overall blood lead levels.

Despite these successes, however, an estimated 3 million children, particularly minority and poor children from inner cities younger than 6 years, have blood lead levels high enough to adversely affect their intelligence, behavior, and development (CDC/National Center for Environmental Health, 1994). As a result, the CDC and National Center For Environmental Health have instituted a multilevel program to screen young children for elevated lead levels; identify possible sources of exposure; monitor the medical management of children with elevated blood lead levels; provide health professionals, policy-makers, and the public with educational information on preventing lead poisoning; and support community programs to eliminate childhood lead poisoning.

Lead-based paint in homes and buildings built before 1960 has been identified as the major source of lead poisoning. Chipping or peeling lead-based paint is of concern because it can easily be ingested by children or inhaled through lead-contaminated dust. Anemia, central nervous system disorders, and renal involvement may result from lead exposure. Of particular concern is chronic central nervous system dysfunction, including irreversible deficits in intelligence, behavior, and school performance. Additional concerns relate to children exposed in utero (Landrigan, 1988). The CDC (1991) identifies those at greatest risk for lead poisoning as being children who

1. Live in a house or regularly visit a day care center, preschool, babysitter's home, or other house built before 1960
2. Live in or regularly visit a house built before 1960 with recent, ongoing, or planned renovation
3. Have a brother, sister, or playmate being treated for lead poisoning
4. Live with an adult whose job, hobby, or use of ethnic remedies involves lead
5. Live near an active lead smelter, battery recycling plant, or other industry likely to release lead

Maximum permissible blood levels of lead have been revised downward from 30 μg/dL in 1975. Currently levels greater than 10 μg/dL are denoted as "action" or "intervention levels" (Goyer, 1993). Federal, state, and local efforts to decrease lead exposure should be supported by all health professionals. Table 5–6 contains information for assessment, teaching, counseling, advocacy, and referral for childhood lead exposure useful for nurses practicing in community settings.

ELECTROMAGNETIC FIELDS

Electromagnetic fields (EMFs) are a relatively recently recognized potential environmental health threat. EMFs are produced by electrical currents and consist of "extremely-low-frequency" electromagnetic radio waves. (Ionizing radiation, in comparison, is composed of extremely high frequency waves.) Human exposure to "normal" degrees of EMFs is constant and harmless. However, concern has been expressed regarding exposure to high levels of EMFs, such as those emitted from high-tension power lines or electric blankets, for extended periods.

Questions about potential health threats arose from several research studies, which associated EMFs with certain cancers—specifically brain cancer and leukemia in children (National Institute of Environmental Health Sciences, 1994; National Institute of Environmental Health Sciences/Department of Energy, 1995). Multiple research studies, however, have produced conflicting findings, and a causal relationship is far from conclusive. A number of studies are ongoing. Based on expressed concerns and preliminary research findings, several states have adopted standards to limit permissible magnetic field strength along electrical transmission line easements. Also, federal legislation, as part of the National Energy Policy Act of 1992, supports ongoing EMF research and public information programs (EPA/Office of Radiation and Indoor Air, 1992; National Institute of Environmental Health Sciences, 1994).

The most common recognized sources of poten-

TABLE 5–6 Interventions for Prevention of Childhood Environmental Lead Exposure

Primary Prevention

Individual/Family Interventions

- Encourage parents to keep children away from peeling or chipping paint
- Encourage families to remove lead-based paint from older homes
- Wet mop and wet wipe hard surfaces with a high-phosphate solution
- Do not vacuum hard surfaces, as this might scatter dust
- Wash children's hands and faces before they eat
- Wash toys and pacifiers frequently
- If soil around the home is likely to be lead contaminated (if the house was built before 1960 or is near a major highway), plant bushes next to the house and plant grass or other groundcover to reduce dust
- During remodeling of older homes, be certain children and pregnant women are not in the home until the process is completed; thoroughly clean house before inhabitants return
- Do not use pottery or ceramic ware that was inadequately fired or is meant for decorative use for food storage or service
- Do not store drinks or food in lead crystal
- Make sure children eat regular meals; lead is more readily absorbed on an empty stomach

Community Interventions

- Provide education programs and opportunities to learn about lead poisoning and prevention
- Encourage communities to remove lead-based paint from older homes, particularly in low-income housing
- Support policymakers who encourage funding for programs to reduce lead exposure

Secondary Prevention

Individual/Family Interventions

- Recommend screening of "high-risk" children at age 6 months and *at least* every year
- Recommend screening of *all* children at 12 months and yearly thereafter
- Identify the source of lead exposure for children with serum lead levels above 10 μg/dL
- Refer for treatment if needed: (1) if blood lead levels are greater than 20 μg/dL, the child should receive environmental evaluation and remediation and a medical evaluation; drug therapy may also be indicated; (2) if blood lead levels are greater than 45 μg/dL, medical and environmental intervention and chelation therapy are necessary
- Refer families with identified lead poisoning to local or state-sponsored programs if assistance is needed to remove the source of exposure

Community Interventions

- Encourage community-sponsored testing for lead-based paint for all homes built before 1950
- Promote accessibility of screening services
- Monitor incidence of heavy metal poisoning
- Educate the public on signs and symptoms of lead poisoning
- Support government-sponsored financing of lead paint abatement when individual homeowners cannot afford it

Tertiary Prevention

Individual/Family Interventions

- Monitor progress and effects of treatment
- Provide assistance in dealing with long-term effects of lead poisoning—i.e., referral for special education programs

Community Interventions

- Advocate lead abatement programs in older residential areas
- Educate the public on the hazards of lead
- Promote access to social services needed to manage the effects of lead poisoning

Data from Centers for Disease Control. (1991). *Preventing Lead Poisoning in Young Children.* Atlanta, Centers for Disease Control; Clark, M. J. (1992). Environmental influences on community health. In M. J. Clark (Ed.). *Nursing in the Community.* Norwalk, CT, Appleton & Lange; U. S. Department of Health and Human Services. (1990). *Healthy People 2000. National Health Promotion and Disease Prevention Objectives.* Washington, D. C., Government Printing Office; Clemen-Stone, S., Eigsti, D. G., and McGuire, S. L. (1995). *Comprehensive Community Health Nursing* (4th ed.). St. Louis, MO, Mosby-Year Book.

tially damaging EMF exposure are transmission power lines and household appliances. Power line exposure is particularly relevant for families that live in *close* proximity (e.g., across the street or next to a power-line easement) to power lines or stations and occupational exposure for utility company field workers. Household exposure is relevant to everyone, with particular concern surrounding electric blankets, ceiling fans, and video display terminals.

Again, remember that although some evidence suggests cause for concern, research studies are conflicting and ongoing, and remaining informed about the subject is best. General recommendations to limit exposure to EMFs are discussed in Table 5–7.

Work Risks

An estimated 10 million job-related injuries and illnesses occur each year, with about 3 million being severe enough to result in time lost from work (USDHHS, 1990). Workers face a variety of job hazards. Use of heavy equipment; exposure to chemicals, biohazards, sunlight, heat, cold, and noise; and potential for assault or violence pose risks to workers. Heavy lifting, working at elevations, and performing repetitive tasks, for example, can lead to serious injuries, such as sprains, fractures, and carpal tunnel syndrome. According to the Department of Labor (1995), sprains and strains are by far the leading injury and illness category in every major industry, with back sprains being the most common injury. Interestingly, nurses aides and orderlies had the highest rates of back sprains and lost days from work attributed to "overexertion." Other occupations with relatively higher rates of injury include mining, logging, agriculture, construction, manufacturing, trucking, and warehousing.

The extent of illness and injuries directly attributable to occupational risk can be difficult to de-

TABLE 5–7 **Suggestions to Assess and Limit Exposure to Electromagnetic Fields**

- Find out about the EMF levels produced by the particular sources of concern. If the source is a power line, distances may make EMF levels negligible.
- For specific information about EMFs from a particular power line, contact the utility that operates the line. Most utilities will conduct EMF measurements for customers at no charge. Independent technicians will conduct EMF measurements for a fee and are listed in the yellow pages as "engineers, environmental."
- Recognize that EMFs vary greatly between different types of appliances. Small appliances (e.g., electric can openers, mixers, and vacuum cleaners) tend to emit stronger EMFs than large appliances (e.g., televisions). Note that a great deal of variation exists between different models of the same appliance.
- Recognize that cumulative exposure to small levels of EMFs over an extended period of time (alarm clock at the head of the bed, sleeping under an electric blanket or near a ceiling fan) *might* be more harmful than brief exposure to higher EMFs (e.g., using a can opener).
- Increase the distance from the EMF source. Magnetic fields from appliances drop off dramatically in strength with increased distance from the source (e.g., sit at arm's length from your computer terminal).
- Avoid unnecessary proximity to high-EMF sources (e.g., do not let children play directly under power lines or on top of power transformers for underground lines).
- Reduce time spent around the field—turn off your computer monitor and other electrical appliances when they are not in use.
- Be advised that "low–magnetic field" electric blankets significantly lower magnetic fields because of wiring redesign.
- Follow the EMF issue by reading various sources and talking with people who are working to resolve the issue. (This is particularly important for those individuals living close to transmission lines.) The EMF "Infoline" is 1-800-363-2383.

Data from Environmental Protection Agency/Office of Radiation and Indoor Air. (1992). *EMF in Your Environment: Magnetic Field Measurements of Everyday Electrical Devices.* EPA Publication: 402-R-92-008. Washington, D. C., Government Printing Office; National Institute of Environmental Health Sciences/Department of Energy. (1995). *Questions and Answers About EMF.* DOE Publication: EE-0040. Washington, D. C., Government Printing Office.

fine, as many illnesses may result from prolonged exposure to a noxious substance over decades or a combination of factors. Occupational lung disease, occupational cancers, and noise-induced hearing loss, for example, may take many years to develop. Psychological disorders and cardiovascular changes associated with job stress may be suspected, but are difficult to verify. The National Institute for Occupational Safety and Health (NIOSH) is responsible for research efforts to monitor long-term health risks related to work. Ten common work-related illnesses and injuries identified by NIOSH as priority targets for research to address work risk and prevention efforts are (NIOSH, 1989)

- Occupational lung disease
- Musculoskeletal injuries
- Occupational cancer
- Severe occupational traumatic injuries
- Cardiovascular disease
- Reproductive problems
- Neurotoxic illness
- Noise-induced hearing loss
- Dermatological problems
- Psychological disorders

To improve occupational health and safety, a combination of federal and state regulations have been implemented during the 20th century. Table 5–8 outlines major legislative initiatives that have been written to address occupational risks.

Probably the most far-reaching piece of legislation was the Occupational Health and Safety Act (1970). As shown in Table 5–8, the Occupational Health and Safety Act was responsible for the development of the Occupational Safety and Health Administration (OSHA) and NIOSH. These agencies have been instrumental in setting and enforcing standards to improve worker safety and health and in providing research to address a variety of health issues. Over the last two decades, "OSHA has issued hundreds of occupational health and safety standards covering a wide range of hazards, such as toxic chemicals, hazardous equipment and working conditions. These standards require employers to use appropriate practices, means, methods, operations or processes to protect employees from hazards on the job" (Rogers, 1994, p. 437). The "Bloodborne Pathogens Standard" and "Hazard Communication Standard" described in Table 5–8 are examples of OSHA standards. Table 5–9 describes some of the major responsibilities of OSHA and NIOSH.

Prevention of occupational health hazards includes engineering controls, improving work practices, using personal protective equipment, implementing health promotion strategies (e.g., programs for smoking cessation or stress reduction), and monitoring the workplace for emerging hazards. Nurses in community-based practice should be aware of occupational risks and measures that may be taken to prevent or minimize these risks. Table 5–10 lists examples of primary, secondary, and tertiary prevention strategies to reduce occupational illnesses and injuries appropriate for a variety of settings.

Atmospheric Quality

Air pollution threatens the health of humans and animals. It can harm crops and other vegetation; contributes to the erosion, decay, and economic devaluation of buildings and structures; may possibly diminish the protective ozone layer; and contributes to major climatic changes through the "greenhouse effect" (EPA, 1992a). Exposure to air pollutants is associated with increases in morbidity and mortality. "In humans, air pollution can cause lung cell damage, inflammatory responses, impairment of pulmonary host defenses and acute changes in lung function and respiratory symptoms" (Folinsbee, 1992, p. 45). Major air pollutants are listed in Table 5–11.

In the United States, efforts to detect, monitor, reduce, eliminate, and control air pollution have been in effect since the Clean Air Act was passed in 1963. This legislation set standards for "ambient air quality" (which applies to the air quality in a city or town) and industrial emissions standards. The Clean Air Act was amended most recently in November of 1990. Goals of the 1990 amendments (EPA, 1992a) are to

- Cut acid rain in half through implementation

TABLE 5–8 Occupational Health and Safety Legislation

Workers' Compensation Acts

(dates vary by state—first law passed in New York in 1910)

- "No-fault" insurance system operated by the states, with each state having its own law and program
- Benefits are provided through employer-carried insurance plans
- Estimated 87% of the nation's work force is covered by workers' compensation
- Benefits are awarded to individuals who sustain physical or mental injuries from their employment regardless of who or what was the cause of the injury or illness
- Although they vary by state, workers' compensation laws generally allow for ongoing payment of wages and benefits to the injured or disabled worker or dependent survivor for wages lost, medical care and related costs, funeral and burial costs, and some rehabilitation expenses

The Federal Coal Mine Health and Safety Act (1969)

(updated in Federal Mine Safety and Health Amendments Act of 1977)

- Provided for the establishment of health standards for coal mines and medical examinations for underground coal miners
- Provides benefits for coal miners with pneumoconiosis (black lung disease) through social security
- Includes federal funds to compensate mine victims and their survivors

Occupational Safety and Health Act (P.L. 91-596) (1970)

- Formed OSHA, which sets and enforces standards of occupational safety and health (Department of Labor)
- Formed NIOSH, which researches and recommends occupational safety and health standards to OSHA and funds educational centers for the training of occupational health professionals (Department of Health and Human Services)
- Established the National Advisory Council on Occupational Safety and Health—a consumer and professional council that makes occupational safety and health recommendations to OSHA and NIOSH (Presidential appointees)
- Established federal occupational safety and health standards
- Established the Occupational Safety and Health Review Commission to advise OSHA and NIOSH regarding the legal implications of decisions or actions
- Created a mechanism for imposition of fines and other punitive measures for violation of federal occupational safety and health regulations
- Requires employers to maintain records of work-related deaths, injuries, and illnesses

Hazard Communication Standard ("Right-to-Know" Law) (1986)

- One of OSHA's standards
- Developed as a result of the recognition that ALL potentially toxic materials cannot be eliminated from the working environment
- Requires chemical manufacturers and importers to evaluate chemicals with regard to toxicity, label them, and develop information sheets (Material Safety Data Sheets [MSDSs]) for each agent
- Employers must develop, implement, and maintain a hazard communication program to educate employees about identified toxic materials

Bloodborne Pathogens Standard (1992)

- OSHA standard implemented in response to transmission of acquired immunodeficiency syndrome and other bloodborne diseases
- Applies to all individuals (e.g., physicians, dentists, phlebotomists, nurses, morticians, paramedics, laboratory technologists, housekeeping personnel, public safety personnel, laundry workers) occupationally exposed to blood or other potentially infectious materials
- Requires employers to develop and implement procedures to prevent and control exposure to blood and other potentially infectious materials (e.g., semen, vaginal secretions, saliva, amniotic fluid)

Table continued on following page

TABLE 5–8 **Occupational Health and Safety Legislation** *Continued*

Americans with Disabilities Act (1990)

Designed to protect disabled individuals from discrimination specifically in regard to

- Employment—prohibits discrimination against a qualified individual with a disability in all aspects of employment
- State and local government services—prohibits discrimination against individuals with disabilities in providing government services (e.g., public transportation)
- Public accommodations—requires access to private businesses by individuals with disabilities and mandates certain alterations, modifications, and new construction where needed
- Telecommunications—requires telecommunications services be made available, to the extent possible, to the hearing impaired
- Miscellaneous provision—requires varying provisions for accessibility to recreational and other public areas

Data from Travers, P. H. and McDougall, C. E. (1993). The occupational health nurse: Roles and responsibilities, current and future trends. In J. M. Swanson and M. Albrecht (Eds.). *Community Health Nursing: Promoting the Health of Aggregates.* Philadelphia, W. B. Saunders; Ossler, C. C., Stanhope, M., and Lancaster, J. (1996). Community nurse in occupational health. In M. Stanhope and J. Lancaster (Eds.). *Community Health Nursing: Promoting Health of Aggregates, Families and Individuals* (4th ed). St. Louis, Mosby; Rogers, B. (1994). *Occupational Health Nursing: Concepts and Practice.* Philadelphia, W. B. Saunders.

TABLE 5–9 **Responsibilities of the Occupational Safety and Health Administration and National Institute for Occupational Safety and Health**

OSHA is the regulatory agency responsible for promulgating legally enforceable standards that employers must meet to be in compliance with the Occupational Safety and Health Act (Rogers, 1994, p. 437). OSHA responsibilities are to

- Develop and update mandatory occupational safety and health standards
- Monitor and enforce regulations and standards (including the right to enter and inspect the workplace)
- Require employers to keep records of work-related injuries, illnesses, and hazardous exposures
- Educate employers about occupational health and safety
- Maintain an occupational safety and health database of work-related injuries, illnesses, and deaths (in collaboration with NIOSH)
- Supervise employers and worker education and training to identify and prevent unsafe or unhealthy working conditions (in collaboration with NIOSH)

NIOSH functions as the primary research and educational government agency dealing with occupational health and safety issues. NIOSH responsibilities are to

- Research occupational safety and health problems
- Develop recommendations for OSHA standards
- Develop information on safe levels of exposure to toxic materials, physical agents, and substances
- Fund research and training by other agencies or private organizations through grants, contracts, and other arrangements
- Conduct on-site investigations to determine toxicity of materials
- Train occupational safety and health professionals

Data from Ossler, C. C., Stanhope, M., and Lancaster, J. (1996). Community nurse in occupational health. In M. Stanhope and J. Lancaster (Eds.). *Community Health Nursing: Promoting Health of Aggregates, Families and Individuals* (4th ed.). St. Louis, Mosby; Rogers, B. (1994). *Occupational Health Nursing: Concepts and Practice.* Philadelphia, W. B. Saunders; Spradley, B. W. and Allender, J. A. (1996). *Community Health Nursing: Concepts and Practice* (4th ed.). Philadelphia, Lippincott-Raven.

TABLE 5–10 **Prevention Strategies for Work-Related Illness and Injury**

Primary Prevention—Health Promotion

Health education—individual and group programs on a variety of topics
Promoting healthful nutrition
Encouraging exercise and fitness
Assisting with stress reduction and coping mechanisms
Providing prenatal monitoring for pregnant workers
Teaching parenting skills

Primary Prevention—Illness Prevention

Health risk appraisal
Assisting with modification of identified risk factors
Promoting smoking cessation
Encouraging weight control
Providing appropriate immunization (e.g., hepatitis B for health workers)

Primary Prevention—Injury Prevention

Accident investigation
Promoting use of safety devices
Removal of safety hazards
Teaching good body mechanics
Safety education
Instructing on and monitoring safe handling of hazardous substances

Secondary Prevention—Screening

Preplacement and termination physical examinations
Environmental and ergonomic screening
Periodic screening for workers at risk

Secondary Prevention—Management of Episodic Conditions

Assisting client in seeking professional health care when needed
Serving as an advocate to correct a health problem
Monitoring recovery from minor illness or injury
Acting as a resource for information on illness, prevention, and treatment

Secondary Prevention—Emergency Response

First aid for minor injuries
Establishing and maintaining a triage system for injuries
Injury diagnosis and treatment
Mobilizing the emergency medical system when appropriate

Tertiary Prevention

Monitoring chronic illness
Preventing or minimizing complications of chronic conditions
Serving as case manager for clients with chronic conditions
Assisting the worker in seeking reimbursement of health costs from health insurers
Providing on-site therapy where possible

of systems to reduce sulfur dioxide emissions from power plants

- Reduce smog and other pollutants through upgrading inspection and maintenance programs for motor vehicles, adoption of clean fuel programs, and limiting use of wood stoves and fireplaces
- Reduce air toxins (emissions from chemical plants, steel mills, and other businesses) through employment of stringent regulations to reduce industrial emissions
- Protect the ozone layer through the reduction or elimination of chlorofluorocarbons (CFCs) in automobile air conditioners and residential, commercial, and industrial cooling and refrigeration systems

OZONE DEPLETION

"Ozone is both a blessing and a curse in the environment. In the stratosphere, ozone acts to shield the earth from harmful effects of ultraviolet radiation given off by the sun. However, at ground level, high concentrations of ozone are a major health concern" (EPA, 1989c, p. 4). According to Chafee (1991) evidence is increasing that the Earth's stratospheric ozone layer is being destroyed by CFCs. Theoretically, radiation from the sun elicits a chemical reaction between the CFCs and ozone. In 1985, a significant depletion of ozone about the size of North America was first observed in the southern hemisphere. At that time, it was estimated that between 50 and 90% depletion in the ozone layer had occurred, creating a "hole" over Antarctica.

To reduce the threat posed by the ozone depletion, part of the Clean Air Act Amendment of 1990 initiated the phase-out of CFCs. The major concern from a drop in stratospheric ozone levels is the increase in ultraviolet-B light. Increased incidence of skin cancer and cataracts and alterations in the immune system are linked to ozone depletion. Skin cancer is of particular concern. An increase in melanoma and in basal and squamous cell carcinoma is expected (EPA, 1994; Health and Environment Network, 1988). In addition to

TABLE 5–11 **Major Air Pollutants**

Pollutant	Sources	Effects
Ozone. A colorless gas that is the major constituent of photochemical smog at the Earth's surface. In the upper atmosphere (stratosphere), however, ozone is beneficial, protecting us from the sun's harmful rays.	Ozone is formed in the lower atmosphere as a result of chemical reactions between oxygen, volatile organic compounds, and nitrogen oxides in the presence of sunlight, especially during hot weather. Sources of such harmful pollutants include vehicles, factories, landfills, industrial solvents, and numerous small sources such as gas stations and farm and lawn equipment.	Ozone causes significant health and environmental problems at the earth's surface, where we live. It can irritate the respiratory tract, produce impaired lung function such as inability to take a deep breath, and cause throat irritation, chest pain, cough, lung inflammation, and possible susceptibility to lung infection. Smog components may aggravate existing respiratory conditions like asthma. Ozone can also reduce yield of agricultural crops and injure forests and other vegetation. Ozone is the most injurious pollutant to plant life.
Carbon monoxide. Odorless and colorless gas emitted in the exhaust of motor vehicles and other kinds of engines where incomplete fossil fuel combustion occurs.	Automobiles, buses, trucks, small engines, and some industrial processes. High concentrations can be found in confined spaces like parking garages, poorly ventilated tunnels, or along roadsides during periods of heavy traffic.	Reduces the ability of blood to deliver oxygen to vital tissues, affecting primarily the cardiovascular and nervous systems. Lower concentrations have been shown to adversely affect individuals with heart disease (e.g., angina) and to decrease maximal exercise performance in young, healthy men. Higher concentrations can cause symptoms such as dizziness, headaches, and fatigue.
Nitrogen dioxide. Light brown gas at lower concentrations; in higher concentrations, it becomes an important component of unpleasant-looking brown urban haze.	Result of burning fuels in utilities, industrial boilers, cars, and trucks.	One of the major pollutants that causes smog and acid rain. Can harm humans and vegetation when concentrations are sufficiently high. In children, may cause increased respiratory illness such as chest colds and coughing with phlegm. For asthmatics, can cause increased breathing difficulty.
Particulate matter. Solid matter or liquid droplets from smoke, dust, fly ash, and condensing vapors that can be suspended in the air for long periods.	Industrial processes, smelters, automobiles, burning industrial fuels, wood smoke, dust from paved and unpaved roads, construction, and agricultural ground breaking.	These microscopic particles can affect breathing and respiratory symptoms, causing increased respiratory disease and lung damage and possibly premature death. Children, the elderly, and people suffering from heart or lung disease (like asthma) are especially at risk. Also damages paint, soils clothing, and reduces visibility.
Sulfur dioxide. Colorless gas, odorless at low concentrations but pungent at very high concentrations.	Emitted largely from industrial, institutional, utility, and apartment-house furnaces and boilers, as well as petroleum refineries, smelters, paper mills, and chemical plants.	One of the major pollutants that causes smog. Can also, at high concentrations, affect human health, especially among asthmatics (who are particularly sensitive to respiratory tract problems and breathing

		difficulties that sulfur dioxide can induce). Can also harm vegetation and metals. The pollutants it produces can impair visibility and acidify lakes and streams.
Lead. Lead and lead compounds can adversely affect human health through either ingestion of lead-contaminated substances, such as soil, dust, paint, or direct inhalation. This is particularly a risk for young children, whose normal hand-to-mouth activities can result in greater ingestion of lead-contaminated soils and dusts.	Transportation sources using lead in their fuels, coal combustion, smelters, car battery plants, and combustion of garbage containing lead products.	Elevated lead levels can adversely affect mental development and performance, kidney function, and blood chemistry. Young children are particularly at risk because of their greater chance of ingesting lead and the increased sensitivity of young tissues and organs to lead.
Toxic air pollutants. Includes pollutants such as arsenic, asbestos, and benzene.	Chemical plants, industrial processes, motor vehicle emissions and fuels, and building materials.	Known or suspected to cause cancer, respiratory effects, birth defects, and reproductive and other serious health effects. Some can cause death or serious injury if accidentally released in large amounts.
Stratospheric ozone depleters. Chemicals such as CFCs, halons, carbon tetrachloride, and methyl chloroform that are used in refrigerants and other industrial processes. These chemicals last a long time in the air, rising to the upper atmosphere where they destroy the protective ozone layer that screens out harmful ultraviolet radiation before it reaches the earth's surface.	Industrial household refrigeration, cooling and cleaning processes, car and home air conditioners, some fire extinguishers, and plastic foam products.	Increased exposure to ultraviolet radiation could potentially cause an increase in skin cancer, increased cataract cases, suppression of the human immune response system, and environmental damage.
Greenhouse gases. Gases that build up in the atmosphere that may induce global climate change—or the "greenhouse effect." They include carbon dioxide, methane, and nitrous oxide.	The main human-made source of carbon dioxide emissions is fossil fuel combustion for energy use and transportation. Methane comes from landfills, cud-chewing livestock, coal mines, and rice paddies. Nitrous oxide results from industrial processes, such as nylon fabrication.	The extent of the effects of climate change on human health and the environment is still uncertain but could include increased global temperature, increased severity and frequency of storms and other "weather extremes," melting of the polar ice cap, and sea-level rise.

From Environmental Protection Agency. (1992). *What You Can Do to Reduce Air Pollution.* EPA Publication no: 450-K-92-002. Washington, D. C., Government Printing Office.

TABLE 5–12 **What Individuals and Communities Can Do to Reduce Air Pollution**

Driving Tips

- Plan ahead—organize trips to drive fewer miles, combine errands into one trip, avoid driving during peak traffic, walk or bicycle for short errands
- Ride share—participate in carpools or use public transportation
- Use energy-conserving motor oil and "clean" fuels when possible
- Drive at minimum and steady speed; do not idle the engine unnecessarily
- Follow recommendations from the vehicle owner's manual regarding the correct grade of gasoline, shifting gears, and other ways to keep the engine running at maximum efficiency

Car Maintenance

- Do not remove or tamper with pollution controls
- Do not overfill or "top off" the car's gas tank
- Get regular engine tune-ups and car maintenance checks
- Keep car filters and catalytic converters clean
- Consider buying fuel-efficient cars

Reducing Air Pollution at Home and Work

- Conserve electricity—turn off lights and appliances when not in use, raise the temperature level on air conditioners, turn down heaters in the winter, purchase energy-efficient appliances
- Participate in local utilitys' conservation programs
- Use wood stoves and fireplaces wisely and sparingly
- Properly dispose of household paints, solvents, pesticides, and refrigeration and air conditioning equipment

Get Involved in Efforts to Reduce Air Pollution

- Learn about local efforts and issues
- Work with community action groups to improve air quality
- Report air pollution problems to the appropriate local or state agency or the EPA

From Environmental Protection Agency. (1992). *What You Can Do to Reduce Air Pollution.* EPA publication: 450-K-92-002. Washington, D. C., Government Printing Office.

the harmful effects on humans, there is concern over the effects of increased ultraviolet-B light on animals, plants, and marine ecosystems (EPA, 1994b). To combat air pollution, the EPA (1992a) has made a number of suggestions, which are included in Table 5–12.

Water Quality

"The availability of clean, safe water is an absolute necessity in the sustenance of a healthy environment" (Primomo and Salazar, 1995, p. 661). According to the USDHHS (1990), only 80% of the community water systems meet safe drinking water standards established by the EPA. Sewage (containing human waste, detergents), industrial processes and wastes (producing heavy metals, detergents, salts, heat, petrochemicals), and agricultural chemicals (e.g., fertilizer, pesticides) are the main sources of water pollution. To ensure and promote water quality, federal legislation was passed in 1948 and has been amended several times (1972, 1974, 1977, 1986, 1987). The Clean Water Act(s) serve to safeguard the quality of the nation's water supply through setting water standards and maximum allowable water contaminant levels.

MICROBIAL CONTAMINATION

Although surface and groundwater treatment through disinfection and filtration has dramatically reduced the incidence of waterborne diseases in the United States during this century, "annual reports of water-related, microorganism-induced disease continue to number in the thousands" (EPA, 1993a, p. 1). For example, a widely publicized outbreak of cryptosporidiosis in Milwaukee in 1993 affected an estimated 400,000 individuals and prompted measures to determine and address the public health concerns and direct new research on ways to detect and control this organism in community water supplies (CDC, 1995).

Waterborne diseases are those diseases that result from ingestion of contaminated water, inhalation of water vapors, body contact through bathing or swimming, and accidental ingestion of water during recreational activities (e.g., swimming, water skiing). Because symptoms are usually mild and short lived, it is assumed that only a small fraction of waterborne illnesses are recognized, reported, and investigated. Bacteria, viruses, and protozoa are the microorganisms of primary concern in waterborne disease. Table 5–13 lists the most common waterborne diseases found in the United States.

Water treatment processes include filtration, disinfection, and treatment of organic and inorganic contaminants. Removal of solids and microorganisms (e.g., *Giardia* and *Cryptosporidium* species) is accomplished by filtration systems (e.g., sand, diatomaceous earth, membrane, or cartridge filtration). Disinfection techniques include use of chlorine, ozone, and chloramines. Granular or powdered activated carbon column aeration, diffused aeration, oxidation, reverse osmosis, and aeration are also used to remove organic contaminants from water supplies (EPA, 1991).

CHEMICAL AND METAL CONTAMINANTS

Chemical contaminants of surface and ground water include pesticides (e.g., insecticides, fungicides, herbicides), petrochemicals and other organic compounds (e.g., improperly disposed of motor oil, paint, antifreeze), and a variety of industrial wastes (e.g., suspended solids, radionucliotides, asbestos). Metal contaminants include lead, mercury, copper, and iron.

Lead contamination is of particular concern, as a significant number of public water systems in the United States provide drinking water that con-

TABLE 5–13 **Waterborne Diseases of Concern in the United States**

Disease	Microbial Agent	General Symptoms
Amebiasis	Protozoan (*Entamoeba histolytica*)	Abdominal discomfort, fatigue, diarrhea, flatulence, weight loss
Campylobacteriosis	Bacterium (*Campylobacter jejuni*)	Fever, abdominal pain, diarrhea
Cholera	Bacterium (*Vibrio cholerae*)	Watery diarrhea, vomiting, occasional muscle cramps
Cryptosporidiosis	Protozoan (*Cryptosporidium parvum*)	Diarrhea, abdominal discomfort
Giardiasis	Protozoan (*Giardia lamblia*)	Diarrhea, abdominal discomfort
Hepatitis	Virus (hepatitis A)	Fever, chills, abdominal discomfort, jaundice, dark urine
Shigellosis	Bacterium (*Shigella* species)	Fever, diarrhea, bloody stool
Typhoid fever	Bacterium (*Salmonella typhi*)	Fever, headache, constipation, appetite loss, nausea, diarrhea, vomiting, appearance of an abdominal rash
Viral gastroenteritis	Viruses (Norwalk, rotavirus, and other types)	Fever, headache, gastrointestinal discomfort, vomiting, diarrhea

From Environmental Protection Agency. (1993). *Preventing Waterborne Disease.* EPA publication no: 640-K-93-001. Washington, D. C., Government Printing Office.

tains lead levels exceeding the "action level" standard established by the EPA (Urbinato, 1994). Also, lead is particularly harmful to infants, young children, and developing fetuses. Lead contamination is largely caused by widespread use of lead in pipes, brass faucets or fittings, and lead solder and is of most concern in homes that are very old *or* very new. Plumbing installed before 1930 is likely to contain lead. In newer plumbing system construction, lead solder and brass faucets and fittings are often used and can leach lead during the first 5 years of use. Thus, "water in buildings less than five years old . . . may have high levels of lead contamination" (EPA, 1993b, p. 2).

Recommendations from the EPA (EPA, 1993b) to reduce lead in drinking water include the following:

- Flush pipes before drinking. Run cold water through pipes for 5 to 30 seconds, particularly if the water has been in contact with plumbing for more than 6 hours (e.g., overnight or during a workday).
- Use only cold water for consumption. Use only water from the cold water tap for drinking, cooking, and *especially for making baby formula,* as hot water is more likely to contain higher levels of lead.
- Have water tested. Have the amount of lead in household water tested. This is particularly important for apartment dwellers.
- Consider the use of filtering devices. Filters may help in reducing lead levels if properly used (e.g., filters must be changed as specified by the manufacturer).
- Consider bottled water for consumption. Bottled water is regulated by the Food and Drug Administration (FDA) if sold in interstate commerce and is under state regulation if sold within a state.
- Use only lead-free materials in plumbing repairs and installation. Obtain assurance from a qualified plumber—in writing—that only lead-free materials will be used.

COMMUNITY AND NURSING INTERVENTIONS

Research into improving water treatment, as well as detecting, analyzing, and eliminating contamination is ongoing. Efforts to monitor and improve water quality should be supported by all health care providers, as well as by concerned citizens. "Improved public and professional appreciation of the risks of contaminated drinking water and increased willingness of the public to pay for improved drinking water quality" are essential (USDHHS, 1990, p. 327). Suggestions for improving water quality and ensuring safe water include the following:

- Be aware of the community's water source and supplier. How is the water supply treated and tested for contamination? Does the supplier adhere to guidelines and standards set by the EPA?
- Learn about potential contamination sources of ground water and surface water.
- Urge the community water supplier and state and local regulatory and health officials to ensure that the water supply complies with all standards.
- Support efforts to educate the public and elected officials about the need to protect and improve the quality of drinking water.
- Express willingness to pay higher water rates, if necessary, to finance improvements in water quality.
- Support local and state efforts to develop programs and strategies to protect surface and ground water and to develop programs to control contaminating sources and activities.
- Support ongoing research and training efforts to improve water quality.

Food Quality

The FDA and the Department of Agriculture are responsible for setting standards for food safety, inspection of many foods, regulation of restaurants and food sales, and approval of food additives, as well as for oversight of other aspects of food safety. Although safety of food consumed by United States residents is taken for granted, outbreaks of food-related illnesses and threats to health occur occasionally. Food quality and safety concerns include potentially harmful intentional and unintentional additives, as well as biological and chemical contaminants. A variety of other issues related to food, such as genetically engineered foods and misrepresentations of nutrient qualities and substandard inspection, should also be of concern to all nurses.

MICROBIOLOGICAL CONTAMINATION

The USDHHS (1990) lists four foodborne pathogens as being of primary concern with regard to foodborne illnesses. These are *Salmonella enteritidis, Campylobacter jejuni, Escherichia coli* 0157:H7, and *Listeria monocytogenes*. Table 5–14 presents information on each, including symptoms, associated foods, and strategies for prevention. Additionally, Table 5–15 lists the "Seven Commandments of Food Safety" developed by the Department of Agriculture and reported in *Healthy People 2000* (USDHHS, 1990).

INTENTIONAL FOOD ADDITIVES

Intentional food additives are those substances added to food during processing to enhance the nutritional content of foods (e.g., vitamins and minerals), improve flavor (e.g., monosodium glutamate, salt, sugars, "natural flavors"), enhance color (e.g., dyes), improve texture or consistency (e.g., leavening agents, gums, thickening agents), and/or increase the shelf life (e.g., various preservatives).

Food additives have been regulated, to some degree, by the FDA since the passage of the Food, Drug, and Cosmetic Act in 1938. This law requires food manufacturers to list product ingredients on the food label. Subsequent amendments and legislation have resulted in allowing the FDA to establish and enforce standards for the processing of food, including food additives. The "Delaney clause" was added in 1960 and forbids the use of any additive shown to cause cancer in humans or animals (Blumenthal, 1990). The Nutrition Labeling and Education Act was passed in 1990 to require listing of color additives by name and the listing of ingredients in standardized foods (Segal, 1993). The Dietary Supplement Act of 1992 set more stringent guidelines for health claims and nutrition content of foods to ensure that "claims made about the health and nutritional benefits are truthful" (Farley, 1993, p. 2).

Instruction on food additives should be a component of thorough nutrition counseling. Client education should include encouragement to read food labels and to choose foods appropriate for individual nutritional needs.

UNINTENTIONAL (INCIDENTAL) FOOD ADDITIVES

Unintentional food additives refer to those substances that "enter and remain in food as a result of their use as pesticides or herbicides, after being added to animal food, from packaging material, or through chemical changes brought about by processing methods" (Lancaster, 1992, p. 297). Glass chips, insect fragments, mercury and other heavy metals in fish, and residual antibiotics in beef and milk products are examples of food contaminants that have been the source of recent concern (Foulke, 1994; Stevens and Hall, 1993; Wagner, 1992).

To preserve food quality, the FDA has established "food defect action levels," sets and enforces food safety and quality standards, and routinely monitors foods for evidence of "food defects" (Wagner, 1992). Additionally, the EPA and FDA conduct and support research to ensure food safety.

Foulke (1993) summarized FDA findings regarding residual pesticides in food and made recommendations related to these findings. According to this report, an analysis of numerous research studies has shown that residues of pesticide (e.g., herbicides, fungicides, insecticides) were 83 to 99% eliminated from fruits and vegetables through natural means that cause dilution or degradation (e.g., wind, rain, sunlight) and commercial food processing (e.g., washing, blanching, peeling). To further reduce and virtually eliminate ingestion of pesticide residues, the FDA provides the following recommendations (Foulke, 1993):

- Wash fruits and vegetables with large amounts of cold or warm water and scrub

TABLE 5–14 **Selected Foodborne Microorganisms**

Microorganism	Onset, Duration and Frequency	Acute Symptoms	Associated Foods	Prevention
Salmonella species	*Onset of symptoms:* 6–48 hours after ingestion. *Duration of symptoms:* 1–2 days. *Frequency:* 77 reported outbreaks in 1989 involving 2,400 individuals. Most cases, however, go unreported, and the FDA estimates 2–4 million annual cases of salmonellosis in the United States.	Nausea, vomiting, abdominal cramps, diarrhea, fever, and headache.	Meats, poultry, eggs, milk and dairy products, fish, shrimp, frog legs, yeast, salad dressings and sauces, cream-filled desserts and toppings, peanut butter, cocoa, and chocolate.	Raw eggs and foods containing raw eggs (e.g., home-made ice cream, Caesar salad, mayonnaise) may cause Salmonella infections. Eggs and all meats, particularly poultry, should be thoroughly cooked. Buy refrigerated eggs and keep refrigerated at temperatures less than 40°F. Wash hands, utensils, equipment, and work areas with hot soapy water before and after they come in contact with eggs and poultry. Buy only pasteurized milk, and keep refrigerated.
Campylobacter jejuni	*Onset of symptoms:* 2–5 days after ingestion of contaminated food or water. *Duration of symptoms:* 7–10 days, with relapses in about 25% of cases. *Frequency: C. jejuni* is the leading cause of bacterial diarrhea in the United States. Estimates exceed 2–4 million cases per year.	Diarrhea—often bloody and may contain fecal leukocytes—fever, abdominal pain, nausea, headache, and muscle pain.	Raw chicken, raw milk, contaminated water, and raw clams.	Wash and thoroughly cook chicken. Wash hands and cooking utensils that come in contact with raw chicken with hot soapy water. Complete pasteurization of milk and chlorination of drinking water will kill *C. jejuni.*

Escherichia coli 0157:H7 (*E. coli* 0157:H7)	*Onset of symptoms:* 6–48 hours after ingestion. *Duration of symptoms:* approximately 8 days. *Frequency:* appears to be uncommon; however, probably only the most severe cases are reported.	Severe cramping, abdominal pain, and diarrhea that is initially watery but becomes grossly bloody. Occasionally vomiting occurs. Fever is low grade or absent.	Raw and undercooked hamburger meat (ground beef) is the primary source. Has also been traced to processed salami. Raw milk and other meats may contain *E. coli* 0157:H7.	Thoroughly cook all beef, particularly ground beef. Maintain cooked beef at appropriately hot or cold temperatures. Do not drink unpasteurized milk.
Listeria monocytogenes	*Onset of symptoms:* in general, 7–30 days after exposure, although may be 2–3 days after consumption of heavily contaminated foods. Symptoms in infants may appear hours or days after birth. *Frequency:* appears to be relatively rare—about 1,600 cases per year.	Fever, headache, nausea, and vomiting; of particular concern to pregnant women and their unborn children, as infection may lead to fetal death, premature labor, or infections in newborns. Major concern—mortality rate is almost 25%.	Dairy products, particularly soft cheeses; also found in some imported seafood (e.g., frozen crab meat, cooked shrimp, and cooked surimi).	Consume only pasteurized milk and dairy products made from pasteurized milk.

Adapted from Food and Drug Administration. (1992). *Foodborne Pathogenic Microorganisms and Natural Toxins.* Washington, D. C., Government Printing Office.

TABLE 5–15 **Seven Commandments of Food Safety**

1. Wash hands before handling food.
2. Keep it safe—refrigerate.
3. Do not thaw food on the kitchen counter.
4. Wash hands, utensils, and surfaces after contact with raw meat and poultry.
5. Never leave perishable food out over 2 hours.
6. Thoroughly cook raw meat, poultry, and fish.
7. Freeze or refrigerate leftovers promptly.

Data from the Food and Drug Administration.

with a brush when appropriate (do not use soap).

- Throw away the outer leaves of leafy vegetables such as lettuce and cabbage.
- Peel and cook when appropriate, although some nutrients and fiber are lost when produce is peeled.
- Trim fat from meat and fat and skin from poultry and fish. Residues of some pesticides concentrate in animal fat.

OTHER ISSUES IN FOOD QUALITY

Other concerns and issues in food quality include genetically engineered foods; irradiation of foods; and ongoing development of substances, additives, and chemicals to change food. Recent scientific developments have advanced the production of foods with decreased caloric content, increased nutritive value, and improved shelf life. The Department of Agriculture and the FDA set policy for foods produced from new plant varieties and plant breeding, and the FDA must approve new food additives before marketing. Additionally, "all foods are subject to FDA's post-market authority under the 'adulteration' provisions of the act [Food, Drug and Cosmetic Act], and producers have a legal duty to ensure that the foods they place on the market meet the safety standards of these provisions" (Suddeth, 1993, p.3). As a result of these efforts, clients should be reassured that efforts are being made to ensure food safety. However, clients should also be encouraged to stay informed on current developments regarding food quality.

Waste Control

There are two major concerns in the issue of waste control: volume of solid wastes produced in the United States, and concerns over the disposal of toxic and hazardous wastes. Each is discussed briefly.

SOLID WASTE MANAGEMENT

The United States is the world's biggest producer of solid wastes. Burying wastes in landfills, incineration, and recycling are the current available options for management of solid wastes. It is estimated that United States residents throw away 3.5 to 4.0 pounds of garbage per person per day. Figure 5–1 depicts components of America's trash. Besides involving esthetic and practical concerns, effective solid waste management is essential in decreasing pathogen transmission through insect and rodent control and in eliminating potential exposure to toxic and infectious materials.

In response to this growing problem, the EPA has endorsed an "integrated waste management" strategy of source reduction, recycling, waste combustion and landfilling, and community response and activities to produce less waste. Box 5–1 outlines practical ways all citizens can work to manage solid waste more effectively.

TOXIC AND HAZARDOUS WASTE CONTROL

Hazardous materials make up approximately 10% of industrial wastes and include poisons, inflammable materials, infectious contaminants, explosives, and radionuclides (Lancaster, 1992). The EPA regulates hazardous waste under the Resource Conservation and Recovery Act and, together with the Agency for Toxic Substances and

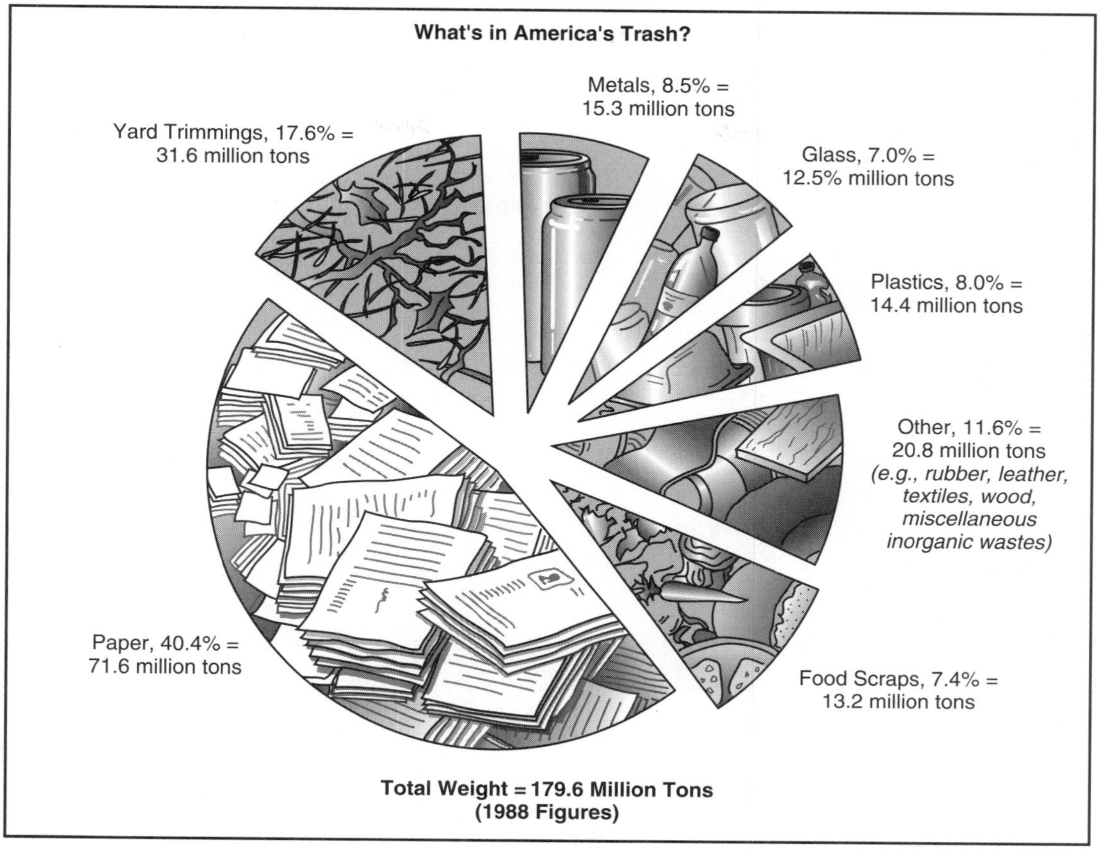

FIGURE 5–1 What's in America's trash? (From the Environmental Protection Agency. [1992]. *The Consumer's Handbook for Reducing Solid Waste.* EPA Publication. 530-K-92-003. Washington, D. C., Government Printing Office.)

Disease Registry, is responsible for oversight of hazardous waste disposal and monitoring potential and actual threats posed to health and safety. According to Breslin (1993), the EPA has identified 1270 sites as being on the "National Priorities List" designated for cleanup under the Comprehensive Environmental Response, Compensation, and Liability Act of 1980 (the Superfund law). This law requires industry to pay for cleaning up the worst hazardous wastes sites, funded by taxes on industries that produce hazardous wastes.

Some of the most common contaminants include lead (e.g., from paint and glass manufacturing and smelting), mercury (e.g., from batteries, paints, pesticides), polychlorinated biphenyls [PCBs] (e.g., from electrical insulation); chromium (e.g., from copy machines, stainless steel manufacturing, chrome plating), trichlolorethane or trichloroethylene (e.g., from dry-cleaning agents), and benzene (e.g., from chemical manufacturing) (EPA, 1994d). To regulate these and other hazardous wastes, the EPA has instituted a tracking system that monitors identified hazardous substances from the time the substance is produced until it reaches an approved site for disposal.

Medical waste, defined by the EPA as cultures and stocks of infectious agents, human blood and blood products, human pathological wastes, contaminated animal carcasses, wastes from patients isolated with highly communicable diseases, and

BOX 5–1 Tips for Reducing Solid Waste

Reduce

Reduce the Amount of Unnecessary Packaging

- When choosing between two similar products, select the one with the least unnecessary packaging
- When possible, consider the purchase of items such as produce or nails, in unpackaged, rather than prepackaged, forms
- Recognize and support store managers when they stock products with no packaging or reduced packaging
- Consider large or economy-size items for household products that are used frequently, as they typically have less packaging per unit of product
- Consider concentrated products, as they often require less packaging

Tip—The Mail Preference Service is a free service that removes names from many national mailing lists. To reduce unwanted advertising mail, contact

Mail Preference Service
Direct Marketing Association
P. O. Box 9008
Farmingdale, NY 11735-9008

Adopt Practices that Reduce Waste Toxicity

- Take actions that use nonhazardous or less hazardous components to accomplish a task; for example, choose reduced mercury batteries or consider nonchemical means to reduce pests in gardens
- Learn about and adopt alternatives to household items containing hazardous substances (e.g., baking soda and steel wool instead of oven cleaner, a plunger or plumber's snake instead of drain cleaner, cedar chips or mint instead of mothballs)
- If products with hazardous components must be used, use only the amount needed and share with neighbors or donate to other groups; recycle motor oil
- Read and follow all directions when using products containing hazardous components, and follow the local community policy on household hazardous waste disposal

Reuse

Consider Reusable Products

- Choose reusable coffee mugs, utensils, tableware, and other items whenever possible, rather than paper, styrofoam, or plastic
- Use cloth napkins, sponges, and dishcloths
- Use items that are available in refillable containers (e.g., detergents, beverages)
- Use rechargeable batteries
- When using single-use items, only take what is needed

Reuse Bags, Containers, and Other Items

- Reuse paper and plastic bags and twist ties
- Reuse scrap paper and envelopes
- Reuse newspaper, boxes, packaging "peanuts," and "bubble wrap" to ship packages
- Wash and reuse empty glass and plastic jars, milk jugs, coffee cans, and butter tubs

Caution: do not reuse containers that originally held products such as motor oil or pesticides, as they may contain potentially harmful residues, and never store anything potentially harmful in containers designed for food or beverages

Borrow, Rent, or Share Items Used Infrequently

- Rent or borrow party decorations and supplies, such as tables, chairs, linens, dishes, and silverware
- Rent or borrow tools, such as ladders, chain saws, floor buffers, rug cleaners
- Share newspapers and magazines with others to extend the lives of the items and reduce waste paper

BOX 5–1 **Tips for Reducing Solid Waste** *Continued*

Sell or Donate Goods Instead of Throwing Them Out

- Donate or resell items to thrift stores or other organizations in need
- Give hand-me-down clothes to family members, neighbors, or the needy
- Conduct a food or clothing drive to help others
- Encourage and support area merchants who donate damaged or other goods or food items to food banks, shelters, and other needy groups

Recycle

Choose Recyclable Products and Containers and Recycle Them

- Consider products made of materials that are collected for recycling locally; glass, aluminum, steel, some paper and cardboard, and certain plastics are routinely collected in many areas
- Participate in community recycling drives, curbside programs, and drop-off collections
- If a recycling program does not exist, participate in establishing one
- Take used car batteries, antifreeze, and motor oil to participating car service centers that collect them for recycling
- Take advantage of businesses and organizations that provide collection opportunities (e.g., used grocery bags)

Select Products Made from Recycled Materials

- Look for items in packages and containers made of recycled materials; many bottles, cans, paper wrappings, bags, boxes, and other cartons are made from recycled materials
- Encourage state and local government agencies, local businesses, and others to purchase recycled products

Compost Yard Trimmings and Some Food Scraps

- Learn how to compost food scraps and yard trimmings through reference materials at the local library or through local agricultural or park services
- Participate in local or regional programs to collect compostable materials
- Allow mown grass clippings to remain on the lawn to decompose rather than bagging and disposing of them

Respond

Educate Others on Source Reduction and Recycling Practice and Make Your Preferences Known to Manufacturers, Merchants and Community Leaders

- Write to companies to encourage them to reduce unnecessary packaging and the use of hazardous components in products and respond positively when they make changes
- Encourage reduction, recycling, and composting programs in the community
- Encourage the use of reusable, recycled, and recyclable materials in the workplace where appropriate
- Urge schools to provide environmental education and to teach about source reduction, recycling, and composting

Be Creative—Find New Ways to Reduce Waste Quantity and Toxicity

- Turn a giant cardboard box into a child's playhouse
- Use an egg carton to plant seedlings
- Select nontoxic inks and art supplies
- Choose beverages such as water, milk, or soda in reusable containers, where appropriate

From EPA. (1992). *The Consumer's Handbook for Reducing Solid Waste.* EPA Publication: 530-K-92-003. Washington D. C., Government Printing Office.

all used sharps, are controlled by the Medical Waste Tracking Act of 1988 and, like other hazardous wastes, are tracked from generation to disposal. Currently, incineration is the method of disposal of choice for medical waste; approximately 70% of hospital waste is currently incinerated on site. An additional 15% is sterilized in autoclaves, and 15% is transported off site for treatment (EPA, 1989b).

Hazardous waste management consists of a combination of treatment to reduce toxicity (e.g., incineration, detoxification), storage, and/or disposal following prescribed methods. Additionally, the EPA strongly encourages "waste minimization" to reduce the volume of hazardous wastes.

LANDFILLS

A landfill is a place where garbage is dumped and covered daily with a layer of soil. The soil cuts down on odor, flies, insects, and animals. Newer landfills, called "sanitary landfills," are lined with clay and strong plastic sheets, which are designed to keep the landfill from leaking into the environment—particularly from contaminating ground water. Although some 70% of the garbage in a landfill is "biodegradable," most garbage, including food and paper, remains intact for decades because of a lack of light, oxygen, and water that prevents composting.

To minimize potential exposure to contaminants from landfills, there are several safeguards of which nurses, as well as all citizens, should be aware. These include

- Maintenance of a "buffer zone" to separate the landfill from surrounding areas
- Surrounding the landfill with a fence
- Installation of gas vents to prevent methane gas build-up
- Installation and maintenance of a system to collect and treat leachate (chemicals that "leach out" of waste in landfills and may contaminate nearby soil and ground water)
- Establishment and ongoing evaluation of a system to monitor the landfill to ensure adherence to state and federal environmental standards and regulations
- Establishment of an emergency action plan that includes readily available equipment to put out fires and manage other crises (Environmental and Occupational Health Sciences Institute [EOHSI], 1989).

INCINERATION

Incineration as a method of solid and hazardous waste management is controversial. Incineration reduces the volume of waste by up to 90% and is effective in destroying most biological contaminants. However, increasing air pollution, particularly with toxic chemicals, and subsequent disposal processes for residual heavy metals are the primary concerns. Commercial waste incinerators are designed to control emissions into the air. A variety of methods and devices, including filters, "scrubbers," and electrostatic precipitators, are employed to collect particulates and neutralize exhausts. Following incineration, residual ash is tested for toxicity and disposed of accordingly. If no toxins are found, the residue is typically dumped into a regular landfill. If toxins are found, the residue is shipped to hazardous waste landfills. A positive byproduct of waste incineration that is gaining in acceptance is energy production. Capturing the energy (i.e., heat) that is produced and "recycling" it is commonplace in newer, "state-of-the-art" incineration plants.

Radiation Risks

Threats to health from ionizing radiation come from several sources. Figure 5–2 illustrates potential sources of exposure to radiation. Unless exposure is occupational in nature (e.g., for radiology technicians, dentists, nuclear plant employees), the most common, and most potentially hazardous, radiation risks come from two sources—radon gas and the sun.

RADON GAS

According to the U. S. Surgeon General, "Indoor radon gas is a national health problem. Radon causes thousands of deaths each year. Millions of

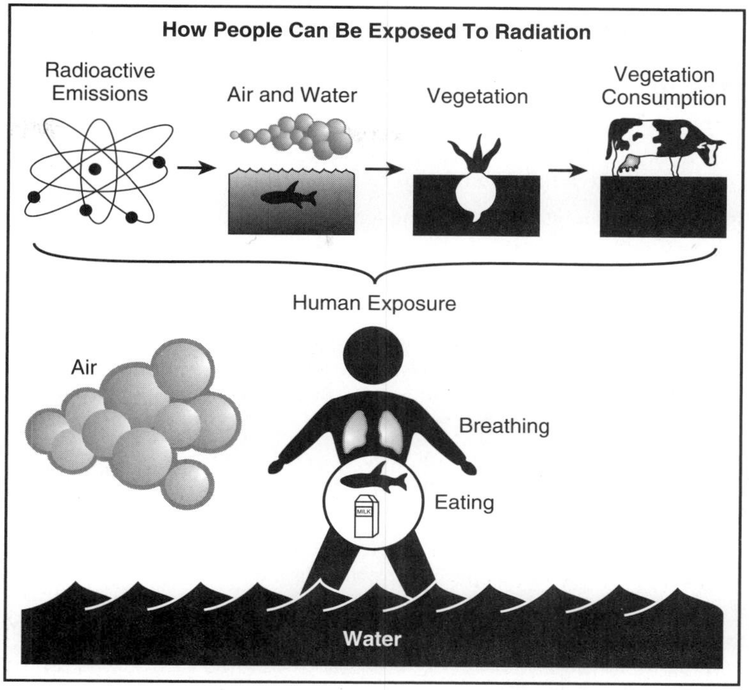

FIGURE 5–2 How people can be exposed to radiation. (From Centers for Disease Control/National Center for Environmental Health. [1993]. *Radiation Studies.* Atlanta, U. S. Department of Health and Human Services, Centers for Disease Control.)

homes have elevated radon levels. Homes should be tested for radon. When elevated levels are confirmed, the problems should be corrected" (USDHHS/EPA, 1994). Radon, an odorless, invisible gas, is a byproduct of the decay of uranium and occurs nearly everywhere in very small amounts. Radon enters buildings through cracks in solid floors, construction joints, cracks in walls, gaps in suspended floors, gaps around service pipes, cavities inside walls, and the water supply (EPA, 1992b). The amount of radon present varies greatly, and dangerously high levels can be found in many homes. As a result, radon is the second leading cause of lung cancer in the United States and is responsible for an estimated 15,000 deaths each year (Anderson, 1994).

Radon is measured in units called picocuries per liter (pCi/L). The average radon level in most houses in the United States is approximately 1 pCi/L. The EPA has established a level of 4 pCi/L or less as desirable.

To measure radon levels, test kits can be purchased through the mail or from hardware stores and other retail outlets. Test kits should stipulate that they "meet EPA requirements" and should be designated "short term" (to remain in the home for 2 to 90 days) or "long term" (to remain in the home for 90 days or more). Because radon levels tend to vary from day to day, a short-term test is less likely to accurately detect radon. If one short-term test records a level of 4 pCi/L or greater, a second test should be conducted. EPA recommendations following radon testing are discussed in Table 5–16.

The EPA recommends employing only trained contractors to perform repairs needed to lower home radon levels. Repair costs range from $500 to $2,500, depending on the house and choice of radon reduction methods. Table 5–17 lists repair options and anticipated costs.

ULTRAVIOLET RADIATION AND SKIN CANCER

Skin cancer is the most common form of cancer in the United States, with 500,000 to 700,000 new

TABLE 5–16 Environmental Protection Agency Recommendations for Radon Testing

Step 1. Take a short-term test. If the result is 4 pCi/L or higher, take a follow-up test to be sure.

Step 2. Follow up with either a long-term test or a second short-term test:

For a better understanding of the year-round average radon level, take a long-term test.

If test results are needed quickly, take a second short-term test. (If the short-term test results are 10 pCi/L or higher, a second short-term test should be conducted immediately.)

Step 3. If the second test was a long-term test: Home repairs are needed if long-term results are 4 pCi/L or greater.

If the second test was a short-term test: Home repairs are needed if the average of both tests is 4 pCi/L or greater.

Adapted from Environmental Protection Agency/U. S. Department of Health and Human Services. (1994). *A Citizen's Guide to Radon* (2nd ed.). EPA publication #402-K92-001. Washington, D. C., Government Printing Office.

cases diagnosed yearly, resulting in approximately 9,000 deaths (Clark, 1994; EOHSI, 1991; USDHHS/Office of Disease Prevention and Health Promotion, 1994). Exposure to the sun is associated with three major types of skin cancer: basal cell carcinoma (80%), squamous cell carcinoma (12%), and malignant melanoma (4.5%) (Clark, 1994). It is acknowledged that "more than 90% of basal and squamous cell carcinomas result from exposure to ultraviolet radiation from the sun" (EOHSI, 1991, p. 1). The correlation between melanoma and sun exposure is less certain.

Rates of skin cancer appear to be rising, and an estimated one in six people will develop skin cancer during his or her lifetime. At highest risk are those individuals with a fair complexion, who sunburn easily, and have blond or red hair and blue eyes. As stated, exposure to ultraviolet radiation, particularly during the early years of life, contributes to skin changes that eventually result in development of skin cancer. According to Clark (1994), "approximately 80% of the ultraviolet radiation damage to the skin occurs by the age of 20 years" (p. 742).

Signs, Symptoms, and Detection of Skin Cancer

Basal and squamous cell carcinoma occurs most frequently in older individuals, and although basal cell carcinoma rarely metastasizes, squamous cell carcinoma produces regional metastasis in approximately 5% of cases. Skin changes that may indicate basal or squamous cell carcinomas most often occur on the face, head, neck, and hands. The National Cancer Institute recommends observation for any of the following conditions on the skin (EOHSI, 1991, p. 2) and examination of any lesions that last longer than 2 weeks by a primary health care provider:

1. A small, smooth, pale, shiny or waxy lump
2. A firm red lump
3. A lump that bleeds or produces a crust
4. A flat, red spot that is rough, dry, or scaly

Malignant melanoma is the most serious and potentially deadly form of skin cancer, developing in about 32,000 individuals and causing approximately 6,800 deaths in the United States annually (Shenefelt, 1994). Melanoma most often occurs in white adults 25 to 29 years of age and develops from pigment-forming cells in the skin, most commonly from preexisting or newly developed nevi. Although melanoma can develop virtually anywhere on the body, intermittently sun-exposed areas, such as the back or calf, are the most common sites in whites. In African-Americans, the palms, soles, and under the nails are the most common sites (American Cancer Society, 1985).

The American Cancer Society (1985) recommends a simple "ABCD" rule to observe for signs of melanoma in preexisting or new moles:

A. ASYMMETRY: One half does not match the other half.

B. BORDER IRREGULARITY: The edges are ragged, notched, or blurred.

C. COLOR: The pigmentation is not uniform. Shades of tan, brown, and black are

TABLE 5–17 **Installation and Operating Costs for Reduction of Radon in Homes**

Technique	Typical Radon Reduction	Typical Range of Installation Costs (Contractor)	Typical Operating Cost Range for Fan Electricity and Heated/Cooled Air Loss (Annual)*	Comments
Subslab suction (subslab depressurization)	80–99%	$800–2,500	$75–175	Works best if air can move easily in material under slab
Passive subslab suction	30–70%	$550–2,250	There may be some energy penalties	May be more effective in cold climates; not as effective as active subslab suction
Draintile suction	90–99%	$800–1,700	$75–175	Works best if draintiles form complete loop around house
Blockwall suction	50–99%	$1,500–3,000	$150–300	Only in houses with hollow blockwalls; requires sealing of major openings
Sump hole suction	90–99%	$800–2,500	$100–225	Works best if air moves easily to sump under slab or if draintiles form complete loop
Submembrane depressurization in a crawl space	80–99%	$1,000–2,500	$70–175	Less heat loss than natural ventilation in cold winter climates
Natural ventilation in a crawl space	0–50%	None $200–500 if additional vents installed	There may be some energy penalties	Costs variable
Sealing of radon entry routes	0–50%	$100–2,000	None	Normally used with other techniques; proper materials and installation required
House (basement) pressurization	50–99%	$500–1,500	$150–500	Works best with tight basement isolated from outdoors and upper floors
Natural ventilation	Variable	None $200–500 if additional vents installed	$100–700	Significant heated/cooled air loss; operating costs depend on utility rates and amount of ventilation
Heat recovery ventilation	25–50% if used for full house; 25–75% if used for basement	$1,200–2,500	$75–500 for continuous operation	Limited use: best in tight house; for full house, use with levels no higher than 8 pCi/L; no higher than 16 pCi/L for use in basement; less conditioned air loss than natural ventilation
Water systems Aeration	95–99%	$3,000–4,500	$40–90	More efficient than granular activated carbon (GAC); requires annual cleaning to maintain effectiveness and to prevent contamination; carefully vent system
Granular activated carbon	85–99%	$1,000–2,000	None	Less efficient for higher levels than aeration; use for moderate levels (around 5,000 pCi/L or less); radon byproducts can build on carbon—may need radiation shield around tank and care in disposal

*__NOTE:__ The fan electricity and house heating/cooling loss cost range is based on certain assumptions regarding climate, your house size, and the cost of electricity and fuel. Your costs may vary. Numbers based upon 1991 data.

From Environmental Protection Agency. (1992). *Consumer's Guide to Radon Reduction: How to Reduce Radon Levels in Your Home.* EPA publication #402-K92-003. Washington, D. C., Government Printing Office.

present. Red, white, and blue may add to the mottled appearance.

D. DIAMETER GREATER THAN 6 MM (about the size of a pencil eraser): Any sudden or continuing increase in size should be of special concern.

With early detection and prompt treatment, most skin cancers, including melanoma, can be treated. Treatment options include excisional surgery, cryosurgery, electrodesiccation, and curettage (Clark, 1994). Recommendations for early detection include skin examination by a primary care provider every 1 to 3 years (depending on the client's age) and teaching and encouraging clients to perform monthly skin self-examination. Guidelines endorsed by the American Cancer Society (1985) for skin self-examination are

1. Using a full-length mirror check any moles, blemishes, or birthmarks from head to toes for anything new—changes in size, shape, or color or a sore that does not heal.
2. Examining the body (front and back) in the mirror, then the right and left sides, with the arms raised. A hand mirror should be used to check the back and buttocks.
3. Bending the elbows and looking carefully at the forearms and upper underarms and palms.
4. Looking at the backs of the legs and feet, including the spaces between the toes and the soles.
5. Examining the back of the neck and the scalp with the help of a hand mirror, parting the hair or using a blow dryer to lift the hair and give a closer look.

Skin Cancer Prevention

Prevention of skin cancer involves limiting exposure to the sun, particularly when ultraviolet radiation is most intense. General guidelines for prevention of skin cancer are listed in Table 5–18.

Environmental Health and Nursing Practice

Nurses, particularly those who work in community settings, must be knowledgeable about actual and potential threats to health from the environment and should adapt their assessment and diagnostic skills to include community environmental health issues. Neufer (1994) states that "in the nursing field, environmental health has traditionally been

TABLE 5–18 **Guidelines for Prevention of Skin Cancer**

- Limit the time spent in the sun. Ultraviolet radiation is most intense between 10:00 am and 3:00 pm and in the months of June to September. Limit outdoor activities during these times when possible.
- Use protective clothing. Long sleeves, long pants, and brimmed hats can protect against ultraviolet radiation.
- Use sunscreen. Sunscreen should be applied at least 30 minutes prior to exposure and should be reapplied every 2–3 hours. Waterproof products with an SPF (sun protection factor) rating of 15 or higher provide the best protection.
- Protect children from overexposure. Studies indicate that about 50% of a person's total lifetime exposure to ultraviolet radiation occurs by age 18.
- Protect skin on hazy days as well as on sunny days. Clouds normally do not screen out ultraviolet rays.
- Be aware that certain foods, medications, and chemicals can worsen the effects of ultraviolet radiation on the skin. Medications, such as some antihypertensive drugs, antibiotics, and antiinflammatory agents, may produce photosensitivity. Some cosmetics, shampoos, and deodorants may also enhance photosensitivity.
- Avoid indoor tanning. Ultraviolet-A radiation is emitted by sun lamps and can increase the risk of skin cancer, eye injury, and skin aging.

Adapted from Environmental and Occupational Health Sciences Institute. (1991). The sun and skin: An unhealthy combination. *INFOletter: Environmental and Occupational Health Briefs, 5* (3), 3–5.

TABLE 5–19 **Prevention Interventions for Environmental Safety and Health**

Primary Prevention

- Advocate safer environmental design of products, automobiles, equipment, and buildings
- Teach home safety related to falls and fire prevention, especially to families with children and elderly members
- Counsel women of childbearing age regarding exposure to environmental hazards
- Advocate vehicle protection systems, such as seat belts
- Advocate use of protective devices, such as earplugs for noise
- Immunize occupationally exposed workers for hepatitis B
- Develop work site health and safety programs
- Develop programs to prevent back injuries at work
- Support the development of exposure standards for toxins
- Support disclosure of radon and lead concentrations in homes at time of sale
- Advocate for safe air and water
- Teach avoidance of ultraviolet exposure and use of sunscreen
- Advocate for reduced waste reduction and effective waste management
- Support programs for waste reduction and recycling

Secondary Prevention

- Assess homes, schools, work sites, and communities for environmental hazards
- Routinely obtain occupational health histories for individuals, counsel about hazard reduction, and refer for diagnosis and treatment
- Screen children from 6 months to 5 years for blood lead levels
- Monitor workers for levels of chemical exposure
- Screen at-risk workers for lung disease, cancer, and hearing loss
- Participate in data collection regarding the incidence and prevalence of injury and disability in homes, schools, and work sites

Tertiary Prevention

- Encourage limitation of activity when air pollution is high
- Support cleanup of toxic waste sites and removal of other hazards
- Provide appropriate nursing care at work sites or in the home for persons with chronic lung diseases and injury-related disabilities
- Refer homeowners to approved lead abatement resources

From Smith, C. Cited in Primomo, J. and Salazar, M. K. (1995). Environmental issues: At home, work, and in the community. In C. M. Smith and F. A. Maurer (Eds.). *Community Health Nursing: Theory and Practice.* Philadelphia, W. B. Saunders.

limited to the immediate environment of the individual (e.g., hospitalized patient) or to the family home (e.g., home safety). . . . Addressing environmental health today requires a systematic assessment of air, soil, surface water, and groundwater quality and the related public health implications of toxic chemicals in the environment. . ." (p. 156).

In taking a proactive role in health teaching, counseling, and advocacy regarding actual and potential environmental threats, nurses are indeed able to promote health and prevent illness and disability. To further assist in this, Table 5–19 lists primary, secondary, and tertiary prevention interventions appropriate for all nurses in community-based practice. Finally, Table 5–20 contains a number of resources relevant to each of the issues discussed in this chapter.

TABLE 5–20 Environmental Health Resources

Centers for Disease Control and Prevention
National Center for Environmental Health (NCEH)
Mailstop F28
4770 Buford Highway, NE
Atlanta, GA 30341-3724
(404) 488-7300

CDC/NCEH
Radiation Studies Branch
(404) 488-7040

CDC/NCEH
Lead Poisoning Prevention Branch
(404) 488-7330

CDC—Office on Smoking and Health
(404) 488-5705

CDC—National Center for Injury Prevention and Control
(404) 488-4362

National Institutes of Health/National Institute of Environmental Health Sciences (NIEHS)
P. O. Box 12233
Research Triangle Park, NC 27709
(800) 643-4794
(919) 541-3484

ENVIRO-HEALTH (NIEHS Information Clearinghouse)
(800) 643-4794

Environmental Protection Agency
Public Information Center
401 M Street, SW
Room 3404
Washington, D. C. 20460
(202) 260-2080

EPA—Hazardous Waste Control Program
(800) 424-9346

EPA—Safe Drinking Water Hotline
(800) 426-4791

EPA—Water Resource Center
(202) 260-7786

EPA—Superfund Hotline
(800) 424-9346

EPA—Asbestos Hotline
(202) 554-1404

EPA—Indoor Air Quality Information Clearinghouse
(800) 438-4318

U. S. Department of Agriculture
Food Safety and Inspection Service
14th and Independence Avenue, SW
Room 2925 South
Washington, D. C. 20205
(800) 535-4555

Meat/Poultry Hotline (202) 720-3333

Food and Drug Administration
Office of Consumer Affairs
5600 Fishers Lane
Rockville, MD 20857
(301) 443-3170

FDA—Center for Food Safety and Applied Nutrition
200 C Street, SW
Washington, D. C. 20204
(202) 205-5004

U. S. Department of Health and Human Services
National Institute for Occupational Safety and Health
Office of the Director
Humphrey Building Room 715-H
Washington, D. C. 20201
(202) 401-6997

Office of Information
4676 Columbia Parkway
Cincinnati, OH 45226-1998
(800) 35-NIOSH

National Safety Council
1121 Spring Lake Drive
Itasca, IL 60143-3201
(800) 621-7615

U. S. Department of Labor
Occupational Safety and Health Administration
Publications, Room N-3647
200 Constitution Avenue, NW
Washington, D. C. 20210
(202) 219-8151

Bureau of Labor Statistics
Office of Safety, Health, and Working Conditions
2 Massachusetts Avenue, NE
Room 3180
Washington, D. C. 20212
(202) 606-6180

Key Points

- Environmental factors have a great impact on human development, health, and disease. Public health efforts have been very successful in reducing threats to health through improving the safety of food and water, management of waste disposal and sewage, and control or elimination of vectorborne illnesses. Contemporary environmental health threats come from toxic and ecological effects associated with the use of fossil fuels and synthetic chemicals, as well as other sources.
- Threats related to housing and living patterns include overcrowding, household chemical exposure, and violence. Indoor air quality may be affected by combustion pollutants (e.g., secondhand smoke, exhausts from space heaters), particles (e.g., asbestos, pollen), and living organisms. Lead may be present in peeling paint and in some water pipes. EMFs are present in transmission power lines and some household appliances and may be harmful to some people.
- Millions of illnesses and injuries each year are related to workplace risks and hazards. Use of heavy equipment, exposure to chemicals and biohazards, sunlight, cold, and noise, as well as potential for assault or violence, can threaten workers. OSHA has been given the responsibility for protection of workers and has set and enforces standards to improve worker safety and health.
- Atmospheric quality is threatened by air pollutants that can cause lung damage, inflammatory responses, and respiratory symptoms. Major air pollutants include ozone, carbon monoxide, nitrogen dioxide, particulates, sulfur dioxide, and lead. The burning of fossil fuels (i.e., gasoline, coal, oil) contributes greatly to air pollution.
- Ensurance of a safe, clean water supply is necessary to health. Sewage, industrial processes and wastes, and agricultural chemicals are the main sources of water pollution. Waterborne diseases can be caused by bacteria, viruses, and protozoa. Common chemical contaminants include pesticides, petrochemicals, lead, and other compounds.
- Food quality may be threatened by both intentional and unintentional food additives (e.g., biological and chemical contaminants). Microbiological contamination is usually caused by improper storage, handling, and/or preparation of food. "Intentional" food additives include substances added to food during processing to enhance the nutritional content, improve flavor, enhance color, improve consistency, or increase the shelf life. "Unintentional" food additives are those substances that enter and remain in food as a result of their use as pesticides, after being added to animal food, or from packaging.
- The volume of solid wastes and problems concerning the disposal of toxic and hazardous wastes present threats to the health and well-being of United States residents. Effective solid waste management is essential to decrease pathogen transmission through insect and rodent control and to eliminate potential exposure to toxic and infectious materials.
- Radiation threats to health come from several sources—most commonly, radon gas and the sun. Radon is a colorless, odorless gas that causes thousands of deaths each year—most commonly from lung cancer. Radon enters buildings through cracks in

solid floors, construction joints, and other ways, and dangerously high levels can be found in many homes. Skin cancer is the most common form of cancer in the United States, and exposure to the sun is associated with all three major types of skin cancer.

Learning Activities and Application to Practice

In Class

- Discuss each of the "areas of environmental health" presented. Encourage students to give examples of health problems they have encountered related to each area. Discuss prevention efforts for each problem discussed. Give examples of each level of prevention (i.e., primary, secondary, tertiary), if possible.

In Clinical

- Have students observe for illnesses or health conditions or risks associated with environmental health threats encountered during their clinical experiences. For example, in a clinic, a student might care for a toddler who is being screened for lead, an adult with carpal tunnel syndrome associated with using a computer, or an elder with skin cancer. Record these in a clinical log or diary and share with other students in the clinical group. How could the risk(s) be prevented or minimized?
- Encourage students to be prepared to teach clients about environmental threats to health and safety. Have them identify times when health education is appropriate (e.g., teaching a new mother not to use hot tap water to make formula, the ABCDs of skin cancer and skin assessment to all adults, and ways to reduce food contamination to high school students).

REFERENCES

American Cancer Society (1995). *Cancer Facts & Figures—1995.* Atlanta, American Cancer Society.

American Cancer Society. (1985). *Why You Should Know About Melanoma.* Atlanta, American Cancer Society.

American Lung Association. (1992). *Facts About Air Pollution and Your Health.* New York, American Lung Association.

Anderson, L. (1994). A creeping suspicion about radon. *Environmental Health Perspectives, 102* (10), 826–830.

Blumenthal, D. (1990). Red No. 3 and other colorful controversies. *FDA Consumer, May,* 1–4.

Breslin, K. (1993). In our own backyards: The continuing threat of hazardous waste. *Environmental Health Perspectives, 101* (6), 484–489.

Centers for Disease Control. (1993). HIV/AIDS surveillance year end edition. *Morbidity and Mortality Weekly Report, 43* (RR-6). Atlanta, Centers for Disease Control.

Centers for Disease Control. (1991). *Preventing Lead Poisoning in Young Children.* Atlanta, Centers for Disease Control.

Centers for Disease Control and Prevention. (1995). Assessing the public health threat associated with waterborne cryptosporidiosis: Report of a workshop. *Morbidity and Mortality Weekly Report, 44* (RR-6), 1–20.

Centers for Disease Control and Prevention/National Center for Environmental Health. (1994). *Childhood Lead Poisoning Prevention Program.* Atlanta, U. S. Department of Health and Human Services, Centers for Disease Control and Prevention.

Chafee, J. H. (1991). Stratospheric ozone: The problem. *EPA Journal, Jan/Feb,* 34–35.

Clark, M. J. (1992). Environmental influences on community health. In M. J. Clark (Ed.), *Nursing in the Community.* Norwalk, CT, Appleton & Lange, pp. 341–362.

Clark, R. E. (1994). Cancer of the skin. In R. E. Rakel (Ed.). *Conn's Current Therapy: 1994.* Philadelphia, W. B. Saunders, pp. 742–744.

Clemen-Stone, S., Eigsti, D. G., and McGuire, S. L. (1995). *Comprehensive Community Health Nursing* (4th ed.). St. Louis, MO, Mosby–Year Book.

Environmental and Occupational Health Sciences Institute. (1989). Landfills. *INFOletter: Environmental and Occupational Health Briefs, 3* (1).

Environmental and Occupational Health Sciences Institute. (1991). The sun and skin: An unhealthy combination. *INFOletter: Environmental and Occupational Health Briefs, 5* (3), 1–5.

Environmental Protection Agency. (1989a). Asbestos. *Environmental Backgrounder, March,* United States, Environmental Protection Agency.

Environmental Protection Agency. (1989b). Medical Waste. *Environmental Backgrounder, March.* United States, Environmental Protection Agency.

Environmental Protection Agency. (1989c). Ozone. *Environmental Backgrounder, March,* United States, Environmental Protection Agency.

Environmental Protection Agency. (1991). *Ensuring Safe Drinking Water.* EPA publication: 600-M-91-001. Washington, D. C., Government Printing Office.

Environmental Protection Agency. (1992a). *What You Can Do to Reduce Air Pollution.* EPA publication: 450-K-92-002. Washington, D. C., Government Printing Office.

Environmental Protection Agency (1992b). *Consumer's Guide to Radon Reduction: How to Reduce Radon Levels in Your Home.* EPA publication: 402-K92-003. Washington, D. C., Government Printing Office.

Environmental Protection Agency. (1992c). *The Consumer's Handbook for Reducing Solid Waste.* EPA Publication: 530-K-92-003. Washington, D. C., Government Printing Office.

Environmental Protection Agency. (1993a). *Preventing Waterborne Disease.* EPA publication: 640-K-93-001. Washington, D. C., Government Printing Office.

Environmental Protection Agency (1993b). *Lead in Your Drinking Water: Actions You Can Take to Reduce Lead in Drinking Water.* EPA publication: 810-F-93-001. Washington, D. C., Government Printing Office.

Environmental Protection Agency. (1993c). *Secondhand Smoke.* EPA Publication: 402-F-93-004. Washington, D. C., Government Printing Office.

Environmental Protection Agency. (1994a). *Measuring Air Quality: The Pollutant Standards Index.* EPA publication: 451/K-94-001. Washington, D. C., Government Printing Office.

Environmental Protection Agency. (1994b). *Protecting the Ozone Layer: A Checklist for Citizen Action.* EPA publication: 430-94-007. Washington, D. C., Government Printing Office.

Environmental Protection Agency/U. S. Department of Health and Human Services. (1994c). *A Citizen's Guide to Radon* (2nd ed.). EPA publication: 402-K92-001. Washington, D. C., Government Printing Office.

Environmental Protection Agency. (1994d). *The Superfund Emergency Response Program.* EPA publication: 450-F-94-041. Washington, D. C., Government Printing Office.

Environmental Protection Agency/Office of Radiation and Indoor Air. (1992). *EMF in Your Environment: Magnetic Field Measurements of Everyday Electrical Devices.* EPA Publication: 402-R-92-008. Washington, D. C., Government Printing Office.

Farley, D. (1993). Dietary supplements: Making sure hype doesn't overwhelm science. *FDA Consumer, November.* Rockville, MD, Food and Drug Administration.

Folinsbee, L. J. (1992). Human health effect of air pollution. *Environmental Health Perspectives, 100,* 45–56.

Food and Drug Administration. (1992). *Foodborne Pathogenic Microorganisms and Natural Toxins.* Washington, D. C., Government Printing Office.

Food and Drug Administration. (1989). *Pesticides.* Washington, D. C., Government Printing Office.

Foulke, J. E. (1993). FDA reports on pesticides in foods. *FDA Consumer, June,* 29–32.

Foulke, J. E. (1994). Mercury in fish: Cause for concern? *FDA Consumer, September.* FDA 95-2285. Washington, D. C., Government Printing Office.

Goyer, R. A. (1993). Lead toxicity: Current concerns. *Environmental Health Perspectives, 100,* 177–187.

Health and Environment Network. (1988). Chlorofluorocarbons: A valuable chemical threatens the atmosphere. *Health & Environment Digest, 2* (4), 1–7.

International Council of Nurses. (1986). *The nurse's role in safeguarding the human environment: Position statement.* Geneva, Switzerland, International Council of Nurses.

Lancaster, J. (1992). Environmental health and safety. In M. Stanhope and J. Lancaster (Eds.), *Community Health Nursing: Process and Practice for Promoting Health.* St. Louis, MO, Mosby–Year Book, pp. 293–311.

Landrigan, P. J. (1988). Lead: Assessing its health hazards. *Health & Environment Digest, 2* (6), 1–4.

McKeown, T. (1995). Determinants of health. In P. R. Lee and C. L. Estes (Eds.). *The Nation's Health* (4th ed.). Boston, Jones and Bartlett Publishers, pp. 9–17.

National Institute of Environmental Health Sciences. (1994). *Electromagnetic Fields and the Potential Hazard to Man.* Washington, D. C., Government Printing Office.

National Institute of Environmental Health Sciences/Department of Energy. (1995). *Questions and Answers About EMF.* DOE Publication: EE-0040. Washington, D. C., Government Printing Office.

National Institute for Occupational Safety and Health (1989). *National Prevention Strategies for the Ten Leading Work-Related Diseases and Injuries.* Atlanta, Centers for Disease Control.

Neufer, L. (1994). The role of the community health nurse in environmental health. *Public Health Nursing, 11* (3), 1155–1162.

Novello, A. C., Shosky, J., and Froehlke, R. (1992). From the Surgeon General, U. S. Public Health Service. *JAMA, 267,* 3007.

Ossler, C. C., Stanhope, M., and Lancaster, J. (1996). Community nurse in occupational health. In M. Stanhope and J. Lancaster (Eds.). *Community Health Nursing: Promoting*

Health of Aggregates, Families and Individuals (4th ed.). St. Louis, Mosby, pp. 731–746.

Primomo, J. and Salazar, M. K. (1995). Environmental issues: At home, work, and in the community. In C. M. Smith and F. A. Maurer (Eds.). *Community Health Nursing: Theory and Practice.* Philadelphia, W. B. Saunders, pp. 640–667.

Rogers, B. (1994). *Occupational Health Nursing: Concepts and Practice*. Philadelphia, W. B. Saunders.

Segal, M. (1993). Ingredient labeling: What's in a food? *FDA Consumer, April,* 14–18.

Shenefelt, P. D. (1994). Malignant melanoma. In R. E. Rakel (Ed.). *Conn's Current Therapy: 1994.* Philadelphia, W. B. Saunders, pp. 773–778.

Spradley, B. W. and Allender, J. A. (1996). *Community Health Nursing: Concepts and Practice* (4th ed.). Philadelphia, Lippincott-Raven.

Stevens, P. E. and Hall, J. M. (1993). Environmental health. In J. M. Swanson and M. Albrecht (Eds.), *Community Health Nursing: Promoting the Health of Aggregates.* Philadelphia, W. B. Saunders, pp. 567–596.

Suddeth, M. A. (1993). Genetically engineered foods: Fears & facts. *FDA Consumer, May,* 1993.

Urbinato, D. (1994). Monitoring lead in drinking water. *EPA Journal, 20,* 1–2.

U. S. Consumer Product Safety Commission/Environmental Protection Agency. (1994). *A Citizen's Guide to Radon: The Guide to Protecting Yourself and Your Family* (2nd ed.). Publication no. 402-K92-001. Washington, D. C., Government Printing Office.

U. S. Consumer Product Safety Commission/Environmental Protection Agency and American Lung Association. (1993). *What You Should Know About Combustion Appliances and Indoor Air Pollution.* Untied States: U. S. Consumer Product Safety Commission/Environmental Protection Agency and American Lung Association.

U. S. Department of Health and Human Services. (1990). *Healthy People 2000: National Health Promotion and Disease Prevention Objectives.* Washington, D. C., Government Printing Office.

U. S. Department of Health and Human Services/Office of Disease Prevention and Health Promotion. (1994). *Clinician's Handbook of Preventive Services.* Washington, D. C., Government Printing Office.

U. S. Department of Labor. (1995). *Work Injuries and Illnesses By Selected Characteristic, 1993.* Washington, D. C., Bureau of Labor Statistics.

Wagner, B. (1992). FDA keeps antennae out for insect fragments. *FDA Consumer, November,* 19–23.

6

Cultural Influences on Health

Case Study

Trisha Thomas is a Registered Nurse working in a city-sponsored pediatric clinic in a large southwestern city. At the clinic, Trisha primarily sees low-income clients, most of whom are eligible for Medicaid or who have no personal health insurance. More than 75% of the clients seen in the clinic are from minority groups, and almost half are Hispanic. Other racial and ethnic groups seen include African-Americans, Southeast Asian immigrants (Vietnamese, Cambodian, and Laotian), and, increasingly, immigrants from Middle-Eastern and African countries (Iraqi Kurds and refugees from Somalia, Ethiopia, and Tanzania).

Because Trisha has practiced nursing at the clinic for almost 4 years, she has learned to speak Spanish fairly well. She is able to perform assessments, take health histories, and teach effectively in that language. In addition, the clinic has interpreters for several of the most common languages heard at the clinic.

Trisha's experience working with people from many different cultures has given her an awareness of their health practices, beliefs, diet, and religions. This, in turn, has enabled her to conduct more thorough assessments and provide more effective teaching and anticipatory guidance than most of her colleagues.

On Thursday, Trisha saw Carlos Sepulveda for his well-child visit. Carlos is 5 years old and will begin kindergarten this fall. Because Carlos' health care is financed through Medicaid, Trisha performed an early periodic screening, diagnosis, and treatment (EPSDT) examination (see Chapter 13), which includes a complete physical examination; developmental testing; height and weight measurements; and screenings for vision and hearing, lead, and anemia. Review of Carlos' immunization records showed that he was due for his second diphtheria-pertussis-tetanus and polio boosters, and his second measles/mumps/rubella vaccination.

Although Mrs. Sepulveda does not speak English, Trisha was able to gain information about Carlos' diet, sleeping habits, and activity. She learned that the family lives in a subsidized apartment in a "safe" area. The apartment has smoke detectors, and all medications and cleaning products are in cabinets with child-proof latches.

All of the findings from the physical assessment were "normal." However, Carlos was small for his age (< 20th percentile). Knowing that because of financial constraints, as well as cultural preferences, Carlos' diet might be deficient in protein, calcium, and some vitamins, Trisha directed her health teaching to his nutritional *needs. After questioning Mrs. Sepulveda about his daily diet, Trisha gave her information on how to increase these nutrients in the diet and referred her to the Women, Infants, and Children (WIC) program (see Chapter 13) located in their building. Before Mrs. Sepulveda and Carlos left to see the Women, Infants, and Children counselor, Trisha made an appointment for Carlos to return in 6 months for further evaluation.*

The United States is becoming increasingly ethnically diverse. According to U. S. Department of Health and Human Services (USDHHS) reports, members of ethnic minority groups in the United States are disproportionately impoverished and have poorer health outcomes and fewer options for seeking health care (USDHHS, 1990). One of the three broad goals of *Healthy People 2000* is to "Reduce health disparities among Americans," and a number of objectives are specifically directed toward members of various racial and ethnic groups. Table 6–1 provides examples of objectives of *Healthy People 2000* that address the improvement of the health of members of minority groups.

Although the Americas have been a "melting pot" since colonization began in the 1600s, the makeup of the population is changing. Figures 6–1 and 6–2 depict current and estimated year 2025 population breakdowns by racial and ethnic groups. As these graphs show, the percentage of whites is declining, and the greatest growth is being seen in Hispanics and other immigrants, largely from Southeast Asia.

Many of the objectives from *Healthy People 2000* addressing the disparity between people from various ethnic groups cite health problems that lead to differences in morbidity and mortality. For example, alcoholism is more common in Native Americans, resulting in increases in liver disease and accidental injuries. Diabetes is much more prevalent in Native Americans, Hispanics, and African-Americans, contributing to related complications and deaths in those groups. To further illustrate some of the differences between health problems found in racial and ethnic groups, Table 6–2 lists the 10 leading causes of death for whites, Hispanics, African-Americans, Native Americans, and Asians.

Transcultural Nursing

Very often, nurses who practice in community settings are in a position to provide nursing care to clients from diverse racial and ethnic groups. To foster understanding and assist those individuals with nursing and health care needs, the Transcultural Nursing Society was established in 1973 by Madeline Leininger (Andrews, 1992; Leininger, 1991b).

According to Herberg, "Transcultural nursing is concerned with the provision of nursing care in a manner that is sensitive to the needs of individuals, families and groups" where "a thorough assessment of the cultural aspect of a client's lifestyle, health beliefs and health practices will enhance the nurse's decision making and judgment when providing care" (1995, p. 3). Culturally sensitive nursing interventions show appreciation of and respect for differences and attempt to decrease the possibility of stress or conflict arising from cultural misunderstanding.

In 1992, the American Academy of Nursing published a commitment to quality and "culturally competent" nursing care. Their recommendations included

- Promotion of culturally competent care that is equitable and accessible
- Development and maintenance of a disciplinary knowledge base and expertise in culturally competent care
- Synthesis of existing theoretical and research knowledge regarding nursing care of different ethnic or minority, stigmatized, and disenfranchised populations
- Creation of an interdisciplinary knowledge base that reflects heterogeneous health care practices within various cultural groups

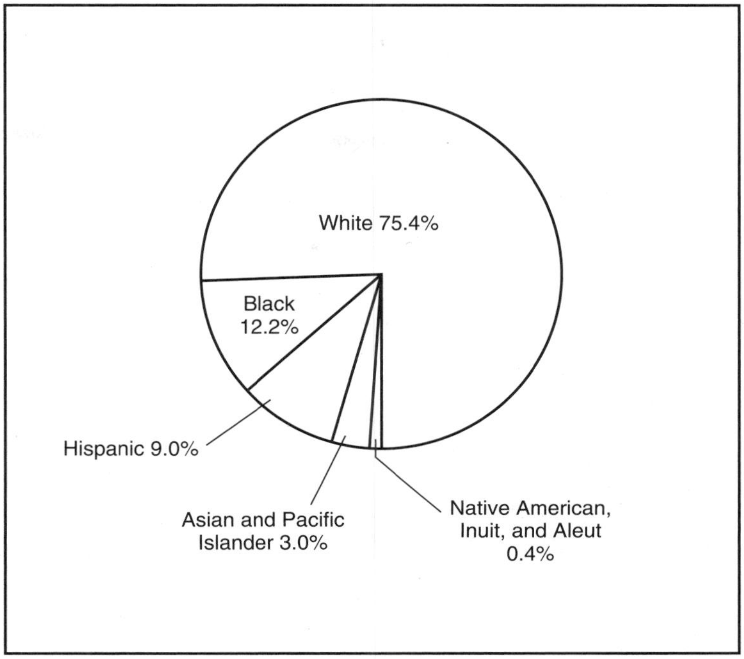

FIGURE 6–1 Population by race/Hispanic origin, 1990. (Data from the U. S. Bureau of the Census. [1993]. *Population Profiles of the U. S., 1993.* CPR, series p-23, No. 185. Washington, D. C., Government Printing Office.)

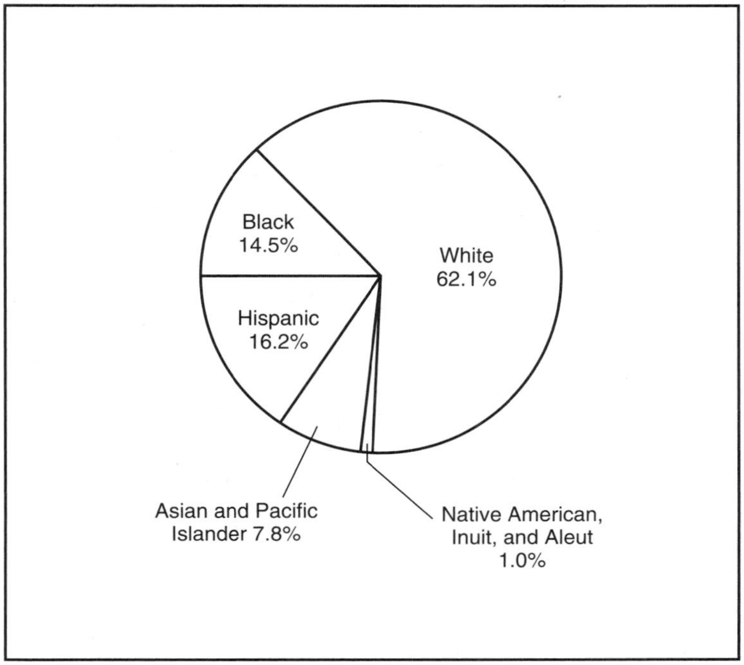

FIGURE 6–2 Population by race/Hispanic origin, 2025 (estimated). (Data from the U. S. Bureau of the Census. [1993]. *Population Profiles of the U. S., 1993.* CPR, series p-23, No. 185. Washington, D. C., Government Printing Office.)

TABLE 6–1 ***Healthy People 2000:* Objectives To Improve the Health of Minority Groups**

2.4—Reduce growth retardation among low-income children 5 years of age and younger to less than 10% (baseline: 11% among low-income children 5 years and younger in 1988)

	Special Population Targets	
Prevalence of Short Stature	***1988 Baseline (%)***	***2000 Target (%)***
2.4a—Low-income black children younger than 1 year	15	10
2.4b—Low-income Hispanic children younger than 1 year	13	10
2.4c—Low-income Hispanic children 1 year of age	16	10
2.4d—Low-income Asian/Pacific Islander children 1 year of age	14	10
2.4e—Low-income Asian/Pacific Islander children 2–4 years of age	16	10

2.10e—Reduce the prevalence of anemia to less than 20% among black low-income pregnant women (baseline: 41% of those 15–44 years of age in their third trimester in 1988)

3.4—Reduce cigarette smoking to a prevalence of no more than 15% among people 20 years and older (baseline: 29% in 1987; 32% for men and 27% for women)

	Special Population Targets	
Cigarette Smoking Prevalence	***1987 Baseline (%)***	***2000 Target (%)***
3.4d—Blacks 20 years or older	34	18
3.4e—Hispanics 20 years or older	33	18
3.4f—Native Americans/Alaska Natives	42–70 (estimates for different tribes)	20
3.4g—Southeast Asian men	55	20

5.1—Reduce pregnancies among girls 17 years and younger to no more than 50 per 1,000 adolescents (baseline: 71.1 pregnancies per 1,000 girls 15–17 years of age in 1985)

	Special Population Targets	
Pregnancies (per 1,000)	***1985 Baseline***	***2000 Target***
5.1a—Black adolescent girls 15–19 years of age	186	120
51.b—Hispanic adolescent girls 15–19 years of age	158	105

- Identification and examination of methods, theories, and frameworks appropriate for utilization in the development of knowledge related to health care of minority, stigmatized, and disenfranchised populations
- Establishment of ways to teach and guide faculty and nursing students to provide culture-specific care and to support the regulation of content reflecting diversity in nursing curricula

In accordance with these recommendations, nurses—particularly those working in community settings—should be knowledgeable of cultural differences and how they influence health and health practices and be prepared to work within these differences to improve health. Nursing care and interventions to address problems related to cultural, hereditary, social, and other factors that contribute to differences in morbidity and mortality are described in this chapter.

TABLE 6–1 ***Healthy People 2000:* Objectives To Improve the Health of Minority Groups** *Continued*

7.1—Reduce homicides to no more than 7.2 per 100,000 people (age-adjusted baseline: 8.5 per 100,000 in 1987)

	Special Population Targets	
Homicide Rate (per 100,000)	***1987 Baseline***	***2000 Target***
7.1c—Black men 15–34 years of age	90.5	72.4
7.1d—Hispanic men 15–34 years of age	53.1	42.5
7.1e—Black women 15–34 years of age	20.0	16.0
7.1f—Native Americans/Alaska Natives on reservations	14.1	11.3

8.1—Increase years of healthy life to at least 65 (baseline: An estimated 64 years in 1990)

	Special Population Targets	
Years of Healthy Life	***1990 Baseline***	***2000 Target***
8.1a—Blacks	56.0	60.0
8.1d—Hispanics	64.8	65.0

9.1—Reduce deaths caused by unintentional injuries to no more than 29.3 per 100,000 people (age-adjusted baseline: 34.7 per 100,000 in 1987)

	Special Population Targets	
Deaths Caused by Unintentional Injuries (per 100,000)	***1987 Baseline***	***2000 Target***
9.1a—Native Americans/Alaska Natives	66.0	53.0
9.1b—Black males	64.9	51.9
9.1d—Hispanic males	53.3	43.0

17.11—Reduce diabetes to an incidence of no more than 2.5 per 1,000 people and a prevalence of no more than 25 per 1,000 people (baselines: 2.9 per 1,000 in 1987; 28 per 1,000 in 1987)

	Special Population Targets	
Prevalence of Diabetes (per 1,000)	***1982–1984 Baseline***	***2000 Target***
17.11a—Native Americans/Alaska Natives	69	62
17.11b—Puerto Ricans	55	49
17.11c—Mexican-Americans	54	49
17.11d—Cuban-Americans	36	32
17.11e—Blacks	36	32

From U.S. Department of Health and Human Services. (1990). *Healthy People 2000: National Health Promotion and Disease Prevention Objectives.* Washington, D.C., Government Printing Office.

Culture and Related Concepts

The terms *race, ethnic group,* and *culture* are frequently confused and may be erroneously used interchangeably, as they refer to different, although sometimes overlapping, concepts. Lack of recognition of the differences and subsequent misuse of the terms may incur confusion or misunderstanding.

RACE

Race refers to classification or grouping of humans primarily based on *physical* characteristics

TABLE 6–2 **Ten Leading Causes of Death for Various Ethnic/Racial Groups**

White Non-Hispanics	African-Americans	Hispanics	Native Americans	Asians/Pacific Islanders
Heart disease	Heart disease	Heart disease	Heart disease	Heart disease
Cancer	Cancer	Cancer	Cancer	Cancer
Stroke	Homicide	Injuries	Injuries	Stroke
COPD	Injuries	Stroke	Stroke	Injuries
Injuries	Stroke	Homicide	Liver disease	Pneumonia
Pneumonia/influenza	HIV/AIDS	Liver disease	Diabetes	COPD
Diabetes	Pneumonia/influenza	Pneumonia/influenza	Pneumonia/influenza	Suicide
Suicide	COPD	Diabetes	Suicide	Diabetes
Atherosclerosis	Diabetes	HIV/AIDS	Homicide	Perinatal conditions
Liver disease	Liver disease	Perinatal conditions	COPD	Liver disease

COPD = chronic obstructive pulmonary disease; HIV = human immunodeficiency virus.
From U.S. Department of Health and Human Services. (1990). *Healthy People 2000: National Health Promotion and Disease Prevention Objectives.* Washington, D.C., Government Printing Office.

(e.g., skin color, hair color and texture, eye shape and color, height). Anthropologically, individuals from a given race have a common, geographic origin of their ancestors. Early anthropologists recognized three races based largely on skin color—Caucasoid (white), Mongoloid (yellow), and Negroid (black). According to Garn (1985), research studies during the 20th century led anthropologists to conclude that nine major geographical races exist, roughly based on continental divisions. These races are (Garn, 1985, p. 53)

- African (Negroid)—collection of related races in sub-Saharan Africa. Members have curly, tightly coiled hair; thick lips; and large amounts of melanin in the skin, hair, and gums. American blacks are mostly of African origin.
- American Indian—earliest inhabitants of the Western Hemisphere, American Indians are related to Asians but have different blood groups. Skin color ranges from light to dark brown, and hair is black and straight.
- Asian (Mongoloid)—populations in continental Asia (except South Asia and the Middle East), including Japan, Taiwan, the Philippines, and parts of Indonesia. Members have straight black hair, inner eyefolds, and pads of fat over their cheekbones. Most have light brown skin and are shorter than Europeans.
- Australian (Australian Aborigine)—groups native to Australia. Members have large teeth, narrow skulls, and very dark skin coloring.
- European (Caucasoid)—groups throughout Europe, the Middle East, and northern Africa. Group members have lighter skin than other peoples. The "whites" of Australia, North and South America, and South Africa are members of the European race.
- Indian—populations in south Asia from the Himalayas to the Indian Ocean. Skin color ranges from light in the north to dark in the south. Blood groups differ somewhat from those of Europeans.
- Melanesian—peoples of New Guinea and Solomon Islands. They resemble Africans in skin color but have different blood group frequencies.
- Micronesian—occupants of islands in the Pacific (e.g., Carolines, Gilberts, Marianas, Marshalls). Members are small and dark skinned and have wavy or woolly hair. They resemble Polynesians somewhat in blood group frequencies.

- Polynesian—Far southern Pacific Islanders, including people from Hawaii, New Zealand, and Easter Island. Members are tall, may be heavy, and have light to moderate skin color.

Although descendants of a given geographical race are similar, variations exist in people from different subgeographical areas, and they may differ quite markedly from other members of the same race. For example, people from Northern Europe usually have very light skin, light hair, and blue eyes, whereas Southern Europeans often have olive skin, dark hair, and dark eyes. Likewise, Alaskan Inuits vary markedly from Southern Native American tribes in height and other characteristics, and members of central and eastern African tribes may vary greatly from the Bushmen of South Africa. Race is largely unchanging, although intermarrying between races and subsequent mixing of races does occur and results in the lessening of some of the distinctive characteristics of each race.

ETHNIC GROUP

An ethnic group is a group of people who share common, distinctive characteristics such as race, ancestry, nationality, language, religion, food preferences, literature, and music and a common history. According to Spector (1996), at least 106 ethnic groups are recognized in the United States, and more than 170 Native American tribes exist.

Although members of ethnic groups share similar cultural patterns, values, beliefs, customs, behavior, and traditions, intraethnic variations usually exist. For example, in the United States, Hispanic-Americans represent a large ethnic group that varies markedly based on country or area of origin; this ethnic group contains Cuban-Americans, Puerto Ricans, Mexican-Americans, and people from Central America, among others. Likewise, African-Americans differ from Caribbean blacks or sub-Saharan Africans, and different tribal groups in Africa may vary greatly from each other.

CULTURE

In 1871, Sir Edward Tylor, an English anthropologist, defined culture as "the complex whole which includes knowledge, belief, art, morals, law, custom, and any other capabilities and habits acquired by man as a member of society" (cited by Andrews, 1993, p. 373 and Herberg, 1995, p. 10). Other definitions of culture include "the acquired knowledge that people use to interpret experience and to generate behavior" (Spradley, 1990, p. 131) and "nonphysical traits, such as values, beliefs, attitudes and customs that are shared by a group of people and passed from one generation to the next" (Spector, 1996, p. 358). Culture, therefore, provides the organizational structure or basis for behavior within the group. Culture is not necessarily tied to race, as members of a given culture may be from different races. Culture, however, is a component of ethnicity.

To illustrate the differences in these concepts, a second-generation Cuban-American who lives in Miami and whose ancestors were African slaves might be classified as follows:

- Race: African
- Ethnicity: Hispanic
- Cultural group: South Floridian/Cuban-American

Another example would be an immigrant from Korea residing in Houston

- Race: Oriental
- Ethnicity: South Korean
- Cultural group: Korean-American/Texan

A number of terms are often used in discussing race, ethnicity, and culture. To clarify some of the differences, Table 6–3 gives definitions of terms commonly used in reference to culture and cultural issues.

Characteristics of Culture

According to Spradley (1990), anthropologists and sociologists have identified a number of characteristics common to all cultures. Some characteristics that are particularly pertinent to the practice of nursing are listed in Table 6–4.

A subculture (see Table 6–3) is a relatively

TABLE 6–3 **Terms Used in Transcultural Nursing Care**

Culture shock—"feelings of bewilderment, confusion, disorganization, frustration, and stupidity, and the inability to adapt to differences in language and word meanings, activities, time, and customs that are part of the new culture" (Zentner and Samiezade'-Yazd, 1993, p. 34)
Cultural blindness—failure to acknowledge or respect cultural differences and behaving as though they do not exist
Dominant value orientation—the basic value orientation that is shared by the majority of its members as a result of early common experiences
Discrimination—the differential treatment of individuals because they belong to a minority group; denying equal opportunity by acting on a prejudice
Enculturation (acculturation)—the process of becoming a member of a cultural group; adapting to another culture
Ethnic group—designated or basic division of groups of individuals distinguished by customs, characteristics, or language; group of persons who possess common physical and mental traits as a result of heredity, cultural traditions, language, customs, and common history
Ethnicity—a classification of individuals based on a shared culture or affiliation, values, perceptions, feelings, and assumptions
Ethnocentrism—the belief that one's own group is superior to others
Minority group—a group of people who, because of their physical or cultural characteristics, are singled out from others in society; minority members may see themselves as recipients of collective discrimination (Andrews, 1993; Herberg, 1995)
Norms—the rules by which human behavior is governed that are the result of the cultural values held by the group
Prejudice—a hostile attitude toward individuals because they belong to a particular racial or ethnic group presumed to have objectionable qualities; negative beliefs or preferences that are generalized about a group that leads to "prejudgment"
Race—a group of individuals who share common biological features
Racism—excessive belief in the superiority of one's own racial group
Stereotyping—the belief or notion that all people from a given group are the same
Subculture—a fairly large aggregate of individuals who share characteristics that are not common to all members of the culture and allow them to be considered a distinguishable subgroup; a group of persons within a culture of the same age, socioeconomic level, ethnic origin, education, or occupation who have an identity of their own but are related to the total culture
Values—personal perceptions of what is good or useful; desirable beliefs and standards

large subsection of the cultural group that has distinctive characteristics that set it apart from the group as a whole. Teenage gangs, professional football players, "hippies," members of the military, and nursing students might be considered subcultures. Based on the characteristics described in Table 6–4, members of each of these groups must "learn" the cultural values, norms, practices, and other characteristics of the group. The soldier must learn terminology, skills, behaviors, and so forth to become a member of the group. In the same way, the beliefs, values, and practices of professional football players are "integrated" into other aspects of their actions, and cultural values beliefs and practices of teenage gang members are "shared." Nursing students (and other health care providers) do not need to explain thoughts, actions, and beliefs to other health care providers—rationale for actions is largely understood or "tacit." Finally, each of the examples listed must remain adaptive and dynamic to subsist and grow.

To illustrate differences in subcultural groups, a white middle-class family from rural Iowa is culturally different from a white middle-class family from Los Angeles. In these two families, variations in values, language, dress, diet, leisure activities,

TABLE 6–4 **Characteristics of Culture**

Culture is learned	Cultural behaviors are acquired—not inherited; enculturation is learned through socialization and language acquisition
Culture is integrated	The various components of a culture are simultaneously interrelated and independent; an integrated web of ideas, beliefs, and practices
Culture is shared	Cultural values, beliefs, and practices are shared by the members of the culture and identify and stabilize the cultural group
Culture is tacit	Much of culture is outside of awareness; members of a culture know how to act and what to expect without need for discussion
Culture is adaptive	Cultures adapt to environmental and technical factors and to the availability of natural resources
Culture is dynamic	Every culture experiences constant change

Data from Spradley, B. W. (1990). *Community Health Nursing: Concepts and Practice* (3rd ed.). Glenview, IL, Scott, Foresman/Little, Brown Higher Education; Herberg, P. (1995). Theoretical foundations of transcultural nursing. In M. M. Andrews and J. S. Boyle (Eds.), *Transcultural Concepts in Nursing Care* (2nd ed.). Philadelphia, J. B. Lippincott, pp. 3–48.

expectations, and so on would exist. Similarly, a working-class Puerto Rican family living in New York City varies markedly from a Mexican family living in the Rio Grande valley.

Cultural Assessment

Nurses who work in community-based settings must recognize the impact of culture on health and health practices, and they should be familiar with the beliefs, values, and practices of the members of cultural groups they may care for. To gain an understanding, pertinent information should be assessed by the nurse. Table 6–5 shows a cultural assessment instrument developed by Andrews and Boyle (1995). As outlined in this assessment guide, some of the components to be considered in cultural assessment are values, socioeconomic status, communication patterns and language, nutrition and dietary habits, religion and religious practices, health beliefs and practices, and biocultural aspects of disease incidence. These are briefly addressed.

CULTURAL VALUES

Values are personal perceptions of what is good or useful and are a universal feature of all cultures (Andrews and Boyle, 1995). Among other purposes, values give meaning to life; provide self-esteem; serve as goals or motivators that direct behaviors; and form the foundation for the individual person on personal, professional, social, political, and philosophical issues (Spector, 1993). Zentner and Samiezade'-Yazd (1993, p. 9) cited a poll of U. S. adults that found that the most prevalent American values are

1. Happy family life (97%)
2. Clean environment (95%)
3. Close friends (85%)
4. Successful career (80%)
5. Satisfying sex life (71%)
6. Good income (60%)

Interestingly, however, these values differed according to economic level. For example, good family life was more important to those with annual income under $25,000 (93%) than those making $40,000 or more (85%). Likewise good physical health was valued by 87% of those in the lower income level, compared with 76% in the upper level.

Much of U. S. culture is shaped by the dominant cultural group (white middle-class), whose values include individuality, material wealth, comfort, humanitarianism, physical beauty, democracy, newness, cleanliness, education, science and technology, achievement, free enterprise, punctuality, rationality, independence, respectability, ef-

Text continued on page 133

TABLE 6–5 Andrews/Boyle Transcultural Nursing Assessment Guide

Cultural Affiliations

With what cultural group(s) does the client report affiliation (e.g., American, Hispanic, Navajo, or combination)? To what degree does the client identify with the cultural group (e.g., "we" concept of solidarity or as a fringe member)?

Where was the client born?

Where has the client lived (country, city) and when (during what years)? *Note:* If a recent relocation to the United States, knowledge of prevalent diseases in country of origin may be helpful. Current residence? Occupation?

Values Orientation

What are the client's attitudes, values, and beliefs about developmental life events such as birth and death, health, illness, and health care providers?

Does culture affect the manner in which the client relates to body image change resulting from illness or surgery (e.g., importance of appearance, beauty, strength, and roles in cultural group)? Is there a cultural stigma associated with the client's illness (i.e., how is the illness or client condition viewed by the larger culture)?

How does the client view work, leisure, education?

How does the client perceive change?

How does the client perceive changes in lifestyle relating to current illness or surgery?

How does the client value privacy, courtesy, touch, and relationships with individuals of different ages, social class (or caste), and gender?

How does the client view biomedical/scientific health care (e.g., suspiciously, fearfully, acceptingly)? How does the client relate to persons outside of his or her cultural group (e.g., withdrawal, verbally or nonverbally expressive, negatively or positively)?

Cultural Sanctions and Restrictions

How does the client's cultural group regard expression of emotion and feelings, spirituality, and religious beliefs? How are dying, death, and grieving expressed in a culturally appropriate manner?

How is modesty expressed by men and women? Are there culturally defined expectations about male-female relationships, including the nurse-client relationship?

Does the client have any restrictions related to sexuality, exposure of body parts, certain types of surgery (e.g., amputation, vasectomy, hysterectomy)?

Are there any restrictions against discussion of dead relatives or fears related to the unknown?

Communication

What language does the client speak at home? What other languages does the client speak or read? In what language would the client prefer to communicate with you?

What is the fluency level of the client in English—both written and spoken use of the language? Remember that the stress of illness may cause clients to use a more familiar language and to temporarily forget some English.

Does the client need an interpreter? If so, is there a relative or friend whom the client would like to interpret? Is there anyone whom the client would prefer did not serve as an interpreter (e.g., member of the opposite sex, a person younger/older than the client, member of a rival tribe or nation)?

What are the rules (linguistics) and modes (style) of communication? How does the client prefer to be addressed?

Is it necessary to vary the technique of communication during the interview and examination to accommodate the client's cultural background (e.g., tempo of conversation, eye contact, sensitivity to topical taboos, norms of confidentiality, and style of explanation)?

How does the client's nonverbal communication compare with that of individuals from other cultural backgrounds? How does it affect the client's relationship with you and with other members of the health care team?

TABLE 6–5 **Andrews/Boyle Transcultural Nursing Assessment Guide** *Continued*

How does the client feel about health care providers who are not of the same cultural background (e.g., black, middle-class nurse and Hispanic of a different social class)?
Does the client prefer to receive care from a nurse of the same cultural background, gender, and/or age?
What are the overall cultural characteristics of the client's language and communication processes?

Health-Related Beliefs and Practices

To what cause(s) does the client attribute illness and disease (e.g., divine wrath, imbalance in hot/cold or yin/yang, punishment for moral transgressions, hex, soul loss, pathogenic organism)?
What are the client's cultural beliefs about ideal body size and shape? What is the client's self-image vis-á-vis the ideal?
What name does the client give to his or her health-related condition?
What does the client believe promotes health (e.g., eating certain foods; wearing amulets to bring good luck; sleep; rest; good nutrition; reducing stress; exercise; prayer, rituals to ancestors, saints, or intermediate deities)?
What is the client's religious affiliation (e.g., Judaism, Islam, Pentacostalism, West African voodooism, Seventh-Day Adventism, Catholicism, Mormonism)? How actively involved in the practice of this religion is the client?
Does the client rely on cultural healers (e.g., curandero, shaman, spiritualist, priest, minister, monk)? Who determines when the client is sick and when he or she is healthy? Who influences the choice/type of healer and treatment that should be sought?
In what types of cultural healing practices does the client engage (e.g., use of herbal remedies; potions; massage; wearing of talismans, copper bracelets, or charms to discourage evil spirits; healing rituals; incantations; prayers)?
How are biomedical/scientific health care providers perceived? How does the client and his or her family perceive nurses? What are the expectations of nurses and nursing care?
What comprises appropriate "sick role" behavior? Who determines what symptoms constitute disease/illness? Who decides when the client is no longer sick? Who cares for the client at home?
How does the client's cultural group view mental disorders? Are there differences in acceptable behaviors for physical versus psychological illnesses?

Nutrition

What nutritional factors are influenced by the client's cultural background? What is the meaning of food and eating to the client?
With whom does the client usually eat? What types of foods are eaten? What is the timing and sequencing of meals?
What does the client define as food? What does the client believe comprises a "healthy" versus an "unhealthy" diet?
Who shops for food? Where are groceries purchased (e.g., special markets or ethnic grocery stores)? Who prepares the client's meals?
How are foods prepared at home (type of food preparation, cooking oil[s] used, length of time foods are cooked [especially vegetables], amount and type of seasoning added to various foods during preparation)?
Has the client chosen a particular nutritional practice such as vegetarianism or abstinence from alcoholic or fermented beverages?
Do religious beliefs and practices influence the client's diet (e.g., amount, type, preparation, or delineation of acceptable food combinations [e.g., kosher diets])? Does the client abstain from certain foods at regular intervals, on specific dates determined by the religious calendar, or at other times?
If the client's religion mandates or encourages fasting, what does the term *fast* mean (e.g., refraining from certain types or quantities of foods, eating only during certain times of the day)? For what period of time is the client expected to fast?
During fasting, does the client refrain from liquids/beverages? Does the religion allow exemption from fasting during illness? If so, does the client believe that an exemption applies to him or her?

Table continued on following page

TABLE 6–5 **Andrews/Boyle Transcultural Nursing Assessment Guide** *Continued*

Socioeconomic Considerations

Who comprises the client's social network (e.g., family, friends, peers, and cultural healers)? How do they influence the client's health or illness status?

How do members of the client's social support network define caring (e.g., being continuously present, doing things for the client, providing material support, looking after the client's family)? What is the role of various family members during health and illness?

How does the client's family participate in the promotion of health (e.g., lifestyle changes in diet, activity level) and nursing care (e.g., bathing, feeding, touching, being present) of the client?

Does the cultural family structure influence the client's response to health or illness (e.g., beliefs, strengths, weaknesses, and social class)? Is there a key family member whose role is significant in health-related decisions (e.g., grandmother in many African-American families or eldest adult son in Asian families)?

Who is the principal wage earner in the client's family? What is the total annual income? (*Note:* This is a potentially sensitive question.) Is there more than one wage earner? Are there other sources of financial support (extended family, investments)?

What insurance coverage (e.g., health, dental, vision, pregnancy) does the client have?

What impact does economic status have on lifestyle, place of residence, living conditions, ability to obtain health care? How does the client's home environment (e.g., presence of indoor plumbing, handicap access) influence nursing care?

Organizations Providing Cultural Support

What influence do ethnic/cultural organizations have on the client's receiving health care (e.g., Organization of Migrant Workers; National Association for the Advancement of Colored People [NAACP]; Black Political Caucus; churches such as African-American, Muslim, Jewish, and others; schools, including those that are church-related; Urban League; community-based health care programs and clinics).

Educational Background

What is the client's highest education level obtained?

Does the client's educational background affect his or her knowledge level concerning the health care delivery system, how to obtain the needed care, teaching-learning, and any written material that he or she is given in the health care setting (e.g., insurance forms, educational literature, information about diagnostic procedures and laboratory tests, admissions forms)?

Can the client read and write English, or is another language preferred? If English is the client's second language, are materials available in the client's primary language?

What learning style is most comfortable/familiar? Does the client prefer to learn through written materials, oral explanation, or demonstration?

Religious Affiliation

How does the client's religious affiliation affect health and illness (e.g., life events such as death, chronic illness, body image alteration, cause and effect of illness)?

What is the role of religious beliefs and practices during health and illness? Are there special rites or blessings for those with serious or terminal illnesses?

Are there healing rituals or practices that the client believes can promote well-being or hasten recovery from illness? If so, who performs these?

What is the role of significant religious representatives during health and illness? Are there recognized religious healers (e.g., Islamic imams, Christian Scientist practitioners or nurses, Catholic priests, Mormon elders, Buddhist monks)?

TABLE 6–5 **Andrews/Boyle Transcultural Nursing Assessment Guide** *Continued*

Cultural Aspects of Disease Incidence

Are there any specific genetic or acquired conditions that are more prevalent for a specific cultural group (e.g., hypertension, sickle cell anemia, Tay-Sachs, G6PD, lactose intolerance)?
Are there socioenvironmental diseases more prevalent among a specific cultural group (e.g., lead poisoning, alcoholism, HIV/AIDS, drug abuse, ear infections, family violence)?
Are there any diseases against which the client has an increased resistance (e.g., skin cancer in darkly pigmented individuals, malaria for those with sickle cell anemia)?

Biocultural Variations

Does the client have distinctive physical features characteristic of a particular ethnic or cultural group (e.g., skin color, hair texture)? Does the client have any variations in anatomy characteristic of a particular ethnic or cultural group (e.g., body structure, height, weight, facial shape and structure [nose, eye shape, facial contour], upper and lower extremities)?
How do anatomical and racial variations affect the physical examination?

Developmental Considerations

Are there any distinct growth and development characteristics that vary with the client's cultural background (e.g., bone density, psychomotor patterns of development, fat folds)?
What factors are significant in assessing children of various ages from the newborn period through adolescence (e.g., expected growth on standard grid, culturally acceptable age for toilet training, introducing various types of foods, gender differences, discipline, socialization to adult roles)?
What is the cultural perception of aging (e.g., is youthfulness or the wisdom of old age more highly valued)?
How are elderly persons handled culturally (e.g., cared for in the home of adult children, placed in institutions for care)? What are culturally acceptable roles for the elderly?
Does the elderly person expect family members to provide care, including nurturance and other humanistic aspects of care?
Is the elderly person isolated from culturally relevant supportive persons or enmeshed in a caring network of relatives and friends?
Has a culturally appropriate network replaced family members in performing some caring functions for the elderly person?

From Andrews, M. M. and Boyle, J. S. (1995). *Transcultural Concepts in Nursing Care* (2nd ed.). Philadelphia, J. B. Lippincott, pp. 439–444.

fort and progress, family unity and stability, pursuit of recreational activities, equality of people, future orientation, economic security for the present and future, sporting events, and cultural arts (Andrews and Boyle, 1995; Zentner and Samiezade'-Yazd, 1993). Because these values are so entrenched in U. S. culture, often members of the dominant cultural group fail to recognize that these values are not universally shared or even understood by members of other cultural groups.

To help nurses recognize differences in cultural values, Table 6–6 describes themes and values present in folklore and literature from several groups. To further assist nurses in understanding difference in values between various cultural groups, Leininger and others have researched a number of different groups. Table 6–7 lists differences in cultural values identified by the research of Leininger (1991a) for several of the most prevalent U. S. cultural groups.

Socioeconomic Class Subculture

In addition to variations based on racial or ethnic groups, cultural variations based on socioeco-

TABLE 6–6 Culture Values in Folklore and Literature

Group	Core Metaphors and Themes
African	Interdependence, flexible kinship, courage in overcoming natural forces and adversity, reliance on spiritual forces
Anglo-American	Rugged individualism, self-reliance, self-determination
Arab	Muslim belief in the Koran, *In Sha'a Allah* (if Allah wills) tradition, admonitions that things take time in life
Chinese	Confucian belief in filial piety, hierarchical affiliation
English	Self-contained, class-determined individualism
German	Correctness, orderliness, discipline
Greek	Honor
Hindu	Purification, immersion, submission, fusion
Irish	Roman Catholic belief in morality, respectability
Japanese	Group harmony, interdependence, politeness, honor
Jewish	Courage in facing adversity and religious persecution, relationship with God, spiritual/religious themes, the Torah
Native American	Harmony with nature, coping with natural and human obstacles encountered in life's journey
Portuguese	Family, voyage of exploration and discovery
Puerto Rican	Respect and personalism
Russian	Hardships, open and closed society, political themes

From Andrews, M. M. and Boyle, J. S. (1995). *Transcultural Concepts in Nursing Care* (2nd ed.). Philadelphia, J. B. Lippincott.

nomic levels, or class, are detectable and influence health and health-seeking behaviors. Like other components of culture, socioeconomic class creates a set of values and role expectations regarding factors such as sex, marriage, parenting, birth, education, dress, housing, reading, occupation, and religion. In the United States, health status is more closely linked to income level than to race or ethnicity (USDHHS, 1990). Poor people are more likely to experience poor health and poor health care. Zentner and Samiezade'-Yazd (1993) describe socioeconomic subcultures as

- **Upper-upper level:** Affluent, or "old rich." A small number of people who have money and power. Values include home, position, lineage, power and prestige, economic achievements, education, possession of art, and philanthropy.
- **Lower-upper level:** "New rich." Possess large incomes and lifestyles that flaunt their money. Have and value an abundance of possessions.
- **Upper-middle level:** "Well off." College educated "professionals" (e.g., doctors, dentists, engineers, lawyers). Children and family stability are highly valued. Other values are education, hard work, career success, responsibility, honesty, security, materialism, various leisure activities, and travel.
- **Middle level:** Includes people who have small or medium-sized businesses, skilled workers, office workers, teachers, and nurses. Usually educated above the high school level. They live in middle-class neighborhoods, have two cars (often a van). Usually a nuclear family and are child oriented. Education, creativity, hard work, thrift, patience, planning ahead, and postponing immediate rewards are valued.
- **Lower-middle (working) level:** Includes high school graduates with industrial or "blue-collar" jobs, clerical workers, technicians, semiskilled workers, and waitresses. Minimal chances of advancement. Live in small homes or apartments and possess one or two cars. Values include patriotism, religion, authority, work ethic, honesty, neatness, respectability, self-reliance, independence, conformity, competition, achievement, education, and saving for the future. Adults are typically less educated and read less. Childrearing is

taken for granted, and parents often rely heavily on the extended family for support.

- **Upper-lower level:** Includes those who work at menial tasks (e.g., fast food workers, domestics, gardeners, maintenance, garbage collectors) but are grateful for employment. Often did not complete high school, were early parents with a rapid succession of children, and may have an early separation or divorce.
- **Poor:** History of being unemployed or underemployed. Currently, about 20% of children live in poverty (17% of white children; 40% of Hispanic children, and 50% of African-American children). Single-parent (usually mother-headed) families are very common. Low self-esteem, mistrust of others, anger, susceptibility to drug and alcohol abuse, teen pregnancy, and incarceration are not uncommon. Frequently, the poor have not finished high school and are unskilled and employed in temporary or seasonal jobs and/or rely on welfare.

Language and Communication

LANGUAGE

Language barriers are among the most frequently encountered problems in working with members of other cultural groups. Ideally, the nurse will speak the client's language, and in areas of high concentration of a minority group, many nurses are bilingual. For example, in South Florida, Southern California, and South Texas, there are a greater percentage of Hispanic and non-Hispanic nurses who are able to speak Spanish. In areas with many immigrants from China, Japan, and Southeast Asia (e.g., San Francisco), nurses who speak one or more Asian languages or dialects are often found. However, it is becoming increasingly common for the nurse and the patient to be unable to speak the same language. This challenge requires the use of an interpreter or attempting to communicate without the use of an interpreter. Tables 6–8 and 6–9 list tips for meeting this challenge.

COMMUNICATION PATTERNS

When caring for clients from culturally diverse backgrounds, the nurse should recognize and identify variations in communication patterns. Communication is transmitted by body cues (e.g., space, distance, position), paralinguistic cues (e.g., voice inflection, tone), as well as words (Andrews and Boyle, 1995). Recognition of variations in communication patterns and familiarity with differences is important to delivering culturally appropriate care.

Nonverbal communication includes pitch, tone, and quality of the voice; use of silence; use of eye contact; posture; facial expression; gestures; object cues (e.g., clothes, jewelry, hair style); touch; and use of territorial space (Andrews, 1993). Wide variations may exist in each of these, and nurses should recognize and appreciate these variations and adapt practice accordingly.

Diet and Nutrition

Diet is one of the most significant contributors to health and illness. It is widely known and accepted that excessive intake of certain nutrients (e.g., saturated fats and calories) or lack of nutrients (e.g., protein, vitamins, minerals) adversely affects health. Heart disease, stroke, certain types of cancer, poor outcomes of pregnancy, growth retardation, and other health problems have been linked to diet. Nurses need to be aware of the dietary practices of members of the cultural groups with which they work to recognize potential threats to health and to attempt to modify them. Reduction of sodium for hypertensive African-Americans; encouraging fruits and vegetables and reducing saturated fats in the diet of overweight, middle-class white cardiac patients, modifying the carbohydrate and fat content of diabetic Hispanics, and increasing protein in pregnant Asians, are examples of frequently encountered dietary challenges.

TABLE 6–7 **Cultural Values, Culture Care Meanings, and Action Modes for Selected Groups**

Cultural Group	Cultural Values
Anglo-American (U.S. middle and upper classes)	1. Individualism—focus on self-reliance 2. Independence and freedom 3. Competition and achievement 4. Materialism 5. Technology dependence 6. Instant time and actions 7. Youth and beauty 8. Equal sex rights 9. Leisure time highly valued 10. Scientific facts highly valued 11. Less respect for authority and the elderly 12. Generous in time of crisis
African-American culture	1. Extended family networks 2. Religion valued (many are Baptists) 3. Interdependence with other African-Americans 4. Focus on daily survival 5. Technology (e.g., radio, car) valued 6. Folk (soul) foods 7. Folk health modes may be employed 8. Music and physical activities
Mexican-American culture	1. Extended family valued 2. Interdependence with kin and social activities 3. Patriarchy 4. Exact time less valued 5. High respect for authority and the elderly 6. Religion valued (many are Catholic) 7. Native foods for well-being 8. Traditional folk care healers 9. Belief in hot/cold theory
Native American culture (cultural variations among all Nations exist)	1. Harmony between land, people, and environment 2. Reciprocity with "Mother Earth" 3. Spiritual inspiration (spirit guidance) 4. Folk healers (e.g., Shamans) 5. Practice of culture rituals and taboos 6. Rhythmicity of life with nature 7. Authority of tribal elders 8. Pride in cultural heritage and "Nation" 9. Respect and value for children
Vietnamese-American culture	1. Harmony and balance in universe 2. Extended kinship family ties (centrality of extended family) 3. Religious and spiritual values (Buddhism and Catholicism) 4. Respect for elderly and authority 5. Folk care practices 6. Food and environment

TABLE 6–7 **Cultural Values, Culture Care Meanings, and Action Modes for Selected Groups** *Continued*

Cultural Group	Cultural Values
Jewish-American culture	1. Maintenance of respect for religious beliefs and practices (Judaism) 2. Keeping of centrality of family with patriarchal rule and mother care 3. Support of education and intellectual achievements 4. Maintenance of continuity of Jewish heritage 5. Generosity and charity to arts, music, and community service 6. Success (financial and education) 7. Persistence and persuasiveness 8. Enjoyment of art, music, and religious rituals
Japanese-American culture	1. Duty and obligation to kin and work group 2. Honor and national pride 3. Patriarchal obligations and respect 4. Systematical group work goals 5. Ambitiousness with achievements 6. Honor and pride toward elders 7. Politeness and ritual 8. Group compliance 9. Maintenance of high educational standards 10. Futurists with worldwide plans

Adapted from Leininger, M. M. (1991). Selected culture care findings of diverse cultures using culture care theory and ethnomethods. In M. M. Leininger (Ed.), *Culture Care Diversity & Universality: A Theory of Nursing.* New York, National League for Nursing Press, pp. 345–372.

TABLE 6–8 **Overcoming Language Barriers: Use of an Interpreter**

- Before locating an interpreter, be sure that you know what language the patient speaks at home, because it may be different from the language spoken publicly (e.g., French is sometimes spoken by aristocratic or well-educated people from certain Asian or Middle Eastern cultures)
- Avoid interpreters from a rival tribe, state, region, or nation (e.g., a Palestinian who knows Hebrew may not be the best interpreter for a Jewish client)
- Be aware of sex differences between interpreter and client to avoid violation of cultural mores related to modesty
- Be aware of age differences between interpreter and client
- Be aware of socioeconomic differences between interpreter and client
- Ask interpreter to translate as closely to verbatim as possible
- An interpreter who is not a relative may seek compensation for services rendered

From Andrews, M. M. (1993). Cultural diversity and community health nursing. In J. M. Swanson and M. Albrecht (Eds.), *Community Health Nursing: Promoting the Health of Aggregates.* Philadelphia, W. B. Saunders, pp. 371–406.

TABLE 6–9 **Overcoming Language Barriers When No Interpreter Is Available**

- Be polite and formal
- Greet the client using the last or complete name; gesture to yourself and say your name; offer a handshake or nod; smile
- Proceed in an unhurried manner; pay attention to any effort by the client or family to communicate
- Speak in a low, moderate voice; avoid talking loudly; remember that people tend to raise the volume and pitch of the voice when the listener appears not to understand, and the listener may think that you are shouting or angry
- Use any words that you might know in the patient's language; this indicates that you are aware of and respect his or her culture
- Use simple words, such as "pain" instead of "discomfort"; avoid medical jargon, idioms, and slang; avoid using contractions such as "don't," "can't," and "won't"; use nouns repeatedly instead of pronouns (for example, say "Does Juan take medicine?" instead of "He has been taking his medicine, hasn't he?")
- Pantomime words and simple actions while you verbalize them
- Give instructions in the proper sequence (for example, say "first wash the bottle; second, rinse the bottle" instead of "Before you rinse the bottle, sterilize it"
- Discuss one topic at a time; avoid using conjunctions (for example, say "Are you cold [while pantomiming]?" "Are you in pain?" instead of "Are you cold and in pain?")
- Validate if the client understands by having the client repeat instructions, demonstrate the procedure, or act out the meaning
- Write out several short sentences in English and determine the client's ability to read them
- Try a third language; many Indo-Chinese speak French; Europeans often know three or four languages; try Latin words or phrases
- Ask who among the client's family and friends could serve as an interpreter
- Obtain phrase books from a library or bookstore, make or purchase flash cards, contact hospitals for a list of interpreters, and use both formal and informal networking to locate a suitable interpreter

From Andrews, M. M. (1993). Cultural diversity and community health nursing. In J. M. Swanson and M. Albrecht (Eds.), *Community Health Nursing: Promoting the Health of Aggregates.* Philadelphia, W. B. Saunders, pp. 371–406.

Table 6–10 addresses food preferences of several cultural groups and describes associated risk factors.

Religion

Having at least a basic understanding of the religious beliefs and practices of clients is extremely important in delivering holistic nursing care. Increasingly, spiritual care is being recognized to be as important as caring for the biological and psychosocial needs of clients. This is particularly evident when working with clients who are very ill or elderly or are at significant developmental stages (e.g., childbirth, puberty, death). Knowledge of religious prohibitions, practices, rules, and rituals can be extremely helpful. For example, awareness of baptism rites, circumcision practices, prayer requirements, and appropriate religious leader (e.g., priest, minister, rabbi) can assist the nurse in providing the most appropriate assistive care for the client, as well as his or her family.

Almost 60% of United States residents are Protestant Christians (e.g., Baptist, Methodist, Presbyterian, Lutheran, Episcopalian). Roman Catholics are the second most common religious group (25% of the general population) and comprise the majority in some areas (e.g., South Louisiana and areas with large concentrations of Hispanics) (Spector, 1996). Other fairly frequently encountered religions, varying greatly by geographic area, include Islam, Judaism, Buddhism, and Hinduism. Table 6–11 describes general information

TABLE 6–10 **Selected Food Preferences and Associated Risk Factors Among Selected Cultural Groups**

Cultural Group	Food Preferences	Nutritional Excess	Risk Factors
African-Americans	Fried foods, greens, bread, lard, pork, and rice	Cholesterol, fat, sodium, carbohydrates, and calories	Coronary heart disease and obesity
Asians	Soy sauce, rice, pickled dishes, and raw fish	Cholesterol, fat, sodium, carbohydrates, and calories	Coronary heart disease, liver disease, cancer of the stomach, and ulcers
Hispanics	Fried foods, beans and rice, chili, carbonated beverages	Cholesterol, fat, sodium, carbohydrates, and calories	Coronary heart disease and obesity
Native Americans	Blue corn meal, fruits, game, and fish	Carbohydrates and calories	Diabetes, malnutrition, tuberculosis, infant and maternal mortality

From Degazon, C. (1996). Cultural diversity and community health nursing practice. In M. Stanhope and J. Lancaster (Eds.), *Community Health Nursing: Promoting Health of Aggregates, Families and Individuals* (4th ed.). St. Louis, Mosby-Year Book. Data from Andrews, M. M. and Boyle, J. S. (1995). *Transcultural Concepts in Nursing Care* (2nd ed.). Philadelphia, J. B. Lippincott; Giger and Davidhizar. (1995). *Transcultural Nursing* (2nd ed.), St. Louis, Mosby-Year Book; Jackson and Broussard. (1987). Cultural challenges in nutrition education among American Indians. *Diabetes Educator, 13* (1), 47–50.

that may affect health and health care for the more commonly encountered religions.

Cultural Variations in Health and Illness

When working with clients from a variety of ethnic and racial groups, nurses working in community settings must also be familiar with biocultural variations in illness and physical assessment findings. Table 6–12 outlines variations in disease manifestations based on biocultural characteristics. All nurses should recognize these differences and plan care accordingly (e.g., provide anticipatory teaching on signs and symptoms of diabetes to clients in high-risk groups, such as Native Americans or Filipino-Americans).

To assist in learning a little about differences in health and illness among different cultural groups, some important characteristics of several groups are described briefly here.

AFRICAN-AMERICANS

In the United States, African-Americans comprise about 12% of the total population and are therefore the largest ethnic or racial minority group. The majority of black Americans are direct descendants of West African slaves brought to the United States during the 17th century (Spector, 1996). More recently, black immigrants have come to the United States from Caribbean countries (predominately Haiti, the Dominican Republic, and Jamaica). Although African-Americans live throughout the country, greater percentages live in certain states (predominately the southern states) and urban areas (e.g., Washington, D. C., Detroit, Chicago). About 25% of blacks live below the poverty level.

Common Health Problems

The life expectancy for blacks born in 1990 is 69.1 years (for whites, it is 76.1 years) (USDHHS/

Text continued on page 147

TABLE 6–11 **Selected Religious Beliefs and Practices and Nursing Implications**

Religion	Title of Religious Representative	Beliefs and Practices	Dietary Practices	Nursing and Health Care Issues	Issues Related to Death and Dying
Buddhism (Buddhist Churches of America)	Priest	Founded in sixth century B.C. in India by S. Gautama (Buddha). The goal of Buddhism is to attain "Nirvana," in which the mind has supreme tranquility, purity, and stability. *Buddha* means "enlightened one." Nirvana is attained through "right" views, intention, speech, action, livelihood, effort, mindfulness, and concentration.	No specified restrictions. Extremes of diet are discouraged.	Emphasis is on the person living now. *Reproduction issues:* Birth control is acceptable. Abortion may be acceptable under certain conditions.	*Prolonging life:* If there is hope for recovery and the continuation of the pursuit of enlightenment, all measures of support are encouraged; if the person cannot continue to seek enlightenment, conditions may permit euthanasia. *Organ donation:* If donation will help another seek enlightenment, it may be encouraged. *Body disposal:* Temple funeral with burial or cremation is common.
Catholicism	Priest	The Roman Catholic Church recognizes seven sacraments: Baptism, Reconciliation, Holy Communion (Eucharist), Confirmation, Matrimony, Holy Orders, and Anointing of the Sick (Extreme Unction).	Fasting and abstaining from meat and meat products may be condoned on certain Holy Days. Alcohol and tobacco may be used in moderation.	*Reproduction issues:* Only "natural" means of birth control (abstinence, "rhythm method") are acceptable. The church teaches the sanctity of life and that abortion is morally wrong.	*Prolonging life:* Ordinary means of preserving life are obligated, but extraordinary means are not. Direct euthanasia is not permitted. *Body disposal:* The body is usually buried following a church service. Cremation may be acceptable in certain circumstances.

Christian (Protestant) There are a number of different denominational groups, with variations in beliefs and practices based on denomination.	Minister Pastor Priest Reverend	Salvation is through faith in the work of Jesus Christ, who was born around 4 B.C. and was crucified about 33 years later.	Usually no dietary restrictions. Many denominations expect abstinence from alcohol and/or tobacco.	*Reproduction issues:* Birth control is usually permitted and decided on by the family. Abortion is prohibited by some denominations and based on individual decisions in others.	*Prolonging life:* Is based on individual decision. *Body disposal:* Burial following a funeral service is typical. Cremation is usually permitted and based on individual decision.
Christian Scientist (Church of Christ, Scientist)	There are no clergy. Practitioners are lay members of the church.	Founded by Mary Baker Eddy in the late 1800s. Christian Scientists believe that God heals through prayer, which results in drawing closer to God in thinking and living.	No dietary restrictions. Alcohol and tobacco are not used. Coffee and tea may also be declined.	Do not normally seek medical care or take medications. A surgeon may be employed to set a broken bone. They seek exemption from immunizations; will allow treatment for minor children if required by law. *Reproduction issues:* Birth control is left to individual judgment. An obstetrician or midwife may be used for delivery.	*Prolonging life:* A Christian Science family is unlikely to seek medical care to prolong life. Euthanasia is contrary to the teaching of Christian Science. *Body disposal:* Burial and burial service are decided on by the individual family.

Table continued on following page

TABLE 6–11 **Selected Religious Beliefs and Practices and Nursing Implications** *Continued*

Religion	Title of Religious Representative	Beliefs and Practices	Dietary Practices	Nursing and Health Care Issues	Issues Related to Death and Dying
Church of Jesus Christ of Latter-Day Saints (Mormonism)	Elder	Founded in the 1820s by Joseph Smith, whose writings included *The Pearl of Great Price* and *The Book of Mormon,* which were given to him by God through visions. There are two sects, the initial church based in Salt Lake City, Utah and the reorganized church, based in Independence, MO. Mormons believe salvation is based on faith in Christ, baptism by immersion, obedience to the teaching of the Mormon Church, good works, and keeping the commandments of God.	Abstinence from tobacco, alcohol, and beverages with caffeine (e.g., coffee, tea, colas) is required. Meat is permitted, but dietary intake of fruits, grains and herbs is encouraged. Fasting one day per month is required.	Cleanliness is very important. A sacred undergarment may be worn at all times and should only be removed in emergencies. *Reproduction issues:* Procreation is one of the major purposes of life, and prevention of conception is contrary to teachings. Abortion is opposed except when the life of the mother is in danger.	*Prolonging life:* When possible medicine and faith are used to reverse conditions that threaten life. If death is inevitable, efforts to promote peaceful and dignified death are encouraged. *Body disposal:* Burial is preferred. A church elder should be informed to assist in preparation of the body.

Hinduism	Priest	The oldest religion in the world, founded in sacred scripture called the *Vedas.* "Brahman" (God) is the source and center of the universe. Reincarnation is a central belief. Following death, one will be reborn into a future life based on the behavior in this life. The goal of life is liberation from the cycle of rebirth and redeath and entrance into "Nirvana." Life is determined by "Karma" (the record of individual behavior).	Most sects are vegetarian.	Illness may be viewed as misuse of the body or a consequence of sins committed in a previous life. Hindus do not oppose medical treatment but view its effect as transitory. *Reproduction issues:* Birth control is acceptable. There is no Hindu policy on abortion.	*Prolonging life:* There is no religious custom or restriction on prolonging life. Life is seen as a perpetual cycle, with death one more step toward "Nirvana." *Body disposal:* Cremation is the most common means of body disposal. Ashes are collected and disposed of in holy rivers.

Table continued on following page

TABLE 6–11 **Selected Religious Beliefs and Practices and Nursing Implications** *Continued*

Religion	Title of Religious Representative	Beliefs and Practices	Dietary Practices	Nursing and Health Care Issues	Issues Related to Death and Dying
Islam	Imam	Monotheistic religion founded between 610 and 631 A.D. by Mohammed. Followers are called "Moslems" or "Muslims." *Islam* means subjection to the will of Allah (God). Good deeds will be rewarded at the last judgment, and evil deeds will be punished in hell. There are five essential practices: acknowledgment of Allah as the one God and Mohammed as his messenger; praying five times daily (dawn, noon, afternoon, sunset, and night) facing Mecca, Saudi Arabia; giving alms to the needy; fasting from dawn until sunset throughout Ramadan (the ninth month of the Islamic calendar); and making one pilgrimage to Mecca if able.	No pork is allowed. "Halal" (permissible) meats must be blessed and slaughtered in a directed manner (Zabihah). Alcohol is prohibited. All adults except pregnant women, nursing mothers, the elderly, and the ill are required to fast during Ramadan.	*Reproduction issues:* Contraception is permitted, but many conservative Muslims do not use contraception because it is viewed as interference in God's will. Abortion is objectionable, although there is no official policy. The husband must sign consent forms regarding family planning. Women are very modest, and this should be respected during examination. Circumcision is practiced on male children at an early age. For adult converts, it is sometimes practiced, although not required.	*Prolonging life:* Any attempt to shorten a life or terminate it is prohibited. *Body disposal:* Donation of body parts or organs is not allowed. Burial of the dead is compulsory and follows a prescribed procedure consisting of ritual washing of the body, wrapping of the body in white cloth, special prayers for the dead, burial as soon as possible with the head facing Mecca. A fetus older than 130 days of gestation is treated as a human and buried in the same manner.

Jehovah's Witnesses	Religious titles are generally not used.	Founded by Charles Taze Russell during the 1870s and 1880s in Pittsburgh, Pennsylvania. He began writing for the Watchtower Bible and Tract Society. Belief that 144,000 servants will rule with Jesus. Every "Minister" of the Watch Tower Bible and Tract Society devotes approximately 10 hours or more each month to proselytizing.	No dietary restrictions. Alcohol and tobacco are discouraged.	Blood transfusions violate God's laws and are not allowed. Some will accept alternatives to blood transfusions (e.g., nonblood plasma expanders, autologous transfusions, and autotransfusion). *Reproduction issues:* Birth control is a personal decision, although sterilization is prohibited. Abortion is opposed.	*Prolonging life:* Right to die is a matter of individual choice, but euthanasia is prohibited. *Body disposal:* Burial or cremation is permitted.

Table continued on following page

TABLE 6–11 **Selected Religious Beliefs and Practices and Nursing Implications** *Continued*

Religion	Title of Religious Representative	Beliefs and Practices	Dietary Practices	Nursing and Health Care Issues	Issues Related to Death and Dying
Judaism	Rabbi	Judaism is a monotheistic religion that dates to the time of the prophet Abraham around 1900 B.C. The laws of God are contained in the Torah and explained in the Talmud and in oral tradition. There are several divisions (i.e., Orthodox, Conservative, Reform, and fundamentalist [Hasidic]). Each *Sabbath* (from sunset Friday to just after sunset Saturday) is a holy day, and there are a number of other holy days.	Dietary laws are very strict, but the degree to which they are observed depends on the sect. In general, pork, predatory fowl, and milk with meat dishes are not eaten. Only fish with fins and scales are permissible (shellfish are prohibited). All animals should be ritually slaughtered to be "kosher" (properly prepared). Wine is part of many religious observances. Alcohol is permitted in moderation. Fasting is required during Yom Kippur.	Medical care is expected according to Jewish law. Circumcision is performed on all Jewish male children on the eighth day following birth. This may be done by a ritual circumciser, by the child's father, or by a pediatrician. *Reproduction issues:* Birth control is permissible, but having children is encouraged. Therapeutic abortion is permitted if the health of the mother is jeopardized.	*Prolonging life:* Death with dignity is a right; euthanasia is strictly prohibited. Jewish beliefs include the need to not be alone when the soul leaves the body, so family or friends should be allowed to stay with dying patients. *Body disposal:* Following death, the body should not be left alone and should not be touched by medical personnel. The body will be ritually washed (usually done at a funeral home). Human remains (including a fetus at any stage of gestation) are to be buried as soon as possible. Cremation is not in keeping with Jewish law.

Data from Andrews, M. M. and Hanson, P. A. (1995). Religion, culture and nursing. In M. M. Andrews and J. S. Boyle (Eds.), *Transcultural Concepts in Nursing Care* (2nd ed.). Philadelphia, J. B. Lippincott; Carson, V. B. (1989). *Spiritual Dimensions of Nursing Practice.* Philadelphia, W. B. Saunders; Keegan, L. (1993). Spirituality. In J. M. Black and E. Matassarin-Jacobs (Eds.). *Luckmann and Sorensen's Medical-Surgical Nursing: A Psychophysiologic Approach* (4th ed.). Philadelphia, W. B. Saunders; and Martin, W. (1985). *The Kingdom of the Cults.* Minneapolis, MN, Betany House Publishers.

TABLE 6–12 **Biocultural Aspects of Disease**

Disease	Remarks
Alcoholism	Native Americans have double the rate of whites; lower tolerance to alcohol among Chinese- and Japanese-Americans
Anemia	High incidence among Vietnamese because of presence of infestations among immigrants and low-iron diets; low hemoglobin and malnutrition found among 18.2% of Native Americans, 32.7% of blacks, 14.6% of Hispanics, and 10.4% of white children under 5 years of age
Arthritis	Increased incidence among Native Americans Blackfoot: 1.4% Pima: 1.8% Chippewa: 6.8%
Asthma	Six times greater for Native American infants <1 year; same as general population for Native Americans ages 1–44 years
Bronchitis	Six times greater for Native American infants <1 year; same as general population for Native Americans ages 1–44 years
Cancer	Nasopharyngeal: High among Chinese-Americans and Native Americans Esophageal: Number two cause of death for black males 35–54 years of age *Incidence:* White males: 3.5/100,000 Black males: 13.3/100,000 Liver: Highest among all ethnic groups are Filipino Hawaiians Stomach: Black males twice as likely to have it as white males; low among Filipinos Cervical: 120% higher in black women than in white women Uterine: 53% lower in black women than white women Most prevalent cancers among Native Americans: biliary, nasopharyngeal, testicular, cervical, renal, and thyroid (female patients) cancer Lung cancer among Navajo uranium miners 85 times higher than among white miners Most prevalent cancers among Japanese-Americans: esophageal, stomach, liver, and biliary cancer Among Chinese-Americans, there is a higher incidence of nasopharyngeal and liver cancer than among the general population
Cholecystitis	*Incidence:* Whites 0.3% Puerto Ricans 2.1% Native Americans 2.2% Chinese 2.6%

National Center for Health Statistics [NCHS], 1994). There is also a marked difference in life expectancy between male and female whites and blacks. White women born in 1990 should expect to live 79.4 years; black women, 73.6 years; white men, 72.7 years; and black men, 64.5 years. Other significant differences are as follows: diabetes is one-third more common among blacks than whites; African-American babies are more than twice as likely as white babies to die in their first year; homicide is the most frequent cause of death for African-American men 15 to 34 years of age (seven times greater than for white men in the same age group); the rate of acquired immunodeficiency syndrome (AIDS) in African-American men is three times as high as that in white men; and almost 80% of AIDS cases in women and children are found in blacks (Spector, 1996).

TABLE 6–12 **Biocultural Aspects of Disease** *Continued*

Disease	Remarks
Colitis	High incidence among Japanese-Americans
Diabetes mellitus	Three times as prevalent among Filipino-Americans as whites; higher among Hispanics than blacks or whites Death rate is three to four times as high among Native Americans 25–34 years of age—especially those in the West, such as Utes, Pimas, and Papagos *Complications:* Amputations: Twice as high among Native Americans vs General U. S. population Renal failure: 20 times as high as general U. S. population, with tribal variation, e.g., Utes have 43 times higher incidence
Glucose-6-phosphate dehydrogenase (G6PD) deficiency	Present among 30% of black males
Hepatitis	12% of Vietnamese refugees are hepatitis-B surface antigen carriers
Influenza	Increased death rate among Native Americans 45 years and older
Ischemic heart disease	Responsible for 32% of heart-related causes of death among Native Americans
Lactose intolerance	Present among 66% of Hispanic women; increased incidence among blacks and Chinese
Myocardial infarction	Leading cause of heart disease in Native Americans, accounting for 43% of deaths from heart disease; low incidence among Japanese-Americans
Otitis media	7.9% incidence among school-aged Navajo children vs 0.5% in whites Up to a third of Inuit children younger than 2 years have chronic otitis media Increased incidence among bottle-fed Native American and Inuit infants
Pneumonia	Increased death rate among Native Americans 45 years and older
Psoriasis	Affects 2–5% of whites but <1% of blacks; high among Japanese-Americans
Renal disease	Lower incidence among Japanese-Americans
Sickle cell anemia	Increased incidence among blacks
Trachoma	Increased incidence among Native Americans and Inuit children (three to eight times greater than general population)
Tuberculosis	Increased incidence among Native Americans Apache: 2.0% Sioux: 3.2% Navajo: 4.6%
Ulcers	Decreased incidence among Japanese-Americans

Based on data reported in Henderson, G. and Primeaux, M. (1981). *Transcultural Health Care.* Menlo Park, CA, Addison-Wesley; Orque, M. S., Bloch, B., and Monrroy, L. S. (1983). *Ethnic Nursing Care: A Multicultural Approach.* St. Louis, C. V. Mosby; Overfield, T. (1985). *Biologic Variation in Health and Illness: Race, Age, and Sex Differences.* Menlo Park, CA, Addison-Wesley.

From Andrews, M. M. and Boyle, J. S. (1995). *Transcultural Concepts in Nursing Care* (2nd ed.). Philadelphia, J. B. Lippincott.

Although coronary artery disease mortality rates are similar in black and white men, women's rates of heart disease are higher in blacks. The most distinctive difference is in cerebrovascular disease, where stroke accounts for most of the excess mortality in blacks compared to whites. This may be in part due to the prevalence of hypertension in blacks, as high blood pressure develops in blacks at a younger age and tends to be more severe than in whites. Although the incidence of cancer is similar between the racial groups, the mortality rates for blacks is significantly higher (182 of 100,000 for blacks and 131.5 of 100,000 for whites), possibly indicating delayed diagnosis and treatment. Finally, sickle cell disease, a serious genetic blood disorder, most commonly occurs in black populations (Spector, 1996).

NATIVE AMERICANS, INCLUDING ALEUTS AND INUITS

Native Americans (including Aleuts and Inuits) comprise just less than 1% of the total U. S. population and are the smallest minority group. Although many Native Americans (approximately one third) live on reservations, most live in urban areas. Income and educational levels tend to be low. Health problems of Native Americans are often the result of poverty, as slightly more than half live below the poverty level.

Common Health Problems

Alcohol abuse and obesity are the two major risk factors affecting Native American populations. Alcohol abuse is a significant health problem that contributes to other health threats, including accidental death, homicide, and suicide, as well as liver disease. It has been observed that unintentional injuries are the leading cause of death for Native American men younger than 44 years, with 75% of the injuries being alcohol related. Likewise, cirrhosis deaths are about three times greater than in the U. S. population as a whole. Diabetes, which is associated with obesity, is extremely prevalent in some tribal groups, affecting as many as 40% of adults in some tribes (USDHHS, 1990).

ASIANS AND PACIFIC ISLANDERS

Asians and Pacific Islanders have immigrated to the United States from Korea, China, Japan, Vietnam, Cambodia, Laos, and other countries and comprise about 3% of the total population. In this group, about 13% live below the poverty level.

Because many Asians are recent immigrants, and their health care customs are based on Eastern rather than Western practices, it is helpful to be aware of some of the basics of Eastern health care. Many Asian health practices are based in Chinese tradition. Chinese philosophy of health and illness is holistic in nature and integrated with the external environment. The onset, evolution, and change of diseases are considered in conjunction with geographical, social, and other environmental factors.

Yin and Yang

The terms *yin* and *yang* refer to powers that regulate the universe, with *yang* representing the male, positive energy, producing light, warmth, and fullness and *yin* representing the female, negative energy and darkness, cold, and emptiness (Spector, 1996). Yin and yang regulate themselves to promote normal activities of life and health. Illness is the result of a disharmony of yin and yang.

Acupuncture is an ancient Chinese practice of using needles inserted at specific points of the body to cure disease and relieve pain. The practice and principles of acupuncture are very complex. The basic treatment goal of acupuncture is to restore the balance of yin and yang through insertion of the needles into meridians (the points on the skin corresponding to a "network" or channel of energy that runs longitudinally throughout the body) to treat the condition (Spector, 1996).

Herbology refers to the use of herbs to heal. The Chinese use many herbs and plants for medicinal and healing reasons. Herbal medicines are categorized according to their properties of yin or yang. *Ginseng root* is an example of an herb used to treat a number of health problems, including anemia, depression, indigestion, and impotence (Spector, 1996). Other herbal remedies include *Jen Shen Lu Jung Wan,* a general tonic used to improve health and improve digestion; *tiger balm,* a salve used for relief of minor aches and pains; and *white flower,* a liquid used to treat colds, influenza, headaches, and coughs (Spector, 1993).

Common Health Problems

Health problems of Asian-American vary greatly based on nation of origin, socioeconomic status, and length of time in the United States. In general, however, Asian-Americans have some distinct health problems. Liver cancer among Southeast Asians is more than 12 times higher than in whites. This is thought to be the result of endemic hepatitis B, which, in chronic carriers, predisposes to the development of hepatocellular carcinoma. Tuberculosis is still the leading cause of death in some Asian countries and is a serious threat, being much more commonly found in Asian-Americans than in white populations (USDHHS, 1990).

CAUCASIANS (AMERICANS OF EUROPEAN DESCENT)

White people make up about 80% of the U. S. population and are descendants of immigrants from Germany, Italy, England, Scotland, Ireland, France, Austria, Russia, and other countries. About 9% live below the poverty level.

Common Health Problems

The leading causes of deaths for whites are heart disease, cancer, stroke, and chronic obstructive pulmonary disease, which are for the most part diseases of aging. However, health habits and lifestyle choices contribute to morbidity and mortality. Diet and activity levels, in particular, as well as use of alcohol and tobacco products and unhealthy sex practices, contribute to disease and death in whites.

HISPANIC, OR LATINO, AMERICANS (ALL RACES)

Hispanic Americans originate from Cuba (5%), Central and South America (14%), Mexico (60+%), Puerto Rico (11%), and other Spanish-speaking countries of the Caribbean (7.5%) and make up about 9% of the total U. S. population. They represent the fastest-growing ethnic group. Although Hispanics live in all states, the greatest concentrations are found in southern "border" states (i.e., California, Arizona, New Mexico, Texas), Florida, and New York. As a rule, the Hispanic population is very young and has a high birth rate. About 24% of Hispanics live below the poverty level (USDHHS, 1990).

Balance of "Hot" and "Cold"

According to Stasiak (1991), Mexican-Americans consider health to be a state of well-being brought on by eating proper foods and maintaining a "hot/cold" balance in the foods eaten. Illness to many Hispanic groups is an imbalance in the body between "hot" and "cold" and "wet" and "dry." The belief is that a hot illness must be treated with a cold substance and vice versa. *Hot* or *cold* does not refer to temperature but to the substance itself, and foods, beverages, animals, and people can be considered hot or cold. Examples of hot conditions are fever, infections, diarrhea, liver problems, and constipation. Cold conditions include cancer, pneumonia, menstrual period, earache, and stomach cramps. Examples of hot foods are chocolate, coffee, corn meal, cheese, eggs, onions, hard liquor, beef, and chili peppers, and cold foods include vegetables, fruits, dairy products, fish, chicken, and honey. Hot medicines and herbs include penicillin, tobacco, garlic, cinnamon, vitamins, and aspirin, and cold medicines and herbs include sage, milk of magnesia, and bicarbonate of soda (Kuipers, 1995; Spector, 1993).

Traditional Illness Management and Healers

Although practices vary greatly depending on the ethnic group, traditional or folk healers and religious rituals are sometimes used by Hispanics to treat illness. The use of religious signs, symbols, rituals, and practices is common. The most popular forms of treatment combine Catholic rituals, such as offerings of money, penance, confession, lighting candles, and laying on of hands, with the medicinal use of teas and herbs (Spector, 1996). Examples of Hispanic folk healers are the *curandero*, the *jerbro,* and the *partera.*

A *curandero* is a holistic healer, who may be "called" by God or be born with a "gift" of healing and/or may serve an apprenticeship (Spector, 1996). A *curandero* develops a very personal relationship with the patient, and the goal of care is to restore harmony with the social, physical, and psychological parts of the person. A central focus of the treatment is relieving clients of their sins, which can cause an imbalance between God and people. Treatment is often provided in a room in the *curandero's* home that is decorated with religious paraphernalia and may include massage, diet, rest, practical advice, herbs, prayers, magic, and/or supernatural rituals (Kuipers, 1995).

A *jerbro* is a folk healer who specializes in using herbs and spices (Kuipers, 1995), and a *partera* is a Mexican-American midwife (Spector, 1993). Nurses should be aware of common folk treatments, such as herbal teas and roots, used by these traditional healers and question clients decorously and not judgmentally. It should be noted that many traditional health practices have been shown to be beneficial (Stasiak, 1991).

Common Health Problems

Hispanics experience the greatest disparity in health and health problems among American minority groups. Infant mortality rates, for example, vary substantially between cultural group (Puerto Ricans have almost twice the infant mortality rate of Cubans). Hispanics have a very high birth rate (22.3 births per 1,000 women, compared with 15.7 births per 1,000 women in the total U. S. population) (USDHHS, 1990). AIDS, unintentional injuries, and homicide affect Hispanics disproportionately. Diabetes is also very prevalent among Mexican-Americans. More Hispanic men and teenagers smoke than do either whites or blacks, and more Hispanic teens report heavy drinking. Obesity is a common problem, particularly among Mexican-American women.

Variations in Physical Assessment Findings Across Cultures

Distinctive variations in physical assessment findings are based on biocultural differences. Two of these variations are described briefly.

MUSCULOSKELETAL VARIATIONS

Variations in height and weight are largely caused by differences in bone length and mass. Generally, white men are slightly taller than African-American men (by about 0.5 inches) and nearly 3 inches taller than Asian men. White and African-American women are about the same height, and Asian women are about 1.5 inches shorter. Bones are denser in African-Americans than in whites; therefore, osteoporosis is less common in African-Americans. Bones of Chinese and Japanese are less dense than whites, often creating problems in those groups. Interestingly, children of immigrants from all areas are very frequently taller than children in their country of origin. This is probably the result of improved nutrition and decreased impact of communicable disease.

Other skeletal distinctions include differences in the number of vertebrae. As many as 11% of African-American women are missing one vertebra, and 12% of Native American men have one extra. This may result in differences in back problems (Andrews and Boyle, 1995).

SKIN

One of the most obvious differences of disparate cultural and racial groups is skin color. Assessment of the skin for symptoms of cyanosis, pallor, jaundice, erythema, and petechiae must include consideration of the normal skin color. Table 6–13 contains guidelines for assessment of the skin for these symptoms or characteristics on light-skinned versus dark-skinned persons.

OTHER DIFFERENCES

Table 6–14 is included to summarize much of the information regarding variations in cultural and racial characteristics described here.

Principles for Nursing Practice in Community Settings

One of the barriers to provision of culturally sensitive nursing care is the failure to recognize and

TABLE 6–13 **Assessment of Skin Color**

Characteristic	White or Light-Skinned Person	Dark-Skinned Person
Pallor		
Vasoconstriction present	Skin takes on white hue, which is color of collagen fibers in subcutaneous connective tissue	Skin loses underlying red tones; brown-skinned person appears yellow-brown; black-skinned person appears ashen-gray Mucous membranes, lips, nailbeds pale or gray
Erythema, Inflammation		
Cutaneous vasodilation	Skin is red	Palpate for increased warmth of skin, edema, tightness, or induration of skin; streaking and redness difficult to assess
Cyanosis		
Hypoxia of tissues	Bluish tinges of skin, especially in earlobes, as well as in lips, oral mucosa, and nailbeds	Lips, tongue, conjunctiva, palms, soles of feet are pale or ashen gray; apply light pressure to create pallor; in cyanosis, tissue color returns slowly by spreading from periphery to the center
Ecchymosis		
Deoxygenated blood seeps from broken blood vessel into subcutaneous tissue	Skin changes color from purple-blue to yellow-green to yellow	Oral mucous membrane or conjunctiva will show color changes from purple-blue to yellow-green to yellow; obtain history of trauma and discomfort; note swelling and induration
Petechiae		
Intradermal or submucosal bleeding	Round, pinpoint purplish red spots on skin	Oral mucosa or conjunctiva show purplish-red spots if person has black skin
Jaundice		
Accumulated bilirubin in tissues	Yellow color in skin, mucous membranes, and sclera of eyes; light-colored stools and dark urine often occur	Sclera of eyes, oral mucous membranes, palms of hand, and soles of feet have yellow discoloration

From Zentner, R. M. J. and Samiezade'-Yazd, C. (1993). Sociocultural influences on the person and family. In R. B. Murray and J. P. Zentner (Eds.). *Nursing Assessment and Health Promotion: Strategies Through the Life Span* (5th ed.). Norwalk, CT, Appleton & Lange, pp. 2–47.

appreciate the impact of the culture of the health-care providers. Health-care providers have been socialized into a given culture (usually the dominant cultural group of middle-class white) and then further socialized into the culture of their profession. "Professional socialization teaches the student a set of beliefs, practices, habits, likes, dislikes, norms and rituals. . . ." Therefore,

Text continued on page 155

TABLE 6–14 **Cross-Cultural Examples of Cultural Phenomena Impacting Nursing Care**

Place of Origin	Environmental Control	Biological Variations*	Social Organization	Communication	Space	Time Orientation
Asian China Hawaii Philippines Korea Japan Southeast Asia (Laos, Cambodia, Vietnam)	Traditional health and illness beliefs Use of traditional medicines Traditional practitioners: Chinese doctors and herbalists	Liver cancer Stomach cancer Coccidioidomycosis Hypertension Lactose intolerance	Family: hierarchical structure, loyalty Devotion to tradition Many religions, including Taoism, Buddhism, Islam, and Christianity Community social organizations	National language preference Dialects, written characters Use of silence Nonverbal and contextual cuing	Noncontact people	Present
African West Coast (as slaves) Many African countries West Indian Islands Dominican Republic Haiti Jamaica	Traditional health and illness beliefs Folk medicine tradition Traditional healer: root-worker	Sickle cell anemia Hypertension Cancer of the esophagus Stomach cancer Coccidioidomycosis Lactose intolerance	Family: many female-headed single-parent households Large, extended family networks Strong church affiliation within community Community social organizations	National languages Dialect: Pidgen, Creole, Spanish, and French	Close personal space	Present over future
Europe Germany England Italy Ireland Other European countries	Primary reliance on modern health care system Traditional health and illness beliefs Some remaining folk medicine tradition	Breast cancer Heart disease Diabetes mellitus Thalassemia	Nuclear families Extended families Judeo-Christian religions Community social organizations	National languages Many learn English immediately	Noncontact people Aloof Distant Southern countries: closer contact and touch	Future over present

Table continued on following page

TABLE 6–14 **Cross-Cultural Examples of Cultural Phenomena Impacting Nursing Care** *Continued*

Place of Origin	Environmental Control	Biological Variations*	Social Organization	Communication	Space	Time Orientation
Native American 170 Native American Tribes Aleuts Inuits	Traditional health and illness beliefs Folk medicine tradition Traditional healer: medicine man	Accidents Heart disease Cirrhosis of the liver Diabetes mellitus	Extremely family oriented Biological and extended families Children taught to respect traditions Community social organizations	Tribal languages Use of silence and body language	Space very important and has no boundaries	Present
Hispanic countries Spain Cuba Mexico Central and South America	Traditional health and illness beliefs Folk medicine tradition Traditional healers: curandero, espiritista, partera, senora	Diabetes mellitus Parasites Coccidioidomycosis Lactose intolerance	Nuclear family Extended families Compadrazzo: godparents Community social organizations	Spanish or Portuguese primary language	Tactile relationships Touch Handshakes Embracing Value physical presence	Present

*Indicates a high morbidity incidence.

From Giger, J. N. Davidhizar, R. E. (1991). *Transcultural Nursing.* St. Louis, Mosby-Year Book.

From Spector, R. E. (1993). Culture, ethnicity and nursing. In P. A. Potter and A. G. Perry (Eds.), *Fundamentals of Nursing: Concepts, Process & Practice.* St. Louis, Mosby-Year Book, p. 101.

TABLE 6–15 **Resources for Cultural Care and Transcultural Nursing**

American Anthropological Association
P. O. Box 91104
Washington, D. C. 20090
(202) 232-8800

Council on Nursing and Anthropology
Dr. Mildred Roberson
Nursing Department
Southeast Missouri State University
Cape Girardeau, MO 63701

International Nursing Center
c/o American Nurses' Association
600 Maryland Avenue, S. W.
Suite 100W
Washington, D. C. 20024
(202) 554-4444

Native American Nurses Association
927 Tredale Lane
Cloquet, MN 55720
(218) 879-1227

National Association of Hispanic Nurses
1501 16th Street, N. W.
Washington, D. C. 20036
(202) 387-2477

National Black Nurses Association
P. O. Box 1823
Washington, D. C. 20012-1823
(202) 393-6870

Transcultural Nursing Society
Madonna University
College of Nursing and Health
36600 Schoolcraft Road
Livonia, MI 48150-1173
(313) 591-8320

U. S. Department of Health and Human Services
U. S. Public Health Service
Indian Health Service
5600 Fishers Lane
Rockville, MD 20852
(301) 443-4242

U. S. Department of Health and Human Services
U. S. Public Health Service
Office of Minority Health
P. O. Box 37337
Washington, D. C. 20013
(800) 444-6472

National Council for International Health
1701 K Street, N. W.
Suite 600
Washington, D. C. 20006
(202) 833-5903

National Association of Community Health Centers
1330 New Hampshire Avenue, N. W.
Suite 122
Washington, D. C. 20036
(202) 659-8008

"health-care providers can be viewed as a foreign culture or ethnic group" (Spector, 1996, pp. 75–76). As a result, it is very important that all nurses seek to realize the impact of their personal culture, as well as the culture of health care providers, on their own behavior, values, and practices. They are then in a position to plan and provide appropriate interventions that accommodate and appreciate cultural differences and not merely impart their own culture on the client.

Spradley (1990) succinctly summarized cultural principles for practice for nurses who work in community settings. These principles are to

- Recognize and appreciate cultural differences
- Understand cultural reasons for client behavior
- Listen and learn before advising
- Empathize with culturally different clients
- Show respect for clients and their culture
- Be patient
- Analyze your behavior

Adherence to these principles promotes culturally competent nursing care. Information on resources for transcultural nursing and for groups and organizations that encourage culture sensitivity are included in Table 6–15.

Key Points

- The United States is becoming increasingly ethnically diverse, and this affects health and health care delivery, particularly for nurses in community-based practice.
- Numerous nursing organizations have recognized the need to provide culturally sensitive and culturally competent nursing care. The Transcultural Nursing Society was established in 1973.
- *Race* refers to classification of humans based on physical characteristics, and there are nine recognized distinct races. An *ethnic group* is a group of people who share common distinctive characteristics, such as race, ancestry, nationality, language, religion, food preferences, literature, music, and a common history. There are more than 100 ethnic groups in the United States. *Culture* is closely tied to ethnicity and refers to values, beliefs, attitudes, and customs that provide the organizational structure or basis for behavior within the group. A *subculture* is a relatively large subsection of a cultural group that has distinctive characteristics that set it apart from the group as a whole.
- Community-based nurses may need to perform a cultural assessment to help recognize the impact of culture on health and health practices. Identification of cultural values should be a component of a cultural assessment.
- Cultural variations based on socioeconomic levels or class can greatly influence health and health-seeking behaviors. Socioeconomic class creates a set of values and role expectations regarding sex, marriage, parenting, birth, education, dress, housing, occupation, and religion.
- Language barriers are frequently encountered when working with members of other cultural groups. Appropriate use of an interpreter and tips for communication without an interpreter can be helpful for nurses working in community-based settings. Familiarity with variations in communication patterns between various cultural groups can also be helpful
- Cultural factors that also contribute significantly to health and illness include diet and nutrition and religion.
- Cultural variations occur in health, illness, physical assessment findings, and health practices. Nurses working with significant numbers of persons from a cultural group should be aware of these variations and practices.

Learning Activities and Application to Practice

In Class

- Encourage students from racial or ethnic minorities to share differences in values, norms, religion, and health beliefs. Have them discuss how these factors influence health practices and might affect health care delivery. Explore how students and nurses can develop sensitivity to other cultural groups.
- Invite a health care provider who works with smaller minority groups, such as

refugees or migrant workers, to speak to the class. Have the speaker provide specific examples of difficulties in planning and providing care for these aggregates.

- Invite a speaker from the Public Health Service, Indian Health Service, or Office of Minority Health to speak to the class regarding health initiatives and research currently underway to improve the health of minority groups.
- Review *Healthy People 2000* objectives that relate to minority health. In small groups, have students discuss interventions to address the objectives. Encourage each group to draft and then share a community care plan related to one or more objectives.
- Have each student complete a cultural self-assessment and share findings. Ask cultural minority members of the class to lead a discussion about perceived and actual differences between their culture and the group majority.

In Clinical

- Assign a group of students to review census data to identify the percentages of persons from non-European origin in the local community and delineate the various countries of origin for those persons. If possible, compare to previous data (e.g., has the percentage increased since 1980? Since 1990?). What are projections for the future?
- Have students identify an individual or family from a cultural minority and perform a cultural assessment. Share findings with the clinical group.
- Encourage students to outline health practices, health problems, and other observations uniquely related to race, culture, or ethnicity encountered in clinical practice in a diary or log. Share these with the clinical group. Were there any assessments or interventions performed based on racial, ethnic, or cultural variations?

REFERENCES

American Academy of Nursing. (1992). AAN expert panel report: Culturally competent health care. *Nursing Outlook, 40* (6), 277–283.

Andrews, M. M. (1993). Cultural diversity and community health nursing. In J. M. Swanson and M. Albrecht (Eds.). *Community Health Nursing: Promoting the Health of Aggregates*. Philadelphia, W. B. Saunders, pp. 371–406.

Andrews, M. M. (1992). Cultural perspectives on nursing in the 21st century. *Journal of Professional Nursing, 8* (1), 1–9.

Andrews, M. M. and Boyle, J. S. (1995). *Transcultural Concepts in Nursing Care* (2nd ed.). Philadelphia, J. B. Lippincott.

Andrews M. M. and Hanson, P. A. (1995). Religion, culture and nursing. In M. M. Andrews and J. S. Boyle (Eds.). *Transcultural Concepts in Nursing Care* (2nd ed.). Philadelphia, J. B. Lippincott.

Carson, W. B. (1989). *Spiritual Dimensions of Nursing Practice*. Philadelphia, W. B. Saunders.

Degazon, C. (1996). Cultural diversity and community health nursing practice. In M. Stanhope and J. Lancaster (Eds.). *Community Health Nursing: Promoting Health of Aggregates, Families and Individuals* (4th ed). St. Louis, Mosby–Year Book.

Garn, S. M. (1985). Human races. In *World Book Encyclopedia.* Vol. 16. Chicago, World Book, Inc.

Herberg, P. (1995). Theoretical foundations of transcultural nursing. In M. M. Andrews and J. S. Boyle (Eds.). *Transcultural Concepts in Nursing Care* (2nd ed.). Philadelphia, J. B. Lippincott, pp. 3–48.

Keegan, L. (1993) Spirituality. In J. M. Black and E. Matassarin-Jacobs (Eds.). *Luckmann and Sorensen's Medical-Surgical Nursing: A Psychophysiologic Approach* (4th ed). Philadelphia, W. B. Saunders.

Kuipers, J. (1995). Mexican Americans. In J. N. Giger and R. E. Davidhizar (Eds.). *Transcultural Nursing: Assessment and Intervention* (2nd ed). St. Louis, Mosby–Year Book.

Leininger, M. M. (1991a). Selected culture care findings of diverse cultures using culture care theory and ethnomethods.

In M. M. Leininger (Ed.). *Culture Care Diversity & Universality: A Theory of Nursing*. Publication No. 15–2402. New York, National League for Nursing Press, pp. 345–372.

Leininger, M. M. (1991b). The theory of culture care diversity and universality. In M. M. Leininger (Ed.). *Culture Care Diversity & Universality: A Theory of Nursing*. Publication No. 15–2402. New York, National League for Nursing Press, pp. 5–72.

Spector, R. E. (1996). *Cultural Diversity in Health & Illness* (4th ed). Stamford, CT, Appleton & Lange.

Spector, R. E. (1993). Culture, ethnicity and nursing. In P. A. Potter and A. G. Perry (Eds.). *Fundamentals of Nursing: Concepts, Process & Practice*. St. Louis, Mosby–Year Book, pp. 94–119.

Spradley, B. W. (1990). *Community Health Nursing: Concepts and Practice* (3rd ed.). Glenview, IL, Scott, Foresman/Little, Brown Higher Education.

Stasiak, D. B. (1991). Culture care theory with Mexican-Americans in an urban context. In M. M. Leininger (Ed.). *Culture Care Diversity & Universality: A Theory of Nursing*. Publication No. 15–2402. New York, National League for Nursing Press, pp. 179–202.

Strasser, J. (1995). The cultural context for community health nursing. In C. M. Smith and F. A. Maurer (Eds.). *Community Health Nursing: Theory and Practice*. Philadelphia, W. B. Saunders, pp. 141–151.

U. S. Department of Health and Human Services. (1990). *Healthy People 2000: National Health Promotion and Disease Prevention Objectives*. Publication No (PHS)91–50212. Washington, D. C., Government Printing Office.

U. S. Department of Health and Human Services/National Center for Health Statistics. (1994). *Vital Statistics of the United States, 1990*. DHHS Publication No 94–1104. Hyattsville, MD, U. S. Department of Health and Human Services/National Center for Health Statistics.

Zentner, R. M. J. and Samiezade'-Yazd, C. (1993). Sociocultural influences on the person and family. In R. B. Murray and J. P. Zentner (Eds.). *Nursing Assessment and Health Promotion: Strategies Through the Life Span* (5th ed.). Norwalk, CT, Appleton & Lange, pp. 2–47.

UNIT III

Traditional Settings for Community-Based Nursing Care

7

Home Health Care Nursing

Case Study

Penny Parker has been a home health nurse for 2 years and is employed by a hospital-based agency in a small city. Before taking this position, she worked for 5 years as a staff nurse—primarily in a coronary care unit.

Each day Penny sees four to six clients, mostly elderly, with a variety of health problems. One recent Thursday, she saw four clients: Mr. Carter, who has congestive heart failure, to monitor his blood pressure and weight and perform medication teaching; Mrs. Kirk, who is homebound due to osteoporosis and receives monthly calcitonin injections; Mrs. Thomas, to change her Foley catheter, which her caregiver reported to be leaking; and Mr. Wilson, for admission to home care services following discharge from the hospital yesterday and to initiate dressing changes for a granulating abdominal wound as needed.

Penny prepares for each day by calling her scheduled clients the night before to set up times, outline the services she will be providing, determine if she needs to bring any special supplies, and learn if there are any specific instructions regarding the client's care of which she is not aware. Because Mr. Wilson is a new client and Penny has never been to his home, she is careful to obtain specific directions from his wife. She confirms with Mrs. Kirk that her medication is at her home and that it is not necessary to stop at the pharmacy. She inventories her car stock of dressings, gloves, solutions, and other supplies to identify anything she might need that is not readily available. Finally, she determines what forms will be needed for documentation of each client's care and gathers educational materials that will be beneficial in patient teaching.

Each visit consists of a general assessment followed by implementation of the prescribed skilled nursing services. The clients and their family members or caregivers are given instruction on their illness, treatment regimen, and self-care. Referrals for additional services are made as appropriate, and physicians and/or others involved in the care of each client are called to report findings, clarify orders, and request assistance. Also, the process of admitting new clients, like Mr. Wilson, into agency service necessitates additional assessments (e.g., complete physical assessment, health history, medication, functional, social needs) and explanation and completion of a number of documents related to home health services and Medicare reimbursement.

After she has seen each client and made necessary notifications and referrals,

Penny carefully completes documentation of all findings and services. Her orientation to the agency, 2 years of experience, and several related training sessions have taught her the importance of precise and thorough documentation. Therefore, she painstakingly completes and reviews all documentation and organizes each case folder to return to the agency. Finally, she contacts the agency to give a brief report on each client and receive her assignment for the following day.

With recent and anticipated reforms in health care financing and delivery, hospital occupancy rates have declined dramatically, outpatient surgery has increased markedly, and clients are being discharged "sicker and quicker." This in turn has resulted in a huge increase in home health care. Indeed, home care is the fastest growing specialty of nursing. According to the Public Health Service's Division of Nursing, between 1988 and 1992, the number of nurses working in home health care increased by 50% (U. S. Department of Health and Human Services [USDHHS], 1993). The growth in home health care can also been demonstrated by the rapidly increasing number of Medicare-certified agencies, clients, and visits over the past decade. Table 7–1 illustrates the growth in home health care since 1967.

History of Home Health Care Delivery and Financing

Until very recently, care for the ill and injured was provided almost exclusively in the home by family members, friends, or trained health care providers. In the United States, organized home health nursing services began when the first Visiting Nurse Associations (VNAs) were established in Buffalo, Boston, and Philadelphia during the mid-1880s. The early VNAs were established to care for the poor and disenfranchised suffering from illness or injury. The renowned public health nurse, Lillian Wald, is credited with starting a visiting nursing service for New York City in 1893 and persuading the Metropolitan Life Insurance Company to furnish home nursing services for policyholders in 1909 (Keating and Kelman, 1988). Provision of home health nursing services for insured clients became increasingly common during the following decades. Public health departments, the Red Cross, and philanthropic efforts funded many of the earliest home health agencies.

Initially, home health nursing care services and interventions were determined by the nurse. Teaching on hygiene and infant care; instituting measures to control communicable disease; assistance with self-care; performance of activities of daily living for persons with serious or chronic

TABLE 7–1 **Growth in Medicare-Certified Home Health Care**

Year	Number of Home Health Agencies	Medicare Expenditures (millions)	Number of Clients (1000s)	Number of Visits (1000s)
1967	1,753	$46	N/A	N/A
1980	2,924	$662	957	22,428
1987	5,923	$1,879	1,565	35,591
1992	6,004	$7,878	2,565	135,012
1994	7,521	$13,787	3,345	218,595

Data from National Association for Home Care. (1994). *Basic Statistics About Home Care.* Washington, D. C., National Association for Home Care.

illnesses; and caring for elderly, ill, and dying patients were among the services provided.

Passage of Medicare in 1965 dramatically changed the home health care delivery system. In the early years, home health care was directed and delivered virtually exclusively by nurses; physician guidance and oversight was not required. With Medicare, the payment source, client eligibility, purpose of home care, and provision of home care changed. Medicare developed very stringent requirements for eligibility, services, and physician oversight. Physician-prescribed and -directed care became a necessity, and guidelines for services were defined and requirements for eligibility predetermined. The independent practice of nurses providing care to individuals and families in their homes was greatly altered, and home health care services were determined by physician directives.

Until recently, home health care in the United States was largely provided by "official" (governmental or public) or "voluntary" (private, nonprofit agencies such as VNAs funded by fees-for-service, united community funds, grants, and other sources) agencies. As Table 7–2 depicts, however, the majority of home health agencies now are proprietary or hospital based. This trend also reflects the changes in the health care system. As care moved from acute care institutions, largely because of the advent of diagnoses-related group reimbursement policies, both proprietary and nonprofit hospitals and providers have recognized the need for home care services and the potential for revenue generation (Sereda, 1992; Widmar and Martinson, 1989). Table 7–3 lists current Health Care Financing Administration (HCFA) designations for types of home health agencies.

Definitions

As defined by the USDHHS, *home health care* is "that component of a continuum of comprehensive health care whereby health services are provided to individuals and families in their places of residence for the purpose of promoting, maintaining or restoring health, or maximizing the level of independence, while minimizing the effects of disability and illness, including terminal illness. Services appropriate to the needs of the individual patient and family are planned, coordinated, and made available by providers organized for the delivery of home care through the use of employed staff, contractual arrangements or a combination of the two patterns" (Warhola, 1980, p. 9). Emphasis is placed on the premise that "health care" (not medical care) should be "comprehensive" and designed to "promote, maintain or restore health" with the objective being to "maximize independence."

TABLE 7–2 **Medicare-Certified Home Health Agencies by Sponsor: 1967, 1987, and 1995**

	1967		1987		1995	
Sponsor	***Number***	***Percentage***	***Number***	***Percentage***	***Number***	***Percentage***
VNA	642.0	36.6	561.0	9.5	617.0	7.1
Public	939.0	53.6	1,172.0	19.8	1,161.0	13.3
Proprietary	0.0	0.0	1,882.0	31.8	3,730.0	42.6
Private, not-for-profit	0.0	0.0	803.0	13.6	667.0	7.6
Hospital-based	133.0	7.6	1,382.0	23.3	2,357.0	26.9
Other	39.0	2.2	123.0	2.0	215.0	2.5
Totals	1,753.0	100.0	5,923.0	100.0	8,747.0	100.0

Data from National Association for Home Care. (1995). *Basic Statistics About Home Care.* Washington, D. C., National Association for Home Care.

TABLE 7–3 **Types of Home Health Agencies, as Defined by the Health Care Financing Administration**

Nonprofit agency: an agency exempt from federal income taxation under Section 501 of the Internal Revenue Code of 1954.

Parent home health agency: the agency that is responsible for the services furnished to patients and for implementation of the plan of care.

Proprietary agency: a private profit-making agency licensed by the state.

Public agency: an agency operated by a state or local government.

Subdivision: a component of a multifunction health agency, such as the home care department of a hospital or the nursing division of a health department, which independently meets the conditions of participation for home health agencies. A subdivision that has subunits or branch offices is considered a parent agency.

Subunit: a semiautonomous organization that serves patients in a geographical area different from that of the parent agency and must independently meet the conditions of participation for home health agencies because it is too far from the parent agency to share administration, supervision, and services on a daily basis.

From Health Care Financing Administration. (1991). *Medicare Program: Home Health Agencies—Conditions of Participation and Reductions in Recordkeeping Requirements.* Part 484, Sections 484.1–484.52. Washington, D. C., U. S. Department of Health and Human Services.

Home health nursing combines aspects of community health nursing with selected technical skills from other specialty nursing practices and delivers care for individuals in collaboration with the family and/or designated caregivers. In the *Statement on the Scope of Home Health Nursing Practice,* the American Nurses' Association ([ANA], 1992) published the conceptual model presented in Figure 7–1. This model visually depicts the integration of medical/surgical, community health, parent-child, gerontological, and psychiatric–mental health nursing into home health care nursing practice.

The home health nurse's role is to be "care manager in coordinating and directing all involved disciplines and caregivers to optimize client outcomes. . ." through sharing "knowledge of community health resources with the client and caregivers" (ANA, 1992, p. 2). The home health care nurse must recognize that "influences of family dynamics and the home environment on the physical and emotional state of the client are essential inclusions in the nursing care plan" (ANA, 1992, p. 3). Additionally, a comprehensive knowledge base incorporating aspects of the specialty areas within nursing is required to deliver holistic care in the home.

Unlike other types of nursing practice, home health care nursing is not limited to a particular age group or diagnosis. Depending on the specific client's needs, care may be episodic or continuous and may be primary, secondary, and/or tertiary in nature. Home health nursing should be holistic and focused on the individual client, integrating family/caregiver, environmental, and community resources to promote optimal well-being for the client (American Nurses Credentialing Center [ANCC], 1994). Thus, home care nursing can be defined as "the provision of nursing care to acute and chronically ill clients of all ages in their home while integrating community health nursing principles that focus on the environmental, psychosocial, economic, cultural and personal health factors affecting an individual's and family's health status" (Humphrey and Milone-Nuzzo, 1991, p. 14).

Standards and Credentialing

Similar to other nursing practice standards, the Home Health Nursing standards endorsed by the

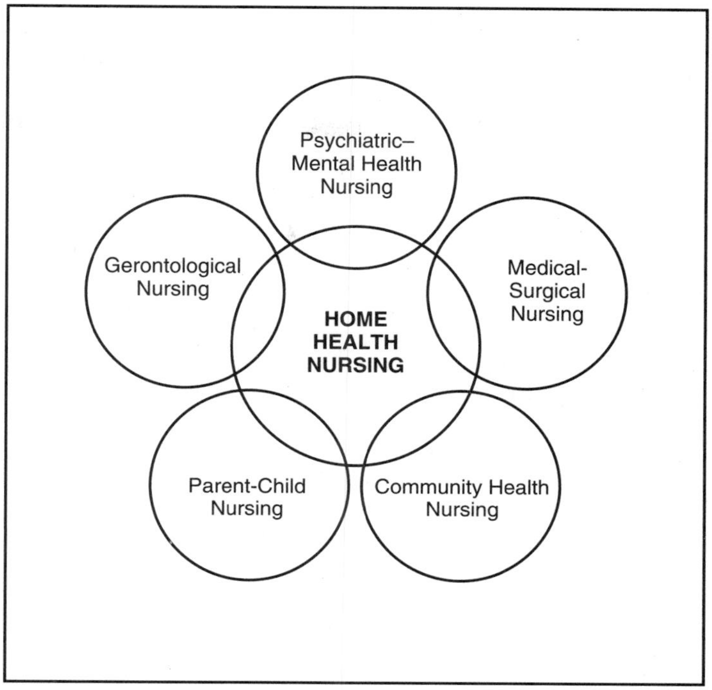

FIGURE 7–1 Conceptual Model of Home Health Nursing. (From American Nurses' Association. 1992. *A Statement on the Scope of Home Health Nursing Practice.* Washington, D. C., American Nurses' Association.)

ANA follow the steps of the nursing process, with separate standards addressing theory, research, ethics, and professional development. Distinctive components of the home health nursing standards are

- Standard I: "Organization of Home Health Services." Requirement that the home care nursing services be planned, organized, and directed by a nurse with a Master's degree.
- Standard VIII: "Continuity of Care." Focus on discharge planning, case management, and coordination of resources.
- Standard IX: "Interdisciplinary Collaboration." Coordination of services delivered by all members of the health care team.

The standards for home health nursing identify two levels of practice: the generalist and the specialist. The roles of the generalist include direct care provision, teaching, resource management, monitoring care, collaboration with other disciplines, and supervision of ancillary personnel. The nurse in the specialist role has a Master's degree and performs consultation with other providers; develops and evaluates agency policy; performs staff development and organizing; and manages, supports, and develops the home health services (ANA, 1986).

Certification in home health nursing is offered by the ANCC (a subsidiary of the ANA) to enhance professional development and recognize professional achievement. Eligibility requirements for certification as a generalist in home health nursing are (1) an active Registered Nurse (RN) license in the United States; (2) a baccalaureate or higher degree in nursing; (3) a minimum of 2 years of practice as an RN; (4) a minimum of 2,000 hours of practice as an RN in home health nursing during the past 2 years; and (5) current practice as an RN in home health nursing for a minimum of 8 hours per week. Following validation that these criteria have been met, the candidate is eligible to sit for the ANCC Board examination (ANCC, 1994).

Home Health Care Reimbursement and Documentation

Public sources (Medicare and Medicaid) finance more than 75% of home health services (Lyon and Stephany, 1993; Nelson, 1989); therefore, the discussion related to financing and documentation is directed toward meeting Medicare requirements. To be reimbursed by Medicare for services rendered to clients, home health agencies must be "Medicare certified." Medicare certification is awarded only to those agencies that have successfully demonstrated that they meet Medicare's "Conditions of Participation" for home health agencies. These conditions are regulations that consist of explicit rules, standards, and requirements established at the federal level of the government and are therefore constant within all states. These regulations outline requirements for virtually all aspects of home health care and detail such areas as personnel qualifications, notifying patients of their rights, acceptance of patients, plan of care and medical supervision, types of services that are offered by the agency, and the duties of each service provider (e.g., skilled nursing, various therapies, home health aide) (HCFA, 1995).

If a home health care agency meets the conditions of participation, it may choose to seek accreditation. Currently, there are two accreditation programs for home health care agencies: the Community Health Accreditation Program and the Home Care Accreditation Program of the Joint Commission on Accreditation of Healthcare Organizations. The accreditation process is very rigorous and includes a thorough self-study and a site visit by a team of professionals from the accrediting agency. If the home health agency is accredited, it is awarded "deemed status" and is eligible to receive Medicare reimbursement (Milone-Nuzzo, 1995).

To process Medicare claims, the HCFA contracts with regional insurance companies, or "fiscal intermediaries." The home health agency sends the fiscal intermediary a bill for services each month accompanied by the required documentation. These materials are reviewed by the intermediary and, if all documentation is included and appropriately meets the coverage criteria for home care, the bill is paid. Often there are questions regarding patient eligibility or appropriateness of services. In these cases, more information may be requested by the intermediary (Clark, 1995).

To qualify for coverage under Medicare guidelines, the following conditions must be met (HCFA, 1995):

- Services must be "reasonable and necessary" in relation to the patient's health status and medical needs, as reflected in the medical records and home health plan of care
- The client's care must require intermittent skilled nursing care, physical therapy, or speech therapy
- The client must be homebound
- The client must be under the care of a physician who develops and monitors a home health plan
- The home health agency must be certified to participate in Medicare

Each home health professional service (e.g., nursing, physical therapy, speech therapy) has guidelines on what Medicare defines as covered services. Table 7–4 lists the skilled nursing services reimbursable by Medicare.

HOME HEALTH CARE DOCUMENTATION

When asked what they like *most* about home health care, nurses often respond: "the autonomy," "being able to spend more time caring for my clients" or "the hours." When asked what they like *least* about home health care, nurses almost always respond: "the paperwork!" Completion of all required documentation has several purposes (Rovinski and Zastocki, 1989), including

- Recording services rendered
- Describing the patient's condition and response to care
- Promoting continuity of care
- Validating reimbursement claims
- Forestalling unjust legal actions

TABLE 7–4 **Medicare-Approved Skilled Nursing Services**

Skilled observation and assessment (e.g., including vital signs, response to medicine)	Teaching of nasogastric feeding
Foley insertion	Reinsertion of nasogastric feeding tube
Bladder instillation	Teaching of gastrostomy feeding
Wound care and dressing	Teaching of parenteral nutrition
Decubitus care (e.g., partial tissue loss with signs of infection of full-thickness tissue loss)	Teaching of care of tracheostomy
Venipuncture	Administration of care of tracheostomy
Restorative nursing	Teaching of inhalation therapy
Post–cataract surgery care	Administration of inhalation therapy
Bowel or bladder training	Teaching of administration of injection
Chest physiotherapy (including postural drainage)	Teaching diabetic care
Administration of vitamin B_{12}	Disimpaction and follow-up after enema
Administration of insulin	Other (specified under physician's orders)
Administration of other intramuscular or subcutaneous injection	Wound care and dressing—closed incision
Administration of intravenous drugs or clysis	Teaching care of any indwelling catheter
Teaching of ostomy or ileostomy conduit care	Management and evaluation of patient care plan
	Teaching and training (other specified under physician's orders)

From Health Care Financing Administration. (1990). *Guidelines for Filing Payment: Completion of the Plan of Care.* (485 Series Forms). Washington, D. C., U. S. Department of Health and Human Services.

For reimbursement by Medicare, documentation of all services and care given must be meticulously completed. To standardize and coordinate reimbursement, the HCFA instituted the requirement of completion of several forms to document home health care. Beginning in 1985, Forms 485, 486, and 487 were used for documentation of the home health care plan of services for Medicare reimbursement. These forms (Figs. 7–2 to 7–4), along with documentation of each skilled nursing visit, must be completed and submitted for reimbursement.

The HCFA form 485 is entitled "Home Health Certification and Plan of Treatment." It contains the signed physician's orders and certifies that the patient meets the eligibility requirements for home health care reimbursement. Orders for specific skilled services and goals are listed. Form 486 updates medical and patient care information and is completed at the time of certification or billing for services or for recertification. Specific instructions on completion of each of these forms are included in orientation to the agency.

To develop the requisite plan of care (HCFA form 485), and provide the information needed to ensure client eligibility certification for home care (form 486), each home health care agency has additional forms to be completed for each client. Individual agencies design forms for documentation that best meet the needs of their particular clientele and nurses' preferences. Documentation of a thorough nursing assessment, including physical, psychosocial, functional, nutritional, and safety components, as well as gathering information on all medications, is necessary. Other materials specified by Medicare include written documentation of notification of patient rights, notification of patient liability for payment and charges, and advisement of a state-established home health hotline for complaints or questions.

Orientation of nurses new to home health care practice or to a new agency demands in-depth instruction on documentation requirements, including specifics on how to complete all forms thoroughly and accurately. Tables 7–5 and 7–6 present information to guide home health nurses in documentation of home health care services.

Text continued on page 171

Department of Health and Human Services
Health Care Financing Administration

Form Approved
OMB No. 0938-0357

HOME HEALTH CERTIFICATION AND PLAN OF TREATMENT

1. Patient's HI Claim No.	2. SOC Date	3. Certification Period From: To:	4. Medical Record No.	5. Provider No.

6. Patient's Name and Address	7. Provider's Name and Address.
8. Date of Birth: 9. Sex ☐ M ☐ F	10. Medications: Dose/Frequency/Route (N)ew (C)hanged
11. ICD-9-CM Principal Diagnosis Date	
12. ICD-9-CM Surgical Procedure Date	
13. ICD-9-CM Other Pertinent Diagnoses Date	
14. DME and Supplies	15. Safety Measures:
16. Nutritional Req.	17. Allergies:

18.A. Functional Limitations

1 ☐ Amputation
2 ☐ Bowel/Bladder (Incontinence)
3 ☐ Contracture
4 ☐ Hearing
5 ☐ Paralysis
6 ☐ Endurance
7 ☐ Ambulation
8 ☐ Speech
9 ☐ Legally Blind
A ☐ Dyspnea With Minimal Exertion
B ☐ Other (Specify)

18.B. Activities Permitted

1 ☐ Complete Bedrest
2 ☐ Bedrest BRP
3 ☐ Up As Tolerated
4 ☐ Transfer Bed/Chair
5 ☐ Exercises Prescribed
6 ☐ Partial Weight Bearing
7 ☐ Independent At Home
8 ☐ Crutches
9 ☐ Cane
A ☐ Wheelchair
B ☐ Walker
C ☐ No Restrictions
D ☐ Other (Specify)

19. Mental Status: 1 ☐ Oriented 2 ☐ Comatose 3 ☐ Forgetful 4 ☐ Depressed 5 ☐ Disoriented 6 ☐ Lethargic 7 ☐ Agitated 8 ☐ Other

20. Prognosis: 1 ☐ Poor 2 ☐ Guarded 3 ☐ Fair 4 ☐ Good 5 ☐ Excellent

21. Orders for Discipline and Treatments (Specify Amount/Frequency/Duration)

22. Goals/Rehabilitation Potential/Discharge Plans

23. Verbal Start of Care and Nurse's Signature and Date Where Applicable:

24. Physician's Name and Address	25. Date HHA Received Signed POT	26. I ☐ certify ☐ recertify that the above home health services are required and are authorized by me with a written plan for treatment which will be periodically reviewed by me. This patient is under my care, is confined to his home, and is in need of intermittent skilled nursing care and/or physical or speech therapy or has been furnished home health services based on such a need and no longer has a need for such care or therapy, but continues to need occupational therapy.
27. Attending Physician's Signature (Required on 485 Kept on File in Medical Records of HHA)	*Date Signed*	

Form HCFA-485 (U4) (4-87)

PROVIDER

FIGURE 7–2 HCFA Form 485—Certification and Plan of Treatment. (From Health Care Financing Administration, Baltimore, MD.)

Department of Health and Human Services
Health Care Financing Administration

Form Approved
OMB No. 0938-0357

MEDICAL UPDATE AND PATIENT INFORMATION

1. Patient's HI Claim No.	2. SOC Date	3. Certification Period From: To:	4. Medical Record No.	5. Provider No.

6. Patient's Name	7. Provider's Name

8. Medicare Covered: ☐ Y ☐ N | 9. Date Physician Last Saw Patient: | 10. Date Last Contacted Physician:

11. Is the Patient Receiving Care in an 1861 (J)(1) Skilled Nursing Facility or Equivalent? ☐ Y ☐ N ☐ Do Not Know | 12. ☐ Certification ☐ Recertification ☐ Modified

13. Specific Services and Treatments

Discipline	Visits (This Bill) Rel. to Prior Cert.	Frequency and Duration	Treatment Codes	Total Visits Projected This Cert.

14. Dates of Last Inpatient Stay: Admission Discharge | 15. Type of Facility:

16. Updated Information: New Orders/Treatments/Clinical Facts/Summary from Each Discipline

17. Functional Limitations (Expand From 485 and Level of ADL) Reason Homebound/Prior Functional Status

18. Supplementary Plan of Treatment on File from Physician Other than Referring Physician: ☐ Y ☐ N
(If Yes, Please Specify Giving Goals/Rehab. Potential/Discharge Plan)

19. Unusual Home/Social Environment

20. Indicate Any Time When the Home Health Agency Made a Visit and Patient was Not Home and Reason Why if Ascertainable

21. Specify Any Known Medical and/or Non-Medical Reasons the Patient Regularly Leaves Home and Frequency of Occurrence

22. Nurse or Therapist Completing or Reviewing Form | Date (Mo., Day, Yr.)

Form HCFA-486 (U3) (4-87)

PROVIDER

FIGURE 7–3 HCFA Form 486—Medical Update and Patient Information. (From Health Care Financing Administration, Baltimore, MD.)

Department of Health and Human Services
Health Care Financing Administration

Form Approved
OMB No. 0938-0357

ADDENDUM TO: ☐ PLAN OF TREATMENT ☐ MEDICAL UPDATE

1. Patient's HI Claim No.	2. SOC Date	3. Certification Period From: To:	4. Medical Record No.	5. Provider No.

6. Patient's Name	7. Provider Name

8. Item No.

9. Signature of Physician	10. Date
11. Optional Name/Signature of Nurse/Therapist	12. Date

Form HCFA-487 (U4) (4-87)

PROVIDER

FIGURE 7–4 HCFA Form 487—Addendum to Plan of Treatment and Medical Update. (From Health Care Financing Administration, Baltimore, MD.)

TABLE 7–5 **Terminology Associated with Favorable Claims Review**

Recommended Terminology When Documenting Skilled Care	Terminology to Avoid When Documenting Skilled Care
Acute	Chronic; stabilized
Assessed; evaluated	Observed; monitored
Instructed	Reviewed; reinforced; retaught; stressed; discussed
Bed confined; chair confined	Stays in bed; sits in chair all day
Requires bodily transfer to move from . . . to . . . ; requires assistive device (specify) to move from . . . to . . .	Independent in room with walker; ambulatory in room/house/apartment only; walks with walker/quad cane, and so forth
Impaired balance	Falls easily; leans for support; unsteady gait
Unable to . . .	Has problems/difficulty with . . .
Symptoms (specify) exhibited after exertion (specify)	Tires easily; very weak; fatigued after activity
Has functional limitation of (specify)	Generalized weakness; frail
Transported to the physician by (specify)	Went to the doctor's
Homebound	Ambulatory within confines of home
Per the physician's order/request	At the patient's/family's request
Erythematic/inflamed	Appears red; slightly reddened
Beginning to respond to (specify) interventions	Stabilizing
Amount (specify)	Small; minimal; moderate
Frequency (specify)	Often; sometimes; usually
Parameters of response (specify in measurable exact terms, i.e., able to ambulate 10 feet without dizziness)	Monitor response to activity

From Rovinski, C. A. and Zastocki, D. K. (1989). *Home Care: A Technical Manual for the Professional Nurse.* Philadelphia, W. B. Saunders.

Elements of Home Care Nursing Practice

Home health care nursing practice requires unique skills and knowledge. Marrelli (1994, pp. 3–5) articulately described skills needed in home health care nursing as

- A knowledge of the basic "rules" of home care
- A repertoire of service-driven and patient-oriented interpersonal skills
- The ability to pay incredible attention to detail
- The possession of multifaceted skills, accompanied by flexibility
- The possession of a reliable car and safe, effective driving skills
- The ability to assume responsibility for the patient and the patient's plan of care
- Strong clinical skills and the ability to function as both a specialist and a generalist nurse
- Self-direction and the ability to function autonomously in a nonstructured atmosphere
- The desire to continue learning and to be open to new information and clinical skills
- A sincere appreciation of and for people
- The ability to be open and sincerely accepting of people's unique and chosen lifestyles and of the associated effects that these lifestyles have on their health
- The knowledge that change can be difficult

TABLE 7–6 **Home Health Documentation Hints**

1. Write legibly using blue or black ink
2. Include the patient's name on each page; date all entries
3. Use agency-accepted abbreviations
4. Use verbatim statements when documenting verbal dialogue
5. Record verbal orders from the physician exactly as received
6. Use terms such as
   - Assessment
   - Management
   - Evaluation
   - Instruction
   - Teaching
7. Include specific observations to explain why the visit is necessary, and detail skilled care given
8. Support the requirement of nursing skills based on the condition of the patient, complexity of the care, and/or accepted standards of practice
9. Support the client's or caregiver's inability, or unwillingness, to perform a procedure
10. Support the need of skilled services to promote the client's recovery and safety and to reduce complications
11. Support the need for skilled observation and assessment to change treatment (i.e., modify medication dosage or type/frequency of dressing change)
12. When documenting wound care, be specific regarding
    - Procedure performed
    - Any edema, pain, heat, odor, drainage
    - Amount and type of irrigation solution if used
    - Name of any topical ointments or other medications if applied
    - Measurement and description of wound dimensions
    - Condition of surrounding tissue
    - Description of any packing and type of dressing applied
13. When documenting other skilled procedures, be specific and use details
14. Document facts; be objective, complete, accurate, and concise
15. Document clinical findings related to diagnosis using quantifiable, measurable terms
16. When teaching, document client's and family's progress or lack of progress toward the goal
17. Sign each entry

Data from Rovinski, C. A. and Zastocki, D. K. (1989). *Home Care: A Technical Manual for the Professional Nurse.* Philadelphia, W. B. Saunders; Humphrey, C. J. and Milone-Nuzzo, P. (1991). *Home Care Nursing: An Orientation to Practice.* Norwalk, CT, Appleton & Lange.

- The possession of a kind sense of humor that can help patients and peers get through the rough times

Home health care nursing responsibilities are varied and numerous. A few basic and essential activities that comprise home health care nursing are described here.

DISCHARGE PLANNING

As discussed earlier, continuity of care (Standard VIII) is one of the identified nursing standards for home health nursing. One of the essential components of continuity of care is discharge planning. Discharge planning is the *process* of determining and planning to meet client needs following release from a health care facility. The discharge planning process allows client and family needs to be identified and evaluated, with responsibility for meeting those needs being transferred to the client, the client's caregiver or significant others, or other health care providers. The purposes of discharge planning include promoting continuity of care to improve client health status and coordinating the client's needs with available resources (Clark, 1995; Clemen-Stone *et al.*, 1995). Reduction in average length of service, lower cost, efficient use of resources, fewer requests for additional services, improved communication, and better information on client needs are benefits attributable to discharge planning.

Ideally, the discharge planning process should begin *before the client is hospitalized,* with anticipation of the client's needs during recovery. When the course of recovery is predicted to be difficult for any of several reasons and follow-up care through a home health agency is anticipated or requested, comprehensive discharge planning is beneficial. Discharge planning as a service is performed by different health professionals, including nurses, social workers, physicians, and chaplains (Clark, 1995). Many institutions employ professionals—usually nurses or social workers—for this position. These individuals are responsible for identifying clients in need of ongoing care following discharge, consulting with caregivers (both in the institution and when the client is discharged), educating staff regarding discharge plans, and coordinating activities.

Many health care institutions utilize assessment instruments to identify clients who need more detailed or intensive discharge planning. The Blaylock Risk Assessment Screen was developed to identify patients in need of discharge planning resources and is shown in Figure 7–5. In addition, Figure 7–6 presents an example of a discharge planning tool that can be used to coordinate care following hospitalization and to develop a plan of care for home health nursing.

CASE MANAGEMENT

Case management is a second component of the *Standards of Home Health Nursing Practice's* Standard VIII, "Continuity of Care," as well as an integral part of *Nursing's Agenda for Health Care Reform* (ANA, 1991; see Chapter 1 of this book). Coordination, delegation, referral, and advocacy are very important roles and functions provided by home health nurses and together comprise case management.

Case management has been defined as "the process of ensuring that the services provided are appropriate for the client's needs" (Clark, 1995, p. 65). According to Horn and Horn (1993), in case management, "one professional is responsible for assessing needs, targeting services to meet the needs and monitoring and evaluating client status to ensure that needs are met adequately" (p. 48). The goals of case management are to "provide quality health care, decrease fragmentation, enhance client's quality of life and contain costs" (ANA, 1991).

The case manager's role is comprehensive and includes assessment of the client's needs and resources, outlining a plan of care to meet the identified needs, arranging for the most cost-effective complement of services and providers to meet the identified needs, and coordinating the activities of various health care providers (Clark, 1995). In home health care nursing, *case management* generally refers to the comprehensive supervision of the care given to each patient. The case manager, usually the RN, functions as the team leader who provides or arranges primary care, supervises paraprofessionals, and collaborates with other health professionals (e.g., a physical or occupational therapist or medical social worker). The case manager is responsible for maintaining communication between the disciplines and with the client and monitoring and evaluating client goals.

COORDINATION OF COMMUNITY RESOURCES

Coordination of community resources is the third specified component of Home Health Nursing Standard VIII and requires that the nurse to be knowledgeable about services offered by his or her own agency and any resources available in the community that would benefit clients. In addition to being aware of resources, the home health nurse must understand the referral process.

During the referral process, a client is directed to appropriate agencies or organizations for information or assistance with care. To make effective and appropriate referrals, the nurse must

- Be aware of community services available for needs related to home health nursing practice

Circle all that apply and total. Refer to the Risk Factor Index.*

Age
- 0 = 55 years or less
- 1 = 56 to 64 years
- 2 = 65 to 79 years
- 3 = 80 + years

Living situation/social support
- 0 = Lives only with spouse
- 1 = Lives with family
- 2 = Lives alone with family support
- 3 = Lives alone with friends' support
- 4 = Lives alone with no support
- 5 = Nursing home/residential care

Functional status
- 0 = Independent in activities of daily living and instrumental activities of daily living
- Dependent in:
  - 1 = Eating/feeding
  - 1 = Bathing/grooming
  - 1 = Toileting
  - 1 = Transferring
  - 1 = Incontinent of bowel function
  - 1 = Incontinent of bladder function
  - 1 = Meal preparation
  - 1 = Responsible for own medication administration
  - 1 = Handling own finances
  - 1 = Grocery shopping
  - 1 = Transportation

Cognition
- 0 = Oriented
- 1 = Disoriented to some spheres† some of the time
- 2 = Disoriented to some spheres all of the time
- 3 = Disoriented to all spheres some of the time
- 4 = Disoriented to all spheres all of the time
- 5 = Comatose

Behavior pattern
- 0 = Appropriate
- 1 = Wandering
- 1 = Agitated
- 1 = Confused
- 1 = Other

Mobility
- 0 = Ambulatory
- 1 = Ambulatory with mechanical assistance
- 2 = Ambulatory with human assistance
- 3 = Nonambulatory

Sensory deficits
- 0 = None
- 1 = Visual or hearing deficits
- 2 = Visual and hearing deficits

Number of previous admissions/emergency room visits
- 0 = None in the last 3 months
- 1 = One in the last 3 months
- 2 = Two in the last 3 months
- 3 = More than two inthe last 3 months

Number of active medical problems
- 0 = Three medical problems
- 1 = Three to five medical problems
- 2 = More than five medical problems

Number of Drugs
- 0 = Fewer than three drugs
- 1 = Three to five drugs
- 2 = More than five drugs

Total score: ________

*Risk Factor Index: Score of 10 = at risk for home care resources; score of 11 to 19 = at risk for extended discharge planning; score greater than 20 = at risk for placement other than home. If the patient's score is 10 or greater, refer the patient to the discharge planning coordinator or discharge planning team.

†Spheres = person, place, time, and self.

FIGURE 7–5 Blaylock Discharge Planning Risk Assessment Screen. (From Blaylock, A. and Cason, C.L. Discharge planning predicting patients' needs. 1992. *Journal of Gerontological Nursing* 18 (7), 5–10. Ann Blaylock can be contacted at Baptist Memorial Medical Center, One Pershing Circle, North Little Rock, AR 72114.)

- Determine if the client is eligible for the services offered by the agency or organization
- Have an understanding of *how* to refer a client for a particular service and *who* may refer a client (e.g., some services or service providers require a referral from a physician only)
- Know the costs of services and payment mechanism
- Be aware of the location, telephone number, hours of operation, and contact person

Often, the nurse provides the client or their caregiver with the necessary information for the referral and allows him or her to make initial contact. At other times, it may be appropriate for the nurse to call the individual, agency, or organization directly.

To identify sources for community referrals, the home health nurse may use a directory of community services, which is available in many cities and towns. In addition, home health agencies often provide nurses with a list of available community resources. Experienced home health nurses usually develop a personal listing of service providers that have been helpful for clients in the past. Names of agencies, contact persons, and their telephone numbers are essential. Examples of commonly utilized community resources are various government programs (e.g., Medicaid, Veteran's Affairs, Women, Infants, and Children [WIC] program); Meals on Wheels, adult day care providers; area hospices, if not provided by the nurse's agency; organizations that assist with financial obligations; and transportation providers for the handicapped or elderly.

INTERDISCIPLINARY COLLABORATION

Home Health Nursing Practice Standard IX requires the RN to initiate and maintain a "liaison relationship" with all health care providers working with the client. In health care, collaboration implies joint decision making regarding the plan of care with all professionals involved with the client's care. Interdisciplinary collaboration is integrated within the roles and functions of the home health nurse discussed here and is vitally important in the process of discharge planning and case management. To comply with Medicare requirements and to best direct client care, the nurse must work with the physician to receive orders and outline the plan of care. As the case manager, the nurse must share the plan of care with all involved in the client's care and make recommendations and modifications based on their input. Case conferences should be held regularly, particularly for clients with complicated or prolonged care, to share information among the providers and discuss the client's response to the treatment plan. In addition, the nurse may oversee, evaluate, or supervise the care of others. Professionals involved in home health care planning and delivery include

Nurses: RNs have been the traditional providers of health care in the home. As described, nurses provide skilled nursing services, coordinate care as case managers and referral agents, and act as patient advocates.

Physicians: Most clients are referred for home care services by physicians, and, as stated, physician oversight of the plan of care is required for Medicare reimbursement, as well as for payment from other insurers.

Physical therapists: Most home care agencies employ physical therapists to assess client's needs for assistive devices that will support rehabilitation and safety, evaluate neuromuscular and functional ability and prescribe and administer therapy procedures to meet client needs, and teach the client or caregivers to perform these therapies and related activities.

Occupational therapists: Whereas physical therapists usually concentrate on gross motor skills and rehabilitation, occupational therapists assist the client in restoration of small motor coordination and improving physical tasks related to activities of daily living and reaching the highest level of functioning possible.

Speech therapists/speech pathologists: Speech therapists work with clients with communication problems related to speech, language, and hearing, as well as swallowing difficulties, to treat, manage, or alleviate these problems.

Client name ______________________________

ASSESSMENT OF NEEDS

Date of admission ______________ Anticipated discharge date ______________

Discharge diagnosis ______________________________

Nursing service needs (Check needed services on left; explain on right)

___ 1. Medications: ______________________________

___ 2. Treatments:

___ IV therapy ______________________________

___ Dressings, casts ______________________________

___ Stitch removal ______________________________

___ Oxygen ______________________________

___ Bed care ______________________________

___ Passive exercises ______________________________

___ Other ______________________________

___ 3. Nutritional needs:

___ Special diet ______________________________

___ Assistance with eating ______________________________

___ 4. Activity:

___ Limitations ______________________________

___ Exercises ______________________________

___ Help needed ______________________________

___ 5. Health teaching needed ______________________________

Other services needed:

___ 1. Physical therapy ______________________________

___ 2. Social work ______________________________

___ 3. Occupational therapy ______________________________

___ 4. Dietition ______________________________

___ 5. Pharmacist ______________________________

Other ______________________________

General level of care needed:

___ 1. Skilled nursing ______________________________

___ 2. Custodial care ______________________________

___ 3. Home care with referrals ______________________________

___ 4. Home care ______________________________

FIGURE 7–6 *Figure continues, and legend on facing page.*

EVALUATION OF RESOURCES

Assessment of client strengths and capabilities (Check as applicable on left; explain on right)

___ 1. Capabilities for self-care ______________________________

___ 2. Knowledge deficits ______________________________

___ 3. Other ______________________________

Assessment of family support or support from significant others: ______________________________

____

____

SUMMARY OF NEEDS TO BE ADDRESSED IN THE DISCHARGE PLAN

Discharge plan (Check as applicable on left; explain on right)

___ 1. Plan for teaching ______________________________

____

___ 2. Plan for referrals and arrangements ______________________________

____

___ 3. Other ______________________________

____

IMPLEMENTATION

Teaching done (summary and date) ______________________________

____

Referrals made (list and date) ______________________________

____

EVALUATION

Teaching deficits ______________________________

____

Referral outcomes ______________________________

____

FIGURE 7–6 Discharge Planning Questionnaire. (From Skelly, A. H. 1990. Physical disabilities and rehabilitation: The role of nursing in the community. In Bullough, B. and Bullough, V. (Eds.). *Nursing in the Community.* St. Louis, MO: C. V. Mosby.)

Social workers: Social workers assist clients with social, emotional, and financial needs. In addition, social workers often serve as advocates and refer clients to available community resources.

Registered dietitians/nutritionists: Dietitians provide direct counseling and teaching for clients with special dietary needs and problems. In addition, they may act as consultants or resource persons for nurses and other health care providers.

Home health aides: Home health aides are paraprofessionals who assist in the home with the client's personal care, basic nursing (e.g., vital signs, assistance with self-administered medication), and light housekeeping and related tasks (e.g., shopping, meal preparation). For Medicare reimbursement, home health aides must be supervised by an RN.

Other providers: Other professionals and paraprofessionals that occasionally provide care to clients in the home or might assist home health nurses include pharmacists, phlebotomists, laboratory technicians, respiratory therapists, enterostomal therapists, chaplains, and massage therapists.

Legal and Ethical Considerations in Home Health Care

Care of clients in their homes frequently raises ethical dilemmas and concerns. Use of technology, care of the elderly and dying, financial constraints, questions regarding caregivers' capabilities and willingness to take responsibility for care, and respect for the client's wishes and rights, for example, might produce problems or questions. In the home setting, the nurse is better able to evaluate the long-term consequences of disease, disability, and treatment that may not be recognized, understood, or appreciated in the institutional setting. For example, can the 14-year-old mother of a premature infant needing monitoring for apnea provide the care needed for her baby and respond appropriately in the event of an emergency? Who will help the elderly woman living alone who just had her right leg amputated with her routine self-care needs and with routine tasks such as housecleaning or shopping for groceries? What if a patient wants to forgo extensive treatment for cancer but his family insists he have it? The home care nurse should recognize ethical problems and, when appropriate, intervene. Knowing a patient's rights and responsibilities, as well as the responsibilities of caregivers, is an important component of home health care. Referral to the physician, social worker, or other support groups or agencies for assistance may be appropriate. Reporting of unsafe conditions, care, or practices and/or neglect or abuse may sometimes be necessary.

HOME CARE BILL OF RIGHTS

One of the Medicare funding requirements mandated by HCFA states that "The HHA [Home Health Agency] must provide the patient with a written notice of the patient's rights in advance of furnishing care to the patient or during the initial evaluation visit before the initiation of treatment" (HCFA, 1991, Section 484.10). Thus, before treatment, each home health patient is required to be informed of his or her "right" for health care treatment, and this must be documented on the patient's permanent record. To comply with this requirement, the National Association of Home Care has established a "bill of rights" for clients and their families to inform them of the ethical conduct they can expect form home care agencies. Table 7–7 presents this document.

ADVANCE MEDICAL DIRECTIVES

Home health nurses must be aware of requirements for informed decision making in health care and should therefore assess the client's desires with regard to advance medical directives in compliance with the "Home Care Bill of Rights." The advance medical directive "is a document that indicates the wish of the client regarding various types of medical treatment in representative situations" (Milone-Nuzzo, 1995, p. 792). With the advent of increasing technology in the treatment and management of both acute and chronic illnesses and the desire that all clients make informed decisions regarding treatment options and

TABLE 7–7 **Home Care Bill of Rights***

Home care consumers (clients) have a right to be notified in writing of their rights and obligations before treatment is begun. The client's family or guardian may exercise the client's rights when the client has been judged incompetent. Home care providers have an obligation to protect and promote the rights of their clients, including the following rights.

Clients and Providers Have a Right to Dignity and Respect

Home care clients and their formal caregivers have a right to mutual respect and dignity. Caregivers are prohibited from accepting personal gifts and borrowing from clients.

Clients Have the Right

- To have relationships with home care providers that are based on honesty and ethical standards of conduct
- To be informed of the procedure they can follow to lodge complaints with the home care provider about the care that is, or fails to be, furnished, and regarding a lack of respect from property (to lodge complaints with us call ______________)
- To know about the disposition of such complaints
- To voice their grievances without fear of discrimination or reprisal for having done this
- To be advised of the telephone number and hours of operation of the state's home health comment line. The hours are ______________ and the number is ______________

Decisionmaking

Clients Have the Right

- To be notified in writing of the care that is to be furnished, the types (disciplines) of the caregivers who will furnish the care, and the frequency of the visits that are proposed to be furnished
- To be advised of any change in the plan of care before the change is made
- To participate in the planning of the care and in planning changes in the care, and to be advised that they have the right to do so
- To refuse services or request a change in caregiver without fear of reprisal or discrimination

The home care provider or the client's physician may be forced to refer the client to another source of care if the client's refusal to comply with the plan of care threatens to compromise the provider's commitment to quality care.

Privacy

Clients Have the Right

- To confidentiality with regard to information about their health, social and financial circumstances, and about what takes place in the home
- To expect the home care provider to release information only as required by law or authorized by the client

Financial Information

Clients Have the Right

- To be informed of the extent to which payment may be expected from Medicare, Medicaid, or any other payor known to the home care provider
- To be informed of the charges that will not be covered by Medicare
- To be informed of the charges for which the client may be liable
- To receive this information, orally and in writing, within 15 working days of the date the home care provider becomes aware of any changes in charges
- To have access, upon request, to all bills for service the client has received, regardless of whether they are paid out-of-pocket or by another party

Table continued on following page

TABLE 7–7 **Home Care Bill of Rights*** *Continued*

Quality of Care

Clients Have the Right

- To receive care of the highest quality
- In general, to be admitted by a home care provider only if it has the resources needed to provide the care safely, and at the required level of intensity, as determined by a professional assessment; however, a provider with less than optimal resources may nevertheless admit the client if a more appropriate provider is not available, but only after fully informing the client of its limitations and the lack of suitable alternative arrangements
- To be told what to do in the case of an emergency

Quality of Care

The Home Care Provider Shall Assure That

- All medically related home care is provided in accordance with the physicians' orders and that a plan of care specifies the services to be provided and their frequency and duration
- All medically related personal care is provided by an appropriately trained homemaker-home health aide who is supervised by a nurse or other qualified home care professional

*In 1982, the National Association for Home Care adopted a comprehensive Code of Ethics to which all members subscribed. Among the elements in this Code was a clients' Bill of Rights similar to the rights outlined in this document. In 1987, Congress enacted a provision requiring home care agencies to inform clients of these rights.

From National Association for Home Care. (1990). *Home Care Bill of Rights.* Washington, D. C., National Association for Home Care.

the refusal of medical care, advance medical directives were begun in the early 1990s to assist in the delineation of specified medical care in situations in which the client is unable to make decisions and communicate those decisions to the primary care provider.

There are two types of advance medical directives: living wills and health care proxies (durable power of attorney for health care). Either type of directive explicitly states the patient's desire for health care if he or she is incapacitated and unable to make decisions. It is important to remember that either document can be changed by the patient at any time.

The living will records a patient's decision to decline life-prolonging treatment if that patient becomes hopelessly ill. "The living will indicates the circumstance for its implementation and the care that should be provided if these circumstances arise. A health care proxy (durable power of attorney)" names "someone who will make health care decisions if the client becomes unable to make them" (Milone-Nuzzo, 1995, p. 793).

Although not specifically addressed by Medicare's Conditions of Participation, individual states may have laws and/or regulations may require that all health care providers, whether in institutions or in the home, to be aware of and respect each client's wishes regarding treatment. Agency orientation should include specific directions regarding assessment of, and compliance with, patients' wishes about advanced directives.

SUMMARY

The knowledge base and information necessary for the practice of home health care nursing is vast, and only a small portion has been discussed here. There are many issues and topics that are beyond the scope of this book. The references listed are excellent sources for more information. In addition, Table 7–8 lists national resources for home health care nursing practice. Finally, Chapter 8 presents specific information on the process of home health nursing, and Chapter 9 discusses specialized home health care, including hospice care, high-technology care, postpartum care, and psychiatric home health care.

TABLE 7–8 **National Resources for Home Health Care Nursing**

National Association for Home Care
519 C Street N. E.
Washington, D. C. 20002
(202) 547-7424

Visiting Nurses Association of America
3801 East Florida Avenue
Suite 900
Denver, CO 80210
(303) 753-0218

National Hospice Organization
1901 North Moore Street
Suite 901
Arlington, VA 22209
(703) 938-4449
(800) 658-8898

National League for Nursing
Community Health Accreditation Program
350 Hudson Street
New York, NY 10014
(212) 989-9393

American Cancer Society
90 Park Avenue
New York, NY 10016
(212) 599-3600

American Heart Association
7320 Greenville Avenue
Dallas, TX 75231
(214) 373-6300

Alzheimer's Association
919 North Michigan
Suite 1000
Chicago, IL 60611-1676
(312) 853-3060
(800) 621-0379

American Association of Retired Persons
1909 K Street N. W.
Washington, D. C. 20049
(202) 872-4700

American Diabetes Association
505 8th Avenue
New York, NY 10018
(212) 947-9797

National Multiple Sclerosis Society
205 East 42nd Street
New York, NY 10017
(212) 986-3240

Cystic Fibrosis Foundation
6931 Arlington Road
Bethesda, MD 20814

Public Health Service AIDS Information Hotline
(800) 342-AIDS

Key Points

- Home health nursing integrates medical/surgical, community health, parent-child, gerontological, and psychiatric–mental health nursing into home health care practice. It refers to comprehensive nursing care provided to individuals and families in their place of residence, focusing on the environmental, psychosocial, economic, cultural, and personal health factors affecting health status.
- Although home health care nursing has been present in the United States since the mid-1880s, when the first VNAs were established, it has only recently become one

of the primary sources of delivery of nursing care. Currently, home health care is the fastest growing specialty in nursing.

- With the passage of Medicare in 1965, the practice of home health care nursing changed dramatically. Until recently, home health care was largely provided by "official" (governmental or public) or "voluntary" (private, nonprofit) agencies. This has changed in the past decade, and the majority of home health agencies are now proprietary or hospital based.
- Public sources (Medicare and Medicaid) finance more than 75% of home health services. To be reimbursed by Medicare, home health agencies must be "Medicare certified," follow Medicare's "Conditions of Participation" (explicit rules, standards, and requirements), and be certified by an accreditation organization.
- To qualify for coverage under Medicare, services must be "reasonable and necessary;" the client's care must require intermittent skilled nursing care, physical therapy, or speech therapy; the client must be homebound and under the care of a physician who develops a home health plan; and the agency must be certified to participate in Medicare.
- Thorough and accurate documentation is essential in home health nursing to record services, describe the patient's condition and response to care, promote continuity of care, validate reimbursement claims, and forestall legal action. Completion of the required Medicare forms is necessary for payment.
- Home health care nursing requires unique skills and knowledge. Basic and essential activities include discharge planning (the process of determining the planning to meet client needs following release from a health care facility), case management (the process of ensuring that the services provided are appropriate for the client's needs), coordination of community resources, and interdisciplinary collaboration.
- To address legal and ethical issues in home health care, home health nurses should be aware of the Home Care Bill of Rights and local, state, and national requirements for informed consent and advance medical directives.

Learning Activities and Application to Practice

In Class

- Invite a home health care nurse and/or hospice nurse to speak to the class. Have him or her share information about working with families, independence, pain management, collaboration, and documentation.
- Provide examples of completed forms and other home health care documentation. Discuss the importance of documentation for reimbursement and continuity of care.

In Clinical

- Assign each student to work with a practicing home health care nurse for a minimum of 6 days. Keep a log or a diary recording the types of clients seen.

What skilled nursing interventions were performed? What practical experiences and skills are helpful for nurses considering home health practice? Describe the process of documentation.

REFERENCES

American Nurses' Association. (1991). *Nursing's Agenda For Health Care Reform*. Washington, D. C., American Nurses' Association.

American Nurses' Association. (1986). *Standards for Home Health Nursing Practice*. Kansas City, MO, American Nurses' Association.

American Nurses' Association. (1992). *A Statement on the Scope of Home Health Nursing Practice*. Washington, D. C., American Nurses' Association.

American Nurses Credentialing Center. (1994). *ANCC Certification Catalog*. Washington, D. C., American Nurses' Association.

Blaylock, A. and Cason, C. L. (1992). Discharge planning: Predicting patients' needs. *Journal of Gerontological Nursing, July,* 5–10.

Clark, M. J. (1995). *Nursing in the Community* (2nd ed.). Norwalk, CT, Appleton & Lange.

Clemen-Stone, S., Eigsti, D. G., and McGuire, S. L. (1995). *Comprehensive Community Health Nursing* (4th ed.). St. Louis, MO, Mosby–Year Book.

Health Care Financing Administration. (1991). *Medicare Program: Home Health Agencies—Conditions of Participation and Reductions in Recordkeeping Requirements*. Part 484. Sections 484.1–484.52. Washington, D. C., U. S. Department of Health and Human Services.

Health Care Financing Administration. (1995). *Your Medicare Handbook 1995*. HCFA Publication No. 10050, Baltimore, MD, Health Care Financing Administration.

Horn, B. J. and Horn, B. M. (1993). The health care system. In J. M. Swanson and M. Albrecht (Eds.). *Community Health Nursing: Promoting the Health of Aggregates*. Philadelphia, W. B. Saunders.

Humphrey, C. J. and Milone-Nuzzo, P. (1991). *Home Care Nursing: An Orientation to Practice*. Norwalk, CT, Appleton & Lange.

Keating, S. B. and Kelman, G. B. (1988). *Home Health Care Nursing: Concepts and Practice*. Philadelphia, J. B. Lippincott.

Lyon, J. C. and Stephany, T. M. (1993). Home health care. In J. M. Swanson and M. Albrecht (Eds.). *Community Health Nursing: Promoting the Health of Aggregates*. Philadelphia, W. B. Saunders.

Marrelli, T. M. (1994). *Handbook of Home Health Standards and Documentation Guidelines for Reimbursement*. St. Louis, MO, Mosby-Year Book.

Milone-Nuzzo, P. (1995). Home health care. In C. M. Smith and F. A. Maurer (Eds.). *Community Health Nursing: Theory and Practice*. Philadelphia, W. B. Saunders.

National Association for Home Care. (1994). *Basic Statistics About Home Care*. Washington, D. C., National Association for Home Care.

National Association for Home Care. (1995). *Basic Statistics About Home Care*. Washington, D. C., National Association for Home Care.

Nelson, B. (1989). Reimbursement alternatives and realities. In I. M. Martinson and A. Widmer (Eds.), *Home Health Care Nursing*. Philadelphia, W. B. Saunders.

Rovinski, C. A. and Zastocki, D. K. (1989). *Home Care: A Technical Manual for the Professional Nurse*. Philadelphia, W. B. Saunders.

Sebastian, J. G. (1989). Nutrition in home health. In I. M. Martinson and A. Widmer (Eds.). *Home Health Care Nursing*. Philadelphia, W. B. Saunders.

Sereda, M. M. (1992). Care of clients in the home setting. In M. J. Clark (Ed.). *Nursing in the Community*. Norwalk, CT, Appleton & Lange.

U. S. Department of Health and Human Services, Division of Nursing, Bureau of Health Professions, Public Health Service. (1993). *The Registered Nurse Population: Findings for the National Sample Survey of Registered Nurses, March, 1992*. Washington, D. C., Government Printing Office.

Warhola, C. (1980). *Planning for Home Health Services: A Resource Handbook*. DHHS Publication No. (HRA) 80-14017. Washington, D. C., U. S. Department of Health and Human Services.

Widmar, A. and Martinson, I. M. (1989). The continuum of care: Partners in acute and chronic care. In I. M. Martinson and A. Widmar (Eds.). *Home Health Care Nursing*. Philadelphia, W. B. Saunders.

8

Home Health Nursing: The Process

Case Study

Molly Morgan is employed by the Visiting Nurse Association in a large metropolitan area. Each day Molly sees four to six clients, mostly elderly, with a variety of health problems.

One recent Wednesday, she saw Mrs. Thornton, a 76-year-old client with insulin-dependent diabetes and related peripheral vascular disease. Mrs. Thornton was admitted to a local hospital 3 weeks ago for treatment of ulcerations on her left leg and great toe. While hospitalized, Mrs. Thornton underwent a left femoral-popliteal bypass graft, which improved her circulation; however, her great toe became gangrenous and was amputated 3 days after the bypass surgery. Because of poor arterial blood flow and the extent of the surgical amputation, her foot has not yet healed and requires daily dressing changes. Mrs. Thornton was discharged from the hospital 2 weeks ago and is being seen daily for the dressing changes and diabetes teaching. Although Mrs. Thornton is a widow and lives alone, she has two children in the area who help her on a regular basis.

Mrs. Thornton is receiving several services from the home health agency. In addition to daily skilled nursing visits, a home health aide comes three times per week to help with personal care and light housekeeping, and a physical therapist comes twice weekly for assessment of her home for modifications and equipment (such as hand rails in the bathtub or rearranging furniture) that will assist her in her activities of daily living, as well as instruction on how to use a walker.

Molly arrived at Mrs. Thornton's residence within 15 minutes of her anticipated time. Before leaving her car, Molly quickly reviewed her daily assignment—"V.S./cardiovascular assessment; wet-to-dry dressing change, left foot; diabetes teaching—needs supply of sterile 4 × 4s, normal saline, 4-inch gauze, and sterile gloves." Molly grabbed her large shoulder bag, which contains basic supplies and equipment used in most visits, from the back seat. She then retrieved sufficient supplies from the stock in her trunk to provide care for Mrs. Thornton for a week and approached the front door.

When she scheduled this morning's appointment, Mrs. Thornton had told Molly that the door would be left open and for her to "come on in," as it was still very difficult for Mrs. Thornton to walk. Molly knocked loudly on the door, waited a few seconds, and opened the door. "Hello, Mrs. Thornton. It's Molly from the VNA," she said. Mrs. Thornton answered from the back bedroom and called enthusiastically for Molly to come back.

When she entered the bedroom, Molly found Mrs. Thornton sitting in a recliner with her left foot on a pillow. She was dressed in a loose-fitting house dress, and her hair was neatly combed. Molly used the initiation phase of her visit to begin her assessments. During a few minutes of greeting and small talk, Molly determined that her client's cognitive state was alert, oriented, and appropriate. Psychologically, Mrs. Thornton appeared cheerful, stating that her younger son had brought her grandchildren for a visit last night and had promised to return in a couple of days. She denied having any pain in her left foot and stated she slept well last night.

Molly washed her hands in the adjacent bathroom with antimicrobial soap taken from her bag and dried them with paper towels that she also had brought with her. While questioning Mrs. Thornton about her physical health and related concerns, Molly removed her blood pressure cuff, stethoscope, and thermometer from the bag and then took Mrs. Thornton's vital signs. These were documented in a chart left in the client's home, as well as in the permanent record. Molly noted that all vital signs were consistent with readings charted over the last several days and began a head-to-toe examination, including listening to heart, lung, and bowel sounds; noting skin color, temperature, and turgor; and observing eye movements and hearing ability. Throughout the examination, Molly asked questions eliciting information regarding urinary and bowel habits, appetite, and nutrition. Molly was particularly concerned with assessment of Mrs. Thornton's peripheral pulses and noted moderate (2+) edema in both lower legs. She was able to palpate all pulses and noted that no change had occurred since yesterday. Capillary refill on the toes on Mrs. Thornton's right foot was good, and the skin was warm and dry to touch.

Following the assessment, Molly was ready to change the dressing. First she added the supplies she had brought with her to those on Mrs. Thornton's shelf. She put on nonsterile gloves to remove the soiled dressing, noting a small amount of serous drainage on the dressing, which she carefully placed in a plastic bag along with the gloves. She examined the wound and determined that the edges were pink and granulating; no odor and no sign of infection were present. Molly then set out the needed supplies and performed the dressing change, using careful, sterile technique. Mrs. Thornton reported no unusual pain in her foot and stated that she felt it was slowly improving. Molly quickly disposed of the trash in a designated container in Mrs. Thornton's bathroom and washed her hands again.

Molly then returned to discuss diabetes with her client. Mrs. Thornton tests her blood glucose levels twice each day and records them in a log. Molly reviewed this log and saw that this morning before breakfast, Mrs. Thornton's blood glucose was 120, which was consistent with readings from the past several days. She reported having taken her prescribed insulin prior to a breakfast of a hard-boiled egg, two pieces of toast, and cranberry juice. Molly reviewed Mrs. Thornton's planned meals for the day and determined that they fit well with her 1800-calorie, American Diabetes Association diet.

Molly charted pertinent information on the flow sheet that remained in the home and completed much of the information on her permanent records. She then asked Mrs. Thornton if she needed anything before she left and stated that she would be back at about the same time tomorrow. Molly carefully collected all of her equipment and supplies. As she was leaving, Molly questioned Mrs. Thornton about locking the front door, and they agreed that it would be best if she did, as no other visitors were expected until later that evening.

In her car, Molly reviewed the charting on her nurse's notes to make sure all forms were complete and filled out a requisition for the supplies left in Mrs. Thornton's home. She placed these papers in a folder to return to the agency, glanced at the address for her next scheduled visit, locked her car doors, and drove to her next patient's residence.

As described in Chapter 7, home health nursing involves providing complex, comprehensive, individualized care to individuals and their families in their place of residence. Home health nursing may be specialized and/or generalized and is always detail intensive. Orientation, education, and training of nurses into home health nursing practice should be comprehensive and specific and include significant time spent with preceptors. Chapter 7 introduced the *practice* of home health nursing, including distinctive and essential elements, standards, reimbursement, and related issues, giving an overview of the services provided by home health nurses. This chapter, in contrast, focuses on the *process* of the home health nursing visit and gives specific instructions on how to conduct a home visit and what may be expected and required of the provider.

The process of the home health nursing visit is typically divided into three levels or stages: the previsit/planning stage; the visit, or implementation, stage; and the postvisit stage (Clark, 1995; Humphrey and Milone-Nuzzo, 1991; Smith, 1995). Each of these stages and the home health nurse's activities are described here.

Planning for the Home Health Nursing Visit

To be efficient, safe, and productive, home health care nursing requires a significant amount of previsit planning. Previsit planning involves determining which clients are to be seen during the day and prioritization of the scheduled visits based on a number of factors. For example, one client needs a blood sugar drawn before breakfast, another client needs dressing changes twice a day, and the caregiver of a third client will only be present in the morning to let the nurse into the residence. Other factors to be considered in scheduling include distance between visits, the need to take specimens to the laboratory, the need to coordinate care with other health professionals, and the need to work with physicians. In addition to scheduling, the nurse must be aware of supplies, equipment, medications, teaching materials, and anything else that might be needed and make arrangements for obtaining materials that are not immediately at hand.

The previsit/planning phase consists of those activities that prepare the nurse to accomplish the required tasks of the home visits scheduled. This phase requires a number of considerations as the nurse plans care for all clients to be seen each day. These considerations and activities are outlined here.

CASELOAD SCHEDULING

Assignments and scheduling guidelines for home health clients differ among agencies. The plan of care developed by the admitting nurse and/or "case manager," in collaboration with the physician, determines how often the client will be seen and what services are to be provided during each visit. Often, agencies assign home health nurses a caseload of clients, and each nurse determines which clients to see on which days. In other agencies, all assignments are made from the central office based on individual client needs and available personnel. Typically, the agency assigns nurses based on geographical or distance considerations (e.g., one nurse sees clients in a given area) or based on specialized needs of the client or abilities of the nurse (e.g., infusion therapy or wound care).

Home health nurses usually see four to six patients each day, although this may vary somewhat based on client acuity and prescribed services (e.g., an intravenous infusion may take 2 hours or more) or distances that must be traveled (e.g., in rural areas, the nurse may drive 100 miles or more to see one client). Thus, when planning the day's schedule, the nurse begins with a list of all of clients that will be seen that day. This list should include

- A synopsis of the client's diagnosis(es)
- What services need to be provided during the day's visit
- Any supplies, equipment, or medications needed in the home that are not at hand
- General directions regarding location of each residence (e.g., map coordinates)

From this list, the nurse can begin the process of scheduling client visits. This is typically accomplished during the afternoon or evening before the

TABLE 8–1 **Home Health Nursing Daily Caseload**

Mrs. E. Cooper—Map coordinates, 37G; admit visit; dx—CHF, HTN
Assess: V.S., C/P status, weight, edema—lower extremities, nutrition status, medication compliance
Teaching: HTN, low-Na diet, medication regimen
Special considerations: Daughter to be in the home 09:00–12:00—requests SNV when she is present

Mr. C. McClure—Map coordinates, 38D; return visit; dx—post-CVA (anticoagulant therapy)
Assess: V.S., C/P status, neuro status, weight, nutrition status, medication compliance
Teaching: Anticoagulant therapy (s/sx of complications, medication regimen, safety)
Special considerations: Lab draw—protime—specimen to lab within 30 minutes; call M.D. with results before 14:00.

Mr. T. Johnson—Map coordinates, 23A; return visit; dx—diabetes
Assess: V.S., C/P status, weight, nutrition/diet, blood sugar (fasting), medication compliance
Teaching: IDDM (review materials left in home), observe DFS and self-administration of insulin, ADA diet
Special considerations: Requests SNV around 7:30 to allow breakfast by 8:30

Mrs. M. Charles—Map coordinates, 38M; return visit; dx—wound right foot—BID dressing changes (early A.M. and late afternoon)
Assess: V.S., C/P status, neuro status, nutrition status, medication compliance, wound—right foot
Wound care: Location—right foot; wet-to-dry dressing—cleanse with NS, pack with 2 4 × 4s and secure with 4″ gauze
Teaching: s/sx of infection, safety
Special considerations: Pt had 99.8 temp yesterday—M.D. notified—requests to be called following visit regardless of findings; needs 1 week supply of gauze, NS, sterile gloves, and 4 × 4s

Mrs. G. Grace—Map coordinates, 36A; return visit; dx—urinary incontinence—indwelling catheter
Assess: V.S., C/P status, elimination status, neuro status, nutrition status, skin integrity
Teaching: s/sx of infection, monitoring fluid intake, catheter care
Special considerations: c/g reports catheter leaking—requests change

ADA = American Diabetes Association; BID = twice a day; c/g = caregiver; CHF = congestive heart failure; C/P = cardiopulmonary; CVA = cerebrovascular accident; DFS = diabetic finger stick; dx = diagnosis; HTN = hypertension; IDDM = insulin-dependent diabetes mellitus; lab = laboratory; M.D. = physician; Na = sodium; neuro = neurological; NS = normal saline; pt = patient; s/sx = signs and symptoms; SNV = skilled nursing visit; V.S. = vital signs.

day's visit. Tables 8–1 and 8–2 illustrate examples of typical clients to be seen and scheduling considerations and rationales.

TELEPHONE CONTACT

After the day's preliminary schedule is determined, each client is contacted to inform him or her of the anticipated time for the nursing visit and to briefly explain the purpose of the visit. In addition, the nurse should get specific directions to the residence if this is the first visit and determine if any special additional instructions, requests, or information regarding each client may be needed; for example, scheduling around the presence of a caregiver, or the need to bring additional supplies.

Occasionally, it is impossible to contact the client to schedule the visit. For example, the client may not have a telephone or may not be able to answer it, or he or she may not speak English. In these cases, contacting a relative, neighbor, or other caregiver to establish the time and purpose of the visit should be attempted. Each agency has guidelines on what to do if telephone scheduling is not possible. If no problems (e.g., the client has a physician's appointment or requests an earlier or later time to avoid a conflict) are encountered with the preliminary schedule, the nurse uses this schedule when seeing the day's caseload.

REVIEW OF THE CLIENT'S CHART

Following scheduling, the home health nurse should familiarize himself or herself with the client's plan of care. Chart or case review is a very important step in the care of the home health client. However, this may not be a simple process. Many providers from the home health agency may see the same client. Depending on agency protocols, the client's comprehensive chart may be at the agency or in the possession of the case manager. In many instances, other providers see the client without seeing the master chart and need as much information as possible regarding that client, his or her condition, and the plan of care. Each agency uses different methods to deliver this information. Voice mail or other recorded reports, faxed information, and charts and data left in the home are methods used to manage information about each client and deliver it to health care team members.

TABLE 8–2 **Tentative Schedule—Home Health Nursing Daily Caseload**

Client Prioritization	Rationale
07:30—Mr. Johnson—DFS; IDDM teaching	Pt request and need to take his scheduled insulin and eat breakfast at a prescribed time
08:30—Mrs. Charles—dressing change	BID dressing change should be done as early in the morning as possible to better approximate q12h schedule
09:45—Mrs. McClure—lab draw (protime)	Close proximity to Mrs. Charles; blood may be dropped off on the way to the next client, and the results should be available by 12:00
11:00—Mrs. Cooper—Admit to service; assess CHF and HTN; med teaching	To accommodate daughter's schedule; fairly close proximity to the laboratory and Mr. McClure
12:30—Mrs. Grace—change indwelling catheter	Least pressing with regard to time constraints; near Mrs. Cooper, and the closest to the agency

BID = twice a day; CHF = congestive heart failure; DFS = diabetic finger stick; HTN = hypertension; IDDM = insulin-dependent diabetes mellitus; lab = laboratory; pt = patient; q12h = every 12 hours.

The nurse scheduling the visit should review all available information before seeing the client. If anything is unclear or if the nurse has any questions regarding the care plan, the case manager (if someone other than the scheduled nurse), the physician, the nurse's supervisor, or other appropriate individual should be contacted to answer questions or clarify information, plans, or procedures before the nurse sees the client. This enables the nurse to be prepared for and to better expedite each visit and ensures that all concerns and questions regarding the client's care are addressed.

ASSESSMENT OF PERSONAL SUPPLIES AND EQUIPMENT

Another important step in previsit planning involves daily inventory of the nurse's bag and routine periodic inventory of the car stock of supplies. Table 8–3 lists suggested supplies and equipment that the home health nurse may carry with him or her for all visits, and Table 8–4 suggests supplies that should be readily available in the nurse's car stock. Based on agency guidelines and variations in the nurse's practice (e.g., if he or she is a member of the intravenous team or is a wound specialist), these supplies may vary. The car stock should be checked periodically for expired supplies and to ensure that no supplies are damaged and should be replenished as necessary. The bag should be inventoried and replenished daily.

TABLE 8–3 Suggested Contents of a Home Health Nurse's Bag

Large shoulder bag with multiple compartments and zippered closure

Medical Equipment/Supplies

Antimicrobial soap (preferably liquid) and paper towels; alcohol foam
Stethoscope
Sphygmomanometer
Thermometer (oral and rectal or tympanic) and appropriate covers
Penlight or flashlight
Tape measure and/or small ruler
Alcohol wipes
Nonsterile gloves (dozen pairs)
Nonsterile disposable gown or apron
Nonsterile waterproof pads (chux)
Disposable masks
Goggles
Sterile gloves (three or four pairs)
Dressing supplies (4-inch gauze squares [4 × 4s], 2-inch gauze squares [2 × 2s]), 3-inch and 4-inch dressing gauze, sterile applicators, silk and paper tape, sterile saline, adhesive bandages)
Venipuncture supplies (e.g., assortment of vacutainer needles, tubes, syringes, tourniquet)
Glucometer and strips
Sterile specimen cup, culture tubes
Bandage scissors
Forceps
Biohazard containers and bags

Other Materials

Map
Agency and Medicare required forms and charting materials and information
Laboratory forms and plastic pouches for transporting laboratory specimens
Teaching materials
"Pocket" medication reference book
"Pocket" nursing interventions reference book
Plastic trash bags
Bathroom scale

SAFETY CONCERNS AND PREVISIT PLANNING

It is important to note that several safety concerns apply to home health care nurses. Typically, home health nurses work alone; they may go into questionably "safe" neighborhoods; they may drive many miles in adverse weather conditions; and some encounter threatening situations. To assist in minimizing threats, Table 8–5 provides general information on safety in home health.

To enhance communication between the nurse and the agency and to promote safety, most agencies supply nurses with beepers. Many agencies also supply nurses with cellular telephones.

The final aspect of previsit planning should include notification of the agency of the nurse's anticipated schedule. This allows the agency to trace or monitor the movement of the nurse and, with the use of the beeper or cellular telephone, to contact him or her if necessary.

TABLE 8–4 **Suggested Contents of a Home Health Nurse's "Car Stock"**

Dressing Supplies

Two or three dozen packages of sterile 2 × 2s and 4 × 4s
3-inch and 4-inch gauze dressings (6–12 packages of each)
Sterile abdominal dressing (ABD) pads (box)
Hypertonic dressing gauze
Nonstick dressing gauze (e.g., telfa, adaptic)
Hydrocolloid dressings (several boxes in a variety of sizes)
Adhesive bandages (one box of assorted sizes; "spots" for venipunctures)
Alcohol wipes (one box)
Sterile gloves (one or two boxes)
Nonsterile gloves (one or two boxes)
Assortment of tapes
Sterile scissors (two or three pairs)
Sterile forceps (two or three pairs)
Staple remover (one or two)
Suture removal kit(s)
Steri strips (several sizes)
Sterile saline (several containers)
Hydrogen peroxide (two or three bottles)
Other dressings, ointments, solutions, and supplies based on factors such as client needs, physician preferences

Catheters and Related Equipment and Supplies

Adult briefs (variety of sizes)
Catheter insertion kits (two)
Indwelling catheters (variety of sizes)
Red rubber catheters (variety of sizes)
Catheter drainage bags (two)
Catheter irrigation kit (two)
Sterile water for irrigation (three or four bottles)
Catheter leg bag (two)
Underpads (waterproof pads—chux) (two packages)
Urine specimen containers (sterile; three or four)

Miscellaneous Equipment and Supplies for Routine Visits

Variety of needles and syringes
Lancets and chemstrips for glucometer (if used)
Restraints
Lubricating jelly
Levine tube (two)
Trash bags (one box)
Pill boxes (two)
Disposable masks and aprons or gowns (several of each)

Miscellaneous Equipment and Supplies for Specialized Home Care (When Applicable)

Enterostomal therapy supplies (e.g., colostomy, ileostomy bags, stomahesive)
Infusion therapy supplies (e.g., variety of administration sets, syringes, injectable solutions)
Respiratory therapy or tracheotomy supplies (e.g., suction tubes, suction tips and catheters, tracheotomy care trays)
Gastrointestinal feeding supplies (e.g., variety of bags, tubings)

The Home Visit Activities

Smith (1995) divides the home health visit into three phases: initiation, implementation, and termination. Specific activities for each are described here.

INITIATION PHASE

The initiation phase begins as the nurse knocks on the door and gains entrance into the residence. She or he should identify herself or himself and the agency and briefly review the purpose of the visit. For example, the nurse might say "Good morning, Mrs. Johnson, I'm Mary Smith from the

TABLE 8–5 **Safety Tips for Home Health Nurses**

- Maintain car; keep gas tank at least half full
- Lock all car doors at all times; keep windows rolled up
- Park as close to the entrance to the client's residence as possible
- Use a map; know where clients live; get directions
- Keep purse in the car trunk; carry change and identification in a pocket
- Dress appropriately, conservatively, professionally (according to agency guidelines); wear comfortable shoes, minimal jewelry, and name tag
- Pay attention to uncomfortable, intuitive "feelings"; if the setting or situation seems unsafe, leave at once
- Avoid walking by groups of individuals loitering near building entrances and/or isolated places
- Never walk into a home uninvited; always knock and wait at the door to be "let in" either physically or verbally
- If pets are annoying or threatening, request that they be removed to another room before entering the home
- Know the agency's policy regarding safety; some agencies will provide a security guard, assistant, or escort to accompany providers in questionably safe areas
- Visit only during scheduled hours; if exceptions must be made, notify supervisor

Data from Clark, M. J. (1995). *Nursing in the Community* (2nd ed.). Norwalk, CT, Appleton & Lange; Smith, C. M. (1995). The home visit: Opening the doors for family health. In C. M. Smith and F. A. Maurer (Eds.). *Community Health Nursing: Theory and Practice.* Philadelphia, W. B. Saunders.

Visiting Nurses' Association and am here to change Mr. Johnson's dressing." The nurse should greet all in attendance and determine who is the primary caregiver for the client, if appropriate. (Often, the client lives alone.)

There may a *brief* social phase that can be used to begin assessments and establish rapport. A standard greeting, such as "How are you doing this morning" lets the nurse begin collecting data on the client's physical, psychological, and social well-being. A brief discussion about the weather, holidays, or news events allows the nurse to assess cognitive status, and talking for a few minutes with the caregiver(s) can convey caring and assist with assessment of the family situation, as well as with concerns, abilities, and understanding level of the caregiver. At this point and throughout the visit, the nurse should continually assess the surroundings to determine potential threats to the client's condition or safety.

During this brief social phase, the nurse should review the chart or records left in the home. He or she should make sure that permissions are signed or should obtain them if this is the initial visit. At this time, the nurse may open his or her bag and begin removing needed equipment, such as a blood pressure cuff and stethoscope. The nurse should also remove the soap and paper towels from the bag and excuse himself or herself briefly to the bathroom or kitchen to wash hands. The nurse is now ready to begin the physical assessment and implement the plan of care.

IMPLEMENTATION PHASE

The implementation phase is the "working" component of home health care provision. During this phase, assessments are conducted, skilled nursing care is provided, and teaching is accomplished.

Assessment

Assessment in home health nursing involves a number of different areas. In addition to thorough physical assessment, assessment of psychosocial needs, functional abilities, medication, nutrition, safety issues, and the client's environment is essential. Tables 8–6 through 8–8 give examples of assessment tools that can be used for home health care. Home health agencies typically develop their own assessment tools and provide the requisite forms for documentation of assessment in each of these areas.

Typically, a thorough database is completed during the initial admission visit. From this database, the plan of care is developed to address identified needs and appropriate skilled nursing interventions, as well as other therapies (e.g., physical therapy, occupational therapy) and ancillary assistance (e.g., home health aide assistance

Text continued on page 198

TABLE 8–6 Guidelines for Recording Health History

Client's name ______________________ Date of birth __________ Age _____
ID number ______________________ Race/ethnic origin ______________________
Date of admission ______________________ Date of initial assessment ______________________
Medical diagnosis: Primary ______________________ Secondary ______________________
Attending physician ______________________ Primary nurse ______________________
Rehabilitation team members ______________________
Informant: Client ______________________ Family member ______________________
Reliability of historian: Good ________ Fair ________ Poor ________

Physical/Functional History

1. How would you describe your general health? Excellent ______ Very good ______ Good ______ Fair ______ Poor ______
2. Breathing
   a. Have you had any difficulty breathing before or with this admission? No ________ Yes ________
      If yes, describe the difficulty ______________________
   b. What can be done during your rehabilitation to make breathing easier for you? ______________________
   c. Do you expect any difficulties in breathing when you return home? ______________________
3. Nutrition
   a. How would you describe your nutrition? Excellent ________ Very good ________ Good ________ Fair ________ Poor ________
   b. Describe a typical day's food intake ______________________
   c. What is your weight? ________
   d. What foods do you like the best? ______________________
   e. What foods do you like the least? ______________________
   f. Are you now or have you ever been on a special diet? No ________ Yes ________
      If yes, what was the diet? ______________________
   g. At what times do you usually eat?
   h. Have you needed any assistance to eat? No ________ Yes ________
      If yes, what types of assistance? ______________________
   i. What is the condition of your mouth? Good ________ Cavities ________ Gum disease ________
      Other ________ Specify other ______________________
   j. Do you wear dentures? No ________ Yes ________ Upper ________ Lower ________ Partial ________
4. Elimination
   a. Bladder
      (1) Have you had any difficulty passing urine? No ________ Yes ________
          If yes, what was the problem? ______________________
          what did you do about it? ______________________
          what treatment, if any, did you receive? ______________________
      (2) Do you frequently experience any of the following symptoms?
          Incontinence ________ Foul-smelling urine ________
          Urgency ________ Cloudy urine ________
          Frequency ________ Burning on urination ________
          Pain on urination ________ Bloody urine ________
          If yes, to any of the above problems, what was done about it? ______________________

Table continued on following page

TABLE 8–6 **Guidelines for Recording Health History** *Continued*

Physical/Functional History *Continued*

(3) Do you need any assistance with bladder elimination? No ________ Yes ________
If yes, what type of assistance do you need? ________

b. Bowel
(1) How would you describe your bowel habits? Regular ________ Irregular ________
(2) How often do you usually have a bowel movement? Every day ________ Every other day ________
Twice a week ________ Once a week ________ Other ________
(3) What time of day do you usually have a bowel movement? Morning ________ Afternoon ________
Evening ________
(4) Tell me if you do any of the following things to assist you in having a bowel movement:
Eat certain foods ________ Specify ________
Drink certain fluids ________ Specify ________
Take medications ________ Specify ________
Insert suppositories ________ Specify ________
Perform digital stimulation ________ Perform Valsalva maneuver ________
Specify other ________
(5) Do you frequently experience any of the following problems?
Diarrhea ________ Impaction ________
Constipation ________ Incontinence ________
Specify other ________
If yes to any of the above, what did you do about the problem? ________
____
What treatment, if any, did you receive? ________
____
(6) Do you need any assistance in getting to the bathroom? No ________ Yes ________
If yes, what type of assistance? ________

5. Skin integrity
a. How would you describe the condition of your skin? Excellent ________ Very good ________
Good ________ Fair ________ Poor ________
b. Do you bruise easily? No ________ Yes ________
c. Have you every had open sores or ulcers that are slow to heal? No ________ Yes ________
d. Have you ever had rashes? No ________ Yes ________
e. Have you ever had moles that have grown? No ________ Yes ________
f. Do you sweat easily? No ________ Yes ________
g. Have you ever had itchy skin? No ________ Yes ________
h. If yes to any of the above problems, describe the circumstances and what you did about the problem. ________
____
____

6. Rest/comfort
a. Rest
(1) How would you describe the amount of rest you get? Always enough ________ Enough ________
Sometimes enough ________ Never enough ________
(2) What time do you usually go to bed? ________ Get up in the morning? ________
(3) Do you have any difficulty going to sleep at night? Always ________ Usually ________
Sometimes ________ Never ________
(4) Do you awaken during the night? Always ________ Usually ________ Sometimes ________
Never ________
(5) Do you take naps? No ________ Yes ________ If yes, when? ________
(6) What aids, if any, do you use to go to sleep at night?
Drink warm liquids ________ Read ________
Take an alcoholic beverage ________ Turn night light on in room ________
Watch television ________ Take sleeping pills ________

TABLE 8–6 **Guidelines for Recording Health History** *Continued*

Physical/Functional History *Continued*

b. Comfort

(1) How would you describe your physical comfort? Always very comfortable ________
Usually comfortable ________ Sometimes comfortable ________ Never comfortable ________

(2) Have you experienced discomfort in the past? No ________ Yes ________
If yes, describe ____
____
What did you do about it? ____
Did it help? No ________ Yes ________ Partially ________

(3) If you have discomfort during your rehabilitation program, what would you like the nurse or therapists to do about it? ____
____

7. Personal hygiene/grooming

a. Have you needed the help of another person with
Bathing ________ Shaving ________
Brushing/combing your hair ________ Applying makeup ________
Brushing your teeth ________ Feminine hygiene ________
Applying deodorant ________ Dressing: Uppers ________ Lowers ________ Both ________

b. Have you used any adaptive aids to assist with any personal hygiene or grooming activities?
No ________ Yes ________
If yes, specify ____

8. Communication

a. Vision

(1) How would you describe your vision? Excellent ________ Very good ________ Good ________
Fair ________ Poor ________

(2) Do you wear glasses? All the time ________ For reading ________ Never ________

(3) Do you wear contact lenses? All the time ________ While awake ________ Sometimes ________
Never ________

b. Hearing

(1) How would you describe your hearing?
Right ear: Excellent ________ Very good ________ Good ________ Fair ________ Poor ________
Left ear: Excellent ________ Very good ________ Good ________ Fair ________ Poor ________

(2) Have you ever had pain in either ear? No ________ Yes ________

(3) Have you ever had ringing in your ears? No ________ Yes ________

(4) Have you ever had a discharge from either ear? No ________ Yes ________

(5) If yes to any of these problems, describe ____
____
What did you do about it? ____
What treatment, if any, did you receive? ____
____

c. Sensation/perception

(1) Do you have any difficulties with feeling pain? No ________ Yes ________
With feeling temperature? No ________ Yes ________

(2) Do you have any intolerance to temperature? No ________ Yes ________

(3) If yes to 1 or 2, describe ____
____
What do you do about the problem? ____

Table continued on following page

TABLE 8–6 **Guidelines for Recording Health History** *Continued*

Physical/Functional History *Continued*

d. Speech/language
   (1) How would you describe your ability to express yourself? Excellent ________ Very good ________ Good ________ Fair ________ Poor ________
   (2) How would you describe your ability to understand others? Excellent ________ Very good ________ Good ________ Fair ________ Poor ________
   (3) Have you ever had difficulty expressing yourself? No ________ Yes ________
   If yes, describe the circumstances ________
   (4) Have you ever had difficulty understanding others? No ________ Yes ________
   If yes, describe the circumstances ________

9. Mobility (ask questions appropriate to client's mobility status)
   a. How would you describe your ability to get out of or into a bed or chair? Excellent ________ Very good ________ Good ________ Fair ________ Poor ________
   b. How would you describe your ability to get into the bathtub? Excellent ________ Very good ________ Good ________ Fair ________ Poor ________
   c. How would you describe your ability to walk/navigate a wheelchair? Excellent ________ Very good ________ Good ________ Fair ________ Poor ________
   d. Have you ever had difficulty moving about? No ________ Yes ________
   If yes, describe the difficulty ________
   How did you manage? ________
   e. Do you expect to have any difficulty getting around when you leave the rehabilitation unit?
   No ________ Yes ________
   If yes, what do you expect to do about it? ________

10. Sexuality (ask questions according to client's marital status)
   a. How would you describe your sex life? Very satisfactory ________ Satisfactory ________ Not very satisfactory ________
   b. Has there been or do you expect differences in your ability to be a
   Husband No ________ Yes ________
   Father No ________ Yes ________
   Wife No ________ Yes ________
   Mother No ________ Yes ________
   Significant other No ________ Yes ________
   If yes, describe what you expect the differences to be ________
   ____
   c. Do you expect your sexual functioning to be changed in any way after your rehabilitation?
   No ________ Yes ________
   If yes, describe expected changes ________
   ____
   d. Do you want the nurse to obtain more information about sexual function for you?
   No ________ Yes ________
   If yes, specify interests ________
   Refer you to a sex counselor? No ________ Yes ________

Psychosocial History

1. What is your marital status? Married ________ Divorced ________ Separated ________ Widowed ________ Never married ________
2. Do you have any children? No ________ Yes ________
   If yes, how many? ________ What are their ages? ________
3. What type of housing do you live in? Upper apartment ________ Lower apartment ________ Ranch ________ Two or more story dwelling ________
4. How many people live in your home? ________
5. Where do you sleep? ________

TABLE 8–6 **Guidelines for Recording Health History** *Continued*

Psychosocial History *Continued*

6. Where is the bathroom located? ________
7. How would you describe your relationships with others living in your home? Excellent ____
   Very good ____ Good ____ Fair ____ Poor ____
   If fair or poor, would you like to tell me anything about these relationships? ________
   ____
8. Do you have any interests or hobbies? No ____ Yes ____
   If yes, describe ________
9. How far did you go in school?
   Grammar school ____ College graduate ____
   Some high school ____ Some graduate school ____
   High school graduate ____ Graduate school degree ____
   Some college ____
10. What are your habits?
    Smoking ____ How long? ____ How many packs/day? ____
    Drinking ____ How long? ____ How much? ____
    Drugs ____ How long? ____ How much? ____
    Coffee ____ How many cups/day? ____
    Exercise ____ Type ____ How often? ____ How long? ____
11. Coping
    a. How would you describe your coping abilities? Excellent ____ Very good ____ Good ____
       Fair ____ Poor ____
    b. What do you do when you are upset? ________
       ____
    c. Does it help? No ____ Yes ____
12. Relationships
    a. Who is the most important person to you? ________
    b. How many close friends do you have? ________
    c. What effect has your disability had on your family and friends? ________
       ____
    d. Do you expect your family and friends to visit during your rehabilitation program? ________
    e. Who of your friends or family would you most like to assist with your rehabilitation program? ________
       ____
    f. Who should be notified in case of an emergency? ________
       Telephone number ________
       Address ________

Economic/Vocational History

1. What is your occupation? Present ________ Past ________
   Unemployed ________ If unemployed, are you retired? No ____ Yes ____
2. How would you describe your financial resources? Excellent ____ Very good ____ Good ____
   Fair ____ Poor ____
3. How will you pay for your rehabilitation program?
   Self, family ____ Vocational rehabilitation agency ____
   Insurance plan ____ Medicaid ____
   Worker's compensation ____ Medicare ____
   Specify other ________

Table continued on following page

TABLE 8–6 **Guidelines for Recording Health History** *Continued*

Spiritual History

1. Do you practice a religion? No ________ Yes ________
   If yes, what denomination? Catholic ________ Protestant ________ Jewish ________
   Specify other ____
   a. Do you attend a place of worship regularly? No ________ Yes ________
   b. Do you have any dietary restrictions as part of your religious practices? No ________ Yes ________
   c. Would you like to see a chaplain while you are here? No ________ Yes ________
2. Do you feel your spiritual needs are met? Yes ________ No ________
   If no, is there anything the nurse can do to assist you in meeting your spiritual needs? ____

Other

1. What do you know about your current health concerns? ____
2. Do you have any questions right now about your current health concerns? ____

From Boucher, R. J. (1989). Nursing process. In S. S. Dittmar (Ed.). *Rehabilitation Nursing: Process and Application.* St. Louis, MO, C. V. Mosby.

with activities of daily living) that will be administered as appropriate. During subsequent visits, less comprehensive, more directed assessments are conducted. During each visit, the nurse takes vital signs and performs a routine head-to-toe assessment, including assessment of the respiratory system (e.g., listening to breath sounds, quality of respirations, assessing presence or absence of cough), cardiovascular system (e.g., rate, rhythm, heart sounds, presence or absence of chest pain, peripheral pulses, capillary refill, edema), neurological system (e.g., whether the patient is alert and oriented, reactivity of pupils, ability to move extremities, and equal strength of same), gastrointestinal system (e.g., abdomen; bowel sounds; any distention, masses, or tenderness; nausea, vomiting, or diarrhea; last bowel movement; and appetite), urinary system (e.g., frequency of urination, any burning, unusual odor), and skin integrity (e.g., turgor, temperature, color, any redness, open areas or wounds). Particular attention is given to those areas related to identified problems or potential problems. For example, if the client has diabetes, the nurse should very carefully assess the feet for adequate circulation and evidence of skin breakdown, or if the client has been diagnosed with congestive heart failure, careful attention to cardiovascular and respiratory function, including monitoring of weight and signs of peripheral edema, is essential.

After the home health nurse has washed his or her hands, the assessment is begun. An individual routine is usually established, wherein the nurse develops a pattern to ensure that all systems and areas are covered during the assessment. Most nurses usually begin by taking and charting vital signs. Comparison with previous readings and notation of significant changes may dictate unplanned actions or interventions (e.g., if the client has developed a temperature since yesterday or if the blood pressure is unusually high, the physician may need to be called immediately). While taking

Text continued on page 207

TABLE 8–7 **Assessment of Immediate Living Environment**

Client's name ________________
Date ________________

Parameters	Assessment	Recommendations
Neighborhood	Adequate ___ Inadequate ___	
Amount of physical space	Adequate ___ Inadequate ___	
Cleanliness	Adequate ___ Inadequate ___	
Convenient toilet facilities	Adequate ___ Inadequate ___	
Useable and accessible telephone	Adequate ___ Inadequate ___	
Adequate and safe heating	Adequate ___ Inadequate ___	
Stairways and halls	Adequate ___ Inadequate ___	
Cooking facilities	Adequate ___ Inadequate ___	
Tub, shower, hot water	Adequate ___ Inadequate ___	
Laundry facilities	Adequate ___ Inadequate ___	
Physical barriers in home	Present ___ Absent ___	
Physical barriers to exits from home	Present ___ Not present ___	
Physical hazards	Present ___ Not present ___	
Home accessible to caregivers	Yes ___ No ___	
Use of alcohol or drugs by patient or caregiver	Yes ___ No ___	
Client mobility	Adequate ___ Inadequate ___	
Client safety	Adequate ___ Inadequate ___	
Escort necessary	Yes ___ No ___	
Pets	Yes ___ No ___	

Strengths of physical environment: ________________

Areas of concern: ________________

From A. H. Skelly (1990). Physical disabilities and rehabilitation. The role of the nurse in the community. In B. Bullough and V. Bullough (Eds.). *Nursing in the Community.* St. Louis, MO, Mosby–Year Book.

TABLE 8–8 **Adult Nursing Assessment Database**

Name ____________________
Address ____________________
City, state ____________________
Phone number ____________________
Marital status ____________________
Private physician ____________________

Age ________ Sex ________
Race ____________________
Religion ____________________
Occupation ____________________
Place of employment ____________________
Education ____________________

Health History

Check the problems that you presently have or have had that were diagnosed and treated by a physician.

Yes	***No***	***Problem***
		Alcoholism
		Anemia
		Bleeding trait
		Bronchitis
		Cancer
		Breast
		Cervix
		Lung
		Uterus
		Other
		Cirrhosis
		Colitis
		Depression
		Diabetes
		Emphysema
		Fibrocystic breast
		Heart problems
		Heart attack
		Coronary disease
		Rheumatic heart
		Heart valve problem
		Heart murmur
		Enlarged heart
		Heart rhythm problem
		Other

Yes	***No***	***Problem***
		High blood pressure
		High blood fats
		Cholesterol
		Triglycerides
		Obesity (more than 20 pounds overweight
		Pneumonia
		Polyps in colon
		Rheumatic fever
		Stroke
		Suicide
		Tuberculosis

In the past year have you had

Yes	***No***	
		Chest pain on exertion relieved by rest?
		Shortness of breath lying down, relieved by sitting up?
		Unexplained weight loss of more than 10 pounds?
		Unexplained rectal bleeding?
		Unexplained vaginal bleeding?

Family Medical History

Check items that apply to your blood relatives (parents, grandparents, siblings, children)

Yes	***No***	***Illness***
		Anemia
		Bleeding trait
		Cancer
		Diabetes
		Heart disease

Yes	***No***	***Illness***
		High blood pressure
		Mental illness
		Stroke
		Suicide
		Tuberculosis

TABLE 8–8 **Adult Nursing Assessment Database** *Continued*

Family Medical History *Continued*

Check the items that apply:

Yes	No	
______	______	Father died of heart attack before age 60
______	______	Mother died of heart attack before age 60
______	______	Mother or sister had breast cancer

Surgical History

List any operations and dates ______________________________

____

Females: describe obstetric history (if appropriate) ______________________________

____

____

List childhood illnesses ______________________________

____

____

Immunizations:	Yes	No
Tetanus	______	______
Pertussis	______	______
Diphtheria	______	______
Polio	______	______
Measles	______	______
Rubella (German measles)	______	______
Mumps	______	______
Flu	______	______

List any allergies (food, drugs, other) ______________________________

____

List current medications (if appropriate) ______________________________

____

____

Psychological History

Mark the frequency with which you have the feelings listed by placing a check mark in the appropriate column (*M*—most of the time; *S*—some of the time; *R*—rarely or none)

M	S	R	
______	______	______	Feel sad, depressed?
______	______	______	Wish to end it all?
______	______	______	Feel tense and anxious?
______	______	______	Worry about things generally?
______	______	______	More aggressive and hard driving than friends?
______	______	______	Have an intense desire to achieve?
______	______	______	Feel optimistic about the future?

Table continued on following page

TABLE 8–8 **Adult Nursing Assessment Database** *Continued*

Social History

Family members (parents, siblings, spouse, children, grandparents)
List family members, their ages, and health status or cause of death ______

Educational history (schools attended, diplomas or degrees earned) ______

Marital history (how many years; any past or present difficulties) ______

Work history (types and places of employment) ______

Leisure time activities ______

Financial status (plans for retirement, insurance, medical coverage) ______

Environmental Background

Place of residence: apartment ______ home ______ Do you own? Yes ___ No ___
Travel time to work or school ______
Means of transportation ______
Environmental pollutants in area of residence ______
Place of residence in past and travel history ______

Describe present neighborhood (noisy or quiet; location to shopping, social, cultural, and religious centers) ______

Review of Systems

Head and neck ______
Skin ______
Respiratory ______
Cardiovascular ______
Gastrointestinal ______
Genitourinary ______
Reproductive ______
Musculoskeletal ______
Central nervous ______
Endocrine ______
Circulatory ______

Physical Examination

Height ______ Weight ______
Blood pressure ______ Pulse ______ Respirations ______ Temperature ______

TABLE 8–8 **Adult Nursing Assessment Database** *Continued*

Functional Health Pattern Assessment

The nurse should use these questions as a basis to explore the health patterns listed.

1. Health perception and health management pattern
   How has your general health been?
   Describe the most important things you do to stay healthy.
   Which statement is more like you? "If it's meant to be, I will stay healthy." *or* "If I take care of myself, I will stay healthy."
   Regularly use dental floss?
   Have had dental examination in past 2 years?
   Have had eyes checked in past 2 years?
   Seek professional advice for unusual physical or mental changes?
   Have smoke detector in house?
   Have emergency phone numbers posted?
   (If responsible for children) Keep medicines and cleaning products in locked cabinet?
   Women
   Have had Pap test within a year? Conduct monthly breast self-examinations?
   Men
   Conduct monthly testicular examinations?

   Any concerns about current health practices?
   Behaviors you think you should change? Would like to change?

Strengths and areas for improvement ______________________________
____
____

Weaknesses and problem areas ______________________________
____
____

2. Nutritional and metabolic pattern
   Describe typical daily food and fluid intake.
   Any supplements? Appetite? Discomfort? Diet restrictions?
   Heals well or poorly?
   Skin problems?
   Dental problems?
   Drinks less than three alcoholic beverages (including beer) per week?
   Drinks less than five soft drinks per week?
   Drinks less than three cups of coffee or tea per day?
   Any foods avoided? Why?
   Snacks between meals? What kind?
   Limits intake of refined sugars (junk foods, desserts)
   Adds salt to food? Cooking? At the table?
   Checks ingredients in prepackaged food?
   Adds bran to diet to provide roughage?
   Eats at least one uncooked fruit or vegetable a day?
   Knows ideal weight? Current weight? Recent changes?
   Considers self overweight? Underweight? Ideal weight?
   Any concerns in this area?
   Behaviors you think you should change? Would like to change?

Strengths and areas for improvement ______________________________
____
____

Table continued on following page

TABLE 8–8 **Adult Nursing Assessment Database** *Continued*

Functional Health Pattern Assessment *Continued*

Weaknesses and problem areas ______________________________

3. Elimination pattern
   - Describe bowel elimination pattern.
   - Frequency? Character? Discomfort? Laxatives?
   - Describe urinary elimination pattern.
   - Frequency? Problems with control?
   - Excess perspiration?
   - Odor problem?
   - Any concerns?
   - Behaviors you think you should change? Would like to change?

Strengths and areas for improvement ______________________________

Weaknesses and problem areas ______________________________

4. Activity and exercise pattern
   - Describe daily pattern of activity.
   - Have sufficient energy for desired and required activities?
   - Exercise? Type? How often?
   - Spare time activities?
   - Climb stairs rather than ride elevator?
   - Participate in any strenuous exercise or sports?
   - Engage in warm-up exercises?
   - Participate in sports for competition or enjoyment?
   - Any concerns?
   - Behaviors you think you should change? Would like to change?

Strengths and areas of improvement ______________________________

Weaknesses and problem areas ______________________________

5. Sleep and rest pattern
   - Describe sleep pattern.
   - Generally rested and ready for daily activities after sleeping?
   - Any onset problem? Aids? Dreams? Nightmares? Early awakening?
   - Take time to relax each day? How?
   - Enjoy spending time without planned activities?
   - Any concerns?
   - Behaviors you think you should change? Would like to change?

Strengths and areas for improvement ______________________________

Weaknesses and problem areas ______________________________

6. Cognitive and perception pattern
   - Have hearing difficulties? Aids?

TABLE 8–8 **Adult Nursing Assessment Database** *Continued*

Functional Health Pattern Assessment *Continued*

Have difficulties with vision? Wears glasses? Any pain? Discomfort?
Changes in memory? Describe.
New interest areas?
Easiest way to learn things?
Any difficulty learning?
Any concerns?
Behaviors you think you should change? Would like to change?

Strengths and areas for improvement ______________________________

____

____

Weaknesses and problem areas ______________________________

____

____

7. Self-perception and self-concept pattern
   How would you describe yourself?
   Most of the time, do you feel good or not so good about yourself?
   Perceives self as being well accepted by others?
   Any recent body changes? Changes in the things you do? Is this a problem for you?
   Any changes in the way you feel about your body? Yourself?
   Has an enthusiastic and optimistic outlook?
   Enjoys expressing self through arts, hobbies, or sports?
   Continues to grow and change? Describe.
   Enjoys work or school?
   Member of community group? How active?
   Proud of self?
   Respects own accomplishments?
   Finds it easy to express concern, love, and warmth to others?
   Enjoys meeting and getting to know new people?
   Can accept constructive criticism easily and not react defensively?
   Looks forward to the future?
   Any concerns?
   Behaviors you think you should change? Would like to change?

Strengths and areas for improvement ______________________________

____

____

Weaknesses and problem areas ______________________________

____

____

8. Role and relationship pattern
   Any family problems? Difficulty handling? Describe.
   (If appropriate) problems with children? Difficulty handling? Describe.
   Find it easy or difficult to communicate with others?
   If difficult, with whom? Actions taken to resolve?
   Belong to social groups?
   Enjoy family? Friends?
   Have at least three close friends?
   Things generally go well for you at work or school?
   Enjoy touching other people? Being touched by others?
   Find it easy or difficult to express love, warmth, and concern to those you care about?
   Any concerns?
   Behaviors that you think you should change? Would like to change?

Table continued on following page

TABLE 8–8 **Adult Nursing Assessment Database** *Continued*

Functional Health Pattern Assessment *Continued*

Strengths and areas for improvement ______

Weaknesses and problem areas ______

9. Sexuality and reproductive pattern
   Any problems or changes in sexual relations? Describe.
   (if appropriate) Use of contraceptives? Any problems?
   Any concerns?
   Behaviors you think you should change? Would like to change?

Strengths and areas for improvement ______

Weaknesses and problem areas ______

10. Coping and stress tolerance pattern
    Tense a lot of time? Causes? What helps?
    Who's most helpful when you're distressed? Available now?
    Any big change in your life recently?
    Practice any methods of relaxation? Meditation? Yoga?
    Consider it acceptable to cry, feel sad, angry, or afraid?
    Can laugh at self?
    Able to say no without feeling guilty?
    Any concerns?
    Behaviors you think you should change? Would like to change?

Strengths and areas for improvement ______

Weaknesses and problem areas ______

11. Value and belief pattern
    Generally get things out of life that you want?
    Is religion important? Is it a help when difficulties arise?
    Are you satisfied with how you spend a typical work day? School day? Leisure day?
    Any concerns?
    Behaviors you think you should change? Would like to change?

Strengths and areas for improvement ______

Weaknesses and problem areas ______

Adapted from Koge, N. T. and Bodnar, B. W. (1994). The nursing process. In C. L. Edelman and C. L. Mandel (Eds.). *Health Promotion Throughout the Lifespan* (3rd ed). St. Louis, MO, Mosby-Year Book.

the vital signs and throughout the physical assessment, the nurse can take the opportunity to question the client to obtain additional information (e.g., "When did you have you last bowel movement?" "What did you eat for breakfast?" "Have you noticed any dizziness or pain?"). Follow-up questions to the client's responses of change or identification of possible problems allow the nurse to obtain more information (e.g., "When did you first notice burning when you urinate?" "I see your ankles are a little swollen—have you been up quite a lot?" "Your blood pressure is a little higher than it has been—did you take your medication this morning?"). Any problems should be noted in the visit record and discussed with the physician or case manager as appropriate.

Following the initial visit, much less documentation is required. A revisit summary outlining the routine assessment (described previously) and all findings should be included. This should be followed by narrative description of the purpose of the visit and details of the skilled nursing care given.

Provision of Skilled Nursing Care

Table 7–4 lists Medicare-approved skilled nursing services. The skilled observation and assessment described here is one of the approved services. Others include wound care, venipuncture, administration of medications, tracheotomy, and catheter care, as well as teaching clients and caregivers a variety of skills and services. During each visit, the nurse performs the identified and assigned tasks and documents them according to agency guidelines.

Often, the nursing care performed requires the nurse to use materials carried in his or her bag (e.g., drawing blood, removing sutures or staples) or supplies left in the home (e.g., changing dressings, performing tracheotomy care, administering intravenous medications). As in the acute care setting, the nurse must treat the bag and stock of supplies as "clean" and carefully avoid contamination and cross-contamination. Thus, it is important to remember to remove the supplies and equipment from the bag or stock before beginning the procedures and not to return to the bag without washing hands or removing contaminated gloves. In addition, the nurse should be careful to place the bag on a clean surface (not the floor) and to ensure that children or pets cannot reach it. When leaving equipment and supplies in the home, the same guidelines and procedures should apply, and manufacturer's recommendations regarding storage should be carefully maintained. Dressing supplies, for example, should be placed in a clean cupboard or on a shelf away from the reach of pets and children and away from moisture or extreme heat. Likewise, medications, formulas, and solutions should be stored according to guidelines. If the nurse is unsure of the ability of the client to store supplies properly, he or she should make other arrangements. For example, occasionally a family may not have reliable electricity or a working refrigerator and cannot properly store solutions for total parenteral nutrition. In such a case, the nurse may need to arrange to pick up the prescribed solutions at a pharmacy and bring them with him or her or to store them at a neighbor's residence.

When performing sterile procedures (e.g., dressing changes, insertion of catheters, hanging solutions), it is as important that meticulous technique be followed in the home as in the hospital. In addition, the nurse should ensure that all contaminated materials and waste be disposed of properly. The client and the caregivers should be taught proper management of infectious wastes and the rationale behind such management. Containers for handling sharps should be provided, and methods for appropriate disposal should be taught to the client and the caregiver.

Teaching

In home health care, teaching is one of the most important functions of the nurse. The nurse teaches the client and the caregivers general information about their illness or condition, care or treatment regimen, medications, and identification and reporting of symptoms or complications. In addition, clients and their caregivers may be given specific instructions on a variety of health-related topics, such as self-administration of insulin or other injectable medications, management of an American Diabetic Association diet, self-catheterization, administration of gastrostomy tube feedings, tracheotomy care, bowel training, wound care, or colostomy or ileostomy care.

As discussed in Chapter 2, it is very important to realize that health teaching goes beyond information dissemination. In home health care, the nurse must assess the readiness and ability of the client or caregiver to perform the necessary tasks; present the information in a manner that is understandable to the learner; possibly use several methods, tools, and materials in the instruction process; and carefully, accurately, and thoroughly evaluate the level of understanding and response to the teaching. Observation of the client as he or she performs a sterile dressing change, use of return demonstration in drawing up insulin, and verbalization of principles of infection control are evaluation techniques that the nurse may use to determine how well the client understands the instructions.

Many agencies provide and encourage the use of written materials to assist their nurses in teaching clients and caregivers in home settings. Written instructions are particularly helpful for clients who will be required to perform procedures without the presence of the nurse. Step-by-step guides can be reviewed and discussed with the client and often prove to be very helpful tools. Providing written instruction on areas such as the steps in monitoring blood sugar and self-administration of insulin, the signs and symptoms of complications of anticoagulant therapy and when to notify the physician, the signs and symptoms of urinary tract infection for the client with an indwelling catheter, and the management congestive heart failure can assist in enhancing the client's understanding of his or her health problems; in treating or alleviating symptoms; and in preventing, identifying, or recognizing changes or complications to the condition.

TERMINATION PHASE

Following completion of the skilled nursing interventions and teaching, the home health nurse evaluates the response of the client to care and briefly summarizes the continuing plan of care with the client and caregiver. If care is to be ongoing, the nurse can set up a time for the next home visit. During this phase, the nurse should be careful to gather all equipment and supplies that he or she will take. If any specimens have been collected, these should be placed in appropriate containers, and requisite paperwork completed.

At this point, the nurse should also review potential health emergencies and appropriate actions to take. For example, the nurse might say, "Mrs. Cooper, if you experience any chest pain or shortness or breath or if you gain more than 2 pounds when you weigh yourself in the morning, call your doctor immediately."

Before departure, the nurse should ask the client and caregiver if they have any questions and clarify once more when he or she will return and the purpose of the next visit (e.g., "Good-bye for now, Mrs. Charles. Another nurse will see you this evening, but I will be back about the same time tomorrow to change your dressing" or "Mrs. McClure, I will call your doctor today to report on your laboratory findings. If there are no changes in your Coumadin schedule, I will be back in 2 or 3 weeks to check your clotting times again. I will call you and let you know").

Postvisit Activities

After each visit, several activities must be completed to fulfill the responsibilities of the home health care nurse. These activities include communication of findings to other health care providers (reporting and referral) and documentation (completion of all forms and charting).

COMMUNICATION

Reporting of important assessment and evaluation findings to all appropriate personnel or referral to other providers for follow-up of identified concerns is a very important component of home health care practice. If the nurse seeing the client is the case manager, typically, he or she reports findings or significant changes in the client's condition to the physician. Other providers may also be contacted to refer or initiate services (e.g., occupational therapy, speech therapy). Also, current care providers may be contacted to discuss their assessment of the client (e.g., the nurse might call Mrs. Thornton's physical therapist to discuss whether additional visits might be appropriate to do more in-depth teaching of range of motion exercises.

The home health care nurse should keep the physician informed of the client's condition. Any changes in health status and any significant findings should be reported immediately. If the home health nurse seeing the client is not the case manager, he or she should also report to that nurse, usually following agency guidelines.

Referrals to nonagency providers (e.g., Meals on Wheels, adult day care centers) should be made as appropriate and following agency guidelines. As nurses gain experience in home health care practice, they maintain a list or booklet of community resources to share with their clients. The process of referral is described in Chapter 7.

DOCUMENTATION

The importance of complete, concise, and accurate documentation in home health nursing cannot be overstated. Chapter 7 discussed the purpose and process of documentation in home health care nursing. As described in that chapter, all forms and documents must be completed according to Medicare or other third-party payor guidelines and the home health care agency's requirements. An experienced home health nurse may be able to complete most of the paperwork while in the client's home. However, the nurse should comprehensively review each client's chart at the end of the day.

Documentation should include date and time of reporting to the physician and/or case manager described previously and any actions based on that reporting. For example, "Mrs. Cooper's B/P—160/94; Dr. Black notified @ 13:00; he stated that no changes be made in medication at present, requests that pt's B/P be reevaluated in 2 days. Plan—SNV on Thursday to reevaluate" or "Dr. Brown contacted @ 9:30 and informed that wound edges were reddened, drainage malodorous, and pt reports increased pain. M.D. requested wound C & S be performed and client seen again tomorrow. C & S to lab at 10:30; results available in 24 hrs. Plan—contact lab tomorrow a.m. and schedule p.m. SNV." Often, home health agencies periodically review home care nurses' documentation to ensure comprehensiveness.

SUMMARY

After the home health care nurse has completed the day's visits, the agency should be notified, either in person or by telephone. This includes a brief report of the clients seen that day and any changes or additions to their plans of care. At this time, the nurse can discuss the clients that will need to be seen the next day and/or get the next day's assignment. Agencies vary somewhat on how and when the nurse must return completed papers and charts to the office. Typically, nurses visit the agency every 2 or 3 days to drop off paperwork and replenish supplies. Periodic interdisciplinary team meetings and inservice training classes are scheduled to improve patient care and enhance the nurse's practice, and home care nurses plan agency visits around these meetings.

As this chapter and Chapter 7 have described, home health care is a dynamic, growing field for nursing practice that can be fun, autonomous, flexible, and very rewarding. However, nurses who desire to work in home health care should be experienced and must be well trained and supported by agency management. A comprehensive orientation and ongoing assistance and supervisory support enhance the transition into home health practice and promote highest quality nursing care.

Key Points

- The process of home health nursing is typically divided into three stages—the previsit/planning stage, the visit/implementation stage, and the postvisit stage.
- Previsit planning involves determining which clients are to be seen and prioritization of the scheduled visits. Awareness of supplies, equipment, medications, and teaching materials that might be needed and making arrangements for materials not at hand are important. Planning includes caseload scheduling, making contact by telephone or another method if necessary, review of the client's chart, assessment of supplies and equipment needed and what is on hand, and consideration of safety concerns.
- During the implementation stage, the nurse initiates the visit by identifying himself or herself and reviewing the purpose of the visit. Next, implementation of the scheduled plan of care includes a complete assessment, provision of skilled nursing care, health teaching as necessary, and other interventions. Following completion of the skilled nursing interventions and teaching, the nurse evaluates the response of the client to care, summarizes the continuing plan of care with the client and caregiver, and may set up a time for the next visit.
- Postvisit activities include communication of findings to other health care providers and completing requisite documentation.

Learning Activities and Application to Practice

In Class

- Divide the students into groups of three or four. Encourage them to practice conducting a home visit. One student can act as the patient, one or two can act as caregivers, and one or two can act as the nurses. Practice each stage of the home visit and allow the students to critique each other.

In Clinical

- In a log or diary, have the students list the activities that were accomplished for one home visit within the three stages of a home visit described. Outline what preparations were made during the planning stage, what skilled nursing interventions and teaching were provided during the implementation stage, and describe postvisit activities. If possible, include the rationale chosen for scheduling of the caseload (i.e., what factors were considered in ordering the schedule?).
- Encourage students to review all charts and documentation for at least one client (including forms 485, 486, and 487). If agency policy permits, have students assist in completing the documentation for at least one client.

REFERENCES

Boucher, R. J. (1989). Nursing process. In S. S. Dittmar (Ed.). *Rehabilitation Nursing: Process and Application*. St. Louis, MO, C. V. Mosby, pp. 45–62.

Clark, M. J. (1995). *Nursing in the Community* (2nd ed.). Norwalk, CT, Appleton & Lange.

Humphrey, C. J. and Milone-Nuzzo, P. (1991). *Home Care Nursing: An Orientation to Practice*. Norwalk, CT, Appleton & Lange.

Koge, N. T. and Bodnar, B. W. (1990). The nursing process. In C. L. Edelman and C. L. Mandel (Eds.). *Health Promotion Throughout the Lifespan* (2nd ed.). St. Louis, MO, Mosby–Year Book, pp. 36–64.

Milone-Nuzzo, P. (1995). Home health care. In C. M. Smith and F. A. Maurer (Eds.). *Community Health Nursing: Theory and Practice*. Philadelphia, W. B. Saunders, pp. 776–801.

Skelly, A. H. (1990). Physical disabilities and rehabilitation: The role of nursing in the community. In Bullough, B. and Bullough, V. (Eds.). *Nursing in the Community*. St. Louis, MO, C. V. Mosby.

Smith, C. M. (1995). The home visit: Opening the doors for family health. In C. M. Smith and F. A. Maurer (Eds.). *Community Health Nursing: Theory and Practice*. Philadelphia, W. B. Saunders, pp. 179–204.

9

Specialized Home Health Care

Case Study

Melinda Mitchell is an infusion therapy nurse for a home health care agency in an urban area. Generally, her clients include those with acquired immunodeficiency syndrome (AIDS), who receive a variety of medications for infection control and to improve immune status; those with serious infections that require intravenous antibiotic therapy; and those who are unable to obtain sufficient nutritional intake orally and must have supplemental nutrition. Occasionally, Melinda sees clients diagnosed with cancer to administer chemotherapy.

On a recent Friday, Melinda saw Joe Jefferson, a 75-year-old retired grocer, for administration of intravenous antibiotics. Mr. Jefferson developed a sternal wound infection following coronary artery bypass surgery 3 weeks ago. Intravenous antibiotic therapy was started in the hospital, and Mr. Jefferson was discharged after a 2-week stay. His antibiotic therapy is scheduled to continue for two more weeks. The regimen consists of 1 g vancomycin twice a day, to be administered over 1 hour. In addition to the antibiotic therapy, Mr. Jefferson is scheduled for wet-to-dry dressing changes twice a day for his sternal wound.

Following a brief head-to-toe assessment, Melinda determined that Mr. Jefferson's vital signs were consistent with previous readings, in particular noting that his temperature was 97.6°F. His breath sounds were clear, he had no peripheral edema, and he reported normal bladder and bowel function.

Melinda's agency contracts with an infusion pharmaceutical company to supply the intravenous medications. These are prepared by a pharmacist, following physician's orders, and delivered by the company to the patient's home every 3 days. Melinda retrieved the prepared medication from the refrigerator and checked the label to ensure that the package contained the correct medication and dosage. She collected an infusion set from the supplies kept in the home, then connected and flushed the line.

Because he was scheduled to undergo fairly long-term intravenous therapy, Mr. Jefferson had had a subclavian catheter inserted while he was in the hospital. Following agency protocols and careful sterile technique, Melinda cleaned the infusion port with povidone-iodine, inserted the needle, and began the infusion. She set the drip rate to infuse over 1 hour. While the medication was infusing, Melinda changed the sternal wound dressing using sterile technique. She then assessed Mr. Jefferson's knowledge of his condition and asked if he had any questions or problems. After the medication finished infusing, Melinda again checked the vital signs. As there was no change and no indication of any complications, she prepared to leave. She reminded Mr. Jefferson that another nurse would come at approximately 7:00 pm to infuse the evening dose and change his dressing, and that she would return in the morning.

Home health care, as described in Chapter 7, is rapidly evolving into one of the primary sources for delivery of health care in the United States. Although provision of "traditional" skilled nursing care and health education has been part of home health nursing since the late 1800s, recent advances in health care delivery and changes in health care financing have resulted in dramatic changes in home health care nursing during the past decade. These changes are expected to continue. In addition to traditional skilled care nursing, various therapies (e.g., occupational, physical, speech), and other services offered by home care agencies, specialized services have been added and expanded. For example, infusion therapy, which includes total parenteral nutrition, chemotherapy, and administration of other pharmacotherapeutics, is becoming increasingly common. Other areas of specialized care that are now being provided in the home include care of ventilator-dependent clients, high-risk prenatal clients, routine postpartum clients, clients with chronic mental health problems, and clients with chronic wounds. Hospice, or care of the terminally ill, is also becoming more commonplace. Basic components of each of these areas are described in this chapter.

Infusion Therapy

Home infusion therapy is a very significant component of home health care. With shortened hospital stays, many patients are discharged needing additional or prolonged parenteral medication. Home health care agencies have responded by adding home infusion nurses or teams or incorporating home infusion therapy into specialized orientation or training for their regular home care nurses. In addition, many home health agencies have developed that specialize in infusion therapy.

The growth in home infusion or intravenous therapy programs has been phenomenal since the 1980s. Indeed, home intravenous therapy revenues exceeded $4 billion in 1994 (Geniusz, 1995). Reasons cited for the growth include (Watkins and Rice, 1996)

- Increased complexity of cases
- More aggressive treatments available in the home
- Improved technology (e.g., portable infusion pumps, flexible silicone catheters)
- Efforts to reduce costs through decreasing inpatient hospitalization
- Consumer awareness, whereby patients and their families are more willing to participate in the recovery process

TYPES OF HOME INFUSION THERAPY

Several types of infusion therapy are routinely delivered in homes. Antibiotics, pain medication, total parenteral nutrition (TPN), hydration, and chemotherapy are the most routinely administered home intravenous therapies. Therapies less commonly provided in the home include administration of human growth hormones, cardiac drugs, blood and blood components, and aminophylline (Humphrey and Milone-Nuzzo, 1991). The largest percentage of home infusion involves antibiotics and other antiinfectives (68%); antineoplastics and pain medications account for another 15%, with the remainder being hydration, TPN, and other therapies (Balinsky, 1995). Table 9–1 lists common diagnoses for routine intravenous therapy.

HOME INFUSION THERAPY MANAGEMENT

Home infusion therapy is nursing intensive and can be very complex. Orientation of new nurses

TABLE 9–1 **Home Infusion Therapy**

Type of Infusion Therapy	Examples of Medical Diagnoses
Antibiotic therapy	AIDS-related infections Bacterial endocarditis Cystic fibrosis Osteomyelitis Pneumonia
Parenteral nutrition	AIDS-related enteropathy Colitis Crohn's disease Pancreatitis Various cancers (e.g., colon, liver, stomach)
Chemotherapy	Leukemias Lymphomas Sarcomas Various carcinomas (e.g., breast, lung, pancreas)
Pain management	Chronic intractable pain (secondary to cancer) Various AIDS-related diagnoses
Hydration therapy	Gastroenteritis Hyperemesis gravidarum Intractable diarrhea

Data from Humphrey, C. J. and Milone-Nuzzo, P. (1991). *Home Care Nursing: An Orientation to Practice.* New York, Appleton & Lange.

to home infusion services should be comprehensive and cover specific procedures for each type of care (e.g., TPN, chemotherapy, antibiotic therapy). Resources for assistance, supervision, and consultation should be available at all times, and procedures for complications must be reviewed routinely and followed painstakingly.

In addition to delivering the prescribed medications, the nurse must evaluate the client for complications (e.g., medication reactions or infection) related to the illness or the treatment regimen. Management of the plan of care requires consideration of the drug therapy schedule, presence or absence of other caregivers who may be needed to assist, additional or preliminary medications or therapies, availability or source of the medication; preparation of the medication, use of an infusion pump if prescribed, and assessment and maintenance of the administration port.

EQUIPMENT, SUPPLIES, AND SERVICES FOR HOME INFUSION

Components of home infusion therapy include equipment (pumps and poles), supplies (dressing supplies, infusion sets), drugs and pharmacy services, laboratory services, and physician and nursing care. The IV therapy nurse is usually responsible for ensuring all needed medications, equipment and supplies are available when needed and that ongoing assessment and follow-up care are provided appropriately. For example, if a client is receiving TPN, the nurse will follow the physician's orders or agency protocols regarding monitoring laboratory values. The nurse may be responsible for ordering equipment and supplies and coordinating ancillary services.

SELECTION AND MANAGEMENT OF INTRAVENOUS ADMINISTRATION ACCESS DEVICES

Clients receiving short-term therapy may have standard peripheral venous access using a heparin lock. Peripheral access is appropriate for short-term therapy (e.g., antibiotics and hydration fluids) and should be changed every 48 hours to prevent infiltration, phlebitis, or infection. Monitoring for complications of administration, such as phlebitis and extravasation of drugs, is very important when using a peripheral line.

For intermediate or long-term therapy, a central venous catheter (CVC) or subcutaneous port is used. Central venous catheter lines (e.g., Hickman, Broviac, or Groshong catheters) are used for TPN, chemotherapy, and progressive disease management. The CVC is inserted by a physician into the superior vena cava and threaded into the right atrium during a minor surgical procedure. Externally, the CVC is usually sutured at the exit site. An x-ray is used to determine proper placement. Implantable vascular devices (e.g., Port-a Cath) are inserted similarly; however, the port, a small disc or diaphragm, is implanted into the subcutaneous tissue.

For intermediate infusion therapy (1–6 weeks), a peripherally inserted central catheter (PICC) may be used. PICCs are inserted into the median cephalic basilic, median cubital, or cephalic veins in the upper arm and then advanced into the superior vena cava. A PICC line may be inserted by a Registered Nurse (RN) certified in their insertion, and an x-ray is needed to verify placement. Only trained RNs and physicians may remove PICCs (Steinheiser, 1995; Watkins and Rice, 1996).

Agency policy and physicians' orders direct infection control interventions regarding intravenous site management. CVCs in particular require meticulous evaluation for signs of infection and careful adherence to sterile technique. In general, intravenous gauze dressings should be changed at least three times per week, and transparent or occlusive dressing, often used with CVCs, should be changed one or two times per week. Intravenous tubing should be changed every 48 hours (Watkins and Rice, 1996). Additionally, following heparinization regimens to prevent catheter occlusion, according to agency protocol, is essential.

In addition to intravenous administration of medications, other routes may be used in home infusion therapy. These include intramuscular, subcutaneous, epidural, intrathecal (into the subarachnoid space surrounding the spinal cord), intraperitoneal (into the abdominal cavity), and enteral (into the digestive system) (Watkins and Rice, 1996). Selection of the route of medication administration is based on the type of therapy needed and is determined by the physician.

COMPLICATIONS OF HOME INFUSION THERAPY

As with intravenous therapy in acute care settings, a number of potential complications to home infusion therapy exist. Table 9–2 lists some complications of intravenous therapy, including assessment indicators and suggested nursing interventions. Most agencies have standardized policies and protocols to prevent or manage complications.

PAIN MANAGEMENT

In home health care, pain medications, including narcotics, are used to manage severe pain, usually caused by cancer, AIDS, or neurological or orthopedic conditions. Narcotics may be administered intravenously, intramuscularly, subcutaneously, intrathecally, or epidurally when oral or rectal drug administration is no longer adequate (Watkins and Rice, 1996). In home care, use of patient-controlled analgesia pumps is becoming more common. Pain management is discussed in more detail later in this chapter in the section on hospice care.

TOTAL PARENTERAL NUTRITION

Total parenteral nutrition may be indicated when oral nutrition is not sufficient. TPN requires a physician's order specifying the type of solution, frequency of administration, frequency of vital sign assessment, and periodic serum chemistry assessment. TPN solutions are prepared in a pharmacy and must be refrigerated. An infusion pump is always used to ensure constant flow rates.

ENTERAL NUTRITION THERAPY

Enteral nutrition therapy is indicated for those patients who cannot receive sufficient oral nutrition. Enteral nutrition is the treatment of choice for clients with functioning lower gastrointestinal tract but for whom food intake is not possible, is not adequate, or is too difficult. Home-based enteral nutrition is most commonly seen when providing care to clients with conditions such as pharyngeal or esophageal strictures, neurological disorders resulting in dysphagia, anorexia, and coma (Widmar and Martinson, 1989).

The client's diagnosis, condition, long-term needs, and prognosis determine the type of feeding tube and placement. In acute care facilities, nasogastric or orogastric tubes are often used to insert nutrients directly into the stomach. Surgically implanted feeding tubes (gastrostomy or jejunostomy tubes) are used for clients with long-term nutrition assistance and/or conditions that necessitate bypassing portions of the gastrointestinal system. In

TABLE 9–2 **Troubleshooting Intravenous Therapy in the Home: Patient/Caregiver Education**

Complication	Action
Infusion slows or stops	Observe for swelling, pain, or hardness around needle/catheter site. If any of these are noted, stop the infusion and immediately notify the home health nurse and/or physician. If the above signs and symptoms are not present 1. Check for twisted tubing or pressure on tubing. 2. See if the patient has moved or bent his or her arm. If so, return arm to original position. 3. If the flow rate remains slow or stopped, turn regulator off and contact the home health nurse.
Circulatory overload Occurs when patient has received too much fluid Symptoms Coughing, shortness of breath Increased respirations Headache, facial flushing Rapid pulse rate Dizziness	Stop the infusion and immediately call the home health nurse and/or physician. Call an ambulance directly if the situation is an emergency.
Air embolism Air gets into the bloodstream Symptoms Extreme shortness of breath Anxiety Lips and nailbeds turn blue Rapid pulse rate Loss of consciousness	This is a medical *emergency.* Turn patient on left side with head down. *Immediately* call an ambulance. Stay with the patient.
Pyrogenic reaction May occur with exposure to contaminated equipment or solutions Symptoms Abrupt temperature, chills Complaints of backache, headache Nausea and vomiting Flushed face Dizziness	Discontinue intravenous therapy. Call home health nurse/notify physician. Stay with the patient until arrival of the home health nurse. (If symptoms are severe, take the patient to an emergency department.) Save the equipment/intravenous solution for laboratory analysis.
Severed catheter	Clamp the line and notify the home health nurse/physician.

From Watkins, L. B. and Rice, R. (1996). The patient receiving home infusion therapy. In R. Rice (Ed.). *Home Health Nursing: Concepts and Application* (2nd ed.). St. Louis, MO, Mosby-Year Book, pp. 283–298.

home care, as in institutional settings, the feeding regimen is determined and prescribed by the physician or an interdisciplinary team including a nutritionist, physician, and possibly a pharmacist. Choice of feeding solutions or formulas requires consideration of the metabolic needs of the client, financial limitations, learning ability of the client or caregivers, and other necessary therapies. Instruction for enteral therapy should include the specific supplements, amount, time, route, and procedure. Feedings may be prescribed as continuous, intermittent, or bolus.

As in other areas of home health care, much of the nurse's responsibility lies in teaching the client or caregiver procedures for home nutrition therapy and supporting and monitoring the care. Essential components of client and caregiver education for enteral therapy are outlined in Table 9–3. Orientation to home health nursing agencies should include assessment of the nurse's experience with enteral therapy and training programs and continuing education as appropriate.

Wound Management

Wound care is one of the most common services provided by home health nurses. Rice and Wiersema (1996) estimated that wound care in the United States costs between three and seven billion dollars annually. In the home, nurses typically work with wounds that are difficult to heal, usually because of underlying disease processes (e.g., diabetes, peripheral vascular disease), anemia, poor nutrition, wound contamination, chemical irritants, age, and other factors (Rice and Wiersema, 1996). When wounds do not respond to care or when providing care to a client with an ostomy, nurses with special training or experience may be used.

CHRONIC WOUND CARE

Basic wound care, including frequency of dressing change, type of dressing used, cleaning solutions, and topical medications, is generally determined by the physician. Nurses who specialize in wound care, however, often have latitude to make decisions based on their expertise. Goals for wound treatment and management include (Rice and Wiersema, 1996, p. 222)

"1. Prevention of further tissue destruction by reducing or controlling predisposing causes of tissue destruction
2. Prevention of infection
3. Planning treatments as appropriate for (a) type of wound (pressure, venous, or surgical) and (b) condition and size of the wound (stage, amount of drainage, and related factors)"

In addition to changing dressings, nursing interventions in wound care include assessment of the wound and evaluation of the efficacy of treatment, cleansing and débridement, obtaining cultures when indicated, teaching the patient and/or caregiver how to change the dressing using sterile technique, and teaching caregivers signs and symptoms of infection and how to prevent further tissue breakdown.

A number of wound care products are available and used by home care nurses to treat and prevent wounds. These include transparent dressings, hydrocolloid dressings, nonadherent dressings, and hypertonic saline gauze. The nurse may assist in securing specialized equipment or supplies to prevent pressure sores. Gel pads, foam mattresses, and air support mattresses, for example, may be helpful.

ENTEROSTOMAL CARE

Many home care agencies employ enterostomal nurses or enterostomal therapists to assist clients with a colostomy, an ileostomy, or a urostomy. Client and caregiver education and support and monitoring for complications or side effects are primary functions of enterostomal care.

In addition to providing patient education for ostomy care, enterostomal (ET) nurses are often specialists in wound care and management. Typically, ET nurses case manage clients with ostomies and act as a resource for other home health nurses. Often, the ET nurse is consulted to assist in preventing skin breakdown for high-risk clients

TABLE 9–3 **Components of Patient and Caregiver Education for Enteral Tube Feedings**

Management of Formulas and Solutions

- Proper storage and handling of solutions—include specifics for refrigeration and monitoring of expiration dates
- Mixing of the solutions when necessary; carefully follow printed instructions on formulas or from physician or dietitian
- Proper preparation of solid or blended foods, if permitted
- Optimal temperature for formula—allow to warm to room temperature if solutions have been refrigerated, but do not use formulas that are left opened at room temperature for more than 6 hours (or follow instructions on prepared formulas)

Equipment and Supplies

- Use and maintenance of pumps where prescribed—review and follow the manufacturer's instructions
- Cleaning and maintenance of containers, syringes, or solution sets

Administration

- Importance of correct *clean* technique—stress washing hands and ensuring that equipment and supplies are thoroughly cleaned following each administration
- Checking of tube placement and patency following agency or physician protocols
- Patient positioning—usually semi-Fowler or high-Fowler position unless contraindicated
- Priming of tubing with water if directed
- Administration of feeding using prescribed method (e.g., pump, gravity, bolus)
- Flushing of tubing with water following administration of solution
- Maintenance of position for about 30 minutes

Monitor for Complications or Side Effects

- Importance of hydration and administration of water supplements when ordered or as needed
- Mouth or nostril care if nasogastric or orogastric tube is used
- Care, cleaning, and protection of and observation for signs of infections if patient has a surgically implanted tube
- Performance of blood studies as ordered or needed for electrolyte balance and glucose levels
- Encouragement of observation for and reporting of dehydration, edema, nausea, diarrhea, constipation, bloating, flatulence, cramping, or abdominal distention

(e.g., those who are bed bound, very frail, paraplegic, or quadriplegic) or if a wound is not healing as anticipated.

Care of Ventilator-Dependent Clients

As with areas of specialized care, home health care for ventilator-dependent clients is growing. Individuals with conditions such as severe chronic obstructive pulmonary disease or other chronic lung problems (e.g., cystic fibrosis or complex pneumonia) or spinal cord injuries or defects who are ventilator dependent or need ventilator assistance are sometimes discharged from acute care or long-term institutions into the home. Home health nurses who work with ventilator-dependent clients must have intensive training and consistent agency support. When providing care to ventilator-dependent clients, the home health nurse must work closely with the physician, respiratory therapist, and family members. The nurse's role in the care of ventilator-dependent clients is largely supportive and includes

- Assessing the home situation for availability of 24-hour caregivers who are properly trained, competent, and able to perform cardiopulmonary resuscitation

- Working with the physician and respiratory therapist to outline guidelines for concern (e.g., complications such as infection or respiratory difficulty) and appropriate interventions to teach the caregivers
- Implementing and periodically reviewing emergency plans with the care providers
- Coordinating referrals with social workers, physical or occupational therapists, respite caregivers, support groups, or others as appropriate
- Teaching and monitoring tracheotomy care and suctioning
- Providing skilled nursing care for other needs of the client
- Assisting in monitoring blood gas levels and acid-base balance as ordered or needed

Ventilator-dependent clients are at risk for a number of problems and complications, such as infection, fluid volume overload, impaired skin integrity, and injury (e.g., tracheostomal trauma from suctioning, overinflation of the tracheostomy tube cuff, and tissue adhesions and stricture) (Rice, 1996). Agency policy and physician orders dictate care for these clients. In general, the stoma should be cleaned daily, with the skin being assessed for signs of infection. As-needed suctioning using disposable or properly cleaned catheters should be performed using aseptic technique, and tracheostomy tubes should be changed at least monthly. Knowledge of commonly used equipment and supplies is essential for nurses who work with ventilator-dependent clients. Table 9–4 lists equipment and supplies for home mechanical ventilation.

Perinatal Home Care

Home care for pregnant and postpartum clients has increased dramatically during the past few years. Technologically advanced care for high-risk pregnancies and for neonates with identified breathing difficulties is now delivered in the home under certain conditions. In addition, postpartum care for clients, particularly following shortened hospital stays, is becoming increasingly common and even mandated in some locations. High-tech perinatal home care, apnea monitoring for high-risk infants, and postpartum home care are discussed briefly.

HOME CARE OF HIGH-RISK PERINATAL CLIENTS

One of the newest areas for home health nursing involves the care of high-risk perinatal clients. Until very recently, high-risk maternity clients were hospitalized for extended periods for monitoring or treatment. In many cases, they are now being cared for in the home. Perinatal home care services include

- Uterine monitoring—use of a portable monitor to assess contractions. The monitor may then be taken back to the provider, agency, or institution for evaluation, or the information may be transmitted to a receiving center via telephone lines.
- Fetal monitoring—use of a portable fetal monitor to perform a nonstress test to assess fetal development and condition. Like the uterine monitor, the fetal monitor produces a printed strip that can be transmitted or carried to the institution or agency for interpretation.
- Ultrasound—a portable ultrasound machine is used to perform a biophysical profile to evaluate fetal movement, fetal heart rate, muscle tone, and fluid volume.
- Infusion pump treatment—subcutaneous infusion therapy utilizes a microinfusion pump to deliver continuous or intermittent low doses of a prescribed medication. For example, a medication such as terbutaline can be administered to control uterine contractions associated with preterm labor; an insulin pump may be used to administer insulin subcutaneously for an uncontrolled, brittle diabetic; or heparin may be administered via pump for a pregnant woman prone to developing blood clots.
- Infusion therapy—antibiotics may be needed for severe infection; hydration therapy and TPN may be administered for hyperemesis.

TABLE 9–4 **Principal Equipment and Supplies Used for Home Mechanical Ventilation**

A. Primary ventilator
   1. Ventilator circuits
   2. Ventilator filters
   3. Heated humidifier or cascade
      a. Sterile or distilled water (optional), or tap water boiled for 15 minutes
      b. Condensation drainage bags
      c. Heat and moisture exchangers (optional)
   4. External 12-volt battery with power cord
   5. Volume bag (optional)
   6. Disinfectant
B. Secondary ventilator
   1. Identical backup ventilator (optional)
   2. Ambu bag (manual resuscitator)
C. Oxygen and related supplies
   1. Oxygen source (optional): oxygen concentrator with backup compressed gas cylinder (tank)
   2. Oxygen connecting tubing: pressure-compensated flowmeters are recommended with the use of 50 feet of connecting tubing
   3. Air compressor and aerosol tubing for nebulizer treatments (optional)
D. Tracheostomy equipment and related supplies
   1. Extra tracheostomy tube(s)—keep a tube 1 size smaller in home
   2. Dressings (absorbent and lint free)
   3. Extra tracheostomy tube ties, Velcro collar, or twill tape
   4. Water-soluble lubricant
   5. Syringes
   6. Sterile and nonsterile gloves
   7. Cotton swabs
   8. Stoma ointment (as prescribed by physician)
   9. Sterile unit-dose and bottled normal saline (optional)—may use tap water to rinse suction catheter *after* suctioning is completed
   10. Hydrogen peroxide
   11. Suction machine
      a. Extra collection bottles
      b. Suction catheters (Yankauer catheter—optional)
      c. Extension tubing
E. Home medical equipment
   1. Hospital bed (optional)
   2. Patient communication aid
   3. As needed, equipment to assist with patient bowel/bladder management and personal care
   4. Wheelchair/walker/cane

From Rice, R. (1996). The Ventilator-dependent patient. In R. Rice (Ed.). *Home Health Nursing: Concepts and Application* (2nd ed.). St. Louis, MO, Mosby-Year Book.

- Hypertension monitoring—the nurse can teach the client or family to monitor blood pressure and report findings. As with uterine or fetal monitors, remote blood pressure monitors enable the client to transmit findings to a center or provider for interpretation (Dahlberg et al., 1995).

POSTPARTUM HOME CARE

Increasingly, shortened postpartum hospital stays, attributable to health care reform and cost containment, have led to steady growth in postpartum home care. Evans (1995) reported that during the past decade, hospital stays for women experiencing vaginal delivery have declined from 3 to 4 days to 24 hours or less, and hospital stays for women who have undergone cesarean delivery decreased from 5 to 7 days to 72 hours. Benefits attributable to early discharge are quicker reestablishment of family routines, decreased separation from the family, decreased costs, decreased risk of nosocomial infection, emotional and psychological benefits from familiar surroundings, and increased confidence in learning to care for the neonate in the "normal" setting (Carr, 1989). Disadvantages include decreased educational opportunities; need for increased help at home to provide meals and other home maintenance services; lack of rest for the mother; lack of nursing guidance for breastfeeding and neonatal care; and potential for undiagnosed complications, such as neonatal hyperbilirubinemia, low neonatal temperature, maternal hemorrhage, and excessive maternal pain (Carr, 1989).

Postpartum nursing care, whether in the hospital or home, includes monitoring the physical and emotional well-being of family members; identification of potential or developing complications; and bridging the gap between discharge and ambulatory follow-up for mothers and infants (Lynch et al., 1996).

To meet the educational, physiological, and supportive needs of the childbearing family, a number of different models of postpartum home health care have been developed. In general, postpartum home care services include health promotion and health education activities that have been within the traditional scope and functions of postpartum care. Postpartum home care services described by Evans (1995) include follow-up telephone calls 1 to 3 days after discharge, home visits 1 to 3 days after discharge, new parent information telephone lines staffed by a nurse and available 24 hours a day, lactation consultation to assist with problems encountered with breastfeeding, and organized support groups and outpatient clinics that encourage the first visit 3 to 4 days post discharge to assess both mother and infant and provide relevant teaching and interventions.

Many providers and agencies have programs that offer a combination of these services. For example, Williams and Cooper (1993) describe a program for maternity patients that includes an RN case manager who coordinates care with physicians, discharge planning nurses, and community agencies; home visits 1 to 3 days post discharge for assessment of the mother, infant, and family and provision of interventions as warranted; use of a risk management documentation tool; post visit telephone call(s); and a 24-hour help line.

During postpartum home visitation, the most common concerns of the mother are pain associated with episiotomy or cesarean incision, breast engorgement, backache, and uterine cramping. In addition, teaching regarding nutritional needs and avoidance of infection and constipation is also warranted. Infant concerns and questions are typically related to nutrition—particularly ineffective breastfeeding and bottle-feeding problems—and hyperbilirubinemia (Williams and Cooper, 1993). During the home visit, a comprehensive maternal and infant assessment should be performed. Table 9–5 outlines basic areas for assessment of the postpartum client and infant, and Table 9–6 describes complications that are often seen following childbirth and relevant nursing management.

APNEA MONITORING

Apnea monitoring is most often indicated for premature infants with apnea, infants who have experienced or are at risk for experiencing a life-threatening event, and infants at risk for sudden infant death syndrome (Humphrey and Milone-Nuzzo, 1991). In home care, the primary role of

Text continued on page 227

TABLE 9–5 **Postpartum Home Visit Assessment Guidelines**

Maternal Assessment

Physical Assessment

Vital signs—elevated temperature (>100.4°F) might indicate infection; monitor blood pressure in relation to prepregnancy levels

Breasts—observe for engorgement and symptoms of mastitis (e.g., size, tenderness, tension, color, heat), nipple integrity, use of a well-fitted brassiere

Abdomen—palpate uterine fundus for progression of involution; if post cesarean section, assess incision for signs of infection

Lochia—assess amount, odor, color

Perineum—assess episiotomy, if present, for signs of infection; question mother about perineal hygiene

Elimination pattern—assess urination patterns and frequency, urgency, dysuria, burning, incontinence, or tenderness; determine bowel elimination patterns, including use of stool softeners or laxative and hemorrhoids

Activities of Daily Living

Nutrition/fluid intake—obtain 24-hour diet history (including fluids); if lactating, educate regarding continued use of prenatal vitamins (if prescribed) and increasing fluid intake

Rest/sleep—assess sleep and rest pattern; teaching to promote sufficient uninterrupted sleep periods and inclusion of daytime napping if possible

Maternal activities—assess infant care, household management, and exercise and physical activity

Psychological Assessment

Maternal psychological adaptation—assess mother's progression through Rubin's three stages ("taking in" [passive, dependent, concerned with own needs], "taking hold" [seeks independence, anxious, learning readiness; may have mood swings], and "letting go" [interdependence, realizing role transition, accepts baby as separate, new norms for self])

Postpartum depression—assess for signs of depression ("blues" are fairly common 2 to 10 days after birth); depression may become more serious, producing physical and psychological symptoms or progress to incapacitating depression

Infant Assessment

Physical Assessment

Weight—report weight loss of >10%

Head circumference—may be slightly altered from birth (normal, 33–35 cm).

Chest circumference—(normal, 30.5–33.0 cm).

Vital signs—temperature (axillary preferred; rectal discouraged and tympanic often unreliable in infants); apical pulse (normal, 120–160); heart sounds (irregular rhythms and murmurs should always be reported); respiration (30–60) may be irregular, abdominal—breath should be equal and bilateral

Head—assess fontanels for bulging or retraction

Abdomen—bowel sound should be audible; no masses should be palpable

Umbilical cord—observe for presence of infection; instruct on cord care

Genitalia—female infants' genitals may be swollen; with male infants, if circumcised, inspect for presence of bleeding or swelling, inspect for urethral opening at the tip of the penis; the scrotum may be edematous and testes should be palpable in the scrotal sac; report undescended testes, inguinal hernia, or hydrocele

Skeletal—observe back and spinal column for curves, masses, or openings indicating spina bifida or pilonidal cyst or pilonidal sinus (these should be reported); assess legs for symmetry of gluteal and thigh folds and extremities for abnormalities or malformations

Elimination—question mother about normal voiding and bowel patterns; urine should be clear and nearly odorless; stools vary widely based on whether the infant is breast fed or, if not, the type of formula; frequency can vary from one per feeding to one every few days

Table continued on following page

TABLE 9–5 **Postpartum Home Visit Assessment Guidelines**

Infant Assessment *Continued*

Physical Assessment *Continued*

Neuromuscular—assess flexion and reflexes; listen to the cry
Skin—normal variations include Mongolian spots, milia, and mottling; pallor or generalized cyanosis may indicate cardiovascular compromise and should be referred
Jaundice—common finding in neonates and most common reason for readmission to the hospital after early discharge; visually inspect skin color and extent of progression, time period of development; may require treatment

Nutrition Assessment

General—observe method of feeding; frequency; length of time or amount at each feeding; feeding reflexes (root, suck, swallow, gag); environment during feeding; infant and maternal responses; amount, frequency and character of regurgitation; and use of pacifier
Breastfeeding—lactation education important (encourage feeding on demand initially [8–12 times/day]), suggest altering breasts at each feeding and changing infant's position, discourage use of supplemental bottle feedings and pacifiers
Bottle feeding—assess the type of formula and knowledge of formula preparation, storage, and care of bottles (equipment or techniques for washing and sterilizing equipment)

Behavioral Assessment

Sleep/activity pattern—assess the normal amount of sleep to waking time
Crying—patterns can be very variable; 1–4 hours of crying per day is considered normal
Consolability—assess the infant's ability to self-quiet or to be quieted with assistance

Family Assessment

Family-infant interaction—assess communication patterns, response patterns, interaction with other children
Environmental safety—assess home for proper infant care equipment (e.g., railed bed, car seat, infant seat, latches on doors to cabinets, safety caps)
Infant care abilities of the family—assess family members' ability to bathe, diaper, clothe, and feed the infant and provide cord care and circumcision care as appropriate
Adjustment to parental role—assess changes in financial status, coping patterns; determine the need for referral for social services or community resources
Adjustment of siblings—determine the reactions of siblings through observation and interview

Data from Lynch, A. M., Kordish, R. A. and Williams, L. R. (1996). Maternal-child nursing: Postpartum home care. In R. Rice (Ed.). *Home Health Nursing: Concepts and Application* (2nd ed.). St. Louis, MO, Mosby-Year Book, pp. 379–398.

TABLE 9–6 **Nursing Management of Common Postpartum Complications in the Home**

Complication	Etiology/Symptoms	Nursing Intervention
Maternal Complications		
Urinary retention	From decreased sensation of needing to void and/or trauma during the birth process	Encourage the mother to void every 2–3 hours to avoid overdistention; if having difficulty beginning stream, encourage voiding by pouring warm water over the perineum; straight catheterization PRN; report signs/symptoms of UTI
Bleeding problems	Most commonly caused by uterine atony; other factors include retained placental fragments, vaginal laceration, or rupture of perineal hematoma	Uterine atony—encourage frequent emptying of the bladder; provide gentle uterine massage; encourage frequent nursing of the infant to stimulate oxytocin; retained placental fragments or vaginal or cervical lacerations need referral for further evaluation
Pain	Perineal pain is usually caused by edema, infection, or hematoma; uterine pain is caused by contraction of the uterus to maintain hemostasis	Perineal pain—assess the site for presence of complications; to relieve pain, use ice or heat, sitz baths, medicated sprays, or Kegel exercises; if infection is present, refer for further evaluation; prescribed or OTC analgesics may be used
Breast problems	Breast problems are most often related to engorgement, sore nipples, and/or mastitis; engorgement is caused by overdistention of the breasts with milk; sore nipples are usually caused by inadequate nipple grasp by the nursing baby; mastitis is an infection usually caused by *Staphylococcus aureus* precipitated by obstruction of ducts	Engorgement—if breastfeeding, encourage warm showers, frequent breastfeeding, and/or manual expression and use of a supportive brassiere; if not breastfeeding, lactation suppression includes wearing of a tight-fitting brassiere or binder for 24 hours a day until the breasts become soft, avoiding stimulation of the nipples, and using prescribed lactation suppressants; ice and analgesics may be used for pain; sore nipples—teach the mother to ensure the baby is grasping the areolar tissue when sucking, wash nipples with plain water, and air dry; avoid soap, alcohol, and other drying agents; mastitis—antibiotic treatment is necessary; encourage bed rest, fluids, analgesics, warm compresses, and periodic expression of milk; providers vary on allowing the infant to continue to nurse
Infection	UTI is the most common postpartum infection and is often attributable to catheterization or urinary retention; uterine infection is rare	Referral for diagnosis, antibiotic treatment, and follow-up for infections are essential

Table continued on following page

TABLE 9–6 **Nursing Management of Common Postpartum Complications in the Home** *Continued*

Complication	Etiology/Symptoms	Nursing Intervention
Maternal Complications		
Postpartum depression	Causes include hormonal fluctuation, fatigue, concern about lifestyle changes, body image concerns, conflicting feelings about the baby, stress over finances or career	Assessment of the degree of the depression is vital; be sensitive to maternal concerns and encourage expression of feelings; arrange for assistance with infant care and household maintenance to promote rest and sleep; support groups or psychological or psychiatric evaluation may be necessary
Neonatal Complications		
Respiratory difficulties	May be caused by lack of lung development or birth difficulties or complications (e.g., aspiration)	Refer immediately if infant has over 60 respirations per minute or breath appears labored or if retractions, flared nares, or grunting is present
Temperature instability	Loss of heat may occur because of wet blankets or diapers or if infant is exposed to drafts, fans, or air-conditioning	Observe environment for appropriate temperature and infant for proper clothing; counsel parents regarding use of appropriate clothing and room temperature to avoid hyperthermia or hypothermia
Jaundice	Related to immaturity of the liver commonly observed 2–3 days after birth; observed on skin and mucous membranes	Prevention/management focuses on provision of frequent feeding to stimulate stool and urine production and avoidance of dehydration and hypothermia; if jaundice is observed, serum bilirubin levels may need to be taken; phototherapy may be indicated and must be ordered by a physician
Infection	Infants are at risk because of immaturity of immunological system; infection may be the result of maternal disease (e.g., rubella or syphilis), a result of birth process (e.g., chlamydia, gonococci, herpes, or beta streptococci), or iatrogenic infection	Teach parents to observe for signs of infection, including lethargy, poor feeding, temperature instability, seizure activity; if symptoms develop, refer immediately
Feeding difficulties	Frequent regurgitation/vomiting may be caused by rapid feeding or too much milk at one feeding; if vomiting is excessive or continuous, pyloric stenosis should be suspected; if bottle-fed, the infant may swallow air along with the milk; inadequate feeding may result from insufficient maternal breast milk or a sleepy baby	Encourage parents to feed the infant slowly or decrease the amount of feedings if regurgitation and vomiting are a problem; if pyloric stenosis is suspected, refer immediately; to prevent excessive swallowing of air, encourage slow feeding, frequent burping, and holding the infant upright; if maternal milk supply appears inadequate, encourage additional rest, fluids, and relaxation to improve milk production and let-down reflex

OTC = over-the counter; PRN = as needed; UTI = urinary tract infection.

Adapted from Carr, K. C. (1989). Home care of the new family. In I. M. Martinson and A. Widmer (Eds.). *Home Health Care Nursing*. Philadelphia, W. B. Saunders, pp. 163–182.

the nurse is in educating the parents or caregivers about normal infant breathing patterns, recognition of and response to apnea episodes, infant cardiopulmonary resuscitation, and use and maintenance of the apnea monitor. Additionally, the home care nurse should review the infant's cardiopulmonary status, review teaching, evaluate the parents' level of understanding, and assess the parents' stress. Referral for social services or respite care may be appropriate.

Psychiatric Home Care

Although psychiatric home health care was first recognized as a reimbursable treatment alternative by the Health Care Financing Administration and thereby eligible for Medicare reimbursement in 1979, it has only very recently become widely available for clients (Carson, 1996; Gilkison and Neathery, 1995). Psychiatric home care is appropriate for individuals with diagnosed or suspected mental illness who need psychiatric services but cannot use traditional outpatient mental health services (Dittbrenner, 1994). For example, psychiatric home care can prevent or shorten psychiatric hospitalization, particularly for acutely depressed individuals and those diagnosed as schizophrenic (Hauk, 1996). The goals of psychiatric home health care are to (Gilkison and Neathery, 1995)

- Reduce the need for hospitalization or rehospitalization of clients in psychological crisis
- Promote the client's adjustment to the community and home
- Monitor medication compliance, effectiveness, and side effects
- Provide assistance with problem solving to families
- Reinforce predischarge therapy and treatment
- Provide education to clients and their families regarding issues such as disease process, medication, diet, and community resources
- Provide in-home respite services to the client's family

The elderly, many of whom have been previously hospitalized or institutionalized, make up the largest population served by psychiatric home care (Dittbrenner, 1994). Thus, much of psychiatric home care, like much of home health care in general, is reimbursed by Medicare.

To be eligible for Medicare reimbursement for psychiatric home care services, several criteria must be met regarding the client and the care provider. For example, the client must be homebound and have a diagnosed psychiatric condition. In addition, the plan of care must be directed by a psychiatrist, and the care must be delivered by a "specially trained" or "experienced" nurse. Special training or experience includes a Master's degree in psychiatric nursing or community health nursing, *or* a bachelor's degree in nursing with 1 year of adult or geriatric psychiatric experience, *or* a diploma or associate degree in nursing and 2 years of adult or geriatric psychiatric experience, *or* American Nurses' Association (ANA) certification in psychiatric or community health nursing (Carson, 1996; Hauk, 1996).

Patient conditions or diagnoses in which home care might be beneficial, or even preferable to traditional outpatient or inpatient care, include confusion or disorientation, severe depression, altered perception or cognition, risk for self-harm, vulnerability in the community, requirement of 24-hour supervision, excessive fear or anxiety, agoraphobia, need for assistive devices for mobility, or inability to leave home independently (Carson, 1996). Table 9–7 describes nursing interventions used in psychiatric home health care.

Hospice Care: Home Care of the Terminally Ill

The hospice movement in the United States is relatively recent, beginning in the 1970s (Clemen-Stone et al., 1995). Hospice care is a philosophy intended to provide palliative care to the terminally ill. Most hospice patients have a diagnosis of cancer. Others diagnoses seen in hospice care include AIDS, severe chronic obstructive pulmonary disease, terminal heart conditions, and neu-

TABLE 9–7 **Nursing Interventions and Services in Psychiatric Home Health Care**

- Individual psychotherapy, as appropriate, to improve self-concept, decrease fear or anxiety, decrease hopelessness, increase motivation, increase spiritual well-being, improve eating patterns, improve sleep patterns, increase social interaction, and promote diversional activities
- Ongoing assessment and monitoring of psychiatric and emotional status
- Medication administration and management (including injection of medications such as haloperidol or fluphenazine decanoate) and assessment for medication effectiveness, compliance, and side effects
- Teaching about medication regimens, disease process, communication skills, signs and symptoms of exacerbation of illness
- Crisis and symptom management
- Laboratory services (e.g., medication blood levels, white blood counts for clozapine)
- Case management to link patients and caregivers to community resources
- Assessment of family and community support systems and their effectiveness
- 24-hour on-call nursing support
- Development, implementation, and evaluation of a nursing care plan
- Coordination with other home care services, such as pharmacy, support, therapy, social service, and home care aide services

Data from Lima, B. (1995). In-home psychiatric nursing: The at-home mental health program. *Caring, July,* 14–20; Dittbrenner, H. (1994). Psychiatric home care: An overview. *Caring, June,* 26–30; Carson, V. B. (1996). The journey through home mental health care. In V. B. Carson and E. N. Arnold (Eds.). *Mental Health Nursing: The Nurse-Patient Journey.* Philadelphia, W. B. Saunders; Hauk, D. O. (1996). The mental health patient. In R. Rice (Ed.). *Home Health Nursing: Concepts and Application* (2nd ed.). St. Louis, MO, Mosby-Year Book.

rolgical conditions such as amyotrophic lateral sclerosis or multiple sclerosis.

Hospice programs may be located either at a patient's place of residence or in an inpatient facility. There are five models of hospice care (ANA, 1987):

- the free-standing hospice
- the hospital-affiliated, free-standing hospice
- the hospital-based hospice (with either a centralized team or a specialized hospice team)
- the hospice within an extended care facility
- the home care hospice program (either hospital-, community-, or nursing-based)

Although hospice care is frequently delivered to clients and their families in the home, there are distinctive differences between hospice care and traditional home health care. Table 9–8 presents a contrast between hospice care and conventional home health care. Nurses providing hospice care should be specially trained in all of the areas described.

Hospice care focuses on the patient *and* the family. According to the ANA (1987), hospice care emphasizes

1. Assistance in dealing with emotional, spiritual, and medical problems
2. Support of the family
3. Keeping the patient in his or her home for as long as is feasible while making his or her life as comfortable and as meaningful as possible
4. Coordinated home care; inpatient, acute, and respite care; and bereavement services
5. Coordinated professional services and volunteer services appropriate to the individual client
6. Palliative care focusing on pain management

ELIGIBILITY FOR HOSPICE CARE

Medicare Part A reimburses providers for hospice care. To be eligible for hospice benefits, patients must have life expectancy of 6 months or less, according to a physician's estimate, and they must not be undergoing or contemplating active treatment for their disease. In addition, they must have decided to forgo resuscitative measures at the time of death (Huntley and Rice, 1996).

TABLE 9–8 **Hospice Care Contrasted with Conventional Home Health Care**

Hospice	Conventional
Primary focus on quality of life and palliation	Primary focus on rehabilitation and restoration
Whole family as focus of care; active counseling for family	Patient focus of care with family issues addressed only as they affect patient care
Patient/family choices governing care	Medical condition governing care chosen
Intermittent visits intensifying in frequency until death	Intermittent visits decreasing in frequency until the patient is stable medically
Home care for medical crises and death if patient/family choose	Hospitalization for medical crises
Nurse as case manager until patient dies	Nurse as case manager during period of admission to home care
Emphasis on living in a way chosen by the patient and seen as comforting	Priority on maintaining physical systems (e.g., eating, activity, vital signs, diagnostic monitoring, correcting imbalances)
Expertise in managing terminal symptoms; active effort to try alternative comforting approaches	Common symptoms of terminal illness seen as inevitable and up to the physician to control
Sedatives and narcotics carefully adjusted to maximize comfort	Sedatives and narcotics used with hesitance to reduce but not eliminate suffering
Terminal course of events anticipated; crises avoided	New problems emerging tend to be seen as medical crises, not as a normal expectation with dying
Spiritual dimension of dying is focus of entire team	Patient with religious affiliation may choose support from own clergy
Bereavement care for survivors	At death, no further contact
Staff support process built in	Staff isolation in caring for terminally ill

From Zerwekh, J. V. (1989). Home care of the dying. In I. M. Martinson and A. Widmer (Eds.). *Home Health Care Nursing.* Philadelphia, W. B. Saunders, pp. 217–236.

CAREGIVER SUPPORT

Caregiver support involves teaching about the course and progression of the disease, and pain and symptom management. In addition, reassurance and provision of respite care or relief for the caregivers is very important. The hospice nurse can assist by referring the caregiver to providers of respite care or by instructing other family members or intermediate caregivers how to care for the patient. Reassurance that the care is appropriate and that they are "doing the right thing" is emotionally beneficial. Common reactions seen in caregivers of the dying include grief, loneliness, isolation, feelings of uselessness or helplessness, anxiety, anger, depression, and fatigue. The hospice nurse can anticipate these and be prepared to intervene (Kemp, 1995).

SYMPTOM MANAGEMENT

Control of symptoms is one of the primary goals in caring for hospice patients. Symptoms encountered can be the result of treatment and palliative measures taken (e.g., constipation from pain medications or nausea from radiation therapy) or the disease process and progression. Among the most frequently encountered problems are anorexia, weakness, fatigue, constipation, edema, urinary problems, dyspnea, skin problems, insomnia, dry mouth, dysphasia, and confusion (Huntley and

Rice, 1996). The nurse should anticipate these problems and take preventative measures whenever possible. Teaching the caregivers symptom prevention and/or management is essential.

PAIN MANAGEMENT

According to Kemp (1995), "pain is the most problematic and feared symptom" in terminal care (p. 105). Effective pain management includes accurate assessment of the pain and establishment of an effective, individualized pain management plan. Thorough assessment of a client's pain should include (Matassarin-Jacobs, 1993)

- Location of the pain
- Extension or radiation
- Onset and pattern
- Duration
- Character or quality
- Precipitating, aggravating, or alleviating factors
- Intensity
- Associated symptoms
- Effect on activities of daily living
- Methods of pain relief

Often, pain treatment is inadequate and inconsistent because of failure to routinely assess pain and pain relief; lack of knowledge among nurses and physicians of pain management; social or cultural fears; persistent myths (e.g., that pain is inevitable or use of opioids will result in loss of control or addiction); fear of respiratory depression; social or legal impediments to using opioids; communication problems among patient, caregivers, and professional staff; disease characteristics; and patient characteristics (Kemp, 1995). To assist in developing a pain management plan, Table 9–9 contains basic principles for pain management.

Nurses who care for hospice patients should be very knowledgeable about pain management in general and about pharmacological management in particular. Utilization of appropriate drugs, dosages, and combinations requires experience and may require experimentation (e.g., some drugs or combinations of drugs or routes of administration work better for different patients or for different diagnoses). Hospice nurses must be well informed of the different types of pain medications and adjuvant medications, as well as appropriate dosages and combinations. It is important to note that dosages and schedules may vary dramatically for terminally ill patients, and opioid doses may seem very high to nurses who do not routinely work with patients with severe pain. To assist in understanding the uses of different pain medications, Table 9–10 describes basic pharmacological management of pain, and Figure 9–1 presents the World Health Organization's three-step program to manage cancer pain (Kemp, 1995).

TABLE 9–9 **Principles of Effective Pain Management**

- Use medications or techniques appropriate to the severity and specific type of pain
- Give medications in amounts sufficient to control the pain and at intervals appropriate to the medication's duration of action
- Use oral medications when possible
- Give medications around the clock at regular intervals (prophylactically) to achieve a constant titer
- Use adjuvant medications (nonsteroidal antiinflammatory drugs, corticosteroids, anticonvulsants, antidepressants, phenothiazines)
- Assess and treat side effects or complications
- Anticipate side effects (e.g., constipation from narcotics, nausea)
- Assess for tolerance
- Assess for and intervene in psychosocial and spiritual issues related to pain
- Approach each patient as an individual and assess unique beliefs, strengths, and weaknesses
- Teach the patient and family principles of pain management

Data from Kemp, C. (1995). *Terminal Illness: A Guide to Nursing Care.* Philadelphia, J. B. Lippincott.

PSYCHOLOGICAL AND SPIRITUAL SUPPORT OF THE DYING PATIENT

Addressing the psychological and spiritual needs of the dying patient can be extremely difficult for

TABLE 9–10 **Pharmacological Management of Pain**

Medication	Use/Indication	Potential Side Effects
Mild Analgesics: Nonopioids		
Acetaminophen; nonsteroidal antiinflammatory drugs (NSAIDs): aspirin, indomethacin (Indocin), ibuprofen (Advil, Motrin), naproxen (Naprosyn), naproxen sodium (Voltaren), diflunisal (Dolobid), and piroxicam (Feldene)	Aspirin and acetaminophen are analgesics of first choice for mild pain; NSAIDS added to opioids are used in severe bone pain	Acetaminophen should not be used in patients with liver disease; NSAIDs may cause gastrointestinal, hematopoietic, and renal system side effects, especially with chronic use
Opiates		
Mild opioid analgesics: codeine, oxycodone (Percocet, Percodan), hydrocodone (Lorcet, Lortab, Vicodin), propoxyphene	Used in conjunction with NSAIDs when NSAIDs are not completely effective in controlling mild to moderate pain	Sedation, nausea and vomiting, constipation, confusion, urinary retention, dry mouth, pruritis, respiratory depression, addiction, tolerance, or psychological or physical dependence
Strong opioid analgesics: morphine, hydromorphone (Dilaudid), levorphanol (Levo-Dromoran), meperidine (Demerol), and transdermal fentanyl	Used for moderate to severe pain	
Adjuvant Medications	Used to potentiate the effects of opioids, decrease side effects, and treat associated symptoms, and treat pain that responds poorly to opioids	
Tricyclic antidepressants: amitriptyline (Elavil), desipramine (Norpramin), imipramine (Tofranil), and nortriptyline (Pamelor)	Assist in reducing neuropathic pain and for antidepressant effects	Dryness of the mouth, drowsiness, constipation; contraindications include use of monoamine oxidase inhibitors, recent myocardial infarction, cardiac arrhythmias, glaucoma, and urinary retention
Corticosteroids: Dexamethasone (Decadron), prednisolone, and prednisone	May be used for symptom management and reduction of inflammation, particularly in patients with bone metastases and metastatic arthralgia and to relieve increased intracranial pressure and spinal cord compression; helpful in increasing appetite, strength, and well-being	Sleep disturbances; rapid withdrawal exacerbates pain
Anticonvulsants: carbamazepine (Tegretol), phenytoin (Dilantin), and clonazepam (Klonopin)	Effective in relieving neuropathic pain or tumor invasion of nerves	Monitor serum levels of the medications and complete blood count; neutropenia is a side effect of carbamazepine

Data from Kemp, C. (1995). *Terminal Illness: A Guide to Nursing Care.* Philadelphia, J. B. Lippincott; Mauskop, A. (1994). Symptomatic care pending diagnosis. In R. E. Rakel (Ed.). *Conn's Current Therapy–1994.* Philadelphia, W. B. Saunders, pp. 1–4.

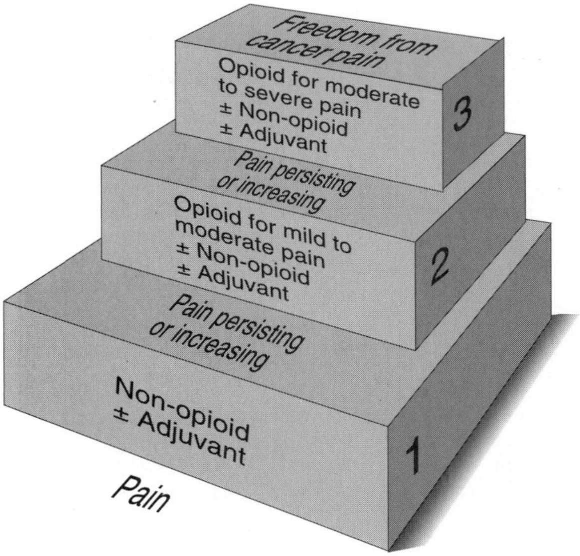

FIGURE 9–1 World Health Organization three-step analgesic ladder. Step 1: Nonopioid ± adjuvant. When pain persists or increases, proceed to Step 2. Step 2: Opioid for mild to moderate pain ± nonopioid ± adjuvant. When pain persists or increases, proceed to Step 3. Step 3: Opioid for moderate to severe pain ± nonopioid ± adjuvant. (Reproduced by permission of WHO, from *Cancer pain relief*, 2nd ed. Geneva, World Health Organization, 1996.)

the nurse and the caregiver. Review of Kubler-Ross's (1969) stages of death and dying (denial, anger, bargaining, depression, and acceptance) can be helpful. Recognition of these stages in the client and the family can assist in determining appropriate interventions. When observing a dying patient, the nurse can expect feelings of loss and grief, loneliness, uselessness, anger, anxiety, fear, and depression.

Spiritual care involves understanding the patient's spiritual beliefs and recognizing spiritual needs. Interventions can include listening to fears and concerns, helping the patient understand the meaning of death, praying with the patient, reading to him or her from the Bible or literature from another religion, expressing hope, and affirming the importance of spiritual concerns at the end of life. Referral to a minister, priest, rabbi, or other spiritual care provider should be offered.

Kemp (1995) describes personal qualities the nurse can demonstrate that are helpful in providing spiritual care at the end of life. These are realism (e.g., death is the end of a life on earth); hopefulness (includes hope of a better life in the present and in the future); truthfulness; faith; resourcefulness (i.e., ability to use the available resources); advocacy; sensitivity (e.g., acceptance of the patient's uniqueness) and openness to the patient's needs. Presence, or simply being near the patient, can also be very comforting.

INTERVENTIONS AT DEATH

Infection, organ failure, lung or heart infarction, electrolyte imbalance, and hemorrhage are the most common causes of death in cancer patients (Kemp, 1995). Teaching the family what to expect as death nears and what to do following death are very important functions of the hospice nurse. Common signs of impending death include progressive anorexia, refusal of fluids, dreams and visions of persons who have died previously, withdrawal, changes in symptoms (e.g., increase or decrease in pain), respiratory symptoms (e.g., increasingly shallow and/or labored respirations, with periods of apnea, dyspnea, increased secretions), increased pulse rate, and changes in consciousness (e.g., drowsiness, unresponsiveness, confusion, agitation) (Kemp, 1995). The patient's skin may become progressively cyanotic, cool, and mottled. The nurse should reassure the family that these signs are expected and manage them appropriately with comfort measures.

As death nears, families are instructed to call the primary hospice nurse or agency and not to call any emergency services. Depending on community or state requirements and agency policy, the nurse usually calls the physician, religious leader, funeral home, or others who have been identified in advance. Following the patient's death, the nurse may bathe the patient, remove all tubes and equipment, cover the body, and stay with the family until all arrangements have been made. It is appropriate for the nurse to cry or express grief with the family if he or she needs to. Frequently, hospice nurses attend the patient's wake, mass, funeral, or memorial service.

SUMMARY

Specialized home health care has been described in this chapter. As health care delivery continues to evolve and become increasingly community based, more and different types of care will be provided in the home. Emerging technology will allow for greater use of telecommunications, which, in turn, may dramatically change the types of care delivered in homes. Other factors, such as the aging of the population and the increasing numbers of AIDS patients, will dictate an increased need for more home health agencies and providers. In particular, those that offer specialized care as described here will be in demand.

Key Points

- Home health care is rapidly evolving into one of the primary sources for delivery of health care in the United States. In addition to traditional skilled care nursing, various specialized home health care services include infusion therapy, hospice care, care of ventilator-dependent clients, care of high-risk prenatal clients, routine postpartum care, and care of clients with chronic mental health problems.
- Home infusion therapy is a very significant component of home health care for a number of reasons, including improved technology, efforts to reduce costs through decreasing inpatient hospitalization, and consumer awareness of options for health care delivery. Home infusion therapy includes delivery of antibiotics, pain medication, total parenteral nutrition, hydration, and chemotherapy.
- Home-based care of clients with chronic wounds is an important component of home health care. Nursing interventions in wound care typically include assessment of the wound and evaluation of the efficacy of treatment, cleaning and débridement, obtaining cultures, and teaching the patient and/or caregiver how to change the dressing using sterile techniques. Enterostomal nurses are specialists in wound care and management, and they provide specialized care for clients with a colostomy, an ileostomy, or a urostomy.
- Home care of ventilator-dependent clients may be necessary for persons with severe chronic obstructive pulmonary disease or other chronic lung problems, spinal cord injuries, or other defects, who have been discharged from acute or long-term institutions into the home.
- Home care for pregnant and postpartum clients has increased dramatically during the past few years. Technologically advanced care for high-risk pregnancies (e.g., uterine monitoring, fetal monitoring, ultrasound, infusion pump treatment and infusion therapy and hypertension monitoring) and care for neonates with complications (e.g., apnea monitoring) are becoming fairly routine. Postpartum care for uncomplicated clients following shortened hospital stays is also growing.
- Psychiatric home care is appropriate for individuals with diagnoses of suspected mental illnesses who need psychiatric services but cannot use traditional outpatient mental health services. Psychiatric home care can prevent hospitalization for clients with diagnoses such as severe depression, schizophrenia, and Alzheimer's disease.
- Hospice care provides palliative care to the terminally ill and is frequently provided in the home. Hospice care focuses on the family, as well as the patient, and provides assistance in dealing with emotional, spiritual, and medical problems; coordinating professional and volunteer services; and making the patient as comfortable as possible through pain and symptom management.

Learning Activities and Application to Practice

In Class

- Invite one or more nurses who routinely work in one of the specialized home health care areas described to speak to the class. Encourage the nurse(s) to describe the types of clients seen, sources of reimbursement, changes in home health care in recent years, and anticipated changes. What professional experience is necessary for this type of practice? What strategies must be used to assist in teaching caregivers to provide the necessary care?

In Clinical

- Have students work with a home health nurse who provides "specialty" care described in the chapter. If possible, assign different students to work with different specialty providers and then share their experiences with the other students.

REFERENCES

American Nurses' Association. (1987). *Standards for Hospice Nursing Practice*. Kansas City, MO, American Nurses' Association.

Balinsky, W. (1995). High-tech homecare. *Caring, May,* 7–9.

Carr, K. C. (1989). Home care of the new family. In I. M. Martinson and A. Widmer (Eds.). *Home Health Care Nursing*. Philadelphia, W. B. Saunders, pp. 163–182.

Carson, V. B. (1996). The journey through home mental health care. In V. B. Carson and E. N. Arnold (Eds.). *Mental Health Nursing: The Nurse-Patient Journey.* Philadelphia: W. B. Saunders, pp. 1151–1170.

Clemen-Stone, S., Eigsti, D. G., and McGuire, S. L. (1995). *Comprehensive Community Health Nursing* (4th ed.). St. Louis, MO, Mosby–Year Book.

Dahlberg, N. L. F., Blazek, D., Wikoff, B., Tuckwell, B. L., and Koloroutis, M. (1995). High-tech, high-touch perinatal home care. *Caring, May,* 36–39.

Dittbrenner, H. (1994). Psychiatric home care: An overview. *Caring, June,* 26–30.

Evans, C. J. (1995). Postpartum home care in the United States. *J Obstet Gynecol Neonatal Nurs 24* (2), 180–186.

Geniusz, G. M. (1995). Future trends affecting the home infusion therapy industry. *Caring, May,* 58–62.

Gilkison, J. R. and Neathery, M. B. (1995). Mental health in the home and community. In D. Antia-Otong (Ed.). *Psychiatric Nursing: Biological and Behavioral Concepts.* Philadelphia, W. B. Saunders, pp. 521–541.

Hauk, D. O. (1996). The mental health patient. In R. Rice (Ed.). *Home Health Nursing: Concepts and Application* (2nd ed.). St. Louis, MO, Mosby-Year Book, pp. 399–420.

Humphrey, C. J. and Milone-Nuzzo, P. (1991). *Home Care Nursing: An Orientation to Practice*. Norwalk, CT, Appleton & Lange.

Huntley, D. and Rice, R. (1996). The hospice patient. In R. Rice (Ed.). *Home Health Nursing: Concepts and Application* (2nd ed.). St. Louis, MO, Mosby-Year Book, pp. 435–450.

Kemp, C. E. (1995). *Terminal Illness: A Guide to Nursing Care*. Philadelphia, J. B. Lippincott.

Kubler-Ross, E. (1969). *On Death and Dying*. New York, Macmillan.

Lima, B. (1995). In-home psychiatric nursing: The at-home mental health program. *Caring, July,* 14–20

Lynch, A. M., Kordish, R. A., and Williams, L. R. (1996). Maternal-child nursing: Postpartum home care. In R. Rice (Ed.). *Home Health Nursing: Concepts and Application* (2nd ed.). St. Louis, MO, Mosby-Year Book, pp. 379–398.

Matassarin-Jacobs, E. (1993). Pain assessment and intervention. In J. M. Black and E. Matassarin-Jacobs (Eds.). *Luckmann and Sorensen's Medical-Surgical Nursing: A Psychophysiologic Approach* (4th ed.). Philadelphia, W. B. Saunders, pp. 311–358.

Mauskop, A (1994). Symptomatic care pending diagnosis. In R. E. Rakel (Ed.). *Conn's Current Therapy—1994*. Philadelphia, W. B. Saunders, pp. 1–4.

Milone-Nuzzo, P. (1995). Home health care. In C. M. Smith and F. A. Maurer (Eds.). *Community Health Nursing: Theory and Practice*. Philadelphia, W. B. Saunders, pp. 776–801.

Rice, R. (1996). The ventilator-dependent patient. In R. Rice (Ed.). *Home Health Nursing Practice: Concepts & Application* (2nd ed.). St. Louis, MO, Mosby-Year Book, pp. 185–210.

Rice, R. and Wiersema, L. A. (1996). The patient with chronic wounds. In R. Rice (Ed.). *Home Health Nursing Practice: Concepts & Application* (2nd ed.). St. Louis, MO, Mosby-Year Book, pp. 211–234.

Sebastian, J. G. (1989). Nutrition in home health. In I. M. Martinson and A. Widmer (Eds.). *Home Health Care Nursing*. Philadelphia, W. B. Saunders.

Steinheiser, M. M. (1995). Vascular access device: choices for home care patients. *Caring, May,* 14–17.

Watkins, L. B. and Rice, R. (1996). The patient receiving home infusion therapy. In R. Rice (Ed.). *Home Health Nursing Practice: Concepts & Application* (2nd ed.). St. Louis, MO, Mosby-Year Book, pp. 283–298.

Widmar, A. and Martinson, I. M. (1989). The continuum of care: Partners in acute and chronic care. In I. M. Martinson and A. Widmar (Eds.). *Home Health Care Nursing*. Philadelphia, W. B. Saunders, pp. 3–12.

Williams, L. R. and Cooper, M. K. (1993). Nurse-managed postpartum home care. *J Obstet Gynecol Neonatal Nurs, 22* (1), 25–31.

10

Ambulatory Care Nursing

Case Study

Bill Barnett is a Registered Nurse (RN) working in a postanesthesia care (recovery) unit (PACU) in a day surgery center. The day surgery center is a freestanding facility located in a small city. The center houses six operating rooms, and 30 to 40 surgical procedures are performed there daily. A variety of surgical procedures are performed at the center involving virtually all surgical specialties. On a typical day, general surgery procedures (e.g., laparoscopic cholecystectomy, inguinal hernia repair), orthopedic procedures (e.g., arthroscopy), gynecological procedures (e.g., laparoscopy, cervical dilatation and curettage), ophthalmic procedures (e.g., cataract extraction, radial keratotomy), plastic surgery (e.g., blepharoplasty, rhinoplasty), otolaryngology procedures (e.g., tonsillectomy, myringotomy/placement of pressure equalization (PE) tubes), and others are performed.

Bill is one of seven PACU RNs employed at the day surgery center and has worked there 5 years. During that time, he has seen the caseload grow dramatically, with many of the procedures becoming increasingly complex. The first surgical cases are scheduled to begin at 07:30 and continue until about 15:00. The RNs work staggered shifts. Bill begins his day at 10:00 and is responsible for recovering patients from the later cases.

On a recent Thursday, Bill cared for Tony Mitchell. Tony is a 17-year-old high school football player who tore his left medial meniscus during practice. The surgeon performed arthroscopic surgery on Tony's left knee and shaved the torn part of the meniscus. The surgery was done under general anesthesia and lasted about an hour.

Tony was beginning to awaken from anesthesia when he was brought into the PACU by the anesthesiologist and the circulating nurse. His endotracheal tube had been removed in the operating room, but he still had an oral airway in place and was breathing without difficulty. Bill placed a blood pressure cuff on Tony's right arm and took his vital signs (blood pressure, 110/56; pulse, 88; respirations, 20; temperature, 97°F). His blood oxygen levels were monitored by a pulse oximeter and remained at 98.

When Bill called Tony's name and instructed him to open his eyes, Tony complied. He gagged slightly and reached toward his mouth to remove the oral airway. Bill assisted him and discarded the airway in a nearby container. Tony responded appropriately to questioning and stated that his left leg hurt a little. The left leg had been wrapped in a heavy dressing and Ace bandage in the operating room and then propped on two pillows. Bill assessed the foot and toes for swelling, color, and capillary refill. All were "normal." When asked, Tony moved his left toes without difficulty.

Bill received a report from the anesthesiologist and circulating nurse, both of whom stated that the procedure was uneventful. The anesthesiologist detailed the medications that had been used during the procedure and gave Bill the anesthesia records and operative report, and both left to prepare for their next cases.

Bill monitored Tony's vital signs and pulse oximeter every 5 minutes for about 20 minutes and then every 10 to 15 minutes for the next hour. By that time, Tony was alert and requested something to drink. Within 2 hours after admittance, Tony was sitting up in a recliner and drinking an iced soft drink; his intravenous line had been removed, and his parents were present. Bill used that time to reinforce the postoperative instructions that Tony and his parents had already been given. They repeated the instructions and stated that they would take Tony to the surgeon's office the next day for postoperative evaluation. They had already filled a prescription for pain medication given to them earlier and correctly verbalized the appropriate dosage. Tony was discharged from the day surgery center about an hour later and left on crutches with his parents.

The term *ambulatory care* refers to "personal health care provided to an individual who is not a bed patient in a health care institution" and generally includes all health services provided to noninstitutionalized patients (Mezey and Lawrence, 1995, p. 122). Today, approximately 60% of all surgical procedures are performed on an outpatient basis. Likewise, chemotherapy, as well as other parenteral medications, are delivered in homes and outpatient centers; diagnostic tests and procedures are performed in freestanding clinics and centers; and health promotion and health education services are provided in convenient settings such as home, work, church, and school.

Many of the objectives of *Healthy People 2000* (U. S. Department of Health and Human Services [USDHHS], 1990) involve health teaching, symptom monitoring and management, and risk reduction activities that are most effectively delivered during primary care office visits, formal or informal health education classes, individual counseling sessions, or other health promotion situations. Table 10–1 lists some of *Healthy People 2000*'s objectives appropriately addressed in ambulatory health care settings.

This chapter explores some of the numerous settings for community-based health care delivery and briefly describes nursing practice in those settings. The settings and descriptions of nursing practice are by no means all inclusive. Settings, clientele, and nursing practice vary greatly by geographical area, population needs, nursing practice guidelines and protocols, and a number of other factors. The purpose of this chapter is to give a general overview of practice opportunities for RNs apart from acute care, long-term care, and home health settings. Included is nursing care in clinics and physicians' offices; schools; work sites; churches, and specialty practices, such as oncology care, surgery, public health, and others.

Nursing Practice in Selected Settings

Community-based nursing practice often involves being a member of a group or practice concerned with the provision of comprehensive, primary care for individuals or families in a geographically or institutionally defined area. In these instances, nursing care is largely focused on health promo-

TABLE 10–1 ***Healthy People 2000*—Examples of Objectives Appropriate for Community-Based Settings (e.g., Clinics, Schools, Work Sites, Churches)**

1.8—Increase to at least 50% the proportion of children and adolescents in first through 12th grade who participate in daily school physical education (baseline: 36% in 1984–86)

1.10—Increase the proportion of work sites offering employer-sponsored physical activity and fitness programs as follows:

Work Site Size	*1985 Baseline (%)*	*2000 Target (%)*
50–99 employees	14	20
100–249 employees	23	35
250–749 employees	32	50
> 750 employees	54	80

2.19—Increase to at least 75% the proportion of the nation's schools that provide nutrition education from preschool to 12th grade, preferably as part of comprehensive school health education (baseline: 60% in 1991)

2.20—Increase to at least 50% the proportion of work sites with 50 or more employees that offer nutrition education and/or with management programs for employees (baseline: 17% offered nutrition education activities, and 15% offered weight control activities in 1985)

3.10—Establish tobacco-free environments and include tobacco use prevention in the curricula of all elementary, middle, and secondary schools, preferably as part of quality school health education (baseline: 17% of school districts totally banned smoking on school premises or at school functions in 1988; antismoking education was provided by 78% of school districts at the high school level, 81% at the middle school level, and 75% at the elementary school level in 1988)

3.11—Increase to at least 75% the proportion of work sites with a formal smoking policy that prohibits or severely restricts smoking at the workplace (baseline: 27% of work sites with 50 or more employees in 1985; 54% of medium and large companies in 1987)

4.13—Provide to children in all school districts and private schools primary and secondary school educational programs on alcohol and other drugs, preferably as part of comprehensive school health education (baseline: 63% provided some instruction, 39% provided counseling, and 23% referred students for clinical assessments in 1987)

6.11—Increase to at least 40% the proportion of work sites employing 50 or more people that provide programs to reduce employee stress (baseline: 26.6% in 1985)

8.4—Increase to at least 75% the proportion of the nation's elementary and secondary schools that provide planned and sequential kindergarten through 12th grade quality school health education (baseline data not available)

8.6—Increase to at least 85% the proportion of workplaces with 50 or more employees that offer health promotion activities for their employees, preferably as part of a comprehensive employee health promotion program (baseline: 65% of work sites with 50 or more employees offered at least one health promotion activity in 1985; 63% of medium and large companies had a wellness program in 1987)

8.8—Increase to at least 90% the proportion of people 65 years and older who had the opportunity to participate during the preceding year in at least one organized health promotion program through a senior center, lifecare facility, or other community-based setting that serves older adults (baseline data unavailable)

8.12—Increase to at least 90% the proportion of hospitals, health maintenance organizations, and large group practices that provide patient education programs and health promotion programs addressing the priority health needs of their communities (baseline: 68% of registered hospitals provided patient education services in 1987; 60% of community hospitals offered community health promotion programs in 1989)

9.18—Provide academic instruction on injury prevention and control, preferably as part of comprehensive school health education, in at least 50% of public school systems (grades kindergarten through 12) (baseline data unavailable)

15.16—Increase to at least 50% the proportion of work sites with 50 or more employees that offer high blood pressure and/or cholesterol education and control activities to their employees (baseline: 16.5% offered high blood pressure activities, and 16.8% offered nutrition education activities in 1985)

Data from U. S. Department of Health and Human Services. (1990). *Healthy People 2000: National Health Promotion and Disease Prevention Objectives.* Washington, D. C., Government Printing Office; U. S. Department of Health and Human Services. (1995). *Healthy People 2000: Midcourse Review and 1995 Revisions.* Washington, D. C., Government Printing Office.

tion, primary prevention, screening for early identification of disease, and assisting in treatment regimens for both acute and chronic illnesses (e.g., colds, influenza, ear infection, hypertension, diabetes). Care is usually ongoing and comprehensive, rather than concentrating on a specific disease process.

Again, it is important to note that nursing roles and interventions may vary markedly in similar settings by organizational or institutional policy, state practice regulations or requirements, and other factors. For example, in one occupational setting, the nurse's practice may primarily be concerned with monitoring Occupational Safety and Health Association guidelines and workers' compensation cases and providing first aid to injured employees, whereas in another company, the occupational health nurse's practice focuses on health promotion and illness prevention activities, such as conducting screenings and health education classes and providing counseling. This section briefly describes nursing practice in selected settings.

HEALTH CARE PROVIDER OFFICE OR CLINIC

Probably the most familiar role of the nurse in community-based practice is that of the office or clinic nurse. Nurses working in physician-based practices, nurse-based practices, and health maintenance organizations collectively account for the largest group of nurses working outside of hospitals. In the United States, approximately 132,000 RNs (or 7.8% of all RNs) are employed in clinic or office settings (USDHHS/Public Health Service [PHS], 1994, p. 46). The most common types of practice are the physician-based solo practice, group practice or partnership, and the health maintenance organization.

Nursing Practice in Ambulatory Clinics and Offices

As mentioned previously, the roles and responsibilities of the nurse vary greatly between clinics, as the practice, focus, and clients are often very different. Physicians may be general or family practitioners who provide preventative care and diagnose and treat clients of all ages and for all types of health problems. Other general areas of practice include pediatrics, obstetrics and gynecology, and internal medicine. Practitioners in these areas provide "primary care" to more focused groups (i.e., children, women, and adults, respectively), but care is still comprehensive, covering multiple body systems. The many medical and surgical specialists (e.g., surgeons, cardiologists, dermatologists, ophthalmologists, psychiatrists, orthopedists) see clients with more specific health problems.

The roles and interventions that nurses practice in physicians' offices obviously are based on the type of care provided in that office or clinic. For example, a nurse working in a surgeon's office may assist with surgical procedures, provide follow-up through phone calls, remove sutures, and help with preprocedure and postprocedure assessments. A nurse working in a cardiologist's office might assist in monitoring stress tests and perform electrocardiograms and other tests, and a nurse working in a pediatric office may assist in physical and developmental assessment, collect specimens (e.g., finger sticks, strep cultures), teach parents about infant care, and administer immunizations.

The scope of ambulatory nursing practice includes such activities as measurement, specimen collection, client follow-up, assessment, health teaching, provision of comfort measures, coordination of services, and preparation of patients for surgical or nonsurgical procedures (Parrinello and Witzel, 1990). Table 10–2 lists some of the roles and responsibilities in practice in ambulatory care clinics.

Education and Experience Recommendations for Clinic Nurses

There are relatively few requirements for employment in physicians' offices and clinics. Although some physicians prefer that the nurses they employ have at least 1 year of hospital experience, many hire new RNs. In addition, a baccalaureate is usually not required for staff nurse positions.

TABLE 10–2 **Examples of Nursing Practice Roles and Interventions in Ambulatory Care**

Enabling Operations
Maintaining safe work environment
Setting up room
Ordering supplies
Providing emotional support
Taking vital signs

Technical Procedures
Preparing client for procedures
Assisting with procedures
Chaperoning during procedures
Informing client about treatment
Witnessing signing of consent forms
Administering medications
Collecting specimens

Nursing Process
Developing nursing care plan
Using nursing diagnosis
Completing client history
Assessing client learning needs
Evaluating client care outcomes
Charting each client encounter

Telephone Communications
Performing telephone triage
Calling pharmacy with prescription
Calling client with test results

Advocacy
Making clients aware of rights
Acting as a client advocate
Referring client to appropriate provider

Teaching
Instructing client on medical/nursing regimen
Instructing client on home and self-care

Care Coordination
Acting as a resource person
Coordinating client care
Assessing needs and initiating referrals
Finding resources in the community
Instructing on health promotion

Adapted from Hackbarth, D. P., Haas, S. A., Kavanagh, J. A. and Vlasses, F. (1995). Dimensions of the staff nurse role in ambulatory care: Part I—Methodology and analysis of data on current staff nurse practice. *Nursing Economic$, 13* (2), 89–98. Reprinted from *Nursing Economic$,* 1995, Volume 13, Number 2, p. 92. Reprinted with permission of the publisher, Jannetti Publications, Inc., East Holly Avenue, Box 56, Pitman, NJ 08071-0056; Phone (609) 256-2300; Fax (609) 589-7463. (For a sample issue of the journal, contact the publisher.)

SCHOOL

Documentation of efforts to promote student health through school health services began in New York City in the late 1800s. The distinguished public health nurse Lillian Wald is credited with convincing New York City's school board to use a public health nurse to decrease absenteeism. As a result of her support, in 1902 Lina Rogers was employed as the first school nurse. Reportedly, Miss Rogers was so successful that 25 additional nurses were hired over the next several years, and the use of public health nurses in school-based practice spread rapidly to other cities, including Boston, Chicago, and Philadelphia (American School Health Association [ASHA], 1991; Pollitt, 1994). Currently, there are more than 40,000 school nurses practicing in the United States, accounting for about 2.2% of all RNs (USDHHS/PHS, 1994).

The early emphasis in school health programs was on control of communicable diseases such as tuberculosis, smallpox, diphtheria, whooping cough, pediculosis, scabies, and ringworm. As measures to control communicable diseases proved successful, attention moved toward sanitation, safety issues, and early detection and remediation of physical problems (e.g., vision and hearing deficits) that might impede learning. Throughout the next 40 to 50 years, school nursing roles and activities expanded to include assisting the physician with examination of students; counseling of students, parents, and teachers; and developing and implementing health education programs. School nurses also made home visits, provided inservice education for teachers, and served as a resource for school administration.

The roles and practice of school nurses have continued to evolve. Most recently, school health service programs have concentrated on

- Prevention of illness and disease transmission and early detection of possible disease
- Intervention in identified problems such as alcohol and drug use, sexually transmitted diseases (STDs), pregnancy, family violence, and the adaptation of children with special health needs to the school setting
- Promotion of healthy lifestyles
- Health education, both formal and informal

School health programs and the role of school nurses have strengthened and expanded during the past two decades. Currently, school-based teams are used nationwide in numerous ways, including caring for disabled children, investigating suspected child abuse, improving health education, promoting the safety of school children, implementation and management of school-based clinics, and research and evaluation of school health programs.

School Nursing Practice

The practice of school nursing involves numerous roles and functions. Some of the characteristics of school nursing practice, as identified by the National Association of School Nurses ([NASN] 1992), are

- A focus on disease prevention, health promotion, and health maintenance
- Incorporation of concepts from pediatric nursing, maternity nursing, child and adolescent psychiatric nursing, community health nursing, and adult medical-surgical nursing
- Delivery of care to aggregates as well as individuals
- Establishment of long-range plans for students, families, and schools
- Involvement with students, families, and schools to enact long-term change
- Establishment of relationships and networking with other school and community personnel

The school nurse is responsible for maintaining the school health program. Key components of a comprehensive school health program identified by the ASHA (1991) include

- Prevention and control of communicable diseases
- Care of ill or injured students
- Responsibility for administration or oversight of procedures for students with special health needs
- Administration of screening programs
- Provision and monitoring for a safe and healthful environment
- Health promotion
- Health counseling
- Health office management
- School health program evaluation and quality assurance and improvement

Each of these components is discussed briefly.

Prevention and Control of Communicable Diseases. Communicable disease control and prevention in school health programs typically involves monitoring immunization records to ensure student compliance with school district and state requirements; exclusion for communicable disease; and efforts for infection control (e.g., universal precautions for all individuals who contact body fluids, hand washing protocols for cafeteria workers, and monitoring incidence of illness and absenteeism).

Although requirements vary, completion of a basic set of childhood immunizations is necessary for school attendance in all states (Lewis and Thomson, 1986). Exceptions to these requirements are occasionally made for religious or health reasons (e.g., having had a documented case of measles).

It is usually the responsibility of the school nurse to monitor the immunization records of each child to ensure compliance. When a deficiency is observed, the nurse follows school district guidelines to ensure remediation of the deficiency. In some districts, this simply involves gaining parental permission and providing the vaccination at the school. In other settings, the nurse sends a letter to the child's parent or guardian explaining which vaccinations are not current. Often, this letter includes consequences (e.g., exclusion from school) if the immunization is not completed in a timely manner and information on where to go for low-cost or free immunizations.

Exclusion from school of students who contract communicable diseases is based on school district policy and state laws. Therefore, it is essential that the nurse be aware of these requirements and understand under what conditions a child is to be excluded from school and under what conditions he or she may return. Table 10–3 lists illness that often require exclusion from school and guidelines for readmission.

Care of Ill or Injured Students. The school nurse is responsible for monitoring the health of students, providing first aid and emergency care when indicated, and administering treatments and medications when prescribed, following school district procedures and standard protocols. The nurse should maintain a file of basic information, health records, and emergency information for each student.

Providing simple first aid for minor injuries is common in school nursing practice. Normally, each school district develops a set of first aid protocols or instructions to follow when caring for simple problems such as scrapes, blisters, sprains, or stings. A first aid kit should be well stocked and readily available for treatment of minor injuries. When more serious emergencies occur, it is often the school nurse's responsibility to provide first aid, inform the parents, and make arrangements to transport the student to the emergency room or physician's office, if necessary. School districts should also have guidelines for the nurse to follow in emergency situations.

For students with acute or chronic illnesses or conditions, administration of medication or treatments at school may be necessary. School districts maintain policies on who is to administer medications and treatment, the process to be followed, and guidelines for record keeping. Sometimes it is the responsibility of the nurse to perform these services, but often the nurse must train others to perform these tasks and monitor their care, per district policy.

Responsibility for Administration or Oversight of Procedures for Students with Special Health Needs. Public Law 94–142 (the Education for All Handicapped Children Act) was enacted by Congress in 1975. Public Law 94–142 "gives all students between the ages of 6 and 18 years the right to a 'free and appropriate public education' in the least restrictive environment possible regardless of physical or mental disabilities" (Kub and Steel, 1995, p. 752). The law was amended in 1986, expanding the eligible population to include preschool students. This amendment was added to reduce developmental delays, minimize institutionalization, and help families meet the special needs of children with disabilities.

According to Lewis and Thomson (1986), 11 handicapping conditions and definitions are stated in Public Law 94–142. These are

1. Deaf—impairment in processing linguistic information through hearing deficiency that adversely affects education performance
2. Deaf-blind—concomitant hearing and visual impairments that cause communication and developmental and educational problems that do not allow the affected child to be accommodated in special education programs set up solely for deaf or blind children
3. Hard of hearing—permanent or fluctuating hearing impairment that adversely affects the child's educational performance but is not included under the definition of "deaf"
4. Mentally retarded—significantly subaverage general intellectual functioning existing concurrently with deficits in adaptive behavior that adversely affects a child's education performance
5. Multihandicapped—concomitant impairments (e.g., mentally retarded and blind, mentally retarded and orthopedically impaired) that cause such severe educational problems that the child cannot be accommodated in special education programs

TABLE 10–3 **Common Health Conditions Typically Requiring Exclusion From School and Guidelines for Readmission**

Chickenpox	Exclude until after 7 days from onset of rash; immunocompromised individuals should not return until all blisters have crusted over
Common cold	Exclude until fever subsides
Conjunctivitis (bacterial or viral)	Exclude until written permission is issued by a physician or local health authority
Fever	Exclude until fever subsides
Fifth disease (erythema infectiosum)	Exclude until fever subsides
Gastroenteritis, viral	Exclude until diarrhea subsides
Giardiasis	Exclude until diarrhea subsides
Hepatitis (viral, type A)	Exclude until 1 week after onset of illness
Impetigo	Exclude until treatment has begun
Infectious mononucleosis	Exclude until physician decides or fever subsides
Influenza	Exclude until fever subsides
Measles (rubeola)	Exclude until 4 days after rash onset; unimmunized children should be excluded for at least 2 weeks after last rash onset occurs
Meningitis, bacterial	Exclude until written permission and/or permit is issued by a physician or local health authority
Mumps	Exclude until 9 days after the onset of swelling
Pediculosis (head lice)	Exclude until one medicated shampoo or lotion treatment has been given
Pertussis (whooping cough)	Exclude until completion of 5 days of antibiotic therapy
Ringworm of the scalp	Exclude until treatment has begun
Rubella (German measles)	Exclude until 7 days after rash onset; unimmunized children should be excluded for at least 3 weeks after last rash onset occurs
Salmonellosis	Exclude until diarrhea and fever subside
Scabies	Exclude until treatment has begun
Shigellosis	Exclude until diarrhea and fever subside
Streptococcal sore throat and scarlet fever	Exclude until 24 hours from time antibiotic treatment was begun and fever subsides
Tuberculosis (pulmonary)	Exclude until antibiotic treatment has begun and a physician's certificate or health permit is obtained

From Texas Department of Health (1994). *Diseases Requiring Exclusion from Child-Care Facilities and Schools.* Austin, TX, Texas Department of Health.

6. Orthopedically impaired—a severe orthopedic impairment that adversely affects a child's education performance, including impairments caused by congenital anomaly, disease, cerebral palsy, and amputation
7. "Other" health impaired—limited strength, vitality, or alertness due to chronic or acute health problems (e.g., heart condition, tuberculosis, epilepsy) that adversely affects the child's education
8. Seriously emotionally disturbed—refers to an (a) inability to learn that cannot be explained by intellectual, sensory, or health factors; (b) inability to build or maintain interpersonal relationship with peers and teachers; (c) inappropriate types of behavior or feelings under normal circumstances; (d) general, pervasive mood of unhappiness or depression; or (e) tendency to develop physical symptoms or fears associated with personal or school problems; included are children who are diagnosed as schizophrenic or autistic
9. Specific learning disability—a disorder of one or more basic psychological processes in understanding or using language, which

may manifest itself in an imperfect ability to listen, think, speak, read, write, spell, or perform mathematical calculation; included are brain injury, dyslexia, and perceptual handicaps

10. Speech impaired—communication disorders including stuttering, impaired articulation, language impairment, or voice impairment that adversely affect the child's education performance
11. Visually handicapped—visual impairment that adversely affects educational performance, even with correction; includes both partially seeing and blind children

Requirements of Public Law 94–142 that specifically relate to school nursing are (1) a provision that efforts must be made to screen or identify children in need of special education and related services; (2) completion of an "Individualized Education Plan," which is developed by an interdisciplinary team and includes current educational level, goals, and specific services to be provided; and (3) provision of "Designated Instruction and Services" (DIS), which outlines services required to help the child benefit from education. The DIS includes nursing care.

As part of, or in addition to, the activities cited here, the school nurse may be called on to monitor ventilator-dependent children, perform or supervise intermittent catheterization, and administer gastrostomy feedings. As with medication administration, performance of these procedures must be within the state's Nurse Practice Act, follow district policy, be authorized by parents, and be prescribed by a physician (ASHA, 1991).

Administration of Screening Programs. Screening for actual and potential health problems and hindrances to education is a very important component of a school health program. State mandates, staff resources, rate of incidence of certain conditions, resources, time, and facilities determine screening programs and procedures.

In most school health programs, screening includes vision, hearing, height and weight, and scoliosis. Additional screening programs may be required or provided by the state (e.g., Early, Periodic Screening, Diagnosis and Treatment [EPSDT] [see Chapter 13] for Medicaid-eligible children).

Comprehensive vision screening programs should be performed annually or minimally in kindergarten, grades 1, 2 or 3, 4 or 5, 7 or 8, and 10 or 11. Additional evaluation can be performed at the request or recommendation of the child's parents or teachers. Vision screening should test for (NASN, 1985, p. 14)

- "Anomalies or conditions of the external eye
- Defects of visual acuity at distance
- Defects of visual acuity at near points
- Refractive error
- Ocular misalignment
- Binocularity defects
- Color discrimination"

After identification of a suspected vision problem, the school nurse should make a referral following district protocol. As with all school referrals, a follow-up should be made within 4 weeks to ensure that the child has had further evaluation and treatment if indicated.

Hearing screening programs, according to the NASN (1993), are conducted to promote a high level of hearing acuity for all students, minimize the number of students with hearing loss, and provide for individual education needs of students with permanent hearing impairment. Hearing screening should be routinely performed in students in kindergarten, grades 1, 2 or 3, 5 and/or 7, 9 or 11; for those with known hearing loss; following academic failure; after a child has failed previous screenings; when speech patterns suggest a hearing problem; or if the child has a history of recurrent middle ear infections or has risk factors for hearing loss (NASN, 1993).

Hearing screening should be performed by nurses or other professionals (e.g., audiologists) trained in hearing screening and should include visual examination through an otoscope (to detect cerumen, foreign bodies, or a perforation of the tympanic membrane), audiometric testing or pure-tone screening (records the softest level at which a tone can be heard), and acoustic emittance testing (used to measure middle ear pressure). As with vision screening, a referral is made following identification of a possible problem.

Optimally, height and weight of each child should be measured and recorded annually to detect potential problems (Parker, 1992). Recording of growth measurements should be completed and referrals made following district guidelines.

Scoliosis usually develops slowly and may go unrecognized in children. Scoliosis occurs more frequently in girls than boys and often begins during periods of active growth (e.g., 10–16 years) (Lewis and Thomson, 1986). As with vision and hearing screening, screening for scoliosis is largely dependent on school district and state mandates, and as with other screening programs, follow-up for suspected scoliosis is essential.

Providing and Monitoring for a Safe and Healthful Environment. For school nurses, provision of a safe and healthful environment includes being aware of fire codes, sanitation measures for the school, and disaster plans for student evacuation and protection. Knowledge of restrictions, laws, and regulations regarding weapons, illegal substances, and other harmful practices (e.g., smoking) is also an essential component of school nursing practice. The school nurse's participation in setting and enforcing rules is also important in maintaining a healthy environment.

Health Promotion, Education and Counseling. Promoting and encouraging positive health practices through health education is a central component of school nursing. Additionally, the school nurse should be available to perform health counseling for students, parents, staff, and others.

As with all other areas of nursing practice, confidentiality regarding students and staff is essential, and district policies must be known and followed for sensitive issues such as pregnancy, STDs, substance use, child abuse, or threats of suicide. Documentation of confidential information regarding students and staff "should be filed separately but may be shared with appropriate individuals who have a 'need to know' in order to assure student health and safety" (ASHA, 1991, p. 14).

Health Office Management. The school nurse's office should be amply equipped and supplied to allow for comprehensive and appropriate services. Minimally, the health offices should contain a desk and chair, locked filing cabinet for student files, locked cabinet for medications, cots for ill students, hot and cold running water, and private office space for conferences.

School Health Program Evaluation and Quality Assurance and Improvement. School health program evaluation should be conducted periodically to assess the achievement of program objectives, identify program strengths and weaknesses, and monitor the quality of practice. The ASHA (1991) suggests that school health service evaluations should demonstrate the contribution of nursing service to education programs, compare the existing program to standards, improve procedures and practices, identify community needs for resources, involve community members in the school program, and improve communication between the school and the community.

Education and Experience Recommendations for School Nurses

A baccalaureate degree in nursing is recommended by the American Nurses' Association (ANA) and the NASN as the entry level for practice as a school nurse, and many school districts require it. Throughout the United States, however, there are many diploma- or associate degree–prepared school nurses currently practicing (USDHHS/PHS, 1994). Some school districts require a minimum of 1 year of experience, preferably in pediatrics, prior to employment. Certification as a school nurse is encouraged and is offered by both the NASN and the ANA (Kub and Steel, 1995).

OCCUPATIONAL HEALTH

Occupational health (industrial) nursing (OHN) in the United States began in the late 1800s. Reportedly, "a group of coal mining companies in Pennsylvania hired a nurse named Betty Moulder . . . to care for ailing miners and their families" (Rogers, 1994, p. 22). At approximately the same time, Ada Mayo Steward was hired as an "industrial health nurse" by the Vermont Marble Company. By 1912, 38 nurses were employed by businesses and industries, and that number had grown to 11,000 by 1943 (Rogers, 1994; Travers and McDougall, 1993). Currently, between 19,000 and 23,000 occupational health nurses are practicing in the United States (Burgel, 1994; USDHHS/PHS, 1994).

Occupational Health Nursing Practice

The American Association of Occupational Health Nurses (AAOHN) has defined OHN as "the specialty practice that provides for and delivers health care services to workers and worker populations. The practice focus is on promotion, protection, and restoration of workers' health within the context of a safe and healthy work environment. Occupational health nursing practice is autonomous, and occupational health nurses make independent nursing judgments in providing occupational health services. The foundation for occupational health nursing practice is research based with, and emphasis on, optimizing health, preventing illness and injury, and reducing health hazards" (cited in Rogers, 1994, p. 35).

Occupational health nursing practice is a synthesis of knowledge from nursing, medicine, public health, occupational health, social and behavioral sciences, management, and administration and includes legal and regulatory principles. OHN practice is directed by a combination of federal and state regulations, company policy and philosophy, the type of work or setting, worker input, nurse interest and expertise, and available resources.

Specific roles and functions of the OHN include (Rogers, 1994)

- Assessing the work environment for threats to health and safety
- Assessing the health status of workers
- Performing physical examinations, including those for job placement, "return to work," and termination or retirement
- Conducting appropriate laboratory tests
- Providing nursing care for occupational and nonoccupational injuries and illnesses
- Counseling and health education
- Helping the worker set goals and objectives for his or her care plan
- Collaborating, communicating, and consulting with other members of the occupational health team and other health care providers in the community
- Maintaining accurate and complete health records of the workers
- Developing and implementing programs to correct or reduce identified health and safety hazards
- Instituting appropriate personal protection programs (e.g., safety glasses, safety shoes, hearing protection)
- Conducting screening programs
- Developing and implementing health promotion programs
- Evaluating various programs
- Managing workers' compensation claims
- Training for cardiopulmonary resuscitation (CPR) and first aid

Legislation Affecting Occupational Health Nursing Practice

As mentioned, much of the practice of the OHN is directed by or in response to federal legislation and state mandates. Several of the most significant laws affecting OHN practice are described here.

Workers' Compensation Acts (Dates Vary by State). Workers' compensation is an insurance system operated by the states, with each state having its own law and program. The first workers' compensation law was passed in New York in 1910, and subsequently all 50 states and the District of Columbia have enacted workers' compensation laws (Rogers, 1994). An estimated 87% of the nation's work force is covered by workers' compensation (Whitted, 1993).

Workers' compensation insurance is "no fault," and benefits are provided through employer-carried insurance plans. Benefits are awarded to individuals who sustain physical or mental injuries from their employment, regardless of who or what was the cause of the injury or illness. Although they vary by state, workers' compensation laws generally allow for ongoing payment of wages and benefits to the injured or disabled worker or dependent survivor for wages lost, medical care and related costs, funeral and burial costs, and some rehabilitation expenses.

The Federal Coal Mine Health and Safety Act (1969) (Updated in Federal Mine Safety and Health Amendments Act of 1977). The Coal Mine Health and Safety Act provided for the establishment of health standards for coal mines and medical examinations for underground coal miners. This act provides benefits for coal miners with pneumoconiosis (black lung disease) through Social Security and includes federal funds to compensate mine victims and their survivors (Petsonk and Attfield, 1994; Spradley, 1990).

Occupational Safety and Health Act (1970). The Occupational Safety and Health Act (Public Law 91–596) is a comprehensive, multifaceted, and far-reaching piece of legislation. The purpose of the Occupational Safety and Health Act is to "assure so far as possible every working man and women in the Nation safe and healthful working conditions and to preserve our human resources" (Public Law 01–596, 91st Congress, December 29, 1970; cited in Rogers, 1994, p. 433).

To accomplish the stated purpose, the Occupational Safety and Health Act

1. Formed the Occupational Safety and Health Administration (OSHA), which sets and enforces standards of occupational safety and health (Department of Labor)
2. Formed the National Institute for Occupational Safety and Health (NIOSH), which researches and recommends occupational safety and health standards to OSHA and funds educational centers for the training of occupational health professionals (DHHS)
3. Established the National Advisory Council on Occupational Safety and Health, a consumer and professional council that makes occupational safety and health recommendations to OSHA and NIOSH
4. Established federal occupational safety and health standards
5. Established the Occupational Safety and Health Review Commission to advise OSHA and NIOSH regarding the legal implications of decisions or actions
6. Created a mechanism for imposition of fines and other punitive measures for violation of federal occupational safety and health regulations
7. Requires employers to maintain records of work-related deaths, injuries, and illnesses (Travers and McDougall, 1993; Clemen-Stone et al., 1995).

The Occupational Safety and Health Administration is responsible for promulgating legally enforceable standards that employers must meet to be in compliance with the Occupational Safety and Health Act. These standards fall into four major categories: general industry, construction, maritime, and agriculture and require employers to "use appropriate practices, means, methods, operations, or processes to protect employees for hazards on the job" (Rogers, 1994, p. 437). A description of each classification is presented in Table 10–4.

Occupational Safety and Health Administration responsibilities are to (Spradley, 1990)

- Develop and update mandatory occupational safety and health standards
- Monitor and enforce regulations and standards
- Require employers to keep accurate records on work-related injuries, illnesses, and hazardous exposures
- Maintain an occupational safety and health statistics collection and analysis system (in collaboration with NIOSH)
- Supervise employers and worker education and training to identify and prevent unsafe or unhealthy working conditions (in collaboration with NIOSH)
- Provide grants to states to assist in compliance with the Occupational Safety and Health Act

As stated, NIOSH was established by the Occu-

TABLE 10–4 **OSHA's Industry Classifications for Standards**

General Industry Standards
The broadest category of OSHA regulations. Rules generally apply to all industries. Specific standards called vertical standards are applicable for certain industry segments (e.g., pulp, paper, and paperboard mills; textiles; telecommunications) and address unique conditions in these workplaces. Standards that cut across industry boundaries and apply to conditions in many different workplaces (e.g., toxic chemicals; hazardous materials; machine guarding; personal protective equipment) are called horizontal standards. Vertical standards take precedence over horizontal standards.
Construction Standards*
Govern safety and health conditions at building sites. Standards for ladders and scaffolding, excavations and trenches, explosives, and other conditions and equipment found in the building trade are included.
Maritime Standards*
Standards that apply to workplaces involved in waterborne commerce conducted within the United States. Rules pertain to work at shipyards, operations at maritime terminals, longshoring activities, and gear certification.
Agriculture Standards*
Govern safety and health rules for agricultural operations. Rules include standards for roll-over protective structures for tractors, field-sanitation rules for farm laborers, and guarding farm equipment.

*The construction, maritime, and agricultural standards are considered vertical standards and take precedence over general industry rules that cover similar hazards.

From Rogers, B. (1994). *Occupational Health Nursing: Concepts and Practice.* Philadelphia, W. B. Saunders

pational Safety and Health Act and functions as the primary research and educational government agency dealing with occupational health issues. NIOSH responsibilities include (Spradley, 1990, p. 537)

- "Research on occupational safety and health problems
- Hazard evaluation
- Toxicity determinations
- Work force development and training
- Industry-wide studies of chronic or low-level exposures to hazardous substances
- Research on psychological, motivational, and behavioral factors as they relate to occupational safety and health
- Training of occupational safety and health professionals"

A number of OSHA standards are vitally important in OHN practice. Two are discussed here.

Hazard Communication Standard ("Right-to-Know" Law) (1986). The hazard communication standard was developed as a result of the recognition that *all* potentially toxic materials cannot be eliminated from the working environment. This standard requires chemical manufacturers and importers to evaluate chemicals with regard to toxicity, label them, and develop information sheets (Material Safety Data Sheets) for each agent. Additionally, employers must develop, implement, and maintain a hazard communication program to educate employees about identified toxic materials.

Bloodborne Pathogens Standard (1992). The bloodborne pathogens standard was implemented in response to concerns regarding the transmission of acquired immunodeficiency syndrome and other bloodborne diseases. This standard applies to all individuals (e.g., physicians, dentists, phlebotomists, nurses, morticians, paramedics, laboratory technologists, housekeeping personnel, public safety personnel, laundry workers) occupationally exposed to blood or other potentially infectious materials and requires employers to develop and implement procedures to prevent and control exposure to blood and other potentially infectious materials (e.g., semen, vaginal secretions, saliva, amniotic fluid) (Rogers, 1994).

As discussed, OHN practice is multifaceted. It involves a variety of roles and specific knowledge and expertise. To implement and maintain a comprehensive occupational health program that meets the needs of the workers, the OHN must have adequate resources, information, and support. Table 10–5 outlines examples of occupational health nursing services.

Education, Experience, and Certification Recommendations for Occupational Health Nurses

The majority of OHNs received their nursing education in associate degree and diploma programs (USDHHS/PHS, 1994). However, preparation as a baccalaureate degree is recommended for OHN practice. In addition to a baccalaureate degree, the AAOHN recommends a minimum of 2 years of professional nursing experience (preferably in ambulatory, emergency, community health, or critical care) before beginning OHN practice (Clemen-Stone et al., 1995). Certification in OHN is available through the AAOHN, and approximately 25% of practicing OHNs are certified (Ossler et al., 1996).

RURAL HEALTH

Like school nursing, early efforts to develop organized nursing practice in rural areas are traced to Lillian Wald. Miss Wald is credited for helping establish the Rural Nursing Service in 1912. A few years later, in 1925, Mary Breckinridge began the Frontier Nursing Service. These efforts focused on improving public health, primary health care, and midwifery services in rural areas (Weinert and Long, 1991). Currently, approximately 2,000 nurses are employed in rural health centers (USDHHS/PHS, 1994). Many other nurses practice in home health care and county or state public health agencies in rural areas.

The term *rural* is somewhat difficult to define. Typically, *rural* refers to communities having fewer than 2,500 residents and/or to communities with a population density of less than 99 persons per square mile (Bushy, 1996). Conversely, any community having a population of greater than 20,000 is considered "urban." More than 50 million Americans live in what are considered to be "nonurban," or "rural," settings (Bushy, 1995; Hanson, 1996). Bushy (1995) states that "of the total U. S. population, approximately 25% live in rural areas, but only 5% live in towns of 2,500 residents. Less than 2% of the total U. S. population live on a farm" (p. 821).

In 15 states, more than 50% of the counties are designated "rural." The states with the greatest percentage of residents in rural areas are Idaho, Vermont, Montana, South Dakota, Wyoming, Mississippi, Maine, West Virginia, and North Dakota (Lee, 1991). Figure 10–1 shows states by rural designation.

Although significant regional variations occur, there are a number of distinctive characteristics common to rural populations in general that are important to nurses. Table 10–6 compares characteristics of residents of rural and urban settings.

Issues in Rural Health Care

"Distance, isolation, and sparse resources are inherent in rural life and are reflected in residents' independent and innovative coping strategies" (Bushy, 1996, p. 324). As with barriers to health care in other settings and populations, barriers to health care for individuals living in rural settings include availability and accessibility to health care providers and institutions; affordability of health care, as many residents are uninsured or underinsured; and acceptability. These problems are often tied to problems with distance and isolation described previously. Table 10–7 describes other barriers to care and issues unique to rural settings.

One critical issue for rural health care is the shortage of nurses in many areas. Indeed, there is an average of 349 nurses per 100,000 persons in counties with fewer than 10,000 residents, compared with an average of 675 nurses per 100,000 persons in all U. S. counties (Turner and Gunn, 1991). In addition, of the 619 counties designated "nurse shortage counties" in 1990, 92.4% were in nonurban areas (ANA, 1996).

Likewise, the high number of hospital closings and shortage of physicians is of concern in many rural areas. Between 1986 and 1988, more than 50% of hospitals closed were rural hospitals. Some rural communities have a physician-to-population ratio of 53:100,000, versus 163:100,000 for the nation overall. Counties with less than 10,000 inhabitants have about one third of the

TABLE 10–5 **Occupational Health Nursing Services**

Services Mandated by Federal and State Regulations

- Safe and healthful work place
- Emergency medical response
  - First aid responder selection and training
  - First aid space, supplies, protocols, and records
  - Designated medical resources for incident response
- Workers' compensation
- Confidentiality of medical records
- Compliance with medical record retention requirements
- OSHA compliance
  - Medical personnel requirement (29 CFR 1910.15)
  - Injury and illness reporting and recording
  - Accident and injury investigation
  - Cumulative trauma disorder prevention
  - Employee access to medical and exposure records
  - Medical surveillance and hazardous work qualification
  - Personal protective equipment evaluation and training
  - Infection control
  - Employee Right-to-Know notification and training
- Toxic Substances Control Act compliance
- Community Right-to-Know compliance
- Americans With Disabilities Act compliance
- Rehabilitation Act: handicap, preplacement, fitness for duty evaluations, accommodations
- Department of Defense, Department of Transportation, Nuclear Regulatory Commission, Drug-Free Workplace Act compliance
  - Policy development
  - Drug awareness education
  - Drug testing, technical support
  - Employee Assistance Program–type services
- Threat of violence/duty to warn
- VDT local regulations
- State and local public health regulations
- Nursing practice acts
- Board of Pharmacy and Drug Envorcement Agency regulations
- Continuing professional education required for licensure

Services Often Mandated by Company Policy

- Clinical supervision of on-site health services
- Health strategy development
- Health services standards
  - Space, staffing, and operational standards
  - Occupational illness and injury assessment, diagnosis, treatment, and referral
  - Nonoccupational illness and injury assessment, diagnosis, treatment, and referral
- Disability and return-to-work evaluations and accommodations
- Impaired employee fitness for duty evaluation
- Preplacement evaluation and medical accommodation
- Handicap evaluation, placement, and accommodation
- Employee Assistance program standards
- International health: travel, medical advisory, and immunizations
- Data collection and analysis
- Medical consultation
- Pregnancy placement in hazardous environments
- Professional education and development
- Audit and quality assurance

Services that Are Optional

- Health education and health promotion
- Medical screening for early detection and disease prevention
- Physical fitness programs
- Allergy injection programs

From Travers, P. H. and McDougall, C. E. (1993). The occupational health nurse: Roles and responsibilities, current and future trends. In J. M. Swanson and M. Albrecht (Eds.). *Community Health Nursing: Promoting the Health of Aggregates.* Philadelphia, W. B. Saunders.

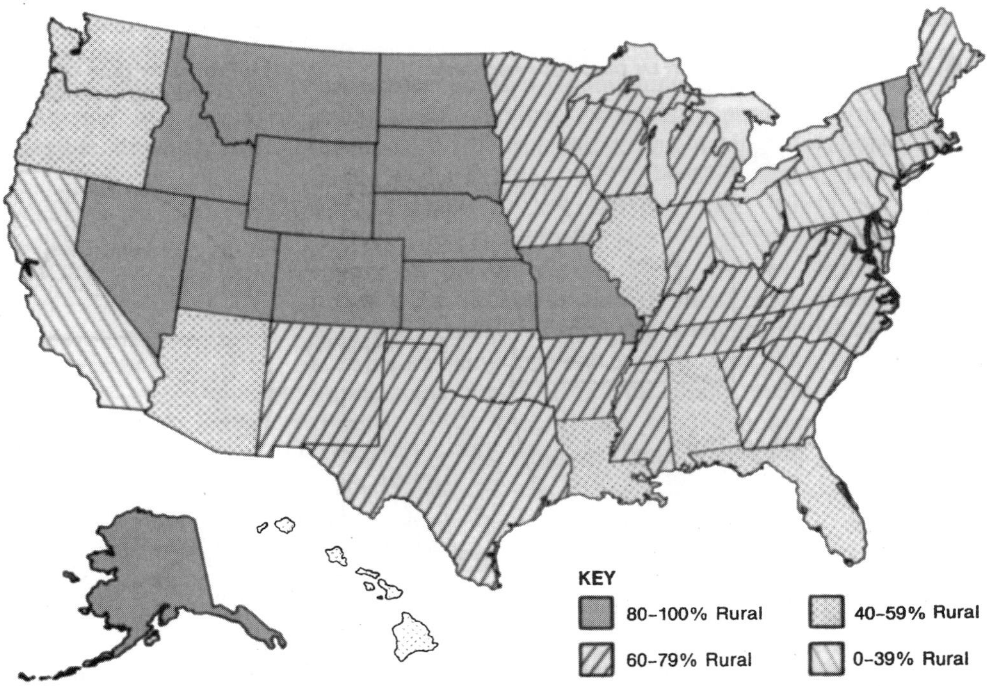

FIGURE 10–1 Percentage of rural counties by state. (From Bushy, A. (1995). Rural Health. In C. M. Smith and F. A. Maurer (Eds.). *Community Health Nursing: Theory and Practice.* Philadelphia, W. B. Saunders. Data from U. S. General Accounting Office. (1989). Rural Development: Federal Programs that Focus on Rural America and Its Economic Development. Pub. No. GAO-RCED-89-56BR. Washington, D. C., U. S. General Accounting Office.)

physician availability of all U. S. counties (Hartwell et al., 1991).

Rural Nursing Practice

Rural nurses most often practice in clinic settings, home health, or a combination. Skills needed by nurses in rural settings include technical and clinical competency; adaptability; flexibility; refined assessment skills; organizational abilities; independence; open attitude about continuing education; good decision-making skills; leadership ability; self-confidence; and skill in handling emergencies, teaching, and public relations. Table 10–8 presents characteristics of nursing practice in rural settings.

It is important that rural health nurses be willing to be cross-trained and educated to acquire competencies outside their primary specialty area. Rural nurses must also be able to remain current and competent in practice in an environment characterized by sparse resources. Furthermore, it is recommended that all nurses in rural settings have advanced clinical training in trauma care and advanced life support, which may be required to assist in the stabilization of emergency cases. Finally, rural nurses need case management skills for transfer, referral, and coordination of care in areas characterized by the lack of specialized health care resources (Turner and Gunn, 1991).

Education and Experience for Rural Nursing Practice

Nurses who practice in rural settings should have experience in a variety of areas, including rehabili-

TABLE 10–6 Comparisons of Rural and Urban Americans

- A higher proportion of Whites live in rural areas (82%) than in urban areas (62%) (however, this varies markedly by region)
- Rural communities have higher percentages of younger and older residents
- Adults in rural areas have fewer years of formal education
- Rural families tend to be poorer (more than 25% of rural Americans live in or near poverty, and nearly 40% of all rural children are impoverished)
- Rural Americans are more likely to be uninsured or underinsured
- Rural residents are more likely to have chronic illnesses (e.g., hypertension, arthritis, diabetes, cardiovascular disease, cancer)
- Rural residents have higher infant and maternal morbidity and mortality rates
- There are a number of health care risks unique to rural occupations (e.g., machinery accidents, skin cancer from exposure to the sun, pulmonary and other problems related to exposure to chemicals and pesticides)
- Rural adults are less likely to have preventative health care (e.g., Papanicolaou smears, breast examinations, prostate specific antigen, cholesterol screenings)

Data from Bushy, A. (1996). Community health nursing in rural environments. In M. Stanhope and J. Lancaster (Eds.). *Community Health Nursing: Promoting the Health of Aggregates, Families and Individuals* (4th ed.). St. Louis, MO, Mosby-Year Book; Bushy, A. (1995). Rural health. In C. M. Smith and F. A. Maurer (Eds.). *Community Health Nursing: Theory and Practice.* Philadelphia, W. B. Saunders, pp. 820–847.

tation, obstetrics, medical-surgical nursing, geriatrics, pediatrics, and emergency care. A knowledge of available resources and ability to coordinate formal and informal services is very important in rural health nursing (Bushy, 1995).

There are no specific educational recommendations for rural nursing practice. Educational preparation, however, should include public health principles, the process of community assessment, as well as content in health promotion and illness prevention, which historically has been a component of baccalaureate nursing education. Recently, nursing authorities have recognized the need to consider changes in nursing education to develop curricula at each education level to address the unique needs of rural nursing. In particular, "schools and colleges of nursing which are situated in rural areas, or whose graduates tend to serve rural residents, have an obligation to structure their programs to include rural content and clinical experiences in rural settings" (ANA, 1996, p. 24).

PARISH NURSING

"Parish nursing is one of the newer, yet older models of health care delivery. The history of nursing is replete with examples of religious orders or congregations providing care for the sick" (Schank et al., 1996). The concept of modern-day parish nursing in the United States is attributed to a Lutheran chaplain, Granger Westberg, who reportedly advanced the role beginning in 1983 (Miskelly, 1995).

The philosophy of parish nursing is "to promote the health of a faith community (churches or synagogues) by working with the pastor and staff to integrate the theological, psychological, sociological, and physiological perspectives of health and healing into the work, sacrament and services of the congregation" (Solari-Twadell et al., 1990, p.

TABLE 10–7 Barriers to Health Care

- Great distances to obtain services
- Lack of personal transportation
- Unavailable public transportation
- Lack of telephone services
- Unavailable outreach services
- Inequitable reimbursement policies for providers
- Unpredictable weather conditions
- Inability to pay for care
- Lack of "know how" to procure entitlements and services
- Providers' attitudes and knowledge levels about rural populations

From Bushy, A. (1996). Community health nursing in rural environments. In M. Stanhope and J. Lancaster (Eds.). *Community Health Nursing: Promoting the Health of Aggregates, Families and Individuals* (4th ed.). St. Louis, MO, Mosby-Year Book, pp. 315–332.

TABLE 10–8 Characteristics of Nursing Practice in Rural Environments

- Variety/diversity in clinical experiences
- Broader/expanding scope of practice
- Generalist skills
- Flexibility/creativity in delivering care
- Sparse resources (e.g., materials, professionals, equipment, fiscal)
- Professional/personal isolation
- Greater independence
- More autonomy
- Role overlap with other disciplines
- Slower pace
- Lack of anonymity
- Increased opportunity for informal interactions with patients and coworkers
- Opportunity for client follow-up on discharge in informal community settings
- Discharge planning allows for integration of formal with informal resources
- Care for clients across the lifespan
- Exposed to clients with a full range of conditions/diagnoses
- Status in the community: viewed as an occupation of prestige
- viewed as a professional "role model"
- Opportunity for community involvement and informal health education

From Bushy, A. (1996). Community health nursing in rural environments. In M. Stanhope and J. Lancaster (Eds.). *Community Health Nursing: Promoting the Health of Aggregates, Families and Individuals* (4th ed.). St. Louis, MO, Mosby-Year Book, pp. 315–332.

51). Parish nursing programs are supported by many different denominations. There are thought to be at least 3,000 parish nurses practicing in the United States (Simington et al., 1996).

The growing interest in parish nursing is attributed to several factors, including (Schank et al., 1996)

- Increasing focus on health promotion, disease prevention, and health and illness management
- Problems of fragmentation of health care and the reemergence of the "wholeness" concept regarding health care
- Increased emphasis on self-care and individual responsibility
- Problems with access and cost
- Increasing numbers of people with chronic illness
- Recognition of the need to identify and work with people in the community, as well as in institutions

Miskelly (1995) describes four models of parish nursing. These are

- Institutional/paid model—the parish nurse is employed by a hospital, community agency, or long-term care facility, which provides salary, benefits, support, and supervision and which contracts with one or more churches to deliver care
- Institutional/volunteer model—a relationship exists between a church and an institution, whereby the institution provides a stipend to the nurse or congregation and/or education and supervision; the nurse(s) are volunteers
- Congregational/paid model—the nurse is employed by the congregation and receives benefits and supervision from the church itself
- Congregational/volunteer model—the parish health care program is supported by nurse(s) volunteering their time

Parish Nursing Practice

The goal of parish nursing is the enhancement of quality of life for all members of the congregation (Schank et al., 1996). Parish nurses coordinate and train volunteers. They organize and facilitate support groups, provide referrals to community resources, provide health education and counseling, and serve as a liaison within the health care system. In addition, parish nurses provide health education, advocacy, counseling, and screenings. Invasive nursing procedures and/or home health care are not usually components of parish nursing programs.

A number of health education needs appropriate for parish nursing care have been identified by research. These include stress management, development of a durable power of attorney and living wills, nutrition, grief support, cancer risk factors and prevention, CPR training, parenting skills, alcohol abuse, and infertility (Miskelly, 1995). Interventions include health counseling and screening (e.g., cholesterol, blood pressure, skin cancer, occult blood screening), support group facilitation (e.g., grief, parenting, caregiver), education (e.g., stress management, nutrition, exercise, CPR), and community resource referrals (e.g., weight control groups, infertility support groups, violence resources, alcohol abuse support groups). Provision and facilitation of information on health-related topics through use of a monthly newsletter and maintenance of a health section in the church library can be used to disseminate timely information on safety tips, home health care, health insurance, prevention of heart disease, and many other topics (Miskelly, 1995).

The parish nurse should develop the practice and program in response to the unique needs and priorities of the congregation and its members. Leadership, organizational, clinical, counseling, and teaching skills are essential.

Education and Experience for Parish Nursing Practice

A baccalaureate degree is recommended for parish nursing practice. Three to five years of experience in nursing practice, spiritual maturity, and ability to practice independently are important attributes for a parish nurse (Schank et al., 1996).

CORRECTIONAL INSTITUTIONS

According to Droes, "The number of individuals incarcerated in the United States is the highest since data were first available in 1925" (1994, p. 201). In the United States, the judicial system has mandated that correctional facilities have the responsibility to provide health care to all individuals confined to their facilities (Hufft and Fawkes, 1994). In many cases, nurses are the primary health care providers in correctional facilities. Currently, there are nearly 9,000 RNs working in correctional institutions, including jails, prisons, and juvenile detention facilities (USDHHS/PHS, 1994).

Issues in Caring for Persons in Correctional Facilities

Residents of correctional institutions experience a higher rate of diseases and disability than the general population. Infectious diseases (e.g., respiratory infections, influenza, gonorrhea, tuberculosis, hepatitis, and human immunodeficiency virus [HIV]), conditions related to the use and abuse of drugs and alcohol, seizure disorders, and acute mental health problems are particularly common. Trauma and chronic problems such as cirrhosis of the liver, gastritis, pancreatitis, and cardiac pathology are also prevalent (Droes, 1994).

One of the many distinctive characteristics of providing health care in correctional facilities is that clients usually have no choice in the selection of the health care providers and may have no choice in the services provided. Likewise, a great deal of professionalism is needed, in that providers in prison settings must have the ability to separate the action of the crime or offense of the individual inmate from his or her illness or health care need (Hufft and Fawkes, 1994).

Practicing within a correctional facility can be made difficult because of the conflicts of perceptions, beliefs, and norms between health care providers and correctional facility personnel. Differences in the two groups are described in Table 10–9. Stevens (1993) advises that nurses working in correctional facilities learn to recognize these differences and work through them to meet the needs of the patient within the requirements of the institution.

Nursing Practice in Correctional Facilities

Health services in correctional settings vary from health screening to full hospital services. In general, the main component of nursing practice in correctional facilities is provision of primary care and emergency services for the inmates. Primary health care in these facilities typically includes

TABLE 10–9 **Values, Beliefs, and Norms in Health Care and Corrections Cultures**

Element	Health Care	Law Enforcement and Corrections
Values	Basic goodness	Evil is present
	All persons are essentially the same	Criminal traits exist
Beliefs	Individuals who say they are sick should receive attention	Individuals who say they are sick are trying to "get out" of something
	People obey the rules	People break rules
	Health care is a right	Health care is a privilege
	Provide the maximum health care possible	Provide the least possible health care
Norms	Respect the patient	Distrust the inmate
	Get the patients well and out	Get the individuals convicted and incarcerated
	Anger and hostility are acceptable ways of behaving when a person is ill; assistance is offered; anger is redirected	Anger and hostility are not acceptable; hostile inmates necessitate higher security; "safekeeping" is a must
	Resisting treatment calls for counseling, with restraints being last resort	Resisting arrest is not tolerated, and restraints are the first resort (e.g., handcuffs)
	Assumption of danger to self is minimal	Assumption of danger to self is ever present
	Certain things are essential for humanitarian reasons (e.g., blankets)	Nothing is essential; punishment may result in removal of essentials (e.g., blankets)

From Stevens, R. (1993). When your clients are in jail. *Nursing Forum, 28* (4), 5–8.

screening activities, direct health care services, analysis of individual health behaviors, teaching and counseling, and assisting individuals in assuming responsibility for their own health (ANA, 1995).

Because of the situation and population encountered in this type of nursing practice, client needs and related nursing interventions in correctional facilities are quite unique. Specific interventions described by the ANA (1985) include

- Health education—promotion of individual and group well-being through health education activities (e.g., health counseling, health teaching, and formal programs in health education)
- Suicide prevention—ongoing assessment of suicide risk, as well as planning and coordination of interventions that prevent suicidal behaviors
- Communicable disease control—promotion of a healthful environment to reduce the incidence of communicable disease within the correctional setting
- Alcohol and drug rehabilitation—collaboration with other members of the health care team to treat inmates who have substance abuse problems
- Medication administration—supervision of the administration of medications in accordance with state regulations and national standards
- Psychosocial counseling—provision of crisis intervention, as well as episodic and ongoing psychosocial counseling
- Emergency care—initiation of emergency care as needed, according to community standards of care
- Environmental health—ongoing monitoring of the environment for conditions that would have a negative impact on health and safety within the facility and reporting of significant findings to the institution's management

Nurses who work in correctional facilities must work toward the goal of preserving and promoting the health of the incarcerated individual within the institution's broader goal of security. However, it is important to note that these nurses should provide only health care services—it is inappropriate for nurses to be involved in the security functions or disciplinary decisions of the setting (e.g., conducting body cavity or strip searches) (ANA, 1995). The institution should have a well-developed and periodically revised set of policies and procedures developed jointly by nurses, physicians, prisoners, and institution personnel (Stevens, 1993).

Education and Experience Recommendations for Nursing Practice in Correctional Facilities

Experience in mental health nursing is desirable for nurses who wish to practice in correctional facilities. Likewise, experience in emergency services, medical/surgical nursing, and community or public health nursing is also very beneficial. Educationally, a baccalaureate degree in nursing is recommended by the ANA for the practice of nursing in correctional facilities (ANA, 1985). Finally, because of the unique characteristics described here, Stevens (1993, p. 6) suggests that "nurses considering this practice setting should first observe a colleague who practices in the setting."

Nursing Practice with Selected Populations

In contrast to the provision of care to individuals and families in geographical settings, organizations, clinics, or agencies, community-based nursing care often involves caring for individuals and/or families undergoing directed care to treat specified illnesses or to prevent certain illnesses or health threats. Practice in these settings is often limited to single encounters to provide treatment or preventative services (e.g., day surgery, immunization clinics, STD clinics) or multiple visits providing care for a chronic illness (e.g., ambulatory oncology, tuberculosis management, renal dialysis). This section describes nursing practice in specialized, community-based settings.

PUBLIC HEALTH

The public health department is "an administrative or service unit of local or state government concerned with health and carrying some responsibility for the health of a jurisdiction smaller than the state" (Maher, 1995, p. 803). Local health departments are given the authority by the state to protect the health and welfare of their residents and are funded through local taxes and fees and grants from their state and federal sources.

Approximately 3,000 local health departments exist in the United States. Of these, 66% serve populations of less than 50,000, 46% have fewer than 10 full-time employees, and 10% have 100 or more employees. Additionally, 90% of local health departments employ RNs (either directly or through contracted services) (Maher, 1995). State, county, and local health departments combined employ approximately 44,000 RNs (about 2.5% of all RNs) (USDHHS/PHS, 1994).

The scope of services provided by public health departments varies considerably across the country. In general, health departments have traditionally been responsible for environmental sanitation, communicable disease surveillance and prevention, and other services to prevent illness and promote health. Public health efforts include a variety of services and interventions, such as regulation of water and air quality; solid waste disposal; supervision of restaurants, grocery stores, and other food processors and handlers; and control of vectors that might spread disease (e.g., mosquitoes, rats).

To control communicable diseases, health departments are required to monitor them (see Chapter 15) and are usually involved in their prevention as well. This often includes provision of immunizations; easily accessible (affordable) treatment for STDs; and screening, diagnosis, and treatment of certain communicable diseases such as tuberculosis, AIDS, and Hansen's disease. In addition to these programs, again varying greatly by area, many public health departments provide prenatal and family planning services, well-baby care, community mental health services, and home health care.

Public Health Nursing Practice

Nursing practice in public health departments varies greatly, depending on the nurse's assigned area. Much of public health nursing practice focusing on control of communicable disease is described in detail in Chapters 15 and 16. Community mental health, home health, and family planning and maternal child health are covered in Chapters 17, 7, and 12, respectively. The reader is referred to those chapters to learn more about public health nursing practice.

Education and Experience Recommendations for Public Health Nurses

Because public health theory and practice are included in baccalaureate nursing programs, a baccalaureate degree in nursing is preferred by most health departments. However, most nurses currently working in public health departments were educated in diploma or associate degree programs (Maher, 1995).

One or more years of nursing experience is often required for employment in public health departments. Practical experience in maternal and child health, primary health care, mental health care, infection control, and management of clients with HIV and AIDS is particularly helpful in public health nursing.

AMBULATORY ONCOLOGY CARE

According to Lin and Martin (1994), "over 80% of all cancer care is delivered in the outpatient setting" (p. 227). Sites for delivery of care and some services offered for patients with cancer include (Lampkin, 1994)

- Physician's offices: Services may include chemotherapy administration, procedures, laboratory and x-ray facilities, counseling, and educational programs.
- Outpatient clinics: Services performed include radiation therapy, chemotherapy, biotherapy, physician and psychosocial services, symptom control, bone marrow transplantation, and rehabilitation.
- Twenty-three–hour and 24-hour clinics and day hospitals: These provide urgent care and may include an emergency room for oncology patients, an outpatient procedure unit, observation, an investigational treatment area, an after-hours telephone triage center, and on-call physician support.

Health care services related to care of oncology patients include (Lamkin, 1994)

1. Prevention, screening, and detection
2. Chemotherapy
3. Radiation therapy
4. Blood component therapy
5. Patient and family education
6. Discharge planning and referral
7. Nutritional support
8. Group or individual counseling
9. Physical therapy and rehabilitation
10. Outpatient surgery
11. Prescription supply and procurement
12. Survivor services
13. Treatment planning
14. Symptom management

Nursing Practice in Ambulatory Oncology Settings

Nursing interventions in ambulatory oncology nursing practice include patient counseling (e.g., patient advocacy, emotional support during visitations and by telephone), health care maintenance (e.g., general assessment of health, assessment of compliance, measurement of physiological indices), primary care (e.g., triage in person or by telephone, obtaining patient history, performing physical examination), patient education (e.g., group educational programs, explanation of plan of care, reinforcement of physician instructions), therapeutic care (e.g., administration of treatments such as irrigations, dressing changes, specimen collection; administration of medications), normative care (e.g., preparing patient for physician, assisting physician, providing follow-up appointment), non–client-centered care (e.g., maintaining supplies and equipment, developing educational materials and standards of care for staff, maintaining knowledge of new care practice), communication (e.g., providing information to other health care providers regarding patient care issues), and documentation and planning (Cooley et al., 1994). Ambulatory oncology nurses often provide telephone triage, including follow-up; symptom management; patient education; scheduling appointments and tests; and contacting physicians to discuss patient care issues. Well-defined assessment skills, incorporating physical, psychosocial, and financial aspects, are the cornerstone of practice (Cooley et al., 1994).

Patient and family education is essential to accomplish one important goal of outpatient oncology care: to prepare the patient for self-care. Patient education needs include treatment options, information about specific treatments and diagnostic tests, symptom management, nutrition, pharmacology, accessing social services, technical skills (e.g., caring for catheters, central lines, and self-injection), and how and when to access assistance when needed (Lamkin, 1994).

Education, Certification and Experience Recommendations for Ambulatory Oncology Nurses

Nurses who practice in ambulatory oncology centers should have at least 1 year of clinical experience in oncology or chronic illness. They must have good clinical skills, be certified in CPR, and be able to handle emergency situations. Oncology nursing certification is strongly recommended. Some agencies require baccalaureate-level preparation (Cooley et al., 1994).

AMBULATORY SURGERY

Ambulatory surgery refers to the process in which "patients have surgery, recover, and are discharged home the same day" (Groah, 1996, p. 367). Ambulatory surgery is not a new concept (it reportedly dates back to ancient Egypt), but it has increased dramatically in recent years because of advances in anesthesia and surgical techniques and a desire for convenience (Atkinson and Fortunato, 1995).

Cost containment is one of the primary reasons for the proliferation in same-day surgical procedures. Indeed, many third-party payers require that certain procedures be done on an outpatient basis unless documentation can be provided that this would be unsafe for the patient (Mezey and Lawrence, 1995).

"Approximately 65% of all surgical procedures are performed safely on an ambulatory basis without compromising the quality of care" (Atkinson and Fortunato, 1995, p. 834). To determine eligibility for having a surgical procedure performed on an ambulatory basis, considerations should include general health status (patients should be evaluated to determine possibility of complications during and after the surgical procedure), results of preoperative tests (e.g., laboratory tests, chest x-ray, electrocardiogram), willingness and acceptance by the patient and family (including provision for competent care at home), anticipated recovery period, and reimbursement sources (Atkinson and Fortunato, 1995).

Several terms can be used to describe ambulatory surgical care facilities. These include outpatient surgery centers, same-day surgical units, one-day surgery centers, or ambulatory surgery centers. There are several different organizational structures for ambulatory surgery facilities. These are (Atkinson and Fortunato, 1995; Groah, 1996)

- Hospital-based dedicated unit: Patients are admitted to an autonomous, independent, self-contained unit within or attached to the hospital but physically separated from the inpatient operating room suite.
- Hospital-based integrated unit: Patients share the same operating room suite and other hospital facilities with inpatients but have a separate preoperative hold area.
- Hospital-affiliated satellite surgery center: Patients are cared for at an ambulatory surgery center owned and operated by the hospital but physically separated from it.
- Freestanding ambulatory surgery center: Patients are cared for at a totally independent facility that is privately owned and operated for the purpose of providing surgical care.
- Office-based center: Patients are seen at a physician's office that is equipped for surgery.

Many general surgeons, dermatologists, plastic surgeons, periodontists, podiatrists, and others perform surgical procedures in their offices.

Freestanding postsurgical recovery centers provide short nonhospital stays for less-intensive recovery, for less-complex surgical cases (Williams, 1993). These centers are designed for individuals who are otherwise well but may need monitoring or services that cannot be easily, safely, or economically provided in the home. For example, a patient who has undergone extensive plastic surgery may need to be monitored for a day or two and treated for pain and to prevent complications (e.g., infection) but may not require hospitalization. For this person, a short stay in a recovery center would be appropriate. Likewise, if a day surgery patient has no one to provide care at home, an overnight stay in a recovery center might help avoid otherwise unnecessary hospitalization.

Advantages of ambulatory surgery include decreased cost to the patient and institution, increased bed availability for seriously ill patients, decreased risk of acquiring a nosocomial infection, and less disruption to the patient's personal life (Fairchild, 1996). Disadvantages include increased anxiety of the patient and caregiver, complications (e.g., allergic responses to drugs and anesthetics, prolonged procedures, secondary diagnosis), and unrealistic patient expectations of physical capabilities postoperatively. Occasionally, patients require hospitalization because of prolonged procedures, secondary diagnosis, surgical accident, or other complications (e.g., excessive pain, nausea and vomiting, bleeding, swelling) (Atkinson and Fortunato, 1995). Contraindications to ambulatory surgery include patients who are physically unstable, morbidly obese, or acute substance abusers or individuals who do not have adequate support at home (Groah, 1996). Table 10–10 lists surgical procedures commonly performed on an outpatient basis.

Nursing Practice in Ambulatory Surgery

Nursing care during ambulatory surgery is typically provided in three phases: preoperative care, intraoperative care, and postanesthesia care.

Preoperative Care. In the preoperative phase, the patient is admitted to the facility, given preoperative instructions, and prepared for the procedure. Any tests that have been performed in preparation are reviewed, and other tests may be performed at that time. The nurse conducts a preoperative interview to verify information about past medical and surgical history, the pending procedure(s), current medications, drug allergies, and other pertinent information (e.g., whether the patient wears contact lenses or has dental work or any prostheses). The nurse confirms that any instructions regarding eating or drinking before admission have been followed.

The nurse then allows the patient to change into a gown and escorts him or her to the holding area, where baseline vital signs are taken. In the holding area, the patient may be given preoperative medications and further prepared for the procedure (e.g., the operative site may be shaved or an intravenous line started). Agency protocol determines how the consent forms for surgery and other paperwork are completed and who is responsible. The nurse should ensure that all consent forms are complete and accurate.

Intraoperative Care. As with perioperative nursing care in the hospital, the intraoperative team usually consists of a circulating nurse, a scrub nurse, an anesthesiologist or certified registered nurse-anesthetist (CRNA), and the surgeon. Often the surgeon has an assistant. In most agencies, it is the responsibility of the circulating nurse to ensure that the procedure runs smoothly. The circulating nurse typically retrieves the patient from preoperative holding when the anesthesiologist or CRNA is ready. The circulating nurse assists the scrub nurse and the anesthesiologist or CRNA with their preparatory work while helping reduce the patient's anxiety.

Both the circulating nurse and the scrub nurse assist the surgeon throughout the procedure. At the end of the procedure, the circulating nurse attends the anesthesiologist or CRNA while the patient awakens if general anesthetic is used. The circulating nurse assists the patient to a stretcher (a wheelchair may be used for procedures done under local or regional anesthesia) and take him or her to the postanesthesia care area.

TABLE 10–10 **Commonly Performed Outpatient Procedures**

- Gynecology
  - Conization of cervix
  - Dilation and curettage
  - Salpingectomy
  - Hymenal ring lesion excision
  - Salpingogram
  - Therapeutic abortion
  - Tubal ligation
  - Hymenotomy
  - Examination under anesthesia
  - Culdoscopy
  - Vaginoplasty
  - Minilaparotomy
  - Bartholin cyst excision
- Orthopedic surgery
  - Arthroscopy
  - Nail removal
  - Cast change
  - Ligament repair
  - Metacarpal wire removal
  - Plate (bone) removal
  - Ganglion excision
  - Ulnar nerve transplant
  - Median nerve decompression
  - Release Dequervains hand
  - Release Dupuytren contracture
  - Release trigger thumb
  - Fracture reduction
  - Bunionectomy
  - Excision exostosis
  - Bursa removal
  - Tendon repair
- Ophthalmology
  - Eye cyst excision
  - Examination under anesthesia
  - Cataract procedures
  - Ptosis
  - Tear duct probe
  - Enucleation
  - Eyelid surgery
  - Eye muscle surgery
  - Chalazion
  - Iridectomy
- Thoracic surgery
  - Esophageal dilation
  - Pacemaker battery replacement
- Neurosurgery
  - Carpal tunnel release
  - Median nerve decompression
  - Ulnar nerve transfer
- Dental/oral surgery
  - Dental extraction
  - Curettage of maxilla
  - Intraoral biopsy
  - Closed reduction jaw fracture
- Otolaryngology
  - Nasopharyngoscopy
  - Nasal septum repair
  - Otoplasty
  - Tonsillectomy and adenoidectomy
  - Adenoidectomy
  - Bronchoscopy, laryngoscopy
  - Nasal fracture reduction
  - Foreign body removed from ear
- Plastic surgery
  - Augmental mammoplasty
  - Nose reduction
  - Blepharoplasty
  - Skin grafts
  - Redundant tissue removal
  - Basal cell carcinoma excision
  - Contracture release
  - Ganglionectomy
  - Otoplasty
  - Scar revision
  - Tendon repair
- General surgery
  - Breast biopsy
  - Laryngoscopy
  - Esophagoscopy
  - Gastroscopy
  - Endoscopy
  - Node biopsies
  - Herniorrhaphy
  - Lipoma removal
  - Nevus removal
  - Lesion excision
  - Polyp excision
  - Bronchoscopy
  - Brachial arteriogram
  - Pilonidal cyst excision
  - Débridement
  - Hemorrhoidectomy
  - Abscess incise and drain
  - Sigmoidoscopy
- Urology
  - Cystogram and pyelogram
  - Biopsy bladder tumor
  - Transurethral resection
  - Circumcision
  - Vasectomy
  - Cystoscopy
  - Orchiectomy
  - Prostate biopsy
  - Testicular biopsy

Adapted from Katz, R. (1987). Issues in outpatient surgery, *Seminars in Anesthesiology, 258.* From Fairchild, S. S. (1996). Topics and issues affecting practice. In S. S. Fairchild (Ed.). *Perioperative Nursing: Principles and Practice* (2nd ed.). Boston, Little, Brown & Co.

Postanesthesia Care and Discharge. Following the procedure, the patient is taken to the designated PACU or recovery area for observation; for management of pain, nausea, and vomiting; and to ensure maintenance of fluid and electrolyte balance. In the PACU, the vital signs are taken periodically, and the patient is monitored for complications related to surgery, anesthesia, or the presenting health condition.

Discharge is based on the absence of indications of serious complications (e.g., bleeding, unusual pain) when the patient is alert and able to walk safely and a responsible person is in attendance. Discharge criteria include the patient being alert and oriented and having stable vital signs; no respiratory distress; no hoarseness or cough following endotracheal intubation; a gag reflex; ability to swallow and cough; no dizziness, nausea, or vomiting; no bleeding and minimal swelling or drainage on dressings; ability to tolerate fluids and having been able to void; no excessive pain that will not be alleviated with oral medications at home; ability to ambulate (based on developmental age or physical limitations); and clear vision (corrected if necessary) (Atkinson and Fortunato, 1995).

The PACU nurse is usually responsible for reviewing postprocedure instructions with the patient and the caregiver(s). It is essential that they be aware of signs and symptoms of complications and when to call the surgeon or go to the hospital. Instructions should also include pain management, bathing instructions, wound care (if applicable), activity limitations, diet, and the importance of a follow-up appointment with the surgeon. Instructions should be written and explicit to ensure that they are easily understood (Groah, 1996).

Experience, Education, and Certification for Ambulatory Surgery Nursing Practice

There are no specific educational requirements for RNs practicing in ambulatory care surgery. However, many ambulatory surgery centers require a minimum of 1 year of experience in either the operating room or postanesthesia care.

Certification in operating room nursing or in postanesthesia care is definitely an advantage. The Association of Operating Room Nurses grants certification to qualifying operating room nurses, and the American Society of Post Anesthesia Nurses certifies nurses in postanesthesia care.

CAMP NURSING

"Nurses have been caring for children in camp settings for as long as children have been attending camp" (Maheady, 1991, p. 247). There are numerous summer camps for children throughout the country, and opportunities for nursing employment are readily available.

Children's summer camps my serve healthy children or children with serious health conditions or "special needs." Examples of "special needs" camps available in some locations include camps for children with cystic fibrosis, diabetes, cancer, behavior disorders, sociocultural deprivation, developmental disabilities, asthma, hemophilia, muscular dystrophy, cerebral palsy, post–acute-phase burns, epilepsy, juvenile arthritis, mental retardation, and AIDS (Maheady, 1991; Praeger, 1994).

Important considerations in camp nursing include staffing requirements (one full-time nurse per 100–120 healthy campers is recommended). Staffing needs obviously increase for children with special needs. Depending on the type of "special needs" and the severity of the children's problems, one pediatrician and one RN should be at the camp 24 hours a day for a population of 50 campers, and an additional RN is recommended for any number above 50 campers.

Physician back-up and emergency resources are very important when considering employment at a camp. Other considerations are nursing responsibilities, facilities, living conditions, health status of the children, malpractice insurance, salary, and on-call and time-off schedules (Maheady, 1991).

Camp Nursing Practice

Roles and responsibilities of camp nurses typically include clinic management (e.g., ordering supplies and medications, developing and maintaining policy and procedures manuals, maintenance of a first aid kit). Camp nurses are usually responsible for administration of medications to the campers. Identification of health hazards and risks is another responsibility. Camp nursing responsibilities should include health promotion, health education, accident and illness prevention, assessment and treatment of a wide variety of actual health problems, evaluation of outcomes of care, and collaboration with other health professionals (Faro, 1994).

The most common problems encountered by camp nurses are sore throat; cuts, lacerations, scrapes, and bruises; sprained ankle; headache; stomach ache; cold symptoms; otitis media; poison ivy; and otitis externa. Homesickness (often indicated by headache, stomachache, and other aches and pains; crying; sleep disturbances; withdrawal; and anxiety) is also commonly encountered—most frequently during the first few days of camp.

Experience and Education Recommendations for Camp Nurses

There are usually no specific education requirements for camp nurses. Camp nurses who work with well children ideally have experience in school nursing, pediatric nursing, and emergency care. However, when working at camps for children with chronic health conditions, experience in working with children with the specific diagnosis or condition (e.g., cancer, diabetes, cystic fibrosis) is usually required. Additionally, camp nurses should be certified in provision of first aid.

Nursing Care in "Other" Ambulatory Settings

A number of other settings exist in which nurses are employed in community-based practice. Among these are nursing in poison control centers, ambulatory diagnostic centers (e.g., outpatient imaging and radiology services for diagnosis and treatment), community hotlines (e.g., suicide, AIDS, drug and alcohol abuse, family violence), and migrant health centers. Nurses who desire to practice in non–acute care settings should be alert to the variety of opportunities. For more information, Table 10–11 lists some resources for nurses interested in nursing practice in the ambulatory settings described here.

Key Points

- Ambulatory care refers to personal health care or health services (e.g., outpatient surgery and chemotherapy, diagnostic tests and procedures) provided to noninstitutionalized patients.
- Ambulatory nursing care is largely focused on health promotion, primary prevention, screening for early identification of disease, and assisting in treatment regimens for both acute and chronic illnesses. Care is usually ongoing and comprehensive.
- Almost 8% of all registered nurses practice in a health care office or clinic (with a provider such as a physician, nurse practitioner, or physician assistant). Clinic or office nurses assist with assessments and procedures, provide education, collect specimens, and administering medications. Coordination of services and preparation of patients for procedures are other roles and responsibilities.
- Currently, about 2.2% of all RNs are school nurses. School nurses work to prevent illnesses, intervene in identified problems, promote healthy lifestyles, and provide health education. Caring for students with special health needs (e.g., urinary catheterization, tube feedings, tracheotomy care) is becoming increasingly common.

TABLE 10–11 Resources for Ambulatory Health Care Nursing

Ambulatory Oncology Nursing

Oncology Nursing Society
501 Holiday Drive
Pittsburgh, PA 15220-2749
(412) 921-7373

National Institutes of Health
National Cancer Institute
Cancer Information Service
Building 31, Room 10A16
9000 Rockville Pike
Bethesda, MD 20892
(800) 4-CANCER
(301) 496-5583

National Cancer Institute
Surveillance, Epidemiology and End Results (SEER) Program
Division of Cancer Prevention and Control
6130 Executive Boulevard North
Room 343
Bethesda, MD 20892
(301) 496-6616

American Cancer Society
1599 Clifton Road, NE
Atlanta, GA 30329
(800) ACS-2345

Ambulatory Surgery

Association of Operating Room Nurses
2170 Parker Road, Suite 300
Denver, CO 80231

American Society of Post Anesthesia Nurses
11512 Allecingie Parkway
Richmond, VA 23235
(804) 379-5516

Occupational Health Nursing

American Association of Occupational Health Nurses
50 Lennox Pointe
Atlanta, GA 30324
(404) 262-1162

National Institute for Occupational Safety and Health
Office of the Director
Humphrey Building Room 715-H
Washington, D. C. 20201
(202) 401-6997
Office of Information
4676 Columbia Parkway
Cincinnati, OH 45226-1998
(800) 35-NIOSH

U. S. Department of Labor
Occupational Safety and Health Administration
Publications, Room N-3647
200 Constitution Avenue, NW
Washington, D. C. 20210
(202) 219-8151

Bureau of Labor Statistics
Office of Safety, Health, and Working Conditions
2 Massachusetts Avenue, NE
Room 3180
Washington, D. C. 20212
(202) 606-6180

National Safety Council
1121 Spring Lake Drive
Itasca, IL 60143-3201
(708) 285-1121
(800) 621-7615

Parish Nursing

National Parish Nursing Resource Center
205 Touhy Avenue, Suite 104
Park Ridge, IL 60068
(800) 556-5368

Health Ministries Association
2427 Country Lane
Poland, OH 44514
(800) 852-5613

Marquette University Parish Nurse Institute
530 North 16th Street
Milwaukee, WI 53233

Public Health Nursing

American Public Health Association
1015 15th Street NW
Washington, D. C. 20005
(202) 789-5600

Centers for Disease Control and Prevention
Atlanta, GA 30333
(404) 329-3311

School Nursing

American School Health Association
P. O. Box 708
Kent, OH 44240
(216) 678-1601

TABLE 10–11 **Resources for Ambulatory Health Care Nursing** *Continued*

National Association of School Nurses
P. O. Box 1300
Scarborough, Maine 04090-1300
(207) 883-2117

American School Food Service Association
1600 Duke Street, 7th floor
Alexandria, VA 22314
(703) 739-3900

Rural Nursing

Department of Agriculture
Office of Small Community and Rural Development
Rural Development Administration
14th Street and Independence Avenue
Washington, D. C. 20250
(202) 690-2394

Department of Health and Human Services
Office of Rural Health Policy
5600 Fishers Lane
Rockville, MD 20857
(301) 443-0835

Indian Health Services
Park Lawn Building
5600 Fishers Lane
Rockville, MD 20857
(301) 443-1180

National Rural Health Association
301 E. Armour Boulevard
Suite 420
Kansas City, MO 64111
(816) 756-3140

- There are more than 20,000 occupational health nurses practicing in the United States. Occupational health nurses provide health care services to workers, focusing on health promotion and protection from injury and illness within the context of a safe and healthy work environment. Occupational health nurses provide assessment of the environment for threats to health and safety, assessment of the health status of workers, nursing care for occupational and nonoccupational injuries and illnesses, counseling, and health education. Several laws directly affect the practice of the occupational health nurses. These include Workers' Compensation Acts, the Federal Coal Mine Health and Safety Act, and the Occupational Safety and Health Act.
- Delivery of nursing and health care to clients in rural areas has a number of distinctive characteristics and challenges: Distance, isolation, and sparse resources, combined with shortage of nurses and other health care providers in rural areas, are particular challenges. Rural nurses must be clinically competent in a very broad number of areas and are typically cross-trained to manage client needs in areas including trauma, routine obstetrical care, care of children and elders, and care of clients with mental health needs.
- Parish nurses seek to promote the health of a community (centered in a church or synagogue) by integration of theological, psychological, sociological, and physiological perspectives of health. Parish nurses work to enhance the quality of life for members of a congregation and often the surrounding neighborhood. Parish nursing interventions include organization of support groups, provision of referrals to community resources, health education, counseling, and acting as a liaison within the larger health care system.
- The U. S. government requires health care services for all inmates in correctional facilities. As a result, there are approximately 9,000 RNs working in jails, prisons, and juvenile detention facilities. The main component of nursing practice in

correctional facilities is provision of primary care and emergency services for the inmates.

- There are approximately 44,000 nurses practicing in local, county, and state public health departments. Depending on mandates of the individual locality, health departments are responsible for diverse areas, including environmental sanitation, communicable disease surveillance and prevention, and maternal and child health.
- Ambulatory oncology care allows cancer patients to receive diagnosis and treatment as outpatients. Nurses may care for oncology clients in physicians' offices, outpatient clinics, and day hospitals. Health care services may include prevention, screening, chemotherapy, radiation therapy, education, discharge planning, nutritional support, counseling, and outpatient surgery.
- Approximately 65% of all surgical procedures can be performed on an ambulatory basis; thus, nursing in outpatient surgical centers continues to grow. Nurses who work in outpatient surgical centers may provide preoperative care, intraoperative care, or postanesthesia care. Preoperative care involves giving the patient and family preoperative instructions and preparing them for the procedure. Intraoperative nursing consists of acting as circulating nurse, scrub nurse, or, in some cases, first assistant during the surgical procedure. During postanesthesia care, the nurse observes the patient for complications, manages complications and side effects (e.g., nausea, pain), and prepares him or her for discharge.
- Camp nursing is an opportunity for nurses to work with children in a fun setting. Camps may be for "normal" healthy children, or they may be for children with special needs (e.g., children with chronic illnesses or disabilities). Responsibilities of camp nurses include clinic management, administration of medications, identification of health hazards, health promotion and education, accident and illness prevention, and administration of first aid.

Learning Activities and Application to Practice

In Class

- Invite nurses who currently practice in several of the ambulatory settings described speak to the class in a "panel" format. Allow and encourage the nurses to describe a "typical" day, including what clients are seen, what interventions are given, examples of collaboration with other providers, and what experience or education is needed to practice in the setting.
- Have students individually or in pairs interview a nurse who practices in an ambulatory setting. What roles and responsibilities does the nurse have? What are common interventions? Describe positive and negative aspects of practice. What are education and experience requirements? What are employment opportunities, work hours, and salaries? Share findings with the class.
- Consider offering an elective course in one or more of the specialty areas described. Nursing electives and/or graduate programs are described in the literature for camp nursing, parish nursing, school nursing, occupational health

nursing, and nursing in correctional facilities, among others. Course objectives, content, and evaluation criteria are frequently available and may be modified to meet needs of the school and students.

In Clinical

- As opportunities permit, allow students to spend one or more days in one or more of the ambulatory settings described. If possible, select an acute or chronic care setting (e.g., ambulatory surgery, oncology) and a primary care setting (e.g., physician office, school, parish nursing). In a log or journal, have students compare and contrast nursing practice in the two settings.

REFERENCES

American Nurses' Association. (1996). *Rural/Frontier Nursing: The Challenge to Grow.* Washington, D. C., American Nurses' Association.

American Nurses' Association. (1995). *Scope and Standards of Nursing Practice in Correctional Facilities.* Washington, D. C., American Nurses' Association.

American Nurses' Association. (1985). *Standards of Nursing Practice in Correctional Facilities.* Kansas City, MO, American Nurses' Association.

American School Health Association. (1991). *Implementation Guide for the Standards of School Nursing Practice.* Kent, OH, American School Health Association.

Atkinson, L. J. and Fortunato, N. H. (1995). Ambulatory surgery. In L. J. Atkinson and N. H. Fortunato. *Berry & Kohn's Operating Room Technique.* St. Louis, MO, Mosby-Year Book, pp. 833–839.

Burgel, B. J. (1994). Occupational health: Nursing in the workplace. *Nursing Clinics of North America, 29* (3), 431–441.

Bushy, A. (1996). Community health nursing in rural environments. In M. Stanhope and J. Lancaster (Eds.). *Community Health Nursing: Promoting the Health of Aggregates, Families and Individuals* (4th ed.). St. Louis, MO, Mosby-Year Book, pp. 315–332.

Bushy, A. (1995). Rural health. In C. M. Smith and F. A. Maurer (Eds.). *Community Health Nursing: Theory and Practice.* Philadelphia, W. B. Saunders, pp. 820–847.

Clemen-Stone, S., Eigsti, D. G., and McGuire, S. L. (1995). *Comprehensive Community Health Nursing* (4th ed.), St. Louis, MO, Mosby-Year Book.

Coolely, M. E., Lin, E. M., and Hunter, S. W. (1994). The ambulatory oncology nurse's role. *Seminars in Oncology Nursing 10* (4), 245–253.

Droes, N. S. (1994). Correctional nursing practice. *Journal of Community Health Nursing 11* (4), 201–210.

Fairchild, S. S. (1996). Topics and issues affecting practice. In S. S. Fairchild (Ed.). *Perioperative Nursing: Principles and Practice* (2nd ed.). Boston, Little, Brown & Co., pp. 634–640.

Faro, B. Z. (1994). Summer camp as a clinical placement for graduate students in pediatrics. *Journal of Nursing Education, 33* (2), 91–92.

Groah, L. K. (1996). Ambulatory surgery. In L. K. Groah. *Perioperative Nursing* (3rd ed.). Stamford, CT, Appleton & Lange, pp. 367–375.

Hackbarth, D. P., Haas, S. A., Kavanagh, J. A., and Vlasses, F. (1995). Dimensions of the staff nurse role in ambulatory care: Part I—Methodology and analysis of data on current staff nurse practice. *Nursing Economics, 13* (2), 89–98.

Hanson, C. M. (1996). Care of clients in rural settings. In M. J. Clark (Ed.). *Nursing in the Community* (2nd ed.). Stamford, CT, Appleton & Lange, pp. 625–644.

Hartwell, S., Parker, M., Korn, K., and Polich, C. L. (1991). Rural health care delivery and financing: Results of eight case studies. In A. Bushy (Ed.). *Rural Nursing.* Newbury Park, CA, Sage Publications, pp. 128–140.

Hufft, A. G. and Fawkes, L. S. (1994). Federal inmates: A unique psychiatric nursing challenge. *Nursing Clinics of North America, 29* (1), 35–41.

Kub, J. and Steel, S. A. (1995). School health. In C. M. Smith and F. A. Maurer (Eds.). *Community Health Nursing: Theory and Practice.* Philadelphia, W. B. Saunders, pp. 747–775.

Lamkin, L. (1994). Outpatient oncology settings: A variety of services. *Seminars in Oncology Nursing 10* (4), 229–235.

Lee, H. J. (1991). Definitions of rural: A review of the literature. In A. Bushy (Ed.). *Rural Nursing.* Newbury Park, CA, Sage Publications, pp. 7–20.

Lewis, K. D. and Thomson, H. B. (1986). *Manual of School Health.* Menlo Park, CA, Addison-Wesley.

Lin, E. M. and Martin, V. R. (1994). Introduction. *Seminars in Oncology Nursing 10* (4), 227–228.

Maheady, D. C. (1991). Camp nursing practice in review. *Pediatric Nursing, 17* (3), 247–250.

Maher, L. H. (1995). Local health departments. In C. M. Smith and F. A. Maurer (Eds.). *Community Health Nursing: Theory and Practice.* Philadelphia, W. B. Saunders, pp. 802–819.

Mezey, A. P. and Lawrence, R. S. (1995). Ambulatory care. In A. R. Kovner (Ed.). *Jonas's Health Care Delivery in the United States* (5th ed.). New York, Springer Publishing Co., pp. 122–161.

Miskelly, S. (1995). A parish nursing model: Applying the community health nursing process in a church community. *Journal of Community Health Nursing, 12* (1), 1–14.

National Association of School Nurses (1992). *Guidelines for a Model School Nursing Services Program.* Scarborough, ME, National Association of School Nurses.

National Association of School Nurses (1993). *Hearing Screening Guidelines for School Nurses.* Scarborough, ME, National Association of School Nurses.

National Association of School Nurses. (1985). *Vision Screening Guidelines for School Nurses.* Scarborough, ME, National Association of School Nurses.

Ossler, C. C., Stanhope, M., and Lancaster, J. (1996). Community health nurse in occupational health. In M. Stanhope and J. Lancaster (Eds.), *Community Health Nursing: Process and Practice for Promoting Health* (4th ed.). St. Louis, MO, Mosby-Year Book, pp. 907–928.

Parrinello, K. M. and Witzel, P. A. (1990). Analysis of ambulatory nursing practice. *Nursing Economic$, 8* (5), 322–328.

Petsonk, E. L. and Attfield, M. D. (1994). Coal workers' pneumoconiosis and other coal-related lung disease. In L. Rosenstock and M. R. Cullen (Eds.). *Textbook of Clinical Occupational and Environmental Medicine.* Philadelphia, W. B. Saunders, pp. 274–287.

Pollitt, P. (1994). Lina Rogers Struthers: The first school nurse. *Journal of School Nursing, 10* (1), 34–36.

Praeger, S. G. (1994). Clinical pediatrics: Nursing students go to camp. *Journal of Pediatric Nursing, 9* (3), 211–212.

Rogers, B. (1994). *Occupational Health Nursing: Concepts and Practice.* Philadelphia, W. B. Saunders.

Schank, M. J., Weis, D., and Matheus, R. (1996). Parish nursing: Ministry of healing. *Geriatric Nursing, 17* (1), 11–13.

Simington, J., Olson, J., and Douglass, L. (1996). Promoting well-being within a parish. *The Canadian Nurse, January,* 20–24.

Solari-Twadell, P., Djupe, A., and McDermott, M. (Eds.). (1990). *Parish Nursing: The Developing Practice.* Park Ridge, IL, National Parish Nurse Resource Center.

Spradley, B. W. (1990). Health of the working population. In B. Spradley (Ed.). *Community Health Nursing: Concepts and Practice* (3rd ed.). Glenview, IL, Scott, Foresman/Little, Brown & Co, pp. 528–561.

Stevens, R. (1993). When your clients are in jail. *Nursing Forum, 28* (4), 5–8.

Travers, P. H. and McDougall, C. E. (1993). The occupational health nurse: Roles and responsibilities, current and future trends. In J. M. Swanson and M. Albrecht (Eds.). *Community Health Nursing: Promoting the Health of Aggregates.* Philadelphia, W. B. Saunders, pp. 597–624.

Turner, T. A. and Gunn, I. P. (1991). Issues in rural health nursing. In A. Bushy (Ed.). *Rural Nursing.* Newbury Park, CA, Sage Publications, pp. 107–127.

U. S. Department of Health and Human Services. (1990). *Healthy People 2000: National Health Promotion and Disease Prevention Objectives.* Washington, D. C., Government Printing Office.

U. S. Department of Health and Human Services/Public Health Service/Health Resources and Services Administration. (1994). *The Registered Nurse Population: Findings from the National Sample Survey of Registered Nurses, March 1992.* Rockville, MD, Government Printing Office.

Weinert, C. and Long, K. A. (1991). The theory and research base for rural nursing practice. In A. Bushy (Ed.). *Rural Nursing.* Newbury Park, CA, Sage Publications, pp. 21–38.

Whitted, G. (1993). Private health insurance and employee benefits. In S. J. Williams and P. R. Torrens (Eds.). *Introduction to Health Services* (4th ed.). Albany, NY, Delmar Publishers, pp. 332–360.

Williams, S. J. (1993). Ambulatory health care services. In S. J. Williams and P. R. Torrens (Eds.). *Introduction to Health Services* (4th ed.). Albany, NY, Delmar Publishers, pp. 108–133.

UNIT IV

Community-Based Nursing Care of Children, Adults, and Elders

11

Health Promotion and Illness Prevention for Adults

Case Study

Rebecca Rogers is a staff nurse at a cardiac rehabilitation center in an urban area. The cardiac center provides comprehensive care to clients with heart disease, as well as services to prevent heart disease. At the center, Rebecca's responsibilities involve assisting in prevention, diagnosis, monitoring, and rehabilitation of cardiovascular disease in adults.

On Monday, Rebecca saw Mr. Ryan, a 50-year-old bank vice president. Although he has never had symptoms indicating a heart condition, Mr. Ryan was referred to the center by his internist, because he was determined to be "at risk" for developing coronary artery disease during a recent physical examination.

At the cardiac center, each patient initially completes a health history and questionnaires that assess known risk factors for heart disease. Among the findings from Mr. Ryan's completed assessments are that he is approximately 30 pounds heavier than "ideal" for his height, smokes one to one and a half packs of cigarettes a day (he has cut down from more than two packs a day during the past year), rarely engages in strenuous physical activity, drinks alcohol "occasionally," and reports "moderate" stress in his life. He eats a variety of foods but admits that he probably eats too many snacks and loves sweets. He has no history of hypertension or diabetes, and his serum cholesterol results over the past 5 years have remained steady, ranging from 200 to 220. He has a positive family history for heart disease. At age 65, his mother died from a heart attack, as did both grandfathers (ages at death unknown). His older brother has had no symptoms of heart disease. His father died in an automobile accident at age 45.

At the cardiac center, additional laboratory tests and diagnostic studies were performed to assess risk and determine if Mr. Ryan has evidence of coronary artery disease. Laboratory tests included a lipid profile to assess high-density and low-density lipoprotein values and ratios, an electrocardiogram, and a cardiac stress test. Rebecca assisted the physicians and technicians with these tests.

Fortunately, Mr. Ryan's tests showed no evidence of previous myocardial infarction and no angina. Following the examinations, Rebecca worked with a team composed of a cardiologist, a dietitian, and an exercise therapist to develop a plan of action for Mr. Ryan to reduce his risk of developing heart disease. Their recommendations:

1. *Stop smoking: Written information on methods to stop smoking was provided and discussed.*
2. *Dietary changes: Detailed literature on methods to lose weight and reduce dietary fat intake was provided and reviewed.*
3. *Increase physical activity: A program to improve physical fitness was presented. Detailed instructions to gradually increase daily exercise to at least 40 minutes, 3 to 4 days a week while increasing his heart rate to between 85 and 127 beats per minute were outlined.*
4. *Reduce stress: Stress management literature was provided. Stress avoidance, relaxation techniques, building supportive relationships, fatigue avoidance, and use of support groups, where indicated, were discussed.*
5. *Medications: It was determined that Mr. Ryan would not be put on medication to reduce his cholesterol at this time, as it is hoped that dietary management will be sufficient to reduce his cholesterol levels. His lipid profile will be reassessed in 3 months to see if his total cholesterol and low-density versus high-density lipoprotein ratios are improved. Aspirin, 325 mg/day, was prescribed following determination that Mr. Ryan had no allergies or history of bleeding tendencies.*

Mr. Ryan agreed to these recommendations, and reasonable goals for each area were set. Finally, he made an appointment to return to the cardiac center in 3 months to assess progress toward his goals.

"Health promotion" refers to those activities or actions related to encouraging individual lifestyles or personal choices that positively influence health. Physical activity and fitness, nutrition, and substance (e.g., tobacco, alcohol) use and abuse are examples of controllable behaviors or actions that ultimately affect health (U. S. Department of Health and Human Services [USDHHS], 1990). Pender (1987) states that the nurse-client relationship for health promotion is based on a "dynamic person-environment interactive model rather than on a traditional medical model" in which the nurse "guides clients in the self-assessment of personal health status and in the exploration of their health situations, helping them 'define concerns' rather than 'offering solutions'" (p. 94). In their practice, all nurses, particularly those working in community settings, should be prepared for opportunities to assist clients (whether individuals, families, groups, or communities) by providing information, counseling, advocacy, referral, or other interventions that allow the client to make informed choices to promote health.

Primary and secondary prevention refer to those interventions, such as counseling, screening, immunization, and education, that directly affect health to prevent acute or chronic disease or disability. This chapter contains assessment and teaching tools and information specific to these concepts. Initially, general health promotion strategies such as health risk appraisal, promotion of exercise and physical fitness, improving nutrition, and reduction or elimination of harmful substances are described in the discussion of health promotion. Primary and secondary prevention, specifically with regard to several of the leading causes of death and disability (i.e., heart disease and stroke, cancer, and diabetes), are then considered.

Causes of Death and Disability

Table 11–1 shows the leading causes of death in the United States. As depicted in this table, heart

TABLE 11–1 **Estimated Deaths, Death Rates, and Percentage of Total Deaths for the 15 Leading Causes of Death: United States, 1992***

Rank	Cause of Death (ICD-9)	No.	Death Rate	Total Deaths (%)
	All causes	2,177,000	853.3	100.0
1	Diseases of heart	720,480	282.5	33.1
2	Malignant neoplasms, including neoplasms of lymphatic and hematopoietic tissues	520,090	204.3	23.9
3	Cerebrovascular diseases	143,640	56.3	6.6
4	Chronic obstructive pulmonary diseases and allied conditions	91,440	35.8	4.2
5	Accidents and adverse effects	86,310	33.8	4.0
	Motor vehicle accidents	41,710	16.4	1.9
	All other accidents and adverse effects	44,600	17.5	2.0
6	Pneumonia and influenza	76,120	29.8	3.5
7	Diabetes mellitus	50,180	19.7	2.3
8	Human immunodeficiency virus infection	33,590	13.2	1.5
9	Suicide	29,760	11.7	1.4
10	Homicide and legal intervention	26,570	10.4	1.2
11	Chronic liver disease and cirrhosis	24,830	9.7	1.1
12	Nephritis, nephrotic syndrome, and nephrosis	22,400	8.8	1.0
13	Septicemia	19,910	7.8	0.9
14	Atherosclerosis	16,100	6.3	0.7
15	Certain conditions originating in the perinatal period	15,790	6.2	0.7
	All other causes	298,430	117.0	13.7

From Centers for Disease Control. (1993). Annual summary of births, marriages, divorces, and deaths: United States, 1992. *Monthly Vital Statistics Report.* Vol. 40. No. 13. Washington, D.C., Government Printing Office.

*Data are provisional, estimated from a 10% sample of deaths. Rates per 100,000 population. Figures may differ from those previously published. Due to rounding, figures may not add to totals.

ICD-9 = Ninth revision, International Classification of Diseases, 1975.

disease, cancer, cerebrovascular disease, and chronic obstructive pulmonary disease are the top four causes of death. Smoking—particularly cigarette smoking—is a risk factor strongly associated with each of these conditions. Indeed, according to McGinnis and Foege (1993), tobacco is implicated in almost 20% of the annual deaths in the United States—approximately 400,000 individuals. Additionally, diet and activity patterns were deemed to account for 14% of deaths (about 300,000/year); alcohol contributes to about 5% of all deaths, as it is associated with a significant percentage of accidents, suicides, and homicides, as well as cirrhosis and chronic liver disease.

Health Promotion and Illness Prevention

Pender (1987) states that "health promotion consists of activities directed toward increasing the level of well being and actualizing the health potential of individuals, families, communities, and society" (p. 4). *Healthy People 2000* (USDHHS, 1990) identifies health promotion strategies as those that relate to individual lifestyles, including physical fitness, nutrition, and tobacco and alcohol use. Examples of goals in *Healthy People 2000* for health promotion are included in Table 11–2.

TABLE 11–2 ***Healthy People 2000*—Examples of Objectives for General Health Promotion in Adults**

Physical Activity and Fitness

1.3—Increase to at least 30% the proportion of people 6 years and older who engage regularly, preferably daily, in light to moderate physical activity for at least 30 minutes per day (baseline: 22% of people 18 years and older were active for at least 30 minutes five or more times per week, and 12% were active seven or more times per week in 1985)

1.12—Increase to at least 50% the proportion of primary care providers who routinely assess and counsel their patients regarding the frequency, duration, type, and intensity of each patient's physical activity practices (baseline: physicians provided exercise counseling for about 30% of sedentary patients in 1988)

Nutrition

2.3—Reduce overweight to a prevalence of no more than 20% among people 20 years and older and no more than 15% among adolescents 12 through 19 years of age (baseline: 26% for people 20 through 74 years in 1976–80; 24% for men and 27% for women; 15% for adolescents 12 through 19 years of age in 1976–80)

Special Population Targets

Overweight Prevalence	***1976–80 Baseline (%)***	***2000 Target (%)***
1.2a—Low-income women 20 years and older	37.0	25.0
1.2b—Black women 20 years and older	44.0	30.0
1.2c—Hispanic women 20 years and older	34.0–39.0	25.0
1.2d—Native Americans/Alaska Natives	29.0–75.0 (estimates for different tribes)	42.5
1.2e—People with disabilities	36.0	25.0
1.2f—Women with high blood pressure	50.0	41.0
1.2g—Men with high blood pressure	39.0	35.0

2.5—Reduce dietary fat intake to an average of 30 percent of calories or less and average saturated fat intake to less than 10 percent of total calories among people aged 2 and older. (Baseline: 36 percent of calories from total fat and 13 percent from saturated fat for people aged 20 through 74 in 1976–80; 36 percent and 13 percent for women aged 19 through 50 in 1985)

2.7—Increase to at least 50 percent the proportion of overweight people aged 12 and older who have adopted sound dietary practices combined with regular physical activity to attain an appropriate body weight. (Baseline: 30 percent of overweight women and 25 percent of overweight men for people aged 18 and older in 1985)

2.21—Increase to at least 75 percent the proportion of primary care providers who provide nutrition assessment and counseling and/or referral to qualified nutritionists or dietitians. (Baseline: physicians provided diet counseling for an estimated 40 to 50 percent of patients in 1988)

Tobacco

3.4—Reduce cigarette smoking to a prevalence of no more than 15 percent among people aged 20 and older. (Baseline: 29 percent in 1987, 32 percent for men and 27 percent for women)

Special Population Targets

Cigarette Smoking Prevalence	***1987 Baseline (%)***	***2000 Target (%)***
3.4a—People with a high school education or less 20 years and older	34	20
3.4b—Blue-collar workers 20 years and older	36	20
3.4c—Military personnel	42	20
3.4d—Blacks 20 years and older	34	18
3.4e—Hispanics 20 years and older	33	18
3.4f—Native Americans/Alaska Natives	42–70 (estimates for different tribes)	20
3.4g—Southeast Asian men	55	20
3.4h—Women of reproductive age	29	12
3.4i—Pregnant women	25	10
3.4j—Women who use oral contraceptives	36	10

TABLE 11–2 ***Healthy People 2000*—Examples of Objectives for General Health Promotion in Adults** *Continued*

3.5—Reduce the initiation of cigarette smoking by children and youth so that no more than 15% have become regular cigarette smokers by age 20 (baseline: 30% of youth had become regular cigarette smokers by ages 20 through 24 in 1987)
3.11—Increase to at least 75% the proportion of work sites with a formal smoking policy that prohibits or severely restricts smoking at the workplace (baseline 27% of work sites with 50 or more employees in 1985; 54% of medium and large companies in 1987)
3.16—Increase to at least 75% the proportion of primary care and oral health care providers who routinely advise cessation and provide assistance and follow-up for all of the tobacco-using patients (baseline: about 52% of internists reported counseling more than 75% of their smoking patients about smoking cessation in 1986; about 35% of dentists reported counseling at least 75% of their smoking patients about smoking in 1986)

Clinical Preventive Services

21.2—Increase to at least 50% the proportion of people who have received, as a minimum within the appropriate interval, all of the screening and immunization services and at least one of the counseling services appropriate for their age and gender as recommended by the U. S. Preventive Services Task Force
21.3—Increase to at least 95% the proportion of people who have a specific source of ongoing primary care for coordination of the preventive and episodic health care (baseline: less than 82% in 1986, as 18% reported having no physician, clinic, or hospital as a regular source of care)

Special Population Targets

Percentage With Source of Care	*1986 Baseline (%)*	*2000 Target (%)*
21.3a—Hispanics	70	95
21.3b—Blacks	80	95
21.3c—Low-income people	80	95

21.4—Improve financing and delivery of clinical preventive services so that virtually no American has a financial barrier to receiving, at a minimum, the screening, counseling, and immunization services recommended by the U. S. Preventive Services Task Force (baseline data not available)

Heart Disease and Stroke

15.1—Reduce coronary heart disease deaths to no more than 100 per 100,000 people (age-adjusted baseline: 135 per 100,000 in 1987)
15.2—Reduce stroke deaths to no more than 20 per 100,000 people (age adjusted baseline: 30.3 per 100,000 in 1987)
15.5—Increase to at least 90% the proportion of people with high blood pressure who are taking action to help control their blood pressure (baseline: 79% of aware hypertensives 18 years and older were taking action to control their blood pressure in 1985)
15.7—Reduce the prevalence of blood cholesterol levels of 240 mg/dL or greater to no more than 20% among adults (baseline: 27% for people 20 through 74 years of age in 1976–1980; 29% for women and 25% for men)
15.14—Increase to at least 75% the proportion of adults who have had their blood cholesterol checked within the preceding 5 years (baseline: 59% of people 18 years and older had "ever" had their cholesterol checked in 1988; 52% were checked "within the preceding 2 years" in 1988)
15.15—Increase to at least 75% the proportion of primary care providers who initiate diet and, if necessary, drug therapy at levels of blood cholesterol consistent with current management guidelines for patients with high blood cholesterol (baseline data not available)

Cancer

16.1—Reverse the rise in cancer deaths to achieve a rate of no more than 130 per 100,000 people (age-adjusted baseline: 133 per 100,000 in 1987)
16.3—Reduce breast cancer deaths to no more than 20.6 per 100,000 women (age-adjusted baseline: 22.9 per 100,000 women in 1987)
16.5—Reduce colorectal cancer deaths to no more than 13.2 per 100,000 people (age-adjusted baseline: 14.4 per 100,000 in 1987)

Table continued on following page

TABLE 11–2 ***Healthy People 2000*—Examples of Objectives for General Health Promotion in Adults** *Continued*

Diabetes

17.10—Reduce the most severe complications of diabetes as follows:

Complications Among People with Diabetes	***1988 Baseline***	***2000 Target***
End-stage renal disease	1.5/1,000	1.4/1,000
Blindness	2.2/1,000	1.4/1,000
Lower extremity amputation	8.2/1,000	4.9/1,000
Perinatal mortality	5%	2%
Major congenital malformations	8%	4%

17.11—Reduce diabetes to an incidence of no more than 2.5 per 1,000 people and a prevalence of no more than 25 per 1,000 people (baselines: 2.9 per 1,000 in 1987; 28 per 1,000 in 1987)

Special Population Targets

Prevalence of Diabetes (per 1,000)	***1982–84 Baseline***	***2000 Target***
17.11a—Native Americans/Alaska Natives	69	62
17.11b—Puerto Ricans	55	49
17.11c—Mexican-Americans	54	49
17.11d—Cuban-Americans	36	32
17.11e—Blacks	36	32

From U. S. Department of Health and Human Services. (1990). *Healthy People 2000: National Health Promotion and Disease Prevention Objectives.* Washington, D. C., Government Printing Office.

Assessment of Health Risks and Health Habits

To apply the nursing process to health promotion and illness prevention, nurses should begin with assessment. In addition to individual physical, functional, and cognitive assessments that are routinely accomplished, an assessment of behaviors and habits that influence health is also important. An understanding of the client's health beliefs and knowledge, as well as health habits (both positive and negative), assists in planning appropriate interventions. Figures 11–1 through 11–3 present examples of tools for general assessment of health risks, lifestyles, and beliefs.

As positive health practices and potential threats to health are identified, nurses can assist individuals, families, and groups by developing plans and programs to promote health and prevent illness. Table 11–3 depicts the relationships among various risk factors and the 10 leading causes of death.

The remainder of this chapter describes specific assessments and risk reduction techniques and provides educational materials and tools to equip nurses to assist clients in reducing risk and promoting health.

Physical Activity and Fitness

The health benefits of regular exercise and physical activity have been thoroughly researched and documented. Indeed, according the Cooper Institute for Aerobic Research, "programs of moderate, regular exercise–half an hour each day, three times a week" can "markedly lower death-rates from all-cause mortality, cancer and cardiovascular disease" (cited in The President's Council on Physical Fitness & Sports, 1993). Table 11–4 lists potential benefits from regular physical activity for several diseases.

healthstyle: a self-test

All of us want good health. But many of us do not know how to be as healthy as possible. Health experts now describe *life-style* as one of the most important factors affecting health. In fact, it is estimated that as many as seven of the ten leading causes of death could be reduced through common-sense changes in lifestyle. That's what this brief test, developed by the Public Health Service, is all about. Its purpose is simply to tell you how well you are doing to stay healthy. The behaviors covered in the test are recommended for most Americans. Some of them may not apply to persons with certain chronic diseases or handicaps, or to pregnant women. Such persons may require special instructions from their physicians.

Cigarette Smoking

If you *never smoke*, enter a score of 10 for this section and go to the next section on *Alcohol and Drugs*.

	Almost Always	Sometimes	Almost Never
1. I avoid smoking cigarettes.	2	1	0
2. I smoke only low-tar and -nicotine cigarettes *or* I smoke a pipe or cigars.	2	1	0

Smoking Score: ____________

Alcohol and Drugs

	Almost Always	Sometimes	Almost Never
1. I avoid drinking alcoholic beverages *or* I drink no more than one or two drinks a day.	4	1	0
2. I avoid using alcohol or other drugs (especially illegal drugs) as a way of handling stressful situations or the problems in my life.	2	1	0
3. I am careful not to drink alcohol when taking certain medicines (for example, medicine for sleeping, pain, colds, and allergies), or when pregnant.	2	1	0
4. I read and follow the label directions when using prescribed and over-the-counter drugs.	2	1	0

Alcohol and Drugs Score: ____________

Eating Habits

	Almost Always	Sometimes	Almost Never
1. I eat a variety of foods each day, such as fruits and vegetables, whole grain breads and cereals, lean meats, dairy products, dry peas and beans, and nuts and seeds.	4	1	0
2. I limit the amount of fat, saturated fat, and cholesterol I eat (including fat on meats, eggs, butter, cream, shortenings, and organ meats such as liver).	2	1	0
3. I limit the amount of salt I eat by cooking with only small amounts, not adding salt at the table, and avoiding salty snacks.	2	1	0
4. I avoid eating too much sugar (especially frequent snacks of sticky candy or soft drinks).	2	1	0

Eating Habits Score: ____________

Exercise/Fitness

	Almost Always	Sometimes	Almost Never
1. I maintain a desired weight, avoiding overweight and underweight.	3	1	0
2. I do vigorous exercises for 15–30 minutes at least three times a week (examples include running, swimming, brisk walking).	3	1	0
3. I do exercises that enhance my muscle tone for 15–30 minutes at least three times a week (examples include yoga and calisthenics).	2	1	0
4. I use part of my leisure time participating in individual, family, or team activities that increase my level of fitness (such as gardening, bowling, golf, and baseball).	2	1	0

Exercise/Fitness Score: ____________

Stress Control

	Almost Always	Sometimes	Almost Never
1. I have a job or do other work that I enjoy.	2	1	0
2. I find it easy to relax and express my feelings freely.	2	1	0
3. I recognize early, and prepare for, events or situations likely to be stressful for me.	2	1	0
4. I have close friends, relatives, or others whom I can talk to about personal matters and call on for help when needed.	2	1	0
5. I participate in group activities (such as church and community organizations) or hobbies that I enjoy.	2	1	0

Stress Control Score: ____________

Safety

	Almost Always	Sometimes	Almost Never
1. I wear a seat belt while riding in a car.	2	1	0
2. I avoid driving while under the influence of alcohol and other drugs.	2	1	0
3. I obey traffic rules and the speed limit when driving.	2	1	0
4. I am careful when using potentially harmful products or substances (such as household cleaners, poisons, and electrical devices).	2	1	0
5. I avoid smoking in bed.	2	1	0

Safety Score: ____________

Figure continued on following page

WHAT YOUR SCORES MEAN TO YOU

Scores of 9 and 10

Excellent! Your answers show that you are aware of the importance of this area to your health. More important, you are putting your knowledge to work for you by practicing good health habits. As long as you continue to do so, this area should not pose a serious health risk. It's likely that you are setting an example for your family and friends to follow. Since you got a very high test score on this part of the test, you may want to consider other areas where your scores indicate room for improvement.

Scores of 6 to 8

Your health practices in this area are good, but there is room for improvement. Look again at the items you answered with a "Sometimes" or "Almost Never." What changes can you make to improve your score? Even a small change can often help you achieve better health.

Scores of 3 to 5

Your health risks are showing! Would you like more information about the risks you are facing and about why it is important for you to change these behaviors. Perhaps you need help in deciding how to successfully make the changes you desire. In either case, help is available.

Scores of 0 to 2

Obviously, you were concerned enough about your health to take the test, but your answers show that you may be taking serious and unnecessary risks with your health. Perhaps you are not aware of the risks and what to do about them. You can easily get the information and help you need to improve, if you wish. The next step is up to you.

YOU Can Start Right Now!

In the test you just completed were numerous suggestions to help you reduce your risk of disease and premature death. Here are some of the most significant:

Avoid cigarettes. Cigarette smoking is the single most important preventable cause of illness and early death. It is especially risky for pregnant women and their unborn babies. Persons who stop smoking reduce their risk of getting heart disease and cancer. So if you're a cigarette smoker, think twice about lighting that next cigarette. If you choose to continue smoking, try decreasing the number of cigarettes you smoke and switching to a low tar and nicotine brand.

Follow sensible drinking habits. Alcohol produces changes in mood and behavior. Most people who drink are able to control their intake of alcohol and to avoid undesired, and often harmful, effects. Heavy, regular use of alcohol can lead to cirrhosis of the liver, a leading cause of death. Also, statistics clearly show that mixing drinking and driving is often the cause of fatal or crippling accidents. So if you drink, do it wisely and in moderation. **Use care in taking drugs.** Today's greater use of drugs—both legal and illegal—is one of our most serious health risks. Even some drugs prescribed by your doctor can be dangerous if taken when drinking alcohol or before driving. Excessive or continued use of tranquilizers (or "pep pills") can cause physical and mental problems. Using or experimenting with illicit drugs such as marijuana, heroin, cocaine, and PCP may lead to a number of damaging effects or even death.

Eat sensibly. Overweight individuals are at greater risk for diabetes, gall bladder disease, and high blood pressure. So it makes good sense to maintain proper weight. But good eating habits also mean holding down the amount of fat (especially saturated fat), cholesterol, sugar and salt in your diet. If you must snack, try nibbling on fresh fruits and vegetables. You'll feel better—and look better, too.

Exercise regularly. Almost everyone can benefit from exercise —and there's some form of exercise almost everyone can do. (If you have any doubt, check first with your doctor.) Usually, as little as 15–30 minutes of vigorous exercise three times a week will help you have a healthier heart, eliminate excess weight, tone up sagging muscles, and sleep better. Think how much difference all these improvements could make in the way you feel!

Learn to handle stress. Stress is a normal part of living; everyone faces it to some degree. The causes of stress can be good or bad, desirable or undesirable (such as a promotion on the job or the loss of a spouse). Properly handled, stress need not be a problem. But unhealthy responses to stress—such as driving too fast or erratically, drinking too much, or prolonged anger or grief—can cause a variety of physical and mental problems. Even on a very busy day, find a few minutes to slow down and relax. Talking over a problem with someone you trust can often help you find a satisfactory solution. Learn to distinguish between things that are "worth fighting about" and things that are less important.

Be safety conscious. Think "safety first" at home, at work, at school, at play, and on the highway. Buckle seat belts and obey traffic rules. Keep poisons and weapons out of the reach of children, and keep emergency numbers by your telephone. When the unexpected happens, you'll be prepared.

FIGURE 11–1 Healthstyle: A self-test. (From Office of Disease Prevention and Health Promotion. [1981]. *Healthstyle: A Self-Test.* Pub. No. H0012. Washington, D. C., National Health Information Clearinghouse.)

Where Do You Go From Here?

Start by asking yourself a few frank questions: "Am I really doing all I can to be as healthy as possible?" "What steps can I take to feel better?" "Am I willing to begin now?" If you scored low in one or more sections of the test, decide what changes you want to make for improvement. You might pick that aspect of your lifestyle where you feel you have the best chance for success and tackle that one first. Once you have improved your score there, go on to other areas.

If you already have tried to change your health habits (to stop smoking or exercise regularly, for example), don't be discouraged if you haven't yet succeeded. The difficulty you have encountered may be due to influences you've never really thought about—such as advertising—or to a lack of support and encouragement. Understanding these influences is an important step toward changing the way they affect you.

There's help available. In addition to personal actions you can take on your own, there are community programs and groups (such as the YMCA or the local chapter of the American Heart Association) that can assist you and your family to make the changes you want to make. If you want to know more about these groups or about health risks, contact your local health department or the National Health Information Clearinghouse. There's a lot you can do to stay healthy or to improve your health—and there are organizations that can help you. Start a new HEALTHSTYLE today!

For assistance in locating specific information on these and other health topics: write to the National Health Information Clearinghouse.

National Health Information Clearinghouse
P.O. Box 1133
Washington, D. C. 20013

FIGURE 11–1 *Continued*

The American Heart Association and the National Heart, Lung, and Blood Institute (1993) recommend that individuals work up to moderate-level activities for a minimum of 30 minutes, three to four times a week, depending on age and presence of existing physical problems. Additionally, they advise that a physician should be consulted *before* a person starts an exercise program if he or she

- Has been diagnosed with a heart condition and the doctor recommends only medically supervised physical activity
- Has pain or pressure in the left or mid-chest area, left neck area, shoulder, or arm during or following exercise
- Has developed chest pain within the past month
- Has a tendency to lose consciousness or suffers from dizziness
- Feels extremely breathless after mild exertion
- Takes medication for blood pressure or a heart condition
- Has bone or joint problems that could be worsened by physical activity
- Has a medical condition that might need special attention during an exercise program (e.g., insulin-dependent diabetes mellitus [IDDM])
- Is middle aged or older and has not been physically active

An exercise program should be vigorous enough to increase the heart rate to 50 to 75% of the maximum heart rate (220 minus your age). This is termed the "target heart rate zone." Table 11–5 shows a sample walking program for beginners. It includes instruction on taking a pulse and lists target heart rate zones. Examples of other physical activities that are particularly beneficial in conditioning the heart and lungs include aerobic dancing, bicycling, jogging, jumping rope, rowing, stair climbing, stationary cycling, and swimming.

In addition to the guidelines listed here, the USDHHS' Office of Disease Prevention and Health Promotion (ODPHP, 1994) suggests that physical activity programs should be

1. Medically safe (e.g., following physician's advice if one of the risk factors listed previously is a possibility; increasing activities

Directions: Read the statements for each dimension of wellness; circle the number that most appropriately resembles the importance of each statement to you and your well-being and your current interest in changing your lifestyle, as follows:

1. I am already doing this. (Congratulate yourself!)
2. This is very important to me and I want to change this behavior now.
3. This is important to me, but I'm not ready to change my behavior right now.
4. This is not important in my life right now.

Nutritional Wellness				
I maximize local fresh fruits and uncooked vegetables in my eating plan.	1	2	3	4
I minimize the use of candy, sweets, sugar, and simple carbohydrates.	1	2	3	4
I eat whole foods rather than processed ones.	1	2	3	4
I avoid foods that have color, artificial flavor, or preservatives added.	1	2	3	4
I avoid coffee, tea, cola drinks, or other substances that are high in caffeine or other stimulants.	1	2	3	4
I eat high-fiber foods daily.	1	2	3	4
I have a good appetite, but I eat sensible amounts of food.	1	2	3	4
I avoid crash diets.	1	2	3	4
I eat only when I am hungry and relaxed.	1	2	3	4
I drink sufficient water so my urine is light yellow.	1	2	3	4
I avoid foods high in saturated fat, such as beef, pork, lamb, soft cheese, gravies, bakery items, fried foods, etc.	1	2	3	4
I use bottled water or an activated carbon filtration system to ensure safe drinking water.	1	2	3	4
Fitness and Wellness				
I weigh within 10% of my desired weight.	1	2	3	4
I walk, jog, or exercise vigorously for more than 20 minutes at least three times per week.	1	2	3	4
I seem to digest my food well (no gas, bloating, etc.)	1	2	3	4
I do flexibility or stretching exercises daily and always before and after vigorous exercise.	1	2	3	4
I am satisfied with my sexual activities.	1	2	3	4
When I am ill, I'm resilient and recover easily.	1	2	3	4
When I look at myself nude, I feel good about what I see.	1	2	3	4
I use imagery to picture myself well and healthy every day.	1	2	3	4
I use affirmations and other self-healing measures when ill or injured or to enhance my fitness.	1	2	3	4
I avoid smoking and smoke-filled places.	1	2	3	4
Stress and Wellness				
I sleep well.	1	2	3	4
I have a peaceful expectation about my death.	1	2	3	4
I live relatively free from disabling stress or painful, repetitive thoughts.	1	2	3	4
I laugh at myself occasionally, and I have a good sense of humor.	1	2	3	4
I use constructive ways of releasing my frustration and anger.	1	2	3	4
I feel good about myself and my accomplishments.	1	2	3	4
I assert myself to get what I need instead of feeling resentful toward others for taking advantage of or intimidating me.	1	2	3	4
I can relax my body and mind at will.	1	2	3	4
I feel accepting and calm about people or things I have lost through separation.	1	2	3	4
I get and give sufficient touch (hugs, etc.) daily.	1	2	3	4

FIGURE 11–2 Wellness self-assessment. (From Clark, C. [1996.] *Wellness Practitioner* (2nd ed.). New York, Springer Publishing Co.)

Wellness Relationships and Beliefs

I have at least one other person with whom I can discuss my innermost thoughts and feelings.	1	2	3	4
I keep myself open to new experiences.	1	2	3	4
I listen to others' words and the feelings behind the words.	1	2	3	4
What I believe, feel, and do are consistent.	1	2	3	4
I allow others to be themselves and to take responsibility for their thoughts, actions, and feelings.	1	2	3	4
I allow myself to be me.	1	2	3	4
I live with a sense of purpose.	1	2	3	4

Wellness and the Environment

I have designed a wellness support network of friends, family, and peers.	1	2	3	4
I have designed my personal living, playing, and working environments to suit me.	1	2	3	4
I work in a place that provides adequate personal space, comfort, safety, direct sunlight, and fresh air and limited air, water, or material pollutants; or I use nutritional, exercise, or stress reduction measures to minimize negative effects.	1	2	3	4
I avoid cosmetics and hair dyes that contain harmful chemicals.	1	2	3	4
I avoid pesticides and the use of harmful household chemicals.	1	2	3	4
I avoid x-rays unless serious disease or injury is at stake, and I have dental x-rays for diagnostic purposes only every 3 to 5 years.	1	2	3	4
I wear a good sunscreen ointment when exposed to the sun.	1	2	3	4
I use the earth's resources wisely.	1	2	3	4

Commitment to Wellness

I examine my values and actions to see that I am moving toward wellness.	1	2	3	4
I take responsibility for my thoughts, feelings, and actions.	1	2	3	4
I keep informed on the latest health/wellness knowledge rather than relying on experts to decide what is best for me.	1	2	3	4
I wear seat belts when driving and insist that others who drive with me do so also.	1	2	3	4
I ask pertinent questions and seek second opinions whenever someone advises me.	1	2	3	4
I know which chronic illnesses are prominent in my family, and I take steps to avoid incurring these illnesses.	1	2	3	4
I work toward achieving a balance in all wellness dimensions to enhance my sense of well-being and satisfaction.	1	2	3	4

FIGURE 11–2 *Continued*

gradually; use of stretching exercise to decrease the risk of musculoskeletal injuries)

2. Enjoyable (e.g., varying activities, exercising with friends or family)
3. Convenient (e.g., flexible, nearby, requiring a minimum of special preparation)
4. Realistic (e.g., gradual increase in intensity, frequency, and duration)
5. Minimally structured (schedules and goals should be set and maintained when possible, but some flexibility is important, as very structured programs may reduce compliance)

Nutrition and Weight Control

Good nutritional practices and maintenance of a desirable weight are essential for good health. It is estimated that approximately 32 million Americans (24% of men and 27% of women) are overweight (USDHHS/ODPHP, 1994). As a risk factor, obesity (weight 20% or more above desirable weight) is associated with hypertension, non–insulin-dependent diabetes mellitus (NIDDM), hy-

Text continued on page 285

Section ________ Term ________ Date ________ Name ________________________________

Directions: Wellness involves a variety of components that work together to build the total concept. Below are some questions concerning the different aspects of wellness. Using the scale, respond to each question by circling the number that most closely corresponds with your feelings and lifestyle. Remember to complete the Lifestyle Assessment Inventory at the completion of the course to compare the results.

Physical

	Yes/always	Often	Once	Rarely	No/never
1. I exercise aerobically at least three times per week for 20 minutes or more.	10	7	5	3	1
2. When participating in physical activities, I include stretching and flexibility exercises.	10	7	5	3	1
3. I include warm-up and cool-down periods when participating in vigorous activities.	10	7	5	3	1
4. I engage in resistance-type exercises at least two times per week.	10	7	5	3	1
5. My physical fitness level is excellent for my age.	10	7	5	3	1
6. My body composition is appropriate for my gender (men, 10%–18% body fat; women, 18%–25%).	10	7	5	3	1
7. I have appropriate medical check-ups regularly and am able to talk to my doctor and ask questions that concern me.	10	7	5	3	1
8. I keep my immunizations up-to-date.	10	7	5	3	1
9. I keep up with the medical history of close relatives.	10	7	5	3	1
10. I keep records of the time, date, and results of medical tests.	10	7	5	3	1

Physical Assessment Score ________

Alcohol and Drugs Assessment

	Yes/always	Often	Once	Rarely	No/never
1. I avoid smoking.	10	7	5	3	1
2. I avoid using smokeless tobacco products.	10	7	5	3	1
3. I avoid drinking alcohol or restrict my consumption to two drinks or less.	10	7	5	3	1
4. I avoid drinking alcohol to the point of intoxication.	10	7	5	3	1
5. I do not drive when drinking alcoholic beverages or taking medicines that make me sleepy.	10	7	5	3	1
6. I avoid using mood-altering substances.	10	7	5	3	1
7. I follow directions when taking medications.	10	7	5	3	1
8. I thoroughly read labels before taking a nonprescription drug.	10	7	5	3	1
9. I ask about contraindications and side effects of prescription drugs before taking them.	10	7	5	3	1
10. I keep a record of drugs to which I am allergic in my wallet or purse.	10	7	5	3	1

Alcohol and Drugs Assessment Score ________

Nutritional Assessment

	Yes/always	Often	Once	Rarely	No/never
1. I eat at least 3 to 5 servings of vegetables and 2 to 4 servings of fruits each day.	10	7	5	3	1
2. My daily diet includes at least 6 to 11 servings from the bread, cereal, rice, and pasta food group.	10	7	5	3	1

FIGURE 11–3 *See legend on page 285*

Nutritional Assessment *Continued*

	Yes/always	Often	Once	Rarely	No/never
3. I limit my daily intake of dairy products to 2 to 3 servings.	10	7	5	3	1
4. My daily intake of meats, eggs, and nuts is 2 to 3 servings.	10	7	5	3	1
5. I make a conscious effort to choose or prepare foods low in saturated fat.	10	7	5	3	1
6. When purchasing a food item, I read the labels to identify foods high in salt, hidden sugars, tropical oils, and saturated fat.	10	7	5	3	1
7. I avoid adding salt to my food without first tasting it.	10	7	5	3	1
8. I avoid eating unless I'm hungry.	10	7	5	3	1
9. I stop eating before feeling completely full.	10	7	5	3	1
10. I avoid binge eating.	10	7	5	3	1

Nutritional Assessment Score ________

Social Wellness Assessment

	Yes/always	Often	Once	Rarely	No/never
1. I have at least one person in whom I can confide.	10	7	5	3	1
2. I have a good relationship with my family.	10	7	5	3	1
3. I have friends at work or school with whom I gain support and talk with regularly.	10	7	5	3	1
4. I am involved in school activities.	10	7	5	3	1
5. I am involved in my community.	10	7	5	3	1
6. I do something for fun and just for myself at least once a week.	10	7	5	3	1
7. I am able to develop close, intimate relationships.	10	7	5	3	1
8. I engage in activities that contribute to the environment.	10	7	5	3	1
9. I am interested in the views, opinions, activities, and accomplishments of others.	10	7	5	3	1

Social Wellness Score ________

Spiritual Wellness Assessment

	Yes/always	Often	Once	Rarely	No/never
1. I know what my values and beliefs are.	10	7	5	3	1
2. I live by my convictions.	10	7	5	3	1
3. My life has meaning and direction.	10	7	5	3	1
4. I derive strength from my spiritual life daily.	10	7	5	3	1
5. I have life goals that I strive to achieve every day.	10	7	5	3	1
6. I view life as a learning experience and look forward to the future.	10	7	5	3	1
7. I am satisfied with my spiritual life.	10	7	5	3	1
8. I am tolerant of the values and beliefs of others.	10	7	5	3	1
9. I am satisfied with the degree that my campus activities are consistent with my values.	10	7	5	3	1
10. Personal reflection is an important part of my life.	10	7	5	3	1

Spiritual Wellness Assessment Score ________

Emotional Wellness Assessment

	Yes/always	Often	Once	Rarely	No/never
1. I feel positive about myself and my life.	10	7	5	3	1
2. I am able to be the person I choose to be.	10	7	5	3	1
3. I am satisfied that I am performing to the best of my ability.	10	7	5	3	1

Figure continued on following page

Emotional Wellness Assessment Continued

	Yes/always	Often	Once	Rarely	No/never
4. I can cope with life's ups and downs effectively and in a healthy manner.	10	7	5	3	1
5. I am nonjudgmental in my approach to others and take responsibility for my own decisions and actions.	10	7	5	3	1
6. I feel there is appropriate amount of excitement in my life.	10	7	5	3	1
7. When I make mistakes, I learn from them.	10	7	5	3	1
8. I can say "no" without feeling guilty.	10	7	5	3	1
9. I find it easy to laugh.	10	7	5	3	1

Emotional Wellness Assessment Score ________

Stress Control Assessment

	Yes/always	Often	Once	Rarely	No/never
1. I am easily distracted.	1	3	5	7	10
2. I tend to be nervous and impatient.	1	3	5	7	10
3. I prepare ahead of time for events/situations that cause stress.	10	7	5	3	1
4. I schedule enough time to accomplish what I need to do.	10	7	5	3	1
5. I set realistic goals for myself.	10	7	5	3	1
6. I can express my feelings of anger.	10	7	5	3	1
7. I avoid putting off important tasks to the last minute.	10	7	5	3	1
8. When working on tasks, I stay focused on what I'm doing and usually concentrate on them through completion.	10	7	5	3	1
9. When working under pressure, I stay calm and patient.	10	7	5	3	1
10. I can make decisions with a minimum of stress and worry.	10	7	5	3	1

Stress Control Assessment Score ________

Intellectual Wellness Assessment

	Yes/always	Often	Once	Rarely	No/never
1. I believe my education is preparing me for what I would like to accomplish in life.	10	7	5	3	1
2. I am interested in learning just for the sake of learning.	10	7	5	3	1
3. I like to be aware of current social and political issues.	10	7	5	3	1
4. I have interests other than those directly related to my vocation.	10	7	5	3	1
5. I am able to apply what I know to real life situations.	10	7	5	3	1
6. I am interested in the viewpoint of others, even if it is very different from my own.	10	7	5	3	1
7. I seek advice when I am uncertain or uncomfortable with a recommended health or medical treatment.	10	7	5	3	1
8. I ask about the risks and benefits of a medical test before its use.	10	7	5	3	1
9. When seeking medical care, I plan ahead how to describe my problem and what questions I should ask.	10	7	5	3	1
10. I keep abreast of the latest trends and information regarding health matters.	10	7	5	3	1

Intellectual Wellness Assessment Score ________

FIGURE 11–3 *See legend on opposite page*

Wellness Assessment Summary

Transfer the total score for each section to the spaces below. Add the scores and divide by eight to determine your average wellness score.

Physical Assessment Score	________
Alcohol and Drugs Assessment	________
Nutritional Assessment	________
Social Wellness Assessment	________
Spiritual Wellness Assessment	________
Emotional Wellness Assessment.................	________
Stress Control Assessment...........................	________
Intellectual Wellness Assessment	________
TOTAL	________
Average Wellness Score (Divide total score by 8)	________

86–100—Excellent. You are engaging in behaviors and attitudes that can significantly contribute to a healthy lifestyle and a higher quality of life. If you scored in this range, you are an example to many.

70–85—Good. You engage in many health-promoting attitudes and behaviors that should contribute to good health and a more satisfying quality of life. However, there are some areas that could use some upgrading to provide optimal benefits. If you are at this level, you are showing how much you care about yourself and your life.

50–69—Average. You are typical of the average American who tends to act without really considering the consequences of your behaviors. Now is the time to consider your lifestyle and what ramifications it is having on you now and in the future. Maybe there are some positive actions that you can consider taking to improve your quality of life.

30–49—Below average. Perhaps you lack current information about behaviors and attitudes that can enhance your health and quality of life. Now is the time to begin to learn about positive changes that can improve your life.

Less than 30—Needs improvement. It's good that you are concerned enough about your health to take this test, but indications are that your behaviors and attitudes may be having detrimental effects on your health. You can easily begin to take action now to improve your prospects for the future.

FIGURE 11–3 Lifestyle assessment inventory. (From Anspaugh, D. J., Hamrick, M. H. and Rosato, F. D. [1994.] *Wellness: Concepts and Applications* [2nd ed.]. St. Louis, MO, Mosby-Year Book.)

percholesterolemia, coronary artery disease, some types of cancer, and stroke.

Tables 11–6 and 11–7 present recommended height and weight tables for men and women, respectively. These tables were adapted from the Metropolitan Life Insurance Company's tables, which have been the most widely used height and weight standards for several decades. As adapted, the tables contain an easy reference guide to identify "20% overweight," the recognized point at which negative health consequences occur (USDHHS/ODPHP, 1994).

General nutrition guidelines for a healthy diet are as follow:

- Eat a variety of foods
- Maintain healthy weight
- Choose a diet low in total fat (less than 30% of calories), saturated fat (less than 10% of calories), and cholesterol
- Choose a diet with plenty of vegetables, fruits, and grain products (five or more servings daily)
- Use sugars only in moderation
- Use salt and sodium only in moderation
- If you drink alcoholic beverages, do so only in moderation (no more that one drink daily for women or two drinks daily for men); women who are pregnant or planning to become pregnant should not drink at all (U. S. Department of Agriculture [USDA], 1993; USDHHS/ODPHP, 1994)

To assist nurses in nutrition counseling, Figure 11–4 contains the "Food Guide Pyramid," which shows a range of daily "servings" for each of the major food groups and was designed to be a pictorial reminder to encourage a healthful diet. Figure 11–5 gives examples that help define "one serving," and Figure 11–6 provides specific information on daily caloric intake and food group servings based on age, gender, and activity level.

TABLE 11–3 **Percent of Total Deaths and Risk Factors Associated with 10 Leading Causes of Death: United States, 1987**

Cause of Death	Percent of Total Deaths	Smoking*	High-Fat, Low-Fiber Diet†	Sedentary Lifestyle†	High Blood Pressure‡	Elevated Serum Cholesterol‡	Obesity‡	Diabetes‡	Alcohol Abuse*
Heart disease	35.7	x	x	x	x	x	x	x	x
Cancer	22.4	x	x	x			x		x
Stroke	7.0	x	x		x	x	x		
Unintentional injury	4.4	x							x
Chronic obstructive lung diseases	3.7	x							
Pneumonia and influenza	3.2	x							
Diabetes	1.7		x	x			x	x	
Suicide	1.4								x
Chronic liver disease/ cirrhosis	1.2								x
Atherosclerosis	1.1	x	x	x		x		x	
All other causes	18.2								

*Other risk factors
†Diet and exercise
‡Risk factors controlled with diet and exercise
From U. S. Department of Health and Human Services. (1992). *Promoting Healthy Diets and Acitve Lifestyles to Lower-SES Adults: Market Research for Public Education.* Washington, D. C., Government Printing Office; data from *Surgeon General's Report on Nutrition and Health,* 1988 and *Integration of Risk Factor Interventions,* 1986.

TABLE 11–4 **Physical Activity Benefits and Major Lifestyle Diseases**

Disease	Physical Activity Benefit
Heart disease	Healthy heart muscle
	Lower resting heart rate
	More blood pumped with each beat
	Reduced blood pressure in submaximal work
	Healthy arteries
	Less atherosclerosis (deposits in arteries)
	Higher HDL ("good" cholesterol)
	Better blood fat profile (fewer "bad" fats)
	Decreased platelet and less fibrin (related to atherosclerosis)
	Better blood flow
	Better working capacity
	Fewer demands during work
	Greater ability to meet work demands
Stroke	Healthy arteries (see above)
	Lower blood pressure
Peripheral Vascular disease	Improved working capacity
	Higher HDL
	Better blood fat profile
High blood pressure	Reduction in blood pressure among those with high levels
	Reduction in body fatness (associated with high blood pressure)
Diabetes (NIDDM)	Reduced body fatness (may relieve symptoms of adult-onset diabetes)
	Better carbohydrate metabolism (improved insulin sensitivity)
Cancer	Less risk of colon cancer (better transit time of food?)
Obesity	Increases lean body mass
	Decreases body fat percentage
	Less central fat distribution
Depression	Relief from some symptoms
Back pain	Increased muscle strength and endurance
	Improved flexibility
	Improved posture
Osteoporosis	Greater bone density as a result of stressing long bones

From President's Council on Physical Fitness & Sports. (1993). The health benefits of physical activity. In *Physical Activity and Fitness Research Digest.* Vol. 1. No. 1. Washington, D. C., U. S. Department of Health and Human Services/President's Council on Physical Fitness and Sports.

HDL = high-density lipoprotein.

TABLE 11–5 **A Sample Walking Program and Target Heart Rates**

A Sample Walking Program

	Warm Up	*Target Zone Exercising**	*Cool Down Time*	*Total*
Week 1				
Session A	Walk normally 5 minutes	Then walk briskly 5 minutes	Then walk normally 5 minutes	15 minutes
Session B	Repeat above pattern			
Session C	Repeat above pattern			
Continue with at least three exercise sessions during each week of the program. If you find a particular week's pattern tiring, repeat it before going on to the next pattern. You do not have to complete the walking program in 12 weeks.				
Week 2	Walk 5 minutes	Walk briskly 7 minutes	Walk 5 minutes	17 minutes
Week 3	Walk 5 minutes	Walk briskly 9 minutes	Walk 5 minutes	19 minutes
Week 4	Walk 5 minutes	Walk briskly 11 minutes	Walk 5 minutes	21 minutes
Week 5	Walk 5 minutes	Walk briskly 13 minutes	Walk 5 minutes	23 minutes
Week 6	Walk 5 minutes	Walk briskly 15 minutes	Walk 5 minutes	25 minutes
Week 7	Walk 5 minutes	Walk briskly 18 minutes	Walk 5 minutes	28 minutes
Week 8	Walk 5 minutes	Walk briskly 20 minutes	Walk 5 minutes	30 minutes
Week 9	Walk 5 minutes	Walk briskly 23 minutes	Walk 5 minutes	33 minutes
Week 10	Walk 5 minutes	Walk briskly 26 minutes	Walk 5 minutes	36 minutes
Week 11	Walk 5 minutes	Walk briskly 28 minutes	Walk 5 minutes	38 minutes
Week 12	Walk 5 minutes	Walk briskly 30 minutes	Walk 5 minutes	40 minutes

Week 13 on:

Check your pulse periodically to see if you are exercising within your target zone. As you get more in shape, try exercising within the upper range of your target zone. Gradually increase your brisk walking time to 30 to 60 minutes, three or four times a week. Remember that your goal is to get the benefits you are seeking and enjoy your activity.

*Here's how to check if you are within your target heart rate zone:

1. Right after you stop exercising, take your pulse: Place the tips of your first two fingers lightly over one of the blood vessels on your neck, just to the left or right of your Adam's apple. Or try the pulse spot inside your wrist just below the base of your thumb.
2. Count your pulse for 10 seconds and multiply the number by six.
3. Compare the number to the right grouping below: Look for the age grouping that is closest to your age and read the line across. For example, if you are 43, the closest age on the chart is 45; the target zone is 88–131 beats per minute.

AGE	TARGET HEART RATE ZONE	AGE	TARGET HEART RATE ZONE
20 years	100–150 beats per minute	50 years	85–127 beats per minute
25 years	98–146 beats per minute	55 years	83–123 beats per minute
30 years	95–142 beats per minute	60 years	80–120 beats per minute
35 years	93–138 beats per minute	65 years	78–116 beats per minute
40 years	90–135 beats per minute	70 years	75–113 beats per minute
45 years	88–131 beats per minute		

From National Heart, Lung and Blood Institute and American Heart Association (1993). *Exercise and Your Heart: A Guide to Physical Activity.* NIH Publication No. 93–1677 and No. 94–3281. Washington, D. C., National Heart, Lung and Blood Institute and American Heart Association.

TABLE 11–6 **Height and Weight Tables for Men 25 Years and Older**

	Weight (pounds)†			
Height (feet, inches)*	*Small Frame*	*Medium Frame*	*Large Frame*	20% Overweight‡
5, 1	105–113	111–122	119–134	140
5, 2	108–116	114–126	122–137	144
5, 3	111–119	117–129	125–141	148
5, 4	114–122	120–132	128–145	151
5, 5	117–126	123–136	131–149	155
5, 6	121–130	127–140	135–154	160
5, 7	125–134	131–145	140–159	166
5, 8	129–138	135–149	144–163	170
5, 9	133–143	139–153	148–167	175
5, 10	137–147	143–158	152–172	181
5, 11	141–151	147–163	157–177	186
6, 0	145–155	151–168	161–182	191
6, 1	149–160	155–173	168–187	197
6, 2	153–164	160–178	171–192	203
6, 3	157–168	165–183	175–197	209

*Without shoes.
†Without clothing.
‡20% over midpoint of medium frame weight; not in original Metropolitan table.
Adapted from Metropolitan Life Insurance Company. (1983). New weight standards for men and women. *Statistical Bulletin Metropolitan Life Insurance Company, 64,* 2–9.

In 1993, the Food and Drug Administration and the Food Safety and Inspection Service (USDA) introduced a new food label to simplify nutrient content claims (e.g., "low calorie" and "low fat"), provide quick and simplified information about the nutrient qualities of most foods to determine if the food has nutrients desired (e.g., carbohydrates, fiber, vitamins) or is high in those nutrients that the consumer might wish to limit (e.g., fat, saturated fat, cholesterol, sodium) (USDHHS/Food and Drug Association, 1993). Figure 11–7 illustrates and explains the new label. To assist in clarification of food labels, Table 11–8 defines some common label terms.

LOWERING FAT AND CHOLESTEROL INTAKE

One of the purposes of the new food label is to make it easier for the consumer to monitor intake of certain nutrients. Because of the association of dietary fat and cholesterol with heart disease, stroke, obesity, and other problems, limitation of these nutrients is one of the main objectives when counseling on nutrition. Dietary guidelines set by the USDA and USDHHS for fat and cholesterol are to

- Reduce "total dietary fat" to 30% or less of total calories
- Reduce "saturated fat" intake to less than 10% of calories
- Reduce "cholesterol" intake to less than 300 milligrams per day

To assist in food selection to meet these guidelines, Table 11–9 provides information on total fat grams, saturated fat grams, and total calories.

VITAMINS AND MINERALS

Nutrition counseling should include information on essential nutrients, including vitamins and min-

TABLE 11–7 **Height and Weight Tables for Women 25 Years and Older**

	Weight (pounds)†			
Height (feet, inches)*	*Small Frame*	*Medium Frame*	*Large Frame*	20% Overweight‡
4, 9	90–97	94–106	102–118	120
4, 10	92–100	97–109	106–121	124
4, 11	95–103	100–112	108–124	127
5, 0	98–106	103–116	111–127	131
5, 1	101–109	106–118	114–130	134
5, 2	104–112	109–122	117–134	139
5, 3	107–115	112–126	121–138	141
5, 4	110–119	116–131	125–142	148
5, 5	114–123	120–136	129–146	154
5, 6	118–127	124–139	133–150	158
5, 7	122–131	128–143	137–154	163
5, 8	126–136	132–147	141–159	167
5, 9	130–140	136–151	145–164	172
5, 10	134–144	140–155	149–169	177

*Without shoes.
†Without clothing.
‡20% over midpoint of medium frame weight; not in original Metropolitan table.
Adapted from Metropolitan Life Insurance Company. (1983). New weight standards for men and women. *Statistical Bulletin Metropolitan Life Insurance Company, 64,* 2–9.

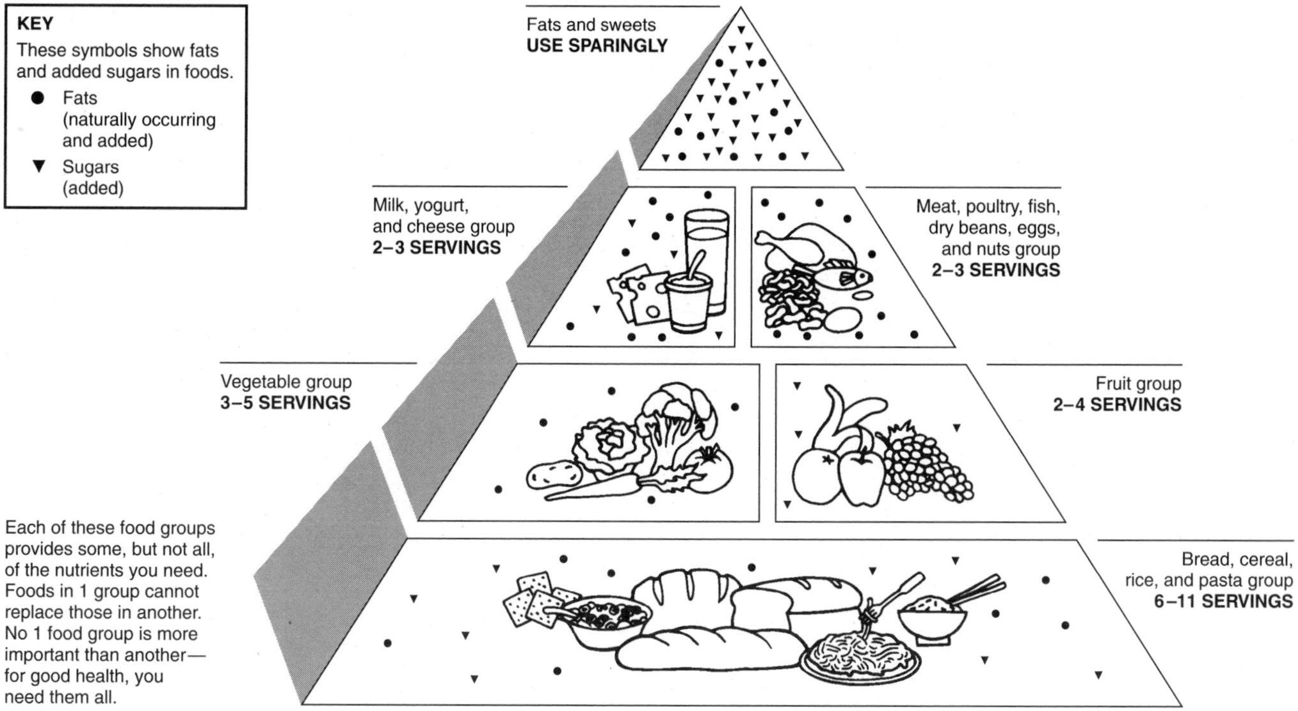

FIGURE 11–4 The food guide pyramid: A guide to daily food choices. (From Human Nutrition Information Service. [1992]. *The Food Guide Pyramid: Beyond the Basic 4.* Washington, D. C., U. S. Department of Agriculture.)

The amount of food that counts as one serving is listed below. If you eat a larger portion, count it as more than one serving. For example, a dinner portion of spaghetti would count as two or three servings of pasta.

Be sure to eat at least the lowest number of servings from the five major food groups listed below. You need them for the vitamins, minerals, carbohydrates, and protein they provide. Just try to pick the lowest fat choices from the food groups. No specific serving size is given for the fats, oils, and sweets group because the message is USE SPARINGLY.

Food Groups

Milk, Yogurt, and Cheese

1 cup of milk or yogurt	1.5 ounces of natural cheese	2 ounces of process cheese

Meat, Poultry, Fish, Dry Beans, Eggs, and Nuts

2–3 ounces of cooked lean meat, poultry, or fish	0.5 cup of cooked dry beans, one egg, or 2 T of peanut butter count as 1 ounce of lean meat

Vegetable

1 cup of raw leafy vegetables	0.5 cup of other vegetables, cooked or chopped raw	0.75 cup of vegetable juice

Fruit

One medium apple, banana, orange	0.5 cup of chopped, cooked, or canned fruit	0.75 cup of fruit juice

Bread, Cereal, Rice, and Pasta

One slice of bread	1 ounce of ready-to-eat cereal	0.5 cup of cooked cereal, rice, or pasta

FIGURE 11–5 What counts as one serving? (From Human Nutrition Information Service. [1992]. *The Food Guide Pyramid: Beyond the Basic 4.* Washington, D. C., U. S. Department of Agriculture.)

	Many Women, Older Adults	Children, Teen Girls, Active Women, Most Men	Teen Boys, Active Men
Calorie Level*	**About 1,600**	**About 2,200**	**About 2,800**
Bread group servings	6	9	11
Vegetable group servings	3	4	5
Fruit group servings	2	3	4
Milk group servings	2–3†	2–3†	2–3†
Meat group servings	2, for a total of 5 ounces	2, for a total of 6 ounces	3, for a total of 7 ounces
Total fat (g)	53	73	93

*These are the calorie levels if you choose low fat, lean foods from the five major food groups and use foods from the fats, oils, and sweets group sparingly.

†Women who are pregnant or breastfeeding, teenagers, and young adults to age 24 need three servings.

FIGURE 11–6 How many servings do you need each day? (From Human Nutrition Information Service. [1992]. *The Food Guide Pyramid: Beyond the Basic 4*. Washington, D. C., U. S. Department of Agriculture.)

erals. Tables 11–10 and 11–11 are included as recommendations and teaching tools and to encourage good dietary habits.

Tobacco Use

"Smoking is the most preventable cause of death in our society. Tobacco use is responsible for nearly one in five deaths in the United States" (American Cancer Society [ACS], 1995, p. 22). It is estimated that about 419,000 deaths each year in the United States and approximately 3 million deaths worldwide are attributable to smoking (ACS, 1995).

In addition to heart disease, lung cancer, and chronic respiratory diseases (e.g., chronic bronchitis and chronic obstructive pulmonary disease), tobacco use is associated with cancers of the mouth, pharynx, larynx, esophagus, pancreas, uterine cervix, kidney, and bladder, as well as intrauterine growth retardation, low birth weight, and birth defects (Centers for Disease Control and Prevention [CDC], 1994a). To put the impact of smoking in perspective, the U. S. Surgeon General "estimates that cigarettes cost Americans $68 billion annually in tobacco-related health care costs and lost productivity. The cost of treating smoking-related diseases and lost productivity amounts to $2.59 for each pack of cigarettes sold in the U. S." (ACS, 1995, p. 22). Thus, the impact of tobacco on the health and the economy of United States residents cannot be overstated.

Per capita cigarette consumption increased annually from 1901 until 1964, when a gradual decline began following the publication of the Surgeon General's Advisory Committee Report on Smoking and Health. Consumption varied somewhat over the next (1964–1974) decade but has declined yearly since 1974 (CDC, 1994b). Table 11–12 profiles trends in smoking between 1965 and 1991.

An estimated 82% of smokers begin smoking before 18 years of age (CDC, 1994a), and approximately 3,000 young persons (mostly children and teenagers) begin smoking each day in the United States. Reportedly, 70% of high school students have tried cigarette smoking, and 28% state that they have smoked cigarettes during the past 30 days (CDC, 1994a). School-based smoking prevention programs have been encouraged to combat the alarming statistics described here. To meet one of the goals for *Healthy People 2000*, the CDC suggests incorporation of tobacco prevention concepts into school health programs. Their recommendations are as follows (CDC, 1994a):

1. Develop and enforce a school policy on tobacco use

2. Provide instruction about the short-term and long-term negative physiological and social consequences of tobacco use, social influences on tobacco use, peer norms regarding tobacco use, and refusal skills

Text continued on page 297

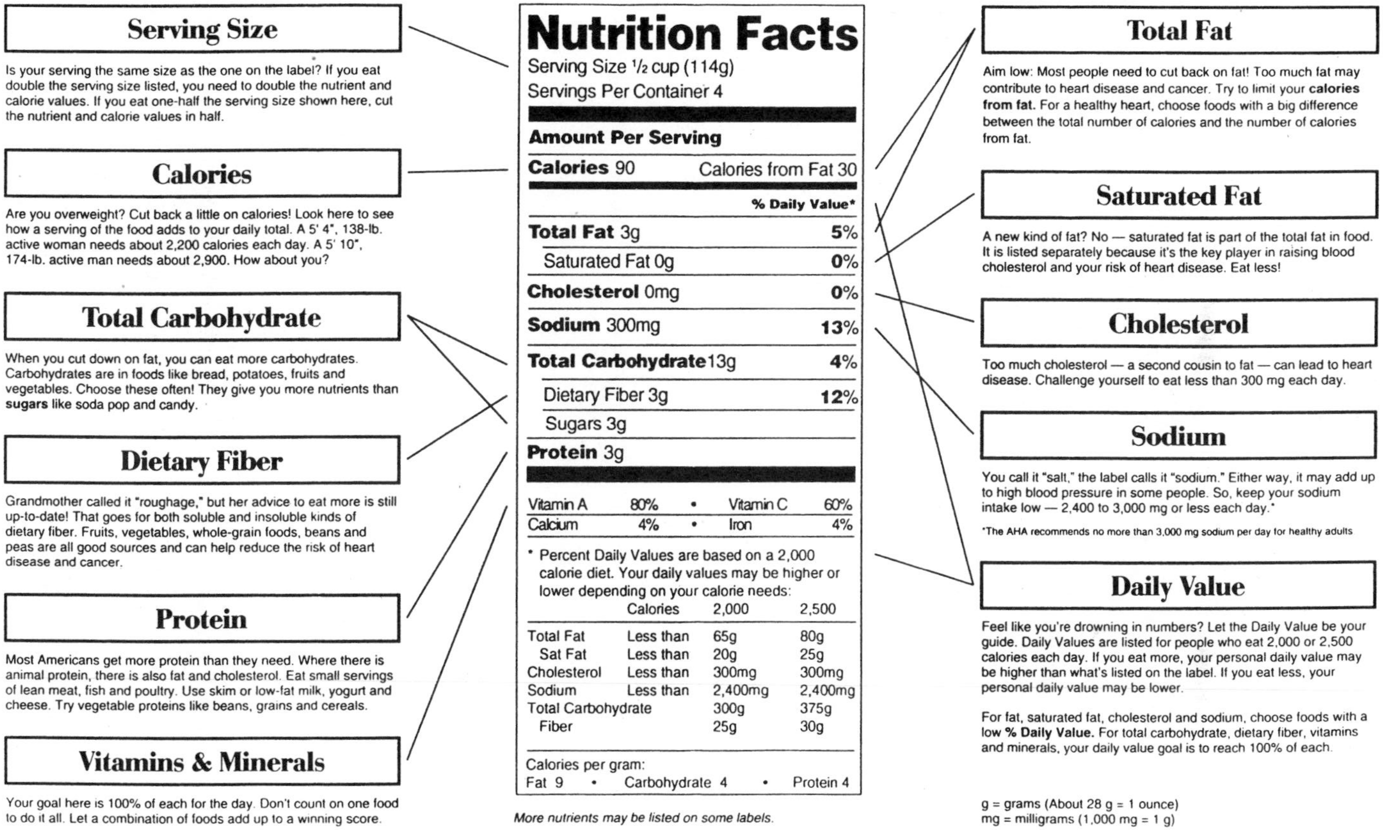
Serving Size
Is your serving the same size as the one on the label? If you eat double the serving size listed, you need to double the nutrient and calorie values. If you eat one-half the serving size shown here, cut the nutrient and calorie values in half.
Calories
Are you overweight? Cut back a little on calories! Look here to see how a serving of the food adds to your daily total. A 5' 4", 138-lb. active woman needs about 2,200 calories each day. A 5' 10", 174-lb. active man needs about 2,900. How about you?
Total Carbohydrate
When you cut down on fat, you can eat more carbohydrates. Carbohydrates are in foods like bread, potatoes, fruits and vegetables. Choose these often! They give you more nutrients than sugars like soda pop and candy.
Dietary Fiber
Grandmother called it "roughage," but her advice to eat more is still up-to-date! That goes for both soluble and insoluble kinds of dietary fiber. Fruits, vegetables, whole-grain foods, beans and peas are all good sources and can help reduce the risk of heart disease and cancer.
Protein
Most Americans get more protein than they need. Where there is animal protein, there is also fat and cholesterol. Eat small servings of lean meat, fish and poultry. Use skim or low-fat milk, yogurt and cheese. Try vegetable proteins like beans, grains and cereals.
Vitamins & Minerals
Your goal here is 100% of each for the day. Don't count on one food to do it all. Let a combination of foods add up to a winning score.
Nutrition Facts
Serving Size 1/2 cup (114g)
Servings Per Container 4
Amount Per Serving
Calories 90 Calories from Fat 30
% Daily Value*
Total Fat 3g 5%
Saturated Fat 0g 0%
Cholesterol 0mg 0%
Sodium 300mg 13%
Total Carbohydrate 13g 4%
Dietary Fiber 3g 12%
Sugars 3g
Protein 3g
Vitamin A 80% • Vitamin C 60%
Calcium 4% • Iron 4%
* Percent Daily Values are based on a 2,000 calorie diet. Your daily values may be higher or lower depending on your calorie needs:
Calories 2,000 2,500
Total Fat Less than 65g 80g
Sat Fat Less than 20g 25g
Cholesterol Less than 300mg 300mg
Sodium Less than 2,400mg 2,400mg
Total Carbohydrate 300g 375g
Fiber 25g 30g
Calories per gram:
Fat 9 • Carbohydrate 4 • Protein 4
More nutrients may be listed on some labels.
Total Fat
Aim low: Most people need to cut back on fat! Too much fat may contribute to heart disease and cancer. Try to limit your calories from fat. For a healthy heart, choose foods with a big difference between the total number of calories and the number of calories from fat.
Saturated Fat
A new kind of fat? No — saturated fat is part of the total fat in food. It is listed separately because it's the key player in raising blood cholesterol and your risk of heart disease. Eat less!
Cholesterol
Too much cholesterol — a second cousin to fat — can lead to heart disease. Challenge yourself to eat less than 300 mg each day.
Sodium
You call it "salt," the label calls it "sodium." Either way, it may add up to high blood pressure in some people. So, keep your sodium intake low — 2,400 to 3,000 mg or less each day.*
*The AHA recommends no more than 3,000 mg sodium per day for healthy adults
Daily Value
Feel like you're drowning in numbers? Let the Daily Value be your guide. Daily Values are listed for people who eat 2,000 or 2,500 calories each day. If you eat more, your personal daily value may be higher than what's listed on the label. If you eat less, your personal daily value may be lower.
For fat, saturated fat, cholesterol and sodium, choose foods with a low % Daily Value. For total carbohydrate, dietary fiber, vitamins and minerals, your daily value goal is to reach 100% of each.
g = grams (About 28 g = 1 ounce)
mg = milligrams (1,000 mg = 1 g)

FIGURE 11–7 Guide to using the new food label. (From USDHHS/Food and Drug Administration/USDA. [1993]. *An Introduction to the New Food Label.* DHHS Publication No. [FDA] 94–2271. Washington, D. C., USDHHS/Food and Drug Administration/USDA.)

TABLE 11–8 Clarifying Food Label Claims

Saturated Fat

***Saturated fat free:** Less than 0.5 g saturated fat in a serving; levels of trans fatty acids must be 1% or less of total fat

†**Low saturated fat:** 1 g saturated fat or less in a serving and 15% or less of calories; for a meal or main dish (like a frozen dinner): 1 g saturated fat or less in 100 g of food and less than 10% of calories from saturated fat

Cholesterol

***Cholesterol free:** Less than 2 mg cholesterol in a serving; saturated fat content must be 2 g or less in a serving

†**Low cholesterol:** 20 mg cholesterol or less in a serving; saturated fat content must be 2 g or less in a serving; for a meal or main dish: 20 mg cholesterol or less in 100 g of food, with saturated fat content less than 2 g in 100 g of food

Fat

***Fat free:** Less than 0.5 g fat in a serving

†**Low fat:** 3 g total fat or less in a serving; for a meal or main dish: 3 g total fat or less in 100 g of food and not more than 30% calories from fat

Percent fat free: A food with this claim must also meet the low fat claim

Calories

***Calorie free:** Less than 5 calories in a serving

†**Low calorie:** 40 calories or less in a serving

Sodium

***Sodium free:** Less than 5 mg sodium in a serving

†**Low sodium:** 140 mg sodium or less in a serving; for a meal or main dish: 140 mg sodium or less in 100 g of food

Very low sodium: 35 mg sodium or less in a serving

Light

A product has been changed to have half the fat or one-third fewer calories than the regular product; or the sodium in a low-calorie, low-fat food has been cut by 50%; or a meal or main dish is low fat or low calorie

"Light" also may be used to describe things like the color or texture of a food, as long as the label explains this; for example, "light brown sugar" or "light and fluffy"

Reduced/Less/Lower/Fewer

A food (like a lower-fat hot dog or a lower-sodium cracker) has at least 25% less of something like calories, fat, saturated fat, cholesterol, or sodium than the regular food or a similar food to which it is compared

Lean/Extra Lean

Terms used to describe the fat content of meat, poultry, fish, and shellfish:

Lean: Less than 10 g fat, 4.5 g or less of saturated fat, and less than 95 mg cholesterol in a serving and in 100 g of food

Extra lean: Less than 5 g fat, less than 2 g saturated fat, and less than 95 mg cholesterol in a serving and in 100 g of food

*Words that mean the same thing as "free": "no," "zero," "without," "trivial source of," "negligible source of," and "dietarily insignificant source of."

†Words that mean the same thing as low: "contains a small amount of" and "low source of."

From U. S. Department of Health and Human Services/National Institutes of Health/National Heart, Lung, and Blood Institute. (1994). *Step by Step: Eating to Lower Your High Blood Cholesterol.* NIH Publication No 94-2920. Washington, D. C., U. S. Department of Health and Human Services/National Heart, Lung, and Blood Institute.

TABLE 11–9 **Fat Content of Selected Foods**

Food (Serving Size)	Total Fat (g)	Saturated Fat (g)	Cholesterol (mg)	Calories
Bread (one slice)—white	1	Trace	Trace	70
Bread (one slice)—whole wheat	1	Trace	0	65
Doughnut (one)	14	5	21	245
Rice (0.5 cup)—white	Trace	Trace	0	110
Cookie (one medium)—oatmeal	3	1	5	60
Milk (1 cup)—whole	8	5	33	150
2%	5	3	18	120
Skim	Trace	Trace	4	85
Cheese (1 ounce)—cheddar	9	6	29	115
Mozzarella	5	3	15	80
Processed American	9	6	27	105
Vanilla ice cream (0.5 cup)	7	4	27	135
Potatoes (0.5 cup)—boiled	Trace	Trace	0	65
French fried (10 strips)	8	3	0	160
Chips (1 ounce)	10	3	0	150
Beef (3 ounces)—roasted lean	4	2	59	145
Ground (3-ounce patty)—lean	16	6	73	230
Chicken (3 ounces)—light and dark meat with skin	12	3	74	200
Chicken (3 ounces)—light and dark meat without skin	6	2	75	160
Tuna (3 ounces)—in oil	7	1	25	170
Tuna (3 ounces)—in water	1	Trace	25	115
Two frankfurters (3 ounces)	27	10	47	300
Peanut butter (2 T)	16	3	0	190
Egg (one large)	5	2	213	60
Dry beans, cooked (0.5 cup)	Trace	Trace	0	110
Apple (medium)	Trace	Trace	0	80
Avocado (one half, medium)	15	2	0	160
Banana (one medium)	1	Trace	0	105
Orange (one medium)	Trace	Trace	0	60
Butter (1 T)	12	7	31	100
Margarine (1 T)—stick	12	2	0	100
Salad dressing (1 T)—mayonnaise (regular)	12	2	7	100
Mayonnaise—reduced calorie (1 T)	5	1	5	50
Italian (1 T)	7	1	0	70
Cream (1 T)—sour	33	2	6	30
Nondairy, frozen (1 T)	1	Trace	0	20
Pie—apple (one eighth of 9-inch pie)	22	5	0	455
Milk chocolate bar (1 ounce)	9	5	6	145
Cake, frosted (one twelfth of 8-inch cake)	16	5	32	405

From U. S. Department of Agriculture/Human Nutrition Information Service. (1993). *Choose a Diet Low in Fat, Saturated Fat and Cholesterol.* Washington, D. C., Government Printing Office.

TABLE 11–10 **Facts about Vitamins**

Vitamin	Food Sources	Benefits to Wellness	Deficiency Signs and Symptoms
Water-Soluble Vitamins			
B complex	Meat products (beef, pork, poultry, eggs, fish), milk, cheese, grains, dried beans, nuts, starchy vegetables	Facilitates release of energy from other nutrients Aids in formation of red blood cells, growth and function of the nervous system, and formation of hormones Contributes to good vision and healthy skin Assists in the metabolism of proteins, fats, and carbohydrates	Fatigue, nausea, weakness, irritability, depression, weight loss, inflamed skin, cracked lips, muscle pain, cramps or twitching, low blood sugar, decreased resistance to disease, nerve dysfunction
C (ascorbic acid)	Citrus fruits, strawberries, cantaloupe, honeydew melons, broccoli, brussels sprouts, green peppers, cauliflower, spinach	Contributes to production of collagen Aids in protection against infection Contributes to tooth and bone formation and repair and wound healing Aids in absorption of iron and calcium	Dry, rough, and scaly skin; bleeding gums; slowly healing wounds; listlessness; fatigue; low glucose tolerance
Fat-Soluble Vitamins			
A	Milk; cheese; butter; fat; eggs; liver; dark-green, leafy vegetables; carrots; cantaloupe; yellow squash; sweet potatoes	Is essential for growth of epithelial cells such as hair, skin, and mucous membranes Aids in vision in dim light Contributes to bone growth and tooth development Plays a role in reproduction (sperm production and estrogen synthesis) Increases resistance to infection	Decreased resistance to infection, skin changes, alteration of tooth enamel, night blindness, corneal deterioration
D*	Milk (fortified), butter, cheese, eggs, clams, fish, salmon, tuna	Is essential for bones and teeth Contributes to calcium and phosphorus absorption	Bone softening and fractures, muscle spasms, tooth malformation
E	Vegetable oils; green, leafy vegetables; liver; eggs; whole-grain cereals and breads	Assists in formation of red blood cells and muscle tissue Aids in absorption of vitamin A Serves as an antioxidant, which preserves vitamins and unsaturated fatty acids	Destruction of cell membrane of red blood cells
K	Green, leafy vegetables; liver; cabbage; cauliflower; eggs; tomatoes; peas; potatoes; milk	Aids in normal formation of the liver Contributes to normal blood clotting	Severe bleeding, prolonged coagulation, bruising

*Sunlight also stimulates vitamin D production.

From Anspaugh, D. J., Hamrick, M. H., and Rosato, F. D. (1994). *Wellness: Concepts and Applications* (2nd ed.). St. Louis, MO, Mosby-Year Book.

TABLE 11–11 **Facts about Minerals**

Major (Macro) Minerals

Calcium, phosphorus, potassium, sulfur, sodium chloride, and magnesium

Trace (Micro) Minerals

Iron, iodine, zinc, selenium, manganese, copper, molybdenum, cobalt, chromium, fluorine, silicon, vanadium, nickel, tin, cadmium

Minerals of Special Concern*

Calcium

Wellness benefits: Contributes to bone and tooth formation, general body growth, maintenance of good muscle tone, nerve function, cell membrane function, and regulation of normal heart beat

Food sources: Dairy products, dark-green vegetables, dried beans, shellfish

Deficiency signs and symptoms: Bone pain and fractures, muscle cramps, osteoporosis

Iron

Wellness benefits: Facilitates oxygen and carbon dioxide transport, formation of red blood cells, production of antibodies, synthesis of collagen, and use of energy

Food sources: Red meat (lean), seafoods, eggs, dried beans, nuts, grains, green, leafy vegetables

Deficiency signs and symptoms: Fatigue, weakness

Sodium

Wellness benefits: Is essential for maintenance of proper acid-base balance and body fluid regulation, aids in formation of digestive secretions, assists in nerve transmission

Food sources: Processed foods, meats, table salt

Deficiency signs and symptoms: Rare

*Calcium and iron are of special concern because deficiencies are likely to exist, especially among women and children.

From Anspaugh, D. J., Hamrick, M. H., and Rosato, F. D. (1994). *Wellness: Concepts and Applications* (2nd ed.). St. Louis, MO, Mosby-Year Book.

3. Provide tobacco use prevention education in kindergarten through 12th grade; this instruction should be especially intensive in junior high or middle school and should be reinforced in high school
4. Provide program-specific training for teachers
5. Involve parents or families in support of school-based programs to prevent tobacco use
6. Support cessation efforts among students and all school staff who use tobacco
7. Assess the tobacco use prevention program at regular intervals

SMOKING CESSATION

The CDC reports that 80% of adults who smoke want to quit and that almost half of all living adults who have ever smoked have quit (USDHHS/National Cancer Institute, 1990). Programs, tools, medications, and various interventions abound to help with smoking cessation. Recognized interventions include self-help groups, videos and written materials, nicotine chewing gum, nicotine patches, hypnosis, and acupuncture. However, most people who stop (about 90%), do so on their own. The National Cancer Institute has developed a list of tips for smokers to help them quit (Table 11–13).

Health Task Force Recommendations—Illness Prevention

The U. S. Preventive Services Task Force has published general guidelines or recommendations for periodic individual health examinations based on age. Included in the guidelines is information on the leading causes of death, appropriate screenings, counseling, and immunizations. Special guidelines and frequencies were detailed for those who are identified as being at high risk for a particular health threat or problem. Table 11–14 contains the guidelines for people 25 to 64 years of age. Guidelines and recommendations are also presented in Chapters 12 through 14.

Screening Principles

The tables presented here list a variety of recommended screenings based on age and risk factors. If a screening test is to be performed and the

TABLE 11–12 **Smoking Trends—1965–1991**

Smoking Status	1965	1974	1983	1991
Total population				
Current	42.4	37.1	32.1	25.7
Former	13.6	19.5	21.8	24.1
Never	44.0	43.4	46.1	50.2
Sex—Male				
Current	51.9	43.1	35.1	28.1
Former	19.8	27.7	28.3	29.9
Never	28.3	29.2	36.6	42.1
Sex—Female				
Current	33.9	32.1	29.5	23.5
Former	8.0	12.7	15.9	19.0
Never	58.1	55.2	54.6	57.6
Race—White				
Current	42.1	36.4	31.8	25.5
Former	14.2	20.5	22.8	25.7
Never	43.8	43.1	45.3	48.9
Race—Black				
Current	45.8	44.0	35.9	29.1
Former	8.4	10.8	14.2	14.6
Never	45.8	45.3	49.9	56.2
Race—Hispanic origin				
Current	NA	NA	25.3	20.2
Former	NA	NA	15.7	16.9
Never	NA	NA	59.0	63.0
Age (years)—18–24				
Current	45.5	37.8	34.2	22.9
Former	6.9	9.5	9.3	7.7
Never	47.6	52.7	56.5	69.3
Age (years)—25–44				
Current	51.2	44.5	36.3	30.4
Former	13.6	18.4	19.0	19.4
Never	35.3	37.1	44.7	50.2
Age (years)—45–64				
Current	41.6	37.7	33.3	26.9
Former	16.1	24.8	28.8	32.9
Never	42.3	37.5	37.9	40.2
Age (years)—65+				
Current	17.9	17.3	16.7	13.3
Former	15.0	23.3	30.7	36.4
Never	67.2	59.4	52.6	50.3
Education (years)—<12				
Current	NA	37.8	34.7	31.4
Former	NA	19.8	23.2	25.3
Never	NA	42.4	42.2	43.3
Education (years)—12				
Current	NA	38.8	34.9	30.6
Former	NA	20.9	23.7	26.1
Never	NA	40.4	41.4	43.3
Education (years)—13–15				
Current	NA	37.9	32.1	25.5
Former	NA	24.1	25.1	28.1
Never	NA	37.0	42.8	46.4
Education (years)—≥16				
Current	NA	28.8	20.6	13.9
Former	NA	27.8	26.5	27.6
Never	NA	43.4	52.9	58.5

NA = not applicable.

From Centers for Disease Control and Prevention. (1994). Surveillance for selected tobacco-use behaviors—United States, 1900–1994. *Morbidity and Mortality Weekly Report, 43* (No. SS-3).

resulting information is to be useful, certain guidelines must be followed. Principles for screening, as outlined by the USDHHS/ODPHP (1994), are as follow:

- The condition must have a significant effect on the quality and quantity of life
- Acceptable methods of treatment must be available
- The condition must have an asymptomatic period during which detection and treatment significantly reduce morbidity or mortality
- Treatment in the asymptomatic phase must yield a therapeutic result superior to that obtained by delaying treatment until symptoms appear
- Tests that are acceptable to patients must be

TABLE 11–13 **Tips to Help Smokers Quit**

Tips for Preparing to Stop

- Decide positively that you want to stop. Try to avoid negative thoughts about possible difficulties.
- List all the reasons why you want to stop. Every night before going to bed, repeat one of the reasons 10 times.
- Develop strong personalized reasons for stopping. For example, think of all of the time you waste taking cigarette breaks, rushing out to buy a pack, or hunting for a lighter.
- Begin to condition yourself physically: Start a moderate exercise program, drink more fluids, get plenty of rest, and avoid fatigue.
- Know what to expect: Have realistic expectations—stopping isn't easy, but it is not impossible either. More than 3 million people in the United States stop each year. Understand that withdrawal symptoms are temporary and are healthy signs that the body is repairing itself from its long exposure to nicotine. Know that most relapses occur in the first week or two after stopping. At this time, withdrawal symptoms are strongest and your body is still most dependent on nicotine.
- Involve someone else: Make a bet with a friend, ask your spouse or a friend to stop smoking with you and make a "buddy" system, tell your family and friends that you are stopping.

Tips for Just Before Stopping

- Practice going without tobacco.
- Do not dwell on the fact that you will never use tobacco again: Think of being tobacco free in terms of 1 day at a time.
- Stop carrying tobacco with you at all times.
- Do not empty your ashtrays or the container that you spit into. This will remind you how much you have used each day, and the sight and smell will be very unpleasant.
- Collect all your cigarette butts into one large glass container as a visual reminder of the mess that smoking represents. Occasionally screw off the lid to smell the foul butt and ash odors.

Tips for the Day You Stop

- Throw away all of your tobacco, lighters, ashtrays, spittoons, and other tobacco-related paraphernalia.
- Clean your clothes to rid them of the smell of smoke.
- Develop a clean, fresh, smoke-free environment around yourself—at work and at home.
- Schedule an appointment to have your teeth cleaned.
- Make a list of things you would like to buy for yourself or someone else. Estimate your cost of using tobacco and put the money aside to buy yourself a present.
- Keep very busy during the big day. Go to the movies, exercise, take long walks, or go bike riding.
- Buy yourself a treat or do something to celebrate.
- Stay away from other tobacco users.
- Remember that one cigarette or one chew could ruin a successful attempt.
- Remember that alcohol will weaken your willpower. Avoid it.
- Refuse to allow anything to change your mind.

Tips to Help You Cope with the Periodic Urge to Use Tobacco

- First remind yourself that you have stopped and you are a nonuser. Look closely at your urge to use tobacco and ask yourself: "Where was I when I got the urge?" "What was I doing at the time?" "Who was I with?" "What was I thinking?"
- Think about why you stopped. Repeat to yourself your three main reasons for stopping.
- Anticipate triggers and prepare to avoid them. Keep your hands busy, avoid people who smoke or chew, find activities that make smoking difficult, put something other than tobacco in your mouth (e.g., carrots, sunflower seeds, apples, celery, or sugarless gum), and avoid places where smoking is permitted.
- Change your daily routine to break old habits and patterns. After meals, immediately get up from the table, brush your teeth or take a walk, change your morning routine, do not sit in your favorite chair, eat lunch at a different location.

Table continued on following page

TABLE 11–13 **Tips to Help Smokers Quit** *Continued*

- Use positive thoughts. Remind yourself that you are a nonuser; observe people who do not smoke and remind yourself that they feel normal and healthy without using tobacco and so can you.
- Use relaxation techniques. Breathe in deeply and slowly while you count to five; breathe out slowly, counting to five again.

Tips for Coping with Relapse

- Stop using tobacco immediately.
- Get rid of any tobacco products that you may have.
- Recognize that you have had a slip or small setback and that a small setback does not make you a smoker or a chewer again.
- Do not be too hard on yourself. One slip does not mean that you are a failure or cannot be a nonuser, but it is important to get yourself back on the nonuser track immediately.
- Realize that many successful former tobacco users stop for good only after more than one attempt.
- Identify triggers. Exactly what was it that prompted you to use tobacco? Be aware of your triggers and decide how you will cope with them when they come up again.
- Sign a contract with yourself to remain a nonuser.

Adapted from U. S. Department of Health and Human Services/National Institutes of Health/National Cancer Institute. (1991). *Clearing the Air: How to Quit Smoking and Quit for Keeps.* NIH Publication No. 92-1647. Washington, D. C., U. S. Department of Health and Human Services/National Institutes of Health/National Cancer Institute.

available, at a reasonable cost, to detect the condition in the asymptomatic period

- The incidence of the condition must be sufficient to justify the cost of the screening
- The screening test performed must be reliable and valid (i.e., the test should have good "sensitivity" and "specificity")
- Methods for follow-up tracking for client referrals should be available
- Patients should be clearly informed of the potential cost and morbidity of necessary follow-up testing and treatment

Primary and Secondary Prevention of Selected Conditions

HEART DISEASE AND STROKE

As discussed earlier and presented in Table 11–1, heart disease and stroke are the number one and number three leading causes of death, respectively, in the United States each year. Indeed, each year as many as 1.5 million U. S. residents have a heart attack, and about one third of these die. It is important to note that although heart disease is associated with aging, about 5% of all heart attacks occur in people younger than 40 years, and 45% occur in people younger than 65. Strokes afflict more than 500,000 U. S. residents each year, and stroke is the leading cause of serious disability in the United States (American Heart Association, 1994). Risk factors associated with heart disease and stroke are listed in Table 11–15.

Figures 11–8 and 11–9 give examples of assessment and teaching tools for identification of an individual's risk of heart disease and describe how risks can be lowered or managed. These tools may be used by nurses and others as part of a comprehensive program that includes health teaching and counseling on nutrition, exercise, and smoking cessation, if applicable, to lower risk for all individuals.

CANCER

Cancer, as has been discussed, is the second leading cause of death in the United States. The ACS

TABLE 11–14 **Recommendations of the U. S. Preventive Task Force, Ages 25–64 Years**

Leading Causes of Death

Malignant neoplasms
Heart diseases
Motor vehicle and other unintentional injuries
Human immunodeficiency virus (HIV) infection
Suicide and homicide

Interventions Considered and Recommended for the Periodic Health Examination for the General Population

Screening

Blood pressure
Height and weight
Total blood cholesterol (men ages 35–65; women ages 45–65)
Papanicolaou (pap) test (women)*
Fecal occult blood test† and/or sigmoidoscopy (≥50 years)
Mammogram ± clinical breast exam‡ (women 50–69 years)
Assess for problem drinking
Rubella serology or vaccination history§ (women of childbearing age)

Counseling

Substance use

Tobacco cessation
Avoid alcohol or drug use while performing activities such as driving, swimming, boating||

Diet and exercise

Limit fat and cholesterol; maintain caloric balance; emphasize grains, fruits, vegetables
Adequate calcium intake (women)
Regular physical activity||

Injury prevention

Lap/shoulder belts
Motorcycle/bicycle/all-terrain vehicle helmets||
Smoke detector||
Safe storage/removal of firearms||

Sexual behavior

Sexually transmitted disease (STD) prevention: avoid high-risk behavior;|| condoms/female barrier with spermicide||
Unintended pregnancy: contraception

Dental health

Regular visits to dental care provider||
Floss, brush with fluoride toothpaste daily||

Immunizations

Tetanus-diphtheria (Td) boosters
Rubella§ (women of childbearing age)

Chemoprophylaxis

Multivitamin with folic acid (women planning or capable of pregnancy)
Discuss hormone prophylaxis (peri- and postmenopausal women)

Table continued on following page

estimates that 1,250,000 new cancer cases are diagnosed each year, resulting in about 547,000 deaths (1,500 people each day) (ACS, 1995). Figures 11–10 and 11–11 graphically illustrate trends in cancer death rates for men and women in the United States, and Figure 11–12 shows estimates of newly diagnosed cases and deaths for different types of cancer.

These figures show the dramatic increase in lung cancer deaths that began during the mid-1950s for men and the mid-1960s for women. As stated earlier, these increases are the direct result of smoking and are expected to continue through the next several decades.

Prevention and Diagnosis of Selected Cancers

Early detection and treatment of cancer has resulted in improved survival rates for most cancers. To assist nurses in teaching and counseling regarding cancer prevention, detection, and treatment, Table 11–16 lists the seven warning signs of cancer, and Table 11–17 lists incidence, symptoms, risk factors, and treatment options for several of the most common cancers.

DIABETES

Approximately 14 million U. S. residents have diabetes, and it is estimated that half are not aware of it. Each year, 500,000 to 700,000 people are diagnosed with diabetes; 11,000 to 12,000 of them are children. Ninety to 95% of people with diabetes have NIDDM (type II diabetes), which usually develops in adults older than 40 years. The remainder (5–10%) of patients have IDDM, which most often develops in children and young adults

TABLE 11–14 Recommendations of the U. S. Preventive Task Force, Ages 25–64 Years *Continued*

Interventions for High-Risk Populations

Population	*Potential Interventions (See Detailed High-Risk [HR] Definitions)*¶
High-risk sexual behavior	RPR/VDRL (HR1); screen for gonorrhea (female) (HR2), HIV (HR3), chlamydia (female) (HR4); hepatitis B vaccine (HR5); hepatitis A vaccine (HR6)
Injection or street drug use	RPR/VDRL (HR1); HIV screen (HR3); hepatitis B vaccine (HR5); hepatitis A vaccine (HR6); PPD (HR7); advice to reduce infection risk (HR8)
Low income; tuberculosis (TB) contacts; immigrants; alcoholics	PPD (HR7)
Native Americans/Alaska Natives	Hepatitis A vaccine (HR6); PPD (HR7); pneumococcal vaccine (HR9)
Travelers to developing countries	Hepatitis B vaccine (HR5); hepatitis A vaccine (HR6)
Certain chronic medical conditions	PPD (HR7); pneumococcal vaccine (HR9); influenza vaccine (HR10)
Blood product recipients	HIV screen (HR3); hepatitis B vaccine (HR5)
Susceptible to measles, mumps, or varicella	MMR (HR11); varicella vaccine (HR12)
Institutionalized persons	Hepatitis A vaccine (HR6); PPD (HR7); pneumococcal vaccine (HR9); influenza vaccine (HR10)
Health care/laboratory workers	Hepatitis B vaccine (HR5); hepatitis A vaccine (HR6); PPD (HR7); influenza vaccine (HR10)
Family history of skin cancer; fair skin, eyes, hair	Avoid excess/midday sun, use protective clothing* (HR13)
Previous pregnancy with neural tube defect	Folic acid 4.0 mg (HR14)

*Women who are or have been sexually active and who have a cervix: q ≤ 3 yr.

†Annually.

‡Mammogram q1–2 yr, or mammogram q1–2 yr with annual clinical breast examination.

§Serologic testing, documented vaccination history, and routine vaccination (preferably with MMR) are equally acceptable alternatives.

‖The ability of clinician counseling to influence this behavior is unproven.

PPD = purified protein derivative (a TB test); RPR = Rapid plasma reagin (test for syphilis); VDRL = Venereal Disease Research Laboratory.

¶**HR1** = Persons who exchange sex for money or drugs, and their sex partners; persons with other STDs (including HIV); and sexual contacts of persons with active syphilis. Clinicians should also consider local epidemiology. **HR2** = Women who exchange sex for money or drugs or who have had repeated episodes of gonorrhea. Clinicians should also consider local epidemiology. **HR3** = Men who had sex with men after 1975; past or present injection drug use; persons who exchange sex for money or drugs, and their sex partners; injection drug-using, bisexual, or HIV-positive sex partner currently or in the past; blood transfusion during 1978–1985; persons seeking treatment for STDs. Clinicians should also consider local epidemiology. **HR4** = Sexually active women with multiple risk factors including history of STD; new or multiple sex partners; nonuse or inconsistent use of barrier contraceptives; cervical ectopy. Clinicians should also consider local epidemiology. **HR5** = Blood product recipients (including hemodialysis patients), persons with frequent occupational exposure to blood or blood products, men who have sex with men, injection drug users and their sex partners, persons with multiple recent sex partners, persons with other STDs (including HIV), travelers to countries with endemic hepatitis B. **HR6** = Persons living in, traveling to, or working in areas where the disease is endemic and where periodic outbreaks occur (e.g., countries with high or intermediate endemicity; certain Alaska Native, Pacific Island, Native American, and religious communities); men who have sex with men; injection or street drug users. Consider for institutionalized persons and workers in these institutions, military personnel, and day-care, hospital, and laboratory workers. Clinicians should also consider local epidemiology. **HR7** = HIV positive, close contacts of persons with known or suspected TB, health care workers, persons with medical risk factors associated with TB, immigrants from countries with high TB prevalence, medically underserved low-income populations (including homeless), alcoholics, injection drug users, and residents of long-term care facilities. **HR8** = Persons who continue to inject drugs. **HR9** = Immunocompetent institutionalized persons aged ≥50 years and immunocompetent persons with certain medical conditions, including chronic cardiac or pulmonary disease, diabetes mellitus, and anatomic asplenia. Immunocompetent persons who live in high-risk environments or social settings (e.g., certain Native American and Alaska Native populations). **HR10** = Annual vaccination of residents of chronic care facilities; persons with chronic cardiopulmonary disorders, metabolic diseases (including diabetes mellitus), hemoglobinopathies, immunosuppression, or renal dysfunction; and health care providers for high-risk patients. **HR11** = Persons born after 1956 who lack evidence of immunity to measles or mumps (e.g., documented receipt of live vaccine on or after the first birthday, laboratory evidence of immunity, or a history of physician-diagnosed measles or mumps). **HR12** = Healthy adults without a history of chickenpox or previous immunization. Consider serological testing for presumed susceptible adults. **HR13** = Persons with a family or personal history of skin cancer, a large number of moles, atypical moles, poor tanning ability, or light skin, hair, and eye color. **HR14** = Women with previous pregnancy affected by neural tube defect who are planning pregnancy. From U. S. Preventive Task Force. (1996). *Guide to Clinical Preventive Services.* Washington, D. C., Government Printing Office.

TABLE 11–15 **Risk Factors Associated with Heart Disease and Stroke**

Smoking—Smoking greatly increases the risk of heart attack and stroke

Hypertension—High blood pressure is a major risk factor in heart attack and is *the* most important risk factor in stroke

High blood cholesterol and low high-density lipoprotein cholesterol concentration—High blood cholesterol causes narrowing in the arterial walls, thus increasing the possibility of occlusion in the brain or heart

Diabetes—Diabetes is linked with increased risk of both heart disease and stroke

Obesity—Obesity increases the risk of heart disease, particularly in individuals more than 30% above ideal body weight

Age—Risk of heart disease and stroke increases steadily with age

Sex—Men have three to four times greater risk of heart disease then premenopausal women; after menopause, women's rate of heart disease increases sharply, although elderly men have roughly twice the risk as elderly women

Genetic predisposition—Risk increases if a parent or sibling has had a heart attack or stroke or died of heart disease before age 55

Data from American Heart Association. (1990). *Nurses' Cholesterol Education Handbook.* Dallas, TX, American Heart Association; American Heart Association. (1994). *Fact Sheet on Heart Attack, Stroke and Risk Factors.* Dallas, TX, American Heart Association.

(National Institutes of Health/National Institute of Diabetes and Digestive and Kidney Diseases, 1994).

Diabetes is one of the leading causes of death and disability in the United States, contributing to 200,000 to 250,000 deaths each year. Additionally, diabetes is associated with many severe illnesses and conditions, including blindness, heart disease, stroke, kidney failure, nerve damage, amputations, and birth defects in babies born to women with diabetes.

Risk factors for NIDDM include obesity (about 80% of people with NIDDM are overweight), increasing age, family history, and/or being a member of certain minority groups. African-Americans and Hispanics are at increased risk for developing diabetes, but the prevalence is extremely high among Native Americans—almost 50% of members of certain tribes are known to be diabetic (National Institutes of Health/National Institute of Diabetes and Digestive and Kidney Diseases, 1994).

Individuals, particularly those in high-risk groups, should be taught symptoms of diabetes. These include (USDHHS/CDC, 1992)

- Excessive thirst
- Excessive urination
- Blurred vision
- Sensory nerve damage, particularly in the extremities
- Fatigue
- Weight loss
- Slow healing of skin
- Gum infection
- Urinary tract infection

Whereas IDDM is managed with strict adherence to a prescribed diet, intensive monitoring of blood glucose levels, and administration of insulin (often two to four times daily), NIDDM is primarily controlled through diet and other lifestyle changes. Weight loss is strongly encouraged, as is avoidance of alcohol and smoking, where indicated. Frequently, people with NIDDM must take medication to control blood glucose levels. Usually, oral medications (e.g., oral hypoglycemic/sulfonylureas such as tolbutamide, chlorpropamide, and tolazamide) are sufficient, but many type II diabetics eventually need to take insulin to better control serum glucose levels.

Health teaching and counseling for all individuals with diabetes should focus on closely following the recommended diet; monitoring blood glucose levels as directed by their physician; taking medications, including insulin, as prescribed; and carefully observing for complications. Some relatively common complications, prevention methods, and teaching principles include the following:

- Diabetic ketoacidosis (insulin deficiency resulting in hyperglycemia, osmotic diuresis, and acidosis)—usually caused by failure to adhere to program for insulin management or

Text continued on page 309

Healthy Heart I.Q.

Please answer "true" or "false" to the following questions to test your knowledge of heart disease and its risk factors. Then check the answers and explanations that follow to see how well you do.

1. The risk factors for heart disease that you *can do something about* are high blood pressure, high blood cholesterol, smoking, obesity, and physical inactivity.	T	F
2. A stroke is often the first symptom of high blood pressure, and a heart attack is often the first symptom of high blood cholesterol.	T	F
3. A blood pressure greater than or equal to 140/90 mm Hg is generally considered to be high.	T	F
4. High blood pressure affects the same number of blacks as it does whites.	T	F
5. The best ways to treat and control high blood pressure are to control your weight, exercise, eat less salt (sodium), restrict your intake of alcohol, and take your high blood pressure medicine, if prescribed by your doctor.	T	F
6. A blood cholesterol level of 240 mg/dL is desirable for adults.	T	F
7. The most effective dietary way to lower the level of your blood cholesterol is to eat foods low in cholesterol.	T	F
8. Lowering blood cholesterol levels can help people who have already had a heart attack.	T	F
9. Only children from families at high risk of heart disease need to have their blood cholesterol levels checked.	T	F
10. Smoking is a major risk factor for four of the five leading causes of death including heart attack, stroke, cancer, and lung diseases such as emphysema and bronchitis.	T	F
11. If you have had a heart attack, quitting smoking can help reduce your chances of having a second attack.	T	F
12. Someone who has smoked for 30 to 40 years probably will not be able to quit smoking.	T	F
13. The best way to lose weight is to increase physical activity and eat fewer calories.	T	F
14. Heart disease is the leading killer of men **and** women in the United States.	T	F

1. TRUE High blood pressure, smoking, and high blood cholesterol are the three most important risk factors for heart disease. On the average, each one doubles your chance of developing heart disease. So, a person who has all three of these risk factors is eight times more likely to develop heart disease than someone who has none. Obesity increases the likelihood of developing high blood cholesterol and high blood pressure, which increase your risk for heart disease. Physical inactivity increases your risk of heart attack. Regular exercise and good nutrition are essential to reducing high blood pressure, high blood cholesterol, and overweight. People who exercise are also more likely to cut down or stop smoking.

2. TRUE A person with high blood pressure or high blood cholesterol may feel fine and look great; there are often no signs that anything is wrong until a stroke or heart attack occurs. To find out if you have high blood pressure or high blood cholesterol, you should be tested by a doctor, nurse, or other health professional.

3. TRUE A blood pressure of 140/90 mm Hg or greater is generally classified as high blood pressure. However, blood pressures that fall below 140/90 mm Hg can sometimes be a problem. If the diastolic pressure, the second or lower number, is between 85 and 89, a person is at increased risk for heart disease or stroke and should have his/her blood pressure checked at least once a year by a health professional. The higher your blood pressure, the greater your risk of developing heart disease or stroke. Controlling high blood pressure reduces your risk.

4. FALSE High blood pressure is more common in blacks than in whites. It affects 29 of every 100 black adults compared to 26 of every 100 white adults. Also, with aging, high blood pressure is generally more severe among blacks than among whites, and therefore causes more strokes, heart disease, and kidney failure.

5. TRUE Recent studies show that lifestyle changes can help keep blood pressure levels normal even into advanced age and are important in treating and preventing high blood pressure. Limit high-salt foods, which include many snack foods, such as potato chips, salted pretzels, and salted crackers; processed foods, such as canned soups; and condiments, such as ketchup and soy sauce. Also, it is **extremely important** to take blood pressure medication, if prescribed by your doctor, to make sure your blood pressure stays under control.

6. FALSE A total blood cholesterol level of under 200 mg/dL is **desirable** and usually puts you at a lower risk for heart disease. A blood cholesterol level of 240 mg/dL or above is **high** and increases your risk of heart disease. If your cholesterol level is high, your doctor will want to check your levels of LDL-

FIGURE 11–8 *See legend on opposite page*

cholesterol ("bad" cholesterol) and HDL-cholesterol ("good" cholesterol). A HIGH level of LDL-cholesterol increases your risk of heart disease, as does a LOW level of HDL-cholesterol. A cholesterol level of 200–239 mg/dL is considered **borderline-high** and usually increases your risk for heart disease. If your cholesterol is borderline-high, you should speak to your doctor to see if additional cholesterol tests are needed. All adults 20 years of age or older should have their blood cholesterol level checked at least once every 5 years.

7. FALSE Reducing the amount of cholesterol in your diet is important; however, eating foods **low in saturated fat** is the most effective dietary way to lower blood cholesterol levels, along with eating less total fat and cholesterol. Choose low-saturated fat foods, such as grains, fruits, and vegetables; low-fat or skim milk and milk products; lean cuts of meat; fish; and chicken. Trim fat from meat before cooking; bake or broil meat rather than fry; use less fat and oil; and take the skin off chicken and turkey. Reducing overweight will also help lower your level of LDL-cholesterol as well as increase your level of HDL-cholesterol.

8. TRUE People who have had one heart attack are at much higher risk for a second attack. Reducing blood cholesterol levels can greatly slow down (and, in some people, even reverse) the buildup of cholesterol and fat in the walls of the coronary arteries and significantly reduce the chances of a second heart attack.

9. TRUE Children from "high risk" families, in which a parent has high blood cholesterol (240 mg/dL or above) or in which a parent or grandparent has had heart disease at an early age (at 55 years of age or younger), should have their cholesterol levels tested. If a child from such a family has a cholesterol level that is high, it should be lowered under medical supervision, primarily with diet, to reduce the risk of developing heart disease as an adult. For most children, who are not from high-risk families, the best way to reduce the risk of adult heart disease is to follow a low-saturated fat, low cholesterol eating pattern. All children over the age of 2 years and all adults should adopt a heart-healthy eating pattern as a principal way of reducing coronary heart disease.

10. TRUE Heavy smokers are two to four times more likely to have a heart attack than nonsmokers, and the heart attack death rate among all smokers is 70% greater than that of nonsmokers. Older male smokers are also nearly twice as likely to die from stroke than older men who do not smoke, and these odds are nearly as high for older female smokers. Further, the risk of dying of lung cancer is 22 times higher for male smokers than male nonsmokers and 12 times higher for female smokers than female nonsmokers. Finally, 80% of all deaths from emphysema and bronchitis are directly due to smoking.

11. TRUE One year after quitting, ex-smokers cut their extra risk for heart attack by about half or more, and eventually the risk will return to normal in healthy ex-smokers. Even if you have already had a heart attack, you can reduce your chances of having a second attack if you quit smoking. Ex-smokers can also reduce their risk of stroke and cancer, improve blood flow and lung function, and help stop diseases like emphysema and bronchitis from getting worse.

12. FALSE Older smokers are more likely to succeed at quitting smoking than younger smokers. Quitting helps relieve smoking-related symptoms like shortness of breath, coughing, and chest pain. Many quit to avoid further health problems and take control of their lives.

13. TRUE Weight control is a question of balance. You get calories from the food you eat. You burn off calories by exercising. Cutting down on calories, especially calories from fat, is key to losing weight. Combining this with a regular physical activity, like walking, cycling, jogging, or swimming, not only can help in losing weight but also in maintaining weight loss. A steady weight loss of 0.5 to 1 pound a week is safe for most adults, and the weight is more likely to stay off over the long run. Losing weight, if you are overweight, may also help reduce your blood pressure, lower your LDL-cholesterol, and raise your HDL-cholesterol. Being physically active and eating fewer calories will also help you control your weight if you quit smoking.

14. TRUE Coronary heart disease is the number one killer in the United States. Approximately 489,000 Americans died of coronary heart disease in 1990, and approximately half of these deaths were women.

FIGURE 11–8 Healthy heart I. Q. (From National Heart, Lung and Blood Institute. [1992]. *Healthy Heart I. Q.* NIH Pub. No. 92–2724. Washington, D. C., National Heart, Lung and Blood Institute.)

Understanding Heart Disease

Estimates are that almost 500,000 Americans die of coronary heart disease every year. It's the single leading cause of death in the United States—as well as in many other countries.

Scientists have identified certain factors linked with an increased risk of developing coronary heart disease. Some of these factors are unavoidable, like increasing age, being male or having a family history of heart disease. However, many other risk factors can be changed to lower the risk of heart disease. High blood pressure, high blood cholesterol, cigarette smoking and physical inactivity are the four major modifiable risk factors; obesity is a contributing risk factor. Diabetes also strongly influences the risk of heart disease.

This RISKO brochure is a way for you to evaluate your risk of coronary heart disease based upon your risk factors. RISKO scores are based on blood pressure, cholesterol, smoking and weight. Physical inactivity is also an important risk factor but was not part of the statistical base from which RISKO was derived.

Men

1. Systolic blood pressure

SCORE

If you **are not** taking antihypertensive medications and your blood pressure is . . .		
	124 or less	0 points
	between 125 and 134	2 points
	between 135 and 144	4 points
	between 145 and 154	6 points
	between 155 and 164	8 points
	between 165 and 174	10 points
	between 175 and 184	12 points
	between 185 and 194	14 points
	between 195 and 204	16 points
	between 205 and 214	18 points
	between 215 and 224	20 points

If you **are** taking antihypertensive medications and your blood pressure is . . .		
	120 or less	0 points
	between 121 and 127	2 points
	between 128 and 135	4 points
	between 136 and 143	6 points
	between 144 and 153	8 points
	between 154 and 163	10 points
	between 164 and 175	12 points
	between 176 and 190	14 points
	between 191 and 204	16 points
	between 205 and 214	18 points
	between 215 and 224	20 points

2. Blood cholesterol

SCORE

Locate the number of points for your total and HDL cholesterol in the table below.

		HDL							
		25	30	35	40	50	60	70	80
	140	4	2	0	0	0	0	0	0
	160	5	3	2	0	0	0	0	0
	180	6	4	3	1	0	0	0	0
	200	7	5	4	3	0	0	0	0
	220	7	6	5	4	1	0	0	0
TOTAL	240	8	7	5	4	2	0	0	0
	260	8	7	6	5	3	1	0	0
	280	9	8	7	6	4	2	0	0
	300	9	8	7	6	4	3	1	0
	340	9	9	8	7	6	4	2	1
	400	10	9	9	8	7	5	4	3

3. Cigarette smoking

SCORE

If you . . .		
	do not smoke	0 points
	smoke less than a pack a day	2 points
	smoke a pack a day	5 points
	smoke two or more packs a day	9 points

4. Weight

Locate your weight category in the table below. If you are in . . .		
	weight category A	0 points
	weight category B	1 point
	weight category C	2 points

SCORE

FT	IN	A	B	C
5	1	up to 162	163–250	251+
5	2	up to 167	168–257	258+
5	3	up to 172	173–264	265+
5	4	up to 176	177–272	273+
5	5	up to 181	182–279	280+
5	6	up to 185	186–286	287+
5	7	up to 190	191–293	294+
5	8	up to 195	196–300	301+
5	9	up to 199	200–307	308+
5	10	up to 204	205–315	316+
5	11	up to 209	210–322	323+
6	0	up to 213	214–329	330+
6	1	up to 218	219–336	337+
6	2	up to 223	224–343	344+
6	3	up to 227	228–350	351+
6	4	up to 232	233–368	359+
6	5	up to 238	239–365	366+
6	6	up to 241	242–372	373+

TOTAL SCORE

FIGURE 11–9 RISKO: A heart health appraisal. (Reproduced with permission, *RISKO: A Heart Health Appraisal, 1994.* Dallas, TX, American Heart Association. © Copyright American Heart Association.)

Women

1. Systolic blood pressure

			SCORE
If you **are not** taking antihypertensive medications and your blood pressure is . . .	125 or less	0 points	
	between 126 and 136	2 points	
	between 137 and 148	4 points	
	between 149 and 160	6 points	
	between 161 and 171	8 points	
	between 172 and 183	10 points	
	between 184 and 194	12 points	
	between 195 and 206	14 points	
	between 207 and 218	16 points	

If you **are** taking antihypertensive medications and your blood pressure is . . .	117 or less	0 points
	between 118 and 123	2 points
	between 124 and 129	4 points
	between 130 and 136	6 points
	between 137 and 144	8 points
	between 145 and 154	10 points
	between 155 and 168	12 points
	between 169 and 206	14 points
	between 207 and 218	16 points

2. Blood cholesterol

SCORE

Locate the number of points for your total and HDL cholesterol in the table below.

	HDL							
TOTAL	25	30	35	40	50	60	70	80
140	2	1	0	0	0	0	0	0
160	3	2	1	0	0	0	0	0
180	4	3	2	1	0	0	0	0
200	4	3	2	2	0	0	0	0
220	5	4	3	2	1	0	0	0
240	5	4	3	3	1	0	0	0
260	5	4	4	3	2	1	0	0
280	5	5	4	4	2	1	0	0
300	6	5	4	4	3	2	1	0
340	6	5	5	4	3	2	1	0
400	6	6	5	5	4	3	2	2

3. Cigarette smoking

SCORE

If you . . .	do not smoke	0 points
	smoke less than a pack a day	2 points
	smoke a pack a day	5 points
	smoke two or more packs a day	9 points

4. Weight

Locate your weight category in the table below. If you are in . . .	weight category A	0 points
	weight category B	1 point
	weight category C	2 points
	weight category D	3 points

SCORE

FT	IN	A	B	C	D
4	8	up to 139	140–161	162–184	185+
4	9	up to 140	141–162	163–185	186+
4	10	up to 141	142–163	164–187	188+
4	11	up to 143	144–166	167–190	191+
5	0	up to 145	146–168	169–193	194+
5	1	up to 147	148–171	172–196	197+
5	2	up to 149	150–173	174–198	199+
5	3	up to 152	153–176	177–201	202+
5	4	up to 154	155–178	179–204	205+
5	5	up to 157	158–182	183–209	210+
5	6	up to 160	161–186	187–213	214+
5	7	up to 165	166–191	192–219	220+
5	8	up to 169	170–196	197–225	226+
5	9	up to 173	174–201	202–231	232+
5	10	up to 178	179–206	207–238	239+
5	11	up to 182	183–212	213–242	243+
6	0	up to 187	188–217	218–248	249+
6	1	up to 191	192–222	223–254	255+

TOTAL SCORE

What Your Score Means

Note: If you're diabetic, you have a greater risk of heart disease. Add 7 points to your total score.

0–2 You have a low risk of heart disease for a person of your age and sex.

3–4 You have a low-to-moderate risk of heart disease for a person of your age and sex. That's good, but there's room for improvement.

5–7 You have a moderate-to-high risk of heart disease for a person of your age and sex. There's considerable room for improvement in some areas.

8–15 You have a high risk of developing heart disease for a person of your age and sex. There's lots of room for improvement in all areas.

16 & over You have a very high risk of developing heart disease for a person of your age and sex. You should act now to reduce all your risk factors.

FIGURE 11–9 *Continued*

Figure continued on following page

Understanding Heart Disease Continued

Some Words of Caution

- RISKO is a way for adults who don't have signs of heart disease now to measure their risk. If you already have heart disease, it's very important to work with your doctor to reduce your risk.
- RISKO is not a substitute for a thorough physical examination and assessment by your doctor. It's intended to help you learn more about the factors that influence the risk of heart disease, and thus to reduce your risk.
- If you have a family history of heart disease, your risk of heart disease will be higher than your RISKO score shows. If you have a high RISKO score and a family history of heart disease, taking action now to reduce your risk is even more important.
- If you're a woman under 45 years old or a man under 35 years old, your real risk of heart disease is probably lower than your RISKO score.
- If you're overweight, have high blood pressure or high blood cholesterol, or smoke cigarettes, your long-term risk of heart disease is higher even if your risk of heart disease in the next several years is low. To reduce your risk, you should eliminate or control these risk factors.

How To Reduce Your Risk

- **Quit smoking for good.** Many programs are available to help.
- **Have your blood pressure checked regularly.** If your blood pressure is less than 130/85 mmHg, have it rechecked in two years. If it's between 130–139/85–89, have it rechecked in a year. If your blood pressure is 140/90 or higher, you have high blood pressure and should follow your doctor's advice. If blood pressure medication is prescribed for you, remember to take it.
- **Stay physically active.** Physical inactivity, besides being a risk factor for heart disease, contributes to other risk factors including obesity, high blood pressure and a low level of HDL cholesterol. To condition your heart, try to get 30–60 minutes of exercise 3–4 times a week.

  Activities that are especially beneficial when performed regularly include
  Brisk walking, hiking, stair-climbing, aerobic exercise,and calisthenics
  Jogging, running, bicycling, rowing, and swimming
  Tennis, racquetball, soccer, basketball, and touch football
  Even low-intensity activities, when performed daily, can have some long-term health benefits.
  Such activities include
  Walking for pleasure, gardening, and yard work
  Housework, dancing, and prescribed home exercise
- **Lose weight if necessary.** For many people, losing weight is one of the most effective ways to improve their blood pressure and cholesterol levels.
- **Reduce high blood cholesterol through your diet.** If you're overweight or eat lots of foods high in saturated fats and cholesterol (whole milk, cheese, eggs, butter, fatty foods, fried foods), then make changes in your diet. Look for *The American Heart Association Cookbook* at your local bookstore; it can help you.
- **Visit or write your local American Heart Association for more information and copies of free pamphlets.**
  Some subjects covered include:
  Reducing your risk of heart attack and stroke
  Controlling high blood pressure
  Eating to keep your heart healthy
  How to stop smoking
  Exercising for good health

Your contributions to the American Heart Association will support research that helps make publications like this possible.

American Heart Association
National Center
7272 Greenville Avenue
Dallas, Texas 75231

For more information, contact your local American Heart Association or call 1-800-AHA-USA1
(1-800-242-8721).

FIGURE 11–9 *Continued*

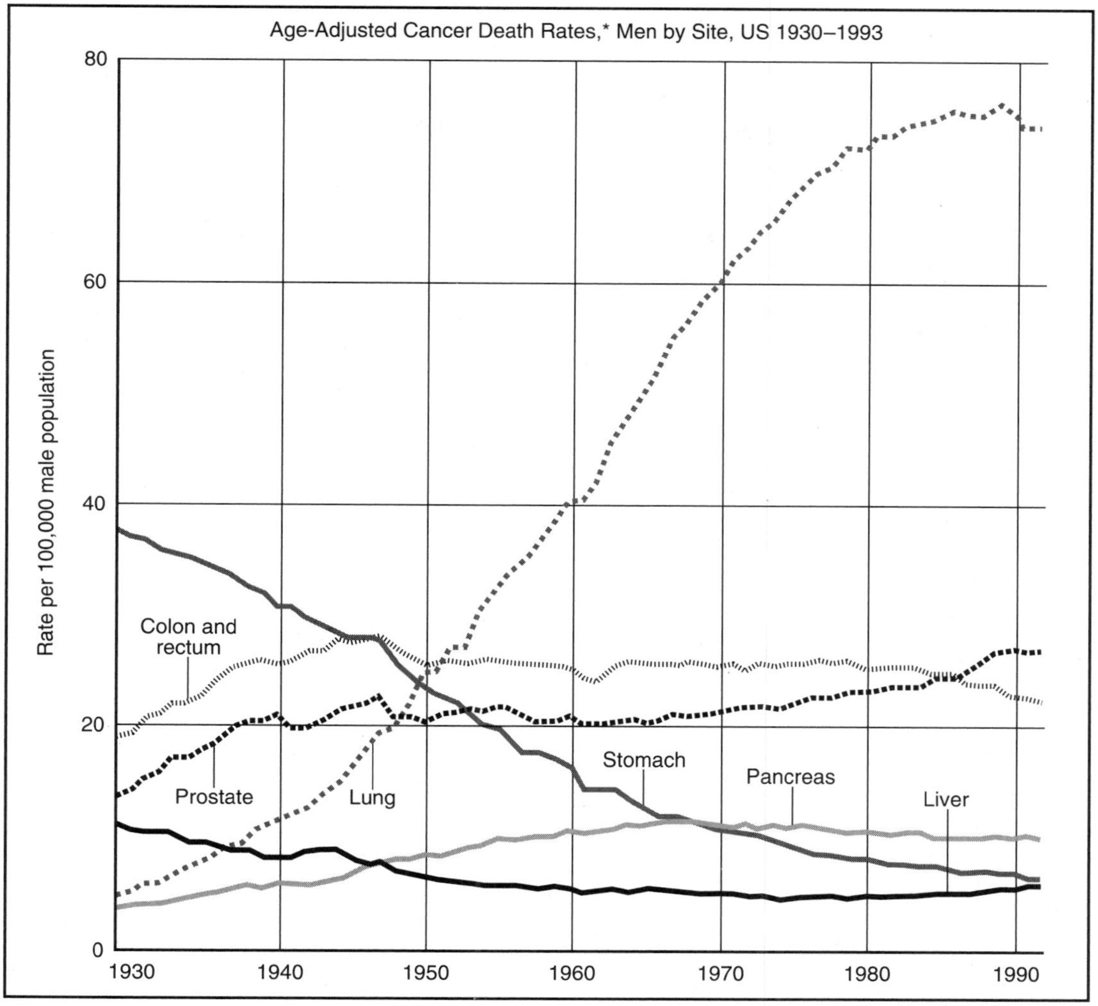

FIGURE 11–10 Cancer death rates by site, males, United States, 1930–93. * Rates are per 100,000 and are age-adjusted to the 1970 U. S. standard population. Note: Due to changes in ICD coding, numerator information has changed over time. Rates for cancers of the liver, lung, and colon and rectum are affected by these coding changes. Denominator information for the years 1930–1959 and 1991–1993 is based on intercensal population estimates, while denominator information for the years 1960–1989 is based on postcensal recalculation of estimates. Rate estimates for 1968–1989 are most likely of a better quality. (From American Cancer Society. [1995]. *Cancer Facts & Figures. 1995.* Atlanta, American Cancer Society. © 1997, American Cancer Society, Inc. Data from Vital Statistics of the United States, 1993.)

failure to alter insulin intake during intercurrent illnesses. Patients should be taught the importance of compliance with the prescribed medication regimen and how to manage serum glucose levels during illness.

- Hypoglycemia—often results from delay or decrease in food intake, vigorous physical activity, or alcohol consumption. Patients should be taught to recognize symptoms of low blood glucose (e.g., apprehension, tremors, sweating,

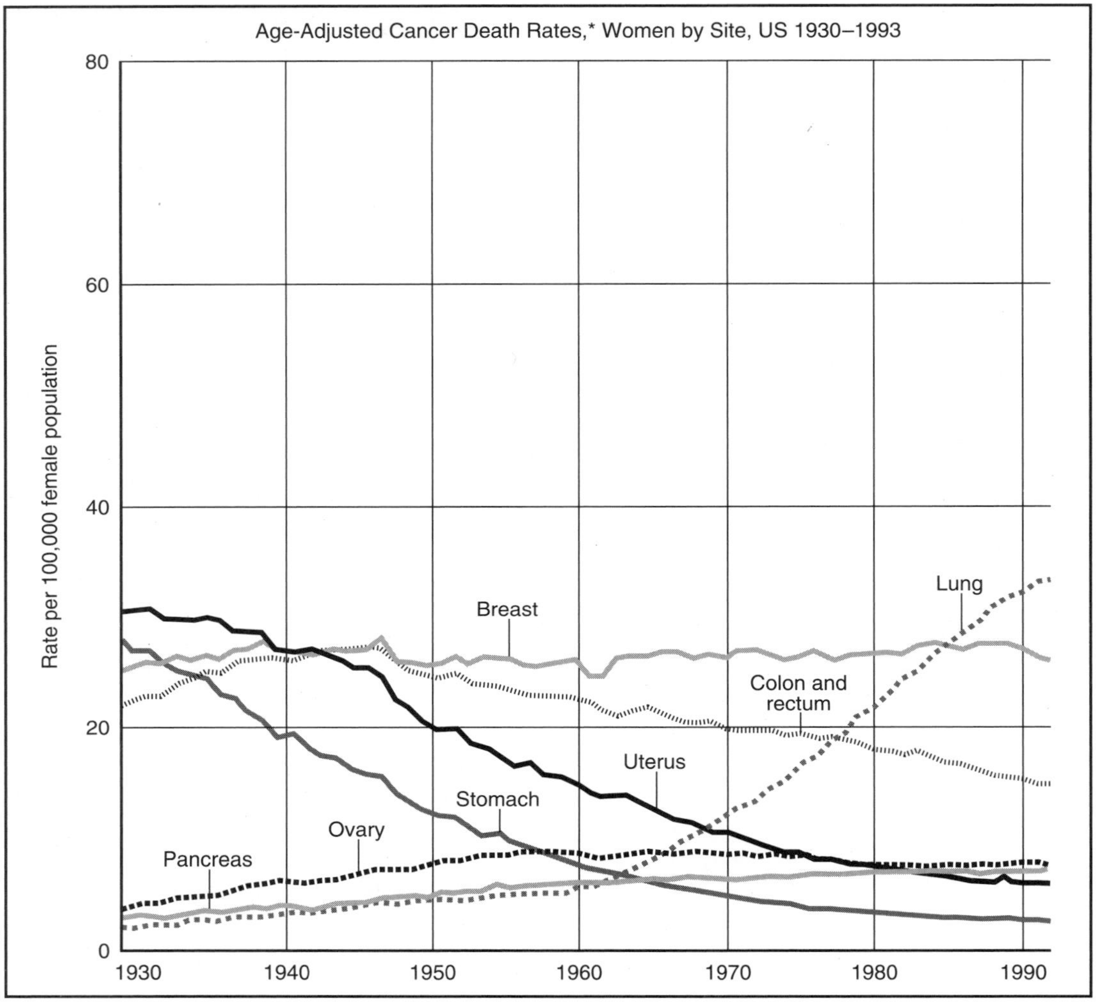

FIGURE 11–11 Cancer death rates by site, females, United States, 1930–93. (From American Cancer Society. [1995]. *Cancer Facts & Figures. 1995.* Atlanta, American Cancer Society.)

palpitations, fatigue, confusion, headache) and treat with rapidly absorbable carbohydrates (e.g., three to five pieces of hard candy, two to three packets of sugar, or 4 ounces of fruit juice). A family member or friend should be taught to administer oral carbohydrates if the patient is unable to treat himself or herself. If this is not possible, the Emergency Medical Service should be notified.

- Periodontal disease—gingivitis and periodontitis are common in diabetics. Instruction on proper brushing and flossing is essential, and preventive dental care, ideally every 6 months, should be encouraged.
- Eye disease—diabetes is a major cause of blindness in the United States. Roughly 70% of people with IDDM develop diabetic retinopathy, and 40% develop macular edema.

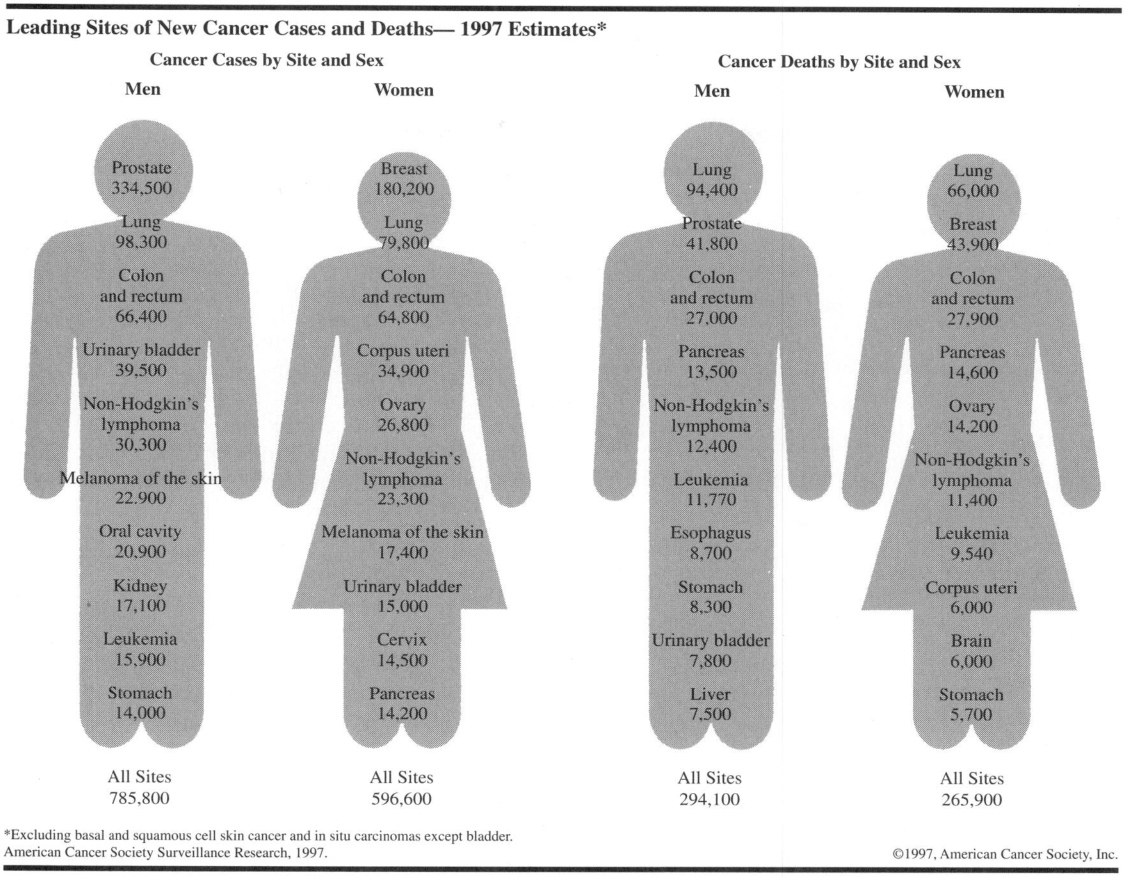

FIGURE 11–12 Leading sites of new cancer cases and deaths—1997 estimates. (From American Cancer Society. [1995]. *Cancer Facts & Figures. 1995.* Atlanta, American Cancer Society.)

Patients with diabetes should be taught to report any changes in vision (e.g., blurred vision, "floaters," and flashing lights) immediately. A yearly eye examination is very important, as early detection of ophthalmic complications and prompt treatment with laser surgery can reduce visual loss significantly.

- Kidney disease—diabetic nephropathy is characterized by albuminuria, hypertension, and progressive renal insufficiency. As a result of chronic renal insufficiency, end-stage renal disease may occur (about a third of end-stage renal disease cases in the United States are attributed to diabetes). To prevent kidney disease, diabetics must be taught to monitor blood pressure and adhere to treatment of hypertension when indicated; closely monitor blood glucose levels; avoid excessive protein intake; and observe for symptoms of urinary tract infection.
- Cardiovascular disease—patients should be told that diabetes increases the risk of developing cardiovascular disease. Maintaining a low-fat, low-sodium diet is very important and should be encouraged. Signs and symptoms of cardiovascular disease can be dis-

TABLE 11–16 **Seven Warning Signs of Cancer**

1. A change in bowel movements or urination
2. A sore that will not heal
3. Sudden bleeding, or discharge
4. A lump or hardening in the breasts or elsewhere
5. Frequent and prolonged indigestion or difficulty when swallowing
6. Any changes in the color or size of moles or warts
7. Hoarseness and persistent cough

Reprinted by the permission of the American Cancer Society, Inc.

cussed and the patient told to report possible symptoms immediately.

- Neuropathy—patients should be informed about the relationship between poor glycemic control and development of diabetic neuropathy. Complications of neuropathy include orthostatic hypotension, constipation, diabetic diarrhea and fecal incontinence, diabetic bladder dysfunction, and sexual dysfunction. Careful monitoring and maintenance of glucose levels can help reduce neuropathy.
- Foot problems—persons with diabetes account for approximately 50% of all nontraumatic amputations performed each year. To prevent foot ulcers and potential complications, diabetics should be taught meticulous foot care. Principles include to wash and inspect feet daily, use foot creams or oils, cut toenails correctly and never cut corns or calluses, avoid extremes of temperature, never walk barefooted, wear appropriate shoes, inspect the inside of shoes daily, and seek medical care for all skin lesions (USDHHS/Public Health Service/CDC, 1991).

To prevent these and other complications, it is vitally important that all diabetics maintain their diets and treatment regimens, monitor illnesses carefully, and report any complications immediately to their primary care providers. Many organizations and resources are available for clients with diabetes. Health care providers should be aware of these resources and refer clients appropriately.

SUMMARY

This chapter has described several issues related to health promotion and illness prevention for adults. For more information on the topics presented here, Table 11–18 lists a number of resources. Additionally, the reader is referred to Chapter 12 for a discussion of women's health issues, Chapter 13 to study health promotion and illness prevention strategies for children, and Chapter 14 for health promotion and illness prevention for older adults.

Key Points

- *Health promotion* refers to activities or actions related to encouraging individual lifestyles or personal choices that positively influence health (e.g., encouraging physical activity and fitness, good nutrition, substance abuse prevention).
- Health benefits of regular exercise and physical activity are well documented. Individuals should work up to moderate-level activities (50–75% of maximum heart rate) for a minimum of 30 minutes, three to four times per week, depending on age and presence of existing physical problems. Walking, aerobic dancing, bicycling, jogging, and swimming are examples of recommended activities.
- Good nutritional practices and maintenance of a desirable weight are essential for good health. In the United States it is estimated that 24% of men and 27% of women are overweight. Obesity is associated with hypertension, NIDDM, hypercholesterolemia, coronary artery disease, some types of cancer, and stroke.

TABLE 11–17 **Incidence, Risk Factors, Symptoms, Early Detection, and Treatment of Selected Cancers**

Cancer Site	Incidence	Risk Factors	Symptoms	Screening/Early Detection	Treatment
Lung	170,000 cases (rate: 80/ 100,000 in men and 42/ 100,000 in women)	Cigarette smoking; exposure to radiation, asbestos and other substances	Persistent cough, sputum streaked with blood, chest pain, recurring pneumonia or bronchitis	Very difficult to detect; chest x-ray, sputum analysis, and fiberoptic examination of the bronchial passages when indicated	Usually a combination of surgery, radiation therapy, and chemotherapy
Colon and rectum	138,200 new cases, with 55,000 deaths	Personal or family history of cancer or polyps of the colon or rectum; inflammatory bowel disease, high-fat diet	Rectal bleeding, blood in the stool, change in bowel habits	Digital rectal examination, stool occult blood examination, proctosigmoidoscopy	Surgery; surgery and radiation therapy
Breast	182,000 new cases, with an estimated 46,000 deaths (less than 1% occur in men)	Increasing age, family history, early menarche, late menopause, never had children or late age at first birth, high-fat diet	Changes on mammogram, lump, thickening, swelling, dimpling, skin irritation, distortion, retraction, pain, nipple discharge	Screening mammogram by age 40; women 40–49 should have a mammogram every 1–2 years, and women 50 years or older, each year; clinical examination of the breast every 3 years to age 40 and every year thereafter; monthly breast self-examination for all women age 20 and older	Lumpectomy, mastectomy, radiation therapy, chemotherapy, hormone manipulation therapy, or a combination of the above
Prostate	244,000 new cases each year, with 40,000 deaths	Age (over 80% are diagnosed in men over age 65); possibly family history; possibly high-fat diet	Weak or interrupted urine flow, inability to urinate, need to urinate frequently, blood in the urine, pain or burning on urination, lower back or pelvic pain	Digital rectal examination for all men 40 years or older; prostate specific antigen (PSA) test for all men over age 50	Surgery, radiation, and/or hormone treatment

Table continued on following page

TABLE 11–17 **Incidence, Risk Factors, Symptoms, Early Detection, and Treatment of Selected Cancers** *Continued*

Cancer Site	Incidence	Risk Factors	Symptoms	Screening/Early Detection	Treatment
Cervix	15,800 invasive and 65,000 carcinoma in situ cases annually, with 4,800 deaths	Early age at first intercourse, multiple sex partners, cigarette smoking, infection with human papillomavirus	Abnormal uterine bleeding or spotting, abnormal vaginal discharge	Papanicolaou test and pelvic examination should be performed annually for women who are sexually active and those age 18 or older	Surgery and or radiation; precancerous (in situ) cases may be treated by cryotherapy or electro-coagulation
Skin cancer	800,000+ cases of basal cell or squamous cell cancer each year; 34,000 cases and 9,300 deaths each year from melanoma	Excessive exposure to ultraviolet radiation, fair complexion	Change in size or color of a mole or pigmented growth or spot; scaliness, oozing, bleeding, or change in appearance of a bump	Skin self-examination once a month and reporting of changes to a physician	Surgery, radiation, cryosurgery, and electro-dessication; for melanoma, wide margin excision and possible lymph node excision
Ovary	Estimated 26,600 new cases, and 14,500 deaths each year	Increase with age, never having had children, family history	Asymptomatic in early stages; enlargement of the abdomen, vague digestive disturbances	Pelvic examination, including palpation each year	Surgery, radiation therapy, and chemotherapy
Oral	Estimated 28,000 new cases, and 8,400 annual deaths	Cigarette, cigar, or pipe smoking; use of smokeless tobacco; excess use of alcohol	Sore that bleeds easily and does not heal; lump or thickening or red or white patch that persists on the mouth, tongue, or gums	Examination of the mouth, lips, tongue, and throat annually by a dentist or primary care provider	Radiation therapy and surgery

Adapted from American Cancer Society. (1995). *Cancer Facts & Figures—1995.* Atlanta, GA, American Cancer Society. Reprinted by the permission of the American Cancer Society, Inc.

TABLE 11–18 Resources for Health Promotion and Illness Prevention

Health Promotion and Illness Prevention

U. S. Department of Health and Human Services
National Center for Chronic Disease Prevention and Health Promotion
4770 Buford Highway, NE
Mailstop K13
Atlanta, GA 30333
(404) 488-5080
National Center for Prevention Services
1600 Clifton Road, NE
Mailstop E07
Atlanta, GA 30333
(404) 639-8008
Office of Disease Prevention and Health Promotion
Switzer Building, Room 2132
330 C Street, SW
Washington, D. C. 20201
(202) 205-8583
Bureau of Primary Health Care
4350 East-West Highway
Room 9-10A2
Bethesda, MD 20857
(301) 594-4420

Physical Fitness/Sports

President's Council on Physical Fitness and Sports
701 Pennsylvania Avenue, NW
Suite 250
Washington, D. C. 20004
(202) 272-3424
American College of Sports Medicine
P. O. Box 1440
Indianapolis, IN 46206
(317) 637-9200
American Heart Association
7272 Greenville Avenue
Dallas, TX 75231-4599
(214) 373-6300
(800) AHA-USA1
YMCA of the USA
Health and Physical Education
101 North Wacker Drive, 14th floor
Chicago, IL 60606
(312) 977-0031
National Recreation and Park Association
2775 South Quincy Street, Suite 300
Arlington, VA 22206
(703) 820-4930

Nutrition

U. S. Department of Agriculture
Food and Nutrition Information Center
10301 Baltimore Boulevard, Room 304
Beltsville, MD 20705
(301) 504-5719
Food and Nutrition Service
3101 Park Center Drive
Alexandria, VA 22302
(703) 305-2276
U. S. Department of Health and Human Services
Food and Drug Administration
Center for Food Safety and Applied Nutrition
200 C Street, SW
Washington, D. C. 20204
(202) 205-5004
National Academy of Science
Food and Nutrition Board
2101 Constitution Avenue, NW
Washington, D. C. 20418
(202) 334-1732

Tobacco Use/Smoking Cessation

U. S. Department of Health and Human Services/ Public Health Service
Office on Smoking and Health
4770 Buford Highway, NE
Mailstop K50
Atlanta, GA 30341
(404) 488-5705
Substance Abuse and Mental Health Services Administration
National Clearinghouse on Alcohol and Drug Information
P. O. Box 2345
Rockville, MD 20852
(800) 729-6686
National Institutes of Health
National Heart, Lung, and Blood Institute
Education Programs Information Center
P. O. Box 30105
Bethesda, MD 20824-0105
(301) 251-1222
National Cancer Institute
Cancer Information Service Building 31, Room 10A16
9000 Rockville Pike
Bethesda, MD 20892
(800) 4-CANCER

Table continued on following page

TABLE 11–18 **Resources for Health Promotion and Illness Prevention** *Continued*

Environmental Protection Agency
Indoor Air Quality Information Clearinghouse
P. O. Box 37133
Washington, D. C. 20013
(800) 438-4318
American Lung Association
1740 Broadway
New York, NY 10019
(212) 315-8700

Heart Disease and Stroke

National Institute of Neurological Disorders and Stroke
9000 Rockville Pike
Building 31, Room 8A06
Bethesda, MD 20892
(301) 496-5924
(800) 352-9424
American Heart Association
7272 Greenville Avenue
Dallas, TX 75231
(800) AHA-USA1
(214) 706-1220
(214) 373-6300
National Stroke Association
8480 East Orchard Road
Suite 1000
Englewood, CO 80110
(303) 771-1700
(800) STROKES (National Stroke Hotline)

Cancer

National Institutes of Health
National Cancer Institute
Cancer Information Service
Building 31, Room 10A16
9000 Rockville Pike
Bethesda, MD 20892
(800) 4-CANCER
(301) 496-5583
National Cancer Institute
Surveillance, Epidemiology, and End Results (SEER) Program
Division of Cancer Prevention and Control
6130 Executive Boulevard North
Room 343
Bethesda, MD 20892
(301) 496-6616
American Cancer Society
1599 Clifton Road, NE
Atlanta, GA 30329
(800) ACS-2345

Diabetes

National Institutes of Health
National Diabetes Information Clearinghouse
Box NDIC
9000 Rockville Pike
Bethesda, MD 20892
(301) 654-3327
National Kidney and Urologic Diseases Information Clearinghouse
Box NKUDIC
Bethesda, MD 20892
(301) 654-4415
American Association of Diabetes Educators
444 North Michigan Avenue, Suite 1240
Chicago, IL 60611
(800) 338-3633
American Diabetes Association
1660 Duke Street
Alexandria, VA 22314
(800) 232-3472
Juvenile Diabetes Foundation
432 Park Avenue South
New York, NY 10016
(800) 223-1138
(212) 889-7575

Nutrition guidelines for a healthy diet include eating a variety of foods; maintaining healthy weight; choosing a diet low in fat, saturated fat, and cholesterol; eating five or more servings daily of vegetables, fruits, and grains; using sugar, salt, and sodium in moderation; and drinking alcoholic beverages in moderation, if at all.

- In the United States, tobacco use is associated with more than 400,000 deaths annually from heart disease; lung cancer; chronic respiratory diseases; cancers of the mouth, pharynx, larynx, pancreas, and other sites; intrauterine growth retardation; low birth weight; and birth defects. More than 80% of smokers began before 18 years of age, and more than 70% of high school students have reportedly tried cigarette smoking. A number of programs, tools, medications, and other interventions are available for clients who want to stop smoking.

- Primary and secondary prevention interventions for heart disease and stroke are essential, as these diseases account for the number one and three causes of death and disability in the United States. Risk factors for heart disease and stroke include smoking, hypertension, hypercholesterolemia, diabetes, obesity, age, sex, and genetic predisposition. Prevention efforts to reduce or eliminate these risk factors include teaching and counseling on nutrition, exercise, and smoking cessation (if applicable).
- Cancer is the second leading cause of death in the United States, resulting in about 550,000 deaths each year. Early detection and treatment of cancer has improved survival rates for most cancers.
- Diabetes affects about 14 million U. S. residents, about half of whom are not aware of it. Diabetes is one of the leading causes of death and disability and is associated with many health conditions, including blindness, heart disease, stroke, renal failure, nerve damage, amputations, and birth defects. Risk factors for NIDDM include obesity, increasing age, family history, and being a member of certain minority groups (African-Americans, Hispanics, and Native Americans).

Learning Activities and Application to Practice

In Class

- Discuss objectives of *Healthy People 2000* related to health promotion and illness prevention of adults (e.g., improving physical activity and nutrition; quitting use of tobacco; and preventing heart disease, stroke, cancer, and diabetes). Analyze baselines and variations in special populations. What objectives should be addressed by nurses working in community-based settings? What health education and anticipatory guidance should be provided?
- Discuss the U. S. Preventive Services Task Force recommendations of clinical preventive services (see Table 11–14). Specifically review recommendations for "high risk" factors and discuss people who have these risk factors.
- Encourage each student to complete one of the assessment tools presented in the chapter (e.g., "Healthstyle: A Self-Test," "Wellness Self-Assessment," or "Lifestyle Assessment Inventory"). Ask several students to share results. What are areas of strength and weakness? How can tools of this type be used in community settings to help improve the health of individuals?
- Divide students into groups of four or five. Have each group review nutritional guidelines and recommendations. Encourage students to develop a menu for 1 week that follows the guidelines and recommendations. Challenge them to follow the

menu and record their food intake in a log. Was the diet difficult to follow? Why or why not? How can findings be applied to clients in community settings?

In Clinical

- Assign each student to use information contained in the chapter, along with materials gathered from related resource organizations (see Table 11–18), to develop a teaching plan or project that addresses primary and secondary prevention activities for one of the areas described (e.g., heart disease and stroke, cancer, diabetes). For example, a student could develop a nutrition education class for persons in an occupational health setting or provide tips for stopping smoking to an individual in a doctor's office. Have students present the information in a class or to an individual as appropriate and record the results in a log or journal.
- Encourage students to observe for opportunities to share health promotion and illness prevention strategies in all settings, particularly as they relate to the leading causes of morbidity and mortality. For example, students working with heart disease, stroke, or diabetes patients in hospitals should provide instruction on minimization and elimination of risk factors and management of the disease process. How is this accomplished? How might health teaching be enhanced?

REFERENCES

American Cancer Society. (1995). *Cancer Facts & Figures—1995.* Atlanta, American Cancer Society.

American Cancer Society. (1997). *Cancer Facts & Figures—1997.* Atlanta, American Cancer Society.

American Heart Association. (1994). *Fact Sheet on Heart Attack, Stroke and Risk Factors.* Dallas, TX, American Heart Association.

American Heart Association. (1990). *Nurses' Cholesterol Education Handbook.* Dallas, TX, American Heart Association.

American Heart Association. (1994). *RISKO: A Heart Health Appraisal.* Dallas, TX, American Heart Association.

American Heart Association and National Heart, Lung and Blood Institute (1993). *Exercise and Your Heart: A Guide to Physical Activity.* Dallas, TX, American Heart Association.

Anspaugh, D. J., Hamrick, M. H., and Rosato, F. D. (1994). *Wellness: Concepts and Applications* (2nd ed.). St. Louis, MO, Mosby-Year Book.

Centers for Disease Control. (1993). Annual summary of births, marriages, divorces and deaths: United States, 1992. In *Monthly Vital Statistics Report.* (CDC/NCHS-PHS, vol. 40, 13). Washington, D. C., Government Printing Office.

Centers for Disease Control and Prevention (1994a). Guidelines for School Health Programs to Prevent Tobacco Use and Addiction. *Morbidity and Mortality Weekly Report, 43,* (No. RR-2).

Centers for Disease Control and Prevention. (1994b). Surveillance for selected tobacco-use behaviors—United States, 1900–1994. *Morbidity and Mortality Weekly Report, 43,* (No. SS-3).

Clark, C. (1986). *Wellness Nursing: Concepts Theory, Research and Practice.* New York, Springer.

Human Nutrition Information Service. (1992). *The Food Guide Pyramid: Beyond the Basic 4.* Washington, D. C., U. S. Department of Agriculture.

McGinnis, M. J. and Foege, W. (1993). Actual causes of death in the United States. *Journal of the American Medical Association, 270,* 2208.

Metropolitan Life Insurance Company. (1983). New weight standards for men and women. *Statistical Bulletin of Metropolitan Life Insurance Company, 64,* 2–9.

National Heart, Lung and Blood Institute. (1992). *Healthy Heart I. Q.* NIH Publication No. 92–2724. Washington, D. C., National Heart, Lung and Blood Institute.

National Institutes of Health/National Institute of Diabetes and Digestive and Kidney Diseases. (1994). *Diabetes Overview.* NIH Publication No. 94–3235. Washington, D. C., National Institutes of Health/National Institute of Diabetes and Digestive and Kidney Diseases.

Office of Disease Prevention and Health Promotion. (1981). *Healthstyle: A Self-Test.* Publication No. H0012. Washington, D. C., National Health Information Clearinghouse.

Pender, N. J. (1987). *Health Promotion in Nursing Practice* (2nd ed.). Norwalk, CT, Appleton & Lange.

President's Council on Physical Fitness & Sports. (1993). The health benefits of physical activity. *Physical Activity and Fitness Research Digest.* Vol. 1. Issue 1. Washington, D. C., USDHHS/President's Council on Physical Fitness and Sports.

U. S. Department of Agriculture/Human Nutrition Information

Service. (1993). *Choose a Diet Low in Fat, Saturated Fat and Cholesterol.* Washington, D. C., Government Printing Office.

U. S. Department of Agriculture/Human Nutrition Information Service. (1993). *Choose a Diet with Plenty of Vegetables, Fruits, and Grain Produces.* Washington, D. C., Government Printing Office.

U. S. Department of Health and Human Services. (1990). *Healthy People 2000: National Health Promotion and Disease Prevention Objectives.* Washington, D. C., Government Printing Office.

U. S. Department of Health and Human Services. (1992). *Promoting Healthy Diets and Active Lifestyles to Lower-SES Adults: Market Research for Public Education.* Washington, D. C., Government Printing Office.

U. S. Department of Health and Human Services/Food and Drug Administration/U. S. Department of Agriculture. (1993). *An Introduction to the New Food Label.* DHHS Publication No. (FDA) 94–2271. Washington, D. C.

U. S. Department of Health and Human Services/National Institutes of Health/National Cancer Institute. (1990). *Self-Guided Strategies for Smoking Cessation: A Program Planners Guide.* NIH Publication 91–3104. Washington D. C., U. S. Department of Health and Human Services/National Institutes of Health/National Cancer Institute.

U. S. Department of Health and Human Services/National Institutes of Health/National Cancer Institute. (1991). *Clearing the Air: How to Quit Smoking and Quit for Keeps.* NIH Publication No. 92–1647. Washington D. C., U. S. Department of Health and Human Services/National Institutes of Health/National Cancer Institute.

U. S. Department of Health and Human Services/Office of Disease Prevention and Health Promotion. (1994). *Clinician's Handbook of Preventive Services.* Washington, D. C., Government Printing Office.

U. S. Department of Health and Human Services/U. S. Preventive Services Task Force. (1996). *Guide to Clinical Preventive Services* (2nd ed.). Washington, D. C., Government Printing Office.

U. S. Department of Health and Human Services/Public Health Service/Centers for Disease Control. (1991). *The Prevention and Treatment of Complications of Diabetes Mellitus: A Guide for Primary Care Practitioners.* Atlanta, U. S. Department of Health and Human Services.

12

Issues in Women's Health Care

Case History *Lisa Lewis is a Registered Nurse (RN) practicing in a public-sponsored, comprehensive obstetrical and family clinic in an urban area. The clinic is staffed by physicians, gynecological nurse practitioners (NPs), certified nurse-midwives, RNs, and social workers. In her role, Lisa performs a variety of services, including health teaching, obtaining health histories, taking vital signs (including fetal heart rate assessment, fundal height), counseling, performing screenings and skilled tasks (e.g., injections, venipuncture), and assisting the primary care providers in other services (e.g., insertion of intrauterine devices [IUDs] and performance of Papanicolaou [Pap] smears, colposcopy, ultrasonography, and biopsies).*

On a recent Friday, Lisa cared for Patty Smith, a 25-year-old mother of two who was being seen for her yearly gynecological examination and to discuss family planning options. While Lisa completed Patty's health history, she learned that Patty's last Pap test was 2 years ago while she was pregnant with her second child. That Pap test and all previous tests have been "normal." Since the birth of her last child, Patty reports that she and her husband have been using condoms and foam to prevent pregnancy, but she would like to explore other forms of contraception. Her vital signs were blood pressure, 110/68; pulse, 76; and respirations, 16, and her weight was appropriate for her height. Patty stated that she smokes approximately one pack of cigarettes each day, as she has for the past 8 years (except during her pregnancies). She reports no serious health problems and states that both of her parents are living and in good health.

Lisa briefly explained the contraceptive options available, including the effectiveness, pros, and cons of each. Lisa explained that because Patty smokes, hormonal contraceptives (e.g., birth control pills, medroxyprogesterone acetate [Depo-Provera] injections, and levonorgestrel implants [Norplant] are contraindicated. Other options would be a diaphragm, IUD, cervical cap, or continuation with condoms and spermicidal preparations. Surgical sterilization for Patty or her husband was also discussed. Patty reported that she and her husband have not yet decided whether they want any more children, so sterilization was not considered. After learning about benefits and potential side effects of each of her options, Patty decided to be fitted for a diaphragm.

Lisa assisted the NP with the general physical examination, breast examination (including instruction on breast self-examination [BSE]), and Pap smear. No abnormalities were noted. The NP carefully fitted Patty for a diaphragm and instructed her on how to insert it properly. The NP allowed Patty to "practice" insertion and removal several times and checked to ensure that Patty could perform the procedure properly. Lisa gave Patty several informational pamphlets on the diaphragm and reminded Patty of the necessity of using spermicidal jelly or cream with each act of intercourse.

Prior to leaving, Lisa informed Patty that she would receive the results of her Pap smear in the mail in about 2 weeks. She was reminded to come back in 2 years if she had no problems.

Nursing practice in community settings encompasses a number of areas concerning women's health, including family planning, pregnancy, childbearing and infant care, cancer detection, detection and prevention of domestic violence, and prevention of osteoporosis. *Healthy People 2000* (U. S. Department of Health and Human Services [USDHHS], 1990, 1995) lists a number of objectives related to women's health, including specific objectives to encourage breastfeeding, discourage smoking, reduce unplanned pregnancies, and improve access to prenatal care. Reducing domestic violence and complications arising from osteoporosis are also among the stated objectives. Table 12–1 presents some examples of *Healthy People 2000* objectives related to women's health.

This chapter discusses a number of topics regarding women's health care. Presented here is information on family planning, including available contraception options; women's health care (e.g., screening for reproductive diseases, breast care); prenatal care; infant care; and infertility. Finally, prevention and intervention in teenage pregnancy and domestic violence are discussed.

Family Planning

Approximately one half (56%) of pregnancies in the United States are unintended (mistimed or unwanted). This is probably because of lack of knowledge, failure to translate knowledge into behavior, or lack of family planning services and information (USDHHS, 1990). Family planning services offer health and medical care and counseling that provide women with information and services they need to make informed choices about whether and when to become parents. Comprehensive family planning includes consideration of a number of factors regarding childbearing, adoption, abstinence from sexual activity outside of a monogamous relationship, use of contraceptives, natural family planning, treatment of infertility, and preconception counseling (USDHHS, 1995).

Without effective contraception, 89% of couples who regularly engage in sexual intercourse will conceive within 1 year (USDHHS, 1990). As stated earlier, an estimated 56% of all pregnancies in the United States are "unintended." African-American women experience much higher rates of unplanned pregnancy; 78% of their pregnancies are unplanned (USDHHS, 1990).

Several suggestions have been made to reduce rates of unintended pregnancy. These include encouraging the postponement of sexual activity (particularly in adolescents) and providing health education to improve the understanding of fertility and to promote the appropriate use of available family planning options. Improved access to providers of family planning services is also essential.

Abstinence education became more widespread in the 1980s to help cut down on initiation of sexual activity among adolescents. The "Just Say 'No' " and related campaigns have been somewhat successful in abstinence education. According to the USDHHS (1995), the number of both adolescent males and females reporting that they have never engaged in sexual intercourse has increased slightly. Counselors and educators who work with adolescents and teenagers should continue to provide abstinence education and to help young people who choose abstinence sustain their choice.

TABLE 12–1 ***Healthy People 2000*—Examples of Objectives for Family Planning, Maternal/Child Health, Domestic Violence, and Women's Health**

Family Planning

5.1—Reduce pregnancies among girls 17 years and younger to no more than 50 per 1,000 adolescents (baseline: 71.1 pregnancies per 1,000 girls 15 through 17 years of age in 1985)

Special Population Targets

Pregnancies (per 1,000)	*1985 Baseline*	*2000 Target*
5.1a—Black adolescent girls 15–19 years of age	186	120
5.1b—Hispanic adolescent girls 15–19 years of age	158	105

5.2—Reduce to no more than 30% the proportion of all pregnancies that are unintended (baseline: 56% of pregnancies in the previous 5 years were unintended—either unwanted or earlier than desired—in 1988)

5.3—Reduce the prevalence of infertility to no more than 6.5% (baseline: 7.9% of married couples with wives 15 through 44 years of age in 1988)

5.4—Reduce the proportion of adolescents who have engaged in sexual intercourse to no more than 15% by age 15 and no more than 40% by age 17 (baseline: 27% of girls and 33% of boys by age 15; 50% of girls and 66% of boys by age 17 reported in 1988)

5.7—Increase the effectiveness with which family planning methods are used, as measured by a decrease to no more than 5% in the proportion of couples experiencing pregnancy despite use of a contraceptive method (baseline: approximately 10% of women using reversible contraceptive methods experienced an unintended pregnancy in 1982)

Maternal and Infant Health

2.11—Increase to at least 75% the proportion of mothers who breastfeed their babies in the early postpartum period and to at least 50% the proportion who continue breastfeeding until their babies are 5 to 6 months old (baseline: 54% at discharge from birth site and 21% at 5 to 6 months in 1988)

Special Population Targets

Mothers Breastfeeding Their Babies: Early Postpartum	*1988 Baseline (%)*	*2000 Target (%)*
2.11a—Low-income mothers	32	75
2.11b—Black mothers	25	75
2.11c—Hispanic mothers	51	75
2.11d—Native Americans/Alaska Native women	47	75
Mothers Breastfeeding Their Babies: Age 5–6 months	*1988 Baseline (%)*	*2000 Target (%)*
2.11a—Low-income mothers	9	50
2.11b—Black mothers	8	50
2.11c—Hispanic mothers	16	50
2.11d—Native Americans/Alaska Native women	28	50

3.7—Increase smoking cessation during pregnancy so that at least 60% of women who are cigarette smokers at the time they become pregnant quit smoking early in pregnancy and maintain abstinence for the remainder of their pregnancy (baseline: 39% of white women 20 through 44 years of age quit at any time during pregnancy in 1985)

14.1—Reduce the infant mortality rate to no more than 7 per 1,000 live births (baseline: 10.1 per 1,000 live births in 1987)

Special Population Targets

Infant Mortality (per 1,000 Live Births)	*1987 Baseline*	*2000 Target*
14.1a—Blacks	17.9	11.0
14.1b—Native Americans/Alaska Natives	12.5	8.5
14.1c—Puerto Ricans	12.9	8.0

14.3—Reduce the maternal mortality rate to no more than 3.3 per 100,000 live births (baseline: 6.6 per 100,000 in 1987 [14.2 per 100,000 in blacks])

14.4—Reduce the incidence of fetal alcohol syndrome to no more than 0.12 per 1,000 live births (baseline: 0.22 per 1,000 live births in 1987)

Table continued on following page

TABLE 12–1 *Healthy People 2000*—Examples of Objectives for Family Planning, Maternal/Child Health, Domestic Violence, and Women's Health *Continued*

Special Population Targets

Fetal Alcohol Syndrome (per 1,000 Live Births)	*1987 Baseline*	*2000 Target*
14.4a—Native Americans/Alaska Natives	4.0	2.0
14.4b—Blacks	0.8	0.4

14.5—Reduce LBW to an incidence of no more than 5% of live births and very LBW to no more than 1% of live births (baseline: 6.9 and 1.2%, respectively, in 1987)

14.6—Increase to at least 85% the proportion of mothers who achieve the minimum recommended weight gain during their pregnancies (baseline: 67% of married women in 1980)

14.11—Increase to at least 90% the proportion of all pregnant women who receive prenatal care in the first trimester of pregnancy (baseline: 76% of live births in 1987)

Special Population Targets

Proportion of Pregnant Women Receiving Early Prenatal Care	*1987 Baseline (Percent of Live Births)*	*2000 Target (Percent of Live Births)*
14.11a—Black women	61.1	90
14.11b—Native Americans/Alaska Natives	60.2	90
14.11c—Hispanic Women	61.0	90

***14.17**—Reduce the incidence of spina bifida and other neural tube defects to 3 per 10,000 live births (baseline: 6 per 10,000 in 1990)

Women's Health

16.3—Reduce breast cancer deaths to no more than 20.6 per 100,000 women (age-adjusted baseline: 23.0 per 100,000 in 1987)

16.4—Reduce deaths from cancer of the uterine cervix to no more than 1.3 per 100,000 women (age-adjusted baseline: 2.8 per 100,000 in 1987)

Special Population Targets

Cervical Cancer Deaths (per 100,000)	*1990 Baseline*	*2000 Target*
16.4a—Black women	5.9	3
16.4b—Hispanic women	3.6	2

17.18—Increase to at least 90% the proportion of perimenopausal women who have been counseled about the benefits and risks of estrogen replacement therapy (combined with progestin, when appropriate) for prevention of osteoporosis

Violence

7.5—Reduce physical abuse directed at women by male partners to no more than 27 per 1,000 couples (baseline: 30 per 1,000 in 1985)

7.15—Reduce to less than 10% the proportion of battered women and their children turned away from emergency housing due to lack of space (baseline: 40% in 1987)

From U. S. Department of Health and Human Services. (1990). *Healthy People 2000: National Health Promotion and Disease Prevention Objectives.* Washington, D. C., Government Printing Office.

*14.17 From U. S. Department of Health and Human Services. (1995). *Healthy People 2000: Midcourse Review and 1995 Revisions.* Washington, D. C., Government Printing Office.

Use of educational materials, counseling, and peer group support should be encouraged.

CONTRACEPTION

At present, several methods are available to prevent pregnancy. Abstinence is the most effective means of avoiding unintended pregnancy and is certainly a key method of contraception for many (e.g., teenagers). Other methods of contraception include barriers (e.g., condoms, diaphragm) and hormonal methods (e.g., oral contraceptives, Depo-Provera, Norplant), IUDs, sterilization, and natural family planning. These methods vary in effectiveness, and each has positive and negative consequences. Table 12–2 compares available contraceptives.

Emergency Contraception

In June 1996, an advisory committee to the Food and Drug Administration recommended approval of the use of high doses of standard birth control pills as postcoital contraception or "morning after pills." Depending on the stage in the woman's reproductive cycle, "emergency contraception" prevents pregnancy by prevention of ovulation or prevention of fertilization of the egg or transportation of the egg to the uterus or may render the uterine lining unfavorable to implantation (Jaroff, 1996).

Recommended doses are two to four pills (depending on the brand) taken up to 72 hours after sex, followed by a repeat of the same dose 12 hours later. If initiated within 72 hours following intercourse, this regimen reduces the risk of pregnancy by 75 to 95% (USDHHS/Office of Disease Prevention and Health Promotion [ODPHP], 1994). Nausea and vomiting are the most common side effects.

Prenatal Care

A country's infant mortality rates and maternal mortality rates are often cited as an indicator of the overall health of the country and the efficacy of its health care system. Although U. S. infant and maternal mortality rates have improved during the past several decades, the United States ranks near the bottom compared with other industrialized countries (Jonas, 1995).

In 1992, the overall infant mortality rate in the United States was 8.5 per 1,000, which demonstrates steady improvement over the past several decades. The infant mortality rate for African-American infants, however, remains problematic, as it is about double the rate for white infants (Jonas, 1995). The higher rate for African-American infants has long been attributed to a number of reasons, including lack of access to health care, poverty, teen pregnancy, and several other factors. Indeed, African-American babies have more than twice the risk of having a low birth weight (LBW) as white babies. In 1990, 13.3% of African-American infants were born with LBW, compared with 5.7% of white infants (Centers for Disease Control [CDC], 1993). Risk factors associated with LBW are younger or older maternal age, high parity, poor reproductive history, low socioeconomic status, low level of education, late entry into prenatal care, low pregnancy weight gain, smoking, and other substance abuse.

Prenatal care is particularly important for women at increased medical and/or social risk. Prenatal care dramatically reduces the likelihood of having a baby with LBW; an expectant mother with no prenatal care is three times more likely to have a baby with LBW than an expectant mother who begins prenatal care during the fist trimester (USDHHS, 1990). Despite this, nearly one fourth of all pregnant women receive no prenatal care during their first trimester. Most of the women who receive delayed or no prenatal care are poor, lack a high school education, or are very young. Table 12–3 outlines barriers to prenatal care.

In addition to LBW, lack of prenatal care has been associated with prematurity, maternal complications, and infant mortality (USDHHS, 1990). Comprehensive and early prenatal care reduces rates of infant death and LBW. Improving prenatal care beginning in the first trimester of pregnancy is one of the objectives cited in *Healthy People 2000* (1990, 1995). This can best be accomplished through removing or lessening barriers.

TABLE 12–2 **Methods of Contraception—Effectiveness, Risks, Benefits, Convenience, and Availability**

Method	Effectiveness (Typical Use)	Potential Complications and Side Effects	Potential Benefits	Convenience/Use	Availability and Cost
Oral contraceptive pills	97–99%	Side effects: water retention, nausea, headaches, spotting, missed periods, breast tenderness, depression, mood changes Complications: blood clots, heart attack, stroke (associated with smoking), hypertension, gallbladder disease, liver tumors; may increase risk of ovarian tumors	May reduce volume and pain associated with menstruation; periods are regular; may protect women from cancer of the ovary and endometrium and benign breast disease; protects against anemia and ectopic pregnancy	Must be taken daily; effectiveness declines when pills are missed	Prescription required; costs vary depending on source—retail, approximately $20.00 per month
Condom	85–88%	Decreases sensation, loss of spontaneity; a few people are allergic to latex or to spermicide; condoms may break	Helps protect both partners against transmission of STDs and HIV if used properly	Must be put onto the erect penis before the penis comes into contact with the vagina; use a new condom for each act of intercourse	Easy availability; minimal costs
IUD	94–98%	Side effects: cramps, bleeding, anemia Complications: pelvic inflammatory disease, infertility, perforation of the uterus (rare)	IUDs with progestin decrease menstrual cramping in some users	Requires no preparation for intercourse; at least once a month (usually after menstruation), user must check in vagina for strings to ensure IUD is in place	Requires insertion by a trained health professional

Implant (Norplant)	99%	Side effects: menstrual irregularity, headaches, nervousness, depression, nausea, dizziness, breast tenderness, weight gain, enlargement of ovaries and/or fallopian tubes, excessive growth of body and facial hair; (side effects may decrease after first year) Complications: infection at insertion site	May decrease menstrual cramps, pain, and blood loss	Effective 24 hours after implantation; effectiveness lasts approximately 5 years; can be removed by a trained health care professional at any time	Requires a prescription and a minor outpatient surgical procedure
Injectables (Depo-Provera)	99%	Side effects: amenorrhea, weight gain, headaches, and others (similar to with implant)	May be used when lactating; may have protective effects against endometrial cancer	Effective almost immediately; requires no preparation for intercourse	Requires prescription; one injection every 3 months
Barriers (diaphragms, cervical caps, sponges)	82% for women who have never had a baby; 64% for women who have borne children	Side effects: cervical, vaginal irritation; pelvic pressure; vaginal discharge if left in too long; difficulty in removal Complications: cervical, vaginal, or bladder infection; toxic shock syndrome (very rare)	Provides some protection against STDs	Requires preparation to insert devices prior to intercourse (diaphragm and cervical cap, up to 6 hours prior to intercourse; sponge up to 24 hours before intercourse); should be left in place for 6–8 (but not more than 24) hours after intercourse. Should not be used by women who have recently given birth.	Diaphragm and cervical cap require a prescription and "fitting" by a trained health care provider; sponge is available without prescription
Periodic abstinence (natural family planning)	Very variable 53–86%	None	Careful monitoring can help determine timing for a planned pregnancy; requires no drugs or "devices"	Requires frequent monitoring of body functions and periods of abstinence	No prescription; obtain instructions from a trained health care provider; basal thermometers and charts available at drugstores and family planning clinics

Table continued on following page

TABLE 12–2 **Methods of Contraception—Effectiveness, Risks, Benefits, Convenience, and Availability** *Continued*

Method	Effectiveness (Typical Use)	Potential Complications and Side Effects	Potential Benefits	Convenience/Use	Availability and Cost
Spermicides (foam, gel, cream)	70–80%	Side effects: allergic reaction	Provides some protection against STDs	Must be inserted immediately prior to intercourse; some find the products messy; no douching for 6–8 hours after intercourse	No prescription necessary; relatively inexpensive
Sterilization	99+%	Side effects: pain at surgical site, psychological reactions Complications: infection, regret that the procedure was performed	No interference with sex drive or sexual functioning	Must be certain there is no desire for future pregnancies; surgery must be done by a trained doctor, and must follow postsurgery instructions; men must return for sperm checks until all sperm have been cleared from the system	Vasectomy—minor surgical procedure for men; usually performed in a physician's office under local anesthesia; tubal ligation—minor surgical procedure for women, under general anesthesia (fairly expensive); most health insurance plans cover sterilization
Abstinence	100%	None	Prevention of STDs and HIV; avoids drugs and devices; safest method of contraception	May be hard to avoid pressure to have intercourse	Prepare responses; talk about decision with partner

STD = sexually transmitted disease.

Data from U. S. Department of Health and Human Services. (1989). *Your Contraceptive Choices For Now, For Later.* Bethesda, MD, U. S. Department of Health and Human Services; Goldberg, M. S. (1994). Choosing a contraceptive. *Current Issues in Women's Health* (2nd ed.). Washington, D. C., Food and Drug Administration; and U. S. Department of Health and Human Services. (1994). *Clinician's Handbook of Preventive Services.* Washington, D. C., Government Printing Office.

TABLE 12–3 **Barriers to Use of Prenatal Care**

I. Sociodemographic

Poverty
Residence: inner city or rural
Minority status
Age: <18 or >39
High parity
Non–English-speaking
Unmarried
Less than high school education

II. System-Related

Inadequacies in private insurance policies (waiting periods, coverage limitations, coinsurance and deductibles, requirements for up-front payments)
Absence of either Medicaid or private insurance coverage of maternity services
Inadequate or no maternity care providers for Medicaid-enrolled, uninsured, and other low-income women (long wait to get appointment)
Complicated, time-consuming process to enroll in Medicaid
Availability of Medicaid poorly advertised
Inadequate transportation services, long travel time to service sites, or both
Difficulty obtaining child care
Weak links between prenatal services and pregnancy testing
Inadequate coordination among such services as Women, Infants, and Children and prenatal care
Inconvenient clinic hours, especially for working women
Long waits to see physician
Language and cultural incompatibility between providers and clients
Poor communication between clients and providers exacerbated by short interactions with providers
Negative attributes of clinics, including rude personnel, uncomfortable surroundings, and complicated registration procedures
Limited information on exactly where to get care (phone numbers and addresses)

III. Attitudinal

Pregnancy unplanned, viewed negatively, or both
Ambivalence
Signs of pregnancy not known or recognized
Prenatal care not valued or understood
Fear of doctors, hospitals, procedures
Fear of parental discovery
Fear of deportation or problems with the Immigration and Naturalization Service
Fear that certain health habits will be discovered and criticized (smoking, eating disorders, drug or alcohol abuse)
Selected lifestyles (drug abuse, homelessness)
Inadequate social supports and personal resources
Excessive stress
Denial or apathy
Concealment

Reproduced with the permission of The Alan Guttmacher Institute from Sarah S. Brown, "Drawing women into prenatal care." *Family Planning Perspectives,* Volume 21, Number 2, March/April 1989.

To reduce the incidence of infants with LBW and other complications, prenatal care should include (Sherwen et al., 1995)

1. Initial and ongoing risk assessment
2. Individualized care based on case management
3. Nutritional counseling
4. Education to reduce or eliminate unhealthy habits
5. Stress reduction
6. Social support services
7. Health education

These are discussed briefly here.

RISK IDENTIFICATION AND CASE MANAGEMENT

Routine health care visits should monitor "normal" progression of the pregnancy, including assessment of fetal growth and development (e.g., measurement of fundal height, listening to fetal heart tones, assessing fetal movement); assessment of maternal response to the pregnancy; and assessment for possible complications such as hypertension, gestational diabetes, or multiple fetuses. Identification of risk factors and developing and implementing interventions to eliminate, reduce, or manage the risk factors is essential in producing good pregnancy outcomes. To help nurses who work with women of childbearing age identify women at risk, Table 12–4 lists some factors that contribute to high-risk pregnancy.

Once a possible risk or complication has been identified, a comprehensive plan of care should be outlined to monitor and minimize risks. This plan or program may include detailed case management if the risk factors are significant. For example, if gestational diabetes is diagnosed, the pregnant woman should receive comprehensive education on this condition and receive ongoing monitoring and intervention as indicated. Likewise, if other complications, such as pregnancy-induced hypertension, multifetal pregnancy, or preexisting maternal health problems dictate the need, a case management plan should be implemented. For pregnant teenagers, a structured case management program should be encouraged to help minimize the risks associated with teenage pregnancy. These are described later in this chapter.

NUTRITION COUNSELING

Maintenance of good nutrition during pregnancy is vital to the health of both the mother and devel-

TABLE 12–4 **Factors Associated with High-Risk Pregnancy**

1. Demographic Factors
- a. Lower socioeconomic status
- b. Disadvantaged ethnic groups
- c. Marital status: unwed mothers
- d. Maternal age
  - (1) Gravida less than 16 years of age
  - (2) Primigravida 35 years of age or older
  - (3) Gravida 40 years of age or older
- e. Maternal weight: nonpregnant weight less than 100 pounds or more than 200 pounds
- f. Stature: height less than 62 inches (1.57 m)
- g. Malnutrition
- h. Poor physical fitness

2. Past Pregnancy History
- a. Grand multiparity: six previous pregnancies terminating beyond 20 weeks' gestation
- b. Antepartum bleeding after 12 weeks of gestation
- c. Premature rupture of membranes, premature onset of labor, premature delivery
- d. Previous cesarean section or mid- or high-forceps delivery
- e. Prolonged labor
- f. Infant with cerebral palsy, mental retardation, birth trauma, central nervous system disorder, or congenital anomaly
- g. Reproductive failure: infertility, repetitive abortion, fetal loss, stillbirth, or neonatal death
- h. Delivery of preterm (less than 37 weeks) or postterm (more than 42 weeks) infant

3. Past or Present Medical History
- a. Hypertension or renal disease or both
- b. Diabetes mellitus (overt or gestational)
- c. Cardiovascular disease (rheumatic, congenital, or peripheral vascular)
- d. Pulmonary disease producing hypoxemia and hypercapnia
- e. Thyroid, parathyroid, and endocrine disorders
- f. Idiopathic thrombocytopenic purpura
- g. Neoplastic disease
- h. Hereditary disorders
- i. Collagen diseases
- j. Epilepsy

4. Additional Obstetrical and Medical Conditions
- a. Toxemia
- b. Asymptomatic bacteriuria
- c. Anemia or hemoglobinopathy
- d. Rh sensitization
- e. Habitual smoking
- f. Drug addiction or habituation
- g. Chronic exposure to any pharmacological or chemical agent
- h. Multiple pregnancy
- i. Rubella or other viral infection
- j. Intercurrent surgery and anesthesia
- k. Placental abnormalities and uterine bleeding
- l. Abnormal fetal lie or presentation, fetal anomalies, oligohydramnios, polyhydramnios
- m. Abnormalities of fetal or uterine growth or both
- n. Maternal trauma during pregnancy
- o. Maternal emotional crisis during pregnancy

Adapted from Clemen-Stone, S., Eigsti, D. G. and McGuire, S. L. (1995). *Comprehensive Community Health Nursing* (4th ed.). St. Louis, MO, Mosby-Year Book; data from Vaughn, V. C., McKay, R. J., and Behrman R. E. (Eds.), and Nelson, W. E. (Senior Ed.). (1979). *Textbook of Pediatrics* (11th ed.). Philadelphia, W. B. Saunders.

oping baby. In general, pregnant women need to increase their caloric intake by about 15% above their normal intake. Basic recommendations include four servings of dairy products, four servings of meat or other protein source, six or more servings of breads and cereals, one serving of dark green or orange/yellow vegetables, two or more servings of other vegetables, and at least one serving of fruit high in vitamin C. Of particular concern in pregnant women is ensuring adequate iron and folic acid. To obtain sufficient vitamins and minerals, most pregnant women are encouraged to take a multivitamin/multimineral supplement.

Iron supplementation is recommend for virtually all pregnant women. According to Boyne (1995), "iron is the one nutrient that cannot be obtained in adequate amounts from dietary sources during pregnancy" (p. 183). Iron is needed to promote fetal and placental growth, increase maternal red blood cell mass, and compensate for basal losses. However, the use of iron supplements may produce unwanted side effects. Abdominal discomfort and constipation are the most common, and nurses who care for pregnant women should counsel them on minimizing these side effects. Suggestions may include taking the supplements at bedtime to decrease nausea and increasing fluids and daily exercise and eating high-fiber foods to reduce constipation.

Research has shown that folic acid is essential to the developing baby, and that supplementation is effective in reducing fetal abnormalities, particularly neural tube defects. Consequently, the benefits of ensuring adequate dietary intake of folic acid should be presented to all women, even before pregnancy. All women of childbearing age should maintain a daily intake of 0.4 mg of folic acid. This may be obtained through the diet or through supplementation. In addition to vitamin and mineral supplements, foods high in folic acid include dark green leafy vegetables (e.g., broccoli, spinach), oranges, bananas, whole wheat products, liver, black beans, pinto beans, peanuts, potatoes, and fortified breads and cereals. Pregnant women should be encouraged to eat these foods in addition to taking their daily vitamins.

A strong correlation exists between weight gain during pregnancy and birth weight of the infant, and low maternal weight gain is a risk factor for having an infant with LBW. An estimated one third of all mothers gain inadequate weight during their pregnancies, a complication particularly common in teenagers and African-American women (USDHHS, 1990). Because of this, pregnant women should be taught the importance of sufficient weight gain. Weight gain should be measured with each prenatal visit and monitored closely for signs that might indicate complications (e.g., sudden weight gain suggestive of pregnancy-induced hypertension or failure to gain) (Boyne, 1995).

General recommendations on total weight gain for pregnant women are 25 to 35 pounds for women who are low to normal prepregnancy weight for height, and 15 to 25 pounds for women who are high weight for height, or obese. The rate of weight gain should be 2 to 4 pounds during the first trimester and about 0.8 pounds per week thereafter (Boyne, 1995).

ELIMINATION OF UNHEALTHY HABITS

The detrimental effects of smoking, alcohol consumption, and use of recreational drugs on the developing fetus have been definitively established. Smoking alone is associated with 20 to 30% of all LBW births in this country (USDHHS, 1990). In addition to LBW, smoking during pregnancy is associated with delayed neurological and intellectual development, spontaneous abortion, bacterial infection, and infant mortality (Sherwen et al., 1995). Therefore, maternal smoking should be *strongly* discouraged throughout pregnancy.

Consumption of alcohol is known to cause defects in developing infants. One of the most serious complications of alcohol use during pregnancy is fetal alcohol syndrome, which is characterized by growth retardation, facial malformations, and central nervous system dysfunction (USDHHS, 1990). Even as little as two drinks per day is associated with developmental delays. As a result, it is recommended that women consume *no* alcohol during pregnancy.

Recreational, or illegal, drug use during pregnancy can cause a number of problems for the infant, as well as for the mother. The potential effects depend on the substance used and the amount. In general, illicit drug use may cause growth retardation, withdrawal symptoms, and physical anomalies (Sherwen et al., 1995). In addition, maternal use of intravenous drugs is associated with human immunodeficiency virus (HIV) infection, which may, in turn, be transmitted to the developing fetus. To eliminate these potential problems, all women who are planning on becoming pregnant or who are pregnant should be counseled to avoid illicit drug use prior to and during pregnancy. Furthermore, testing for HIV is now recommended for all pregnant women (see Chapter 16).

The effect of caffeine on the developing baby has not been determined. Heavy maternal caffeine consumption *may* be associated with intrauterine growth retardation. Therefore, pregnant women should be encouraged to limit their intake of caffeine (Sherwen et al., 1995).

STRESS REDUCTION

Pregnancy and childbirth are stressful for all concerned, as the expectant mother and father must face a number of new experiences and pressures that may produce anxiety. Stress is often higher near the end of pregnancy, and many pregnancy-related concerns are shared with the nurse during the third trimester. Fear of childbirth; effects of birth on the baby, finances, and family; future pregnancies, negative self-concept; previous loss of a fetus; terminating work; major life changes; and concern about pain in labor and delivery are common concerns. Other stressors, more commonly seen in multiparous women, include increased fears for the unborn baby with each successive pregnancy, stress from too much company or interfering relatives, concerns about weight reduction following delivery, concern about housework and family routines, fatigue during the postpartum period, increased depression, fear of not having enough time for self and others, disillusionment with parenting and child care, and concern about her own emotional ability to meet the needs of all family members (Sherwen et al., 1995).

Nurses who work with pregnant women and their families should be alert to signs and comments indicating increased stress and promote adaptive changes related to the pregnancy and impending birth, such as providing information on childbirth and referral to prepared childbirth classes or providing literature on recognizing and managing postpartum depression if that is of concern to the client. Encouraging healthful behaviors, such as getting adequate rest and good nutrition, can help reduce stress. A referral to a psychologist, counselor, or social worker might be necessary to assist with more serious problems (e.g., depression, financial difficulties, or abuse). Nurses should be prepared in advance to provide these referrals by maintaining a list of providers, with their addresses and telephone numbers.

SOCIAL SUPPORT SERVICES

Serving as an advocate and referral source for social programs for eligible mothers and children is one of the most important roles of nurses in community-based practice. Almost 40% of expectant mothers are eligible for at least one social program such as WIC, Medicaid, Aid to Families with Dependent Children, and food stamps. Nurses caring for expectant mothers and infants should be aware of all area social programs for pregnant clients and be prepared to refer those who might need social services.

HEALTH EDUCATION

General health education for pregnant women includes providing anticipatory guidance and health teaching about the normal course of pregnancy, labor and delivery, and the postpartum period. Management of common "discomforts" associated with pregnancy (e.g., nausea and vomiting, constipation, heartburn, urinary frequency, sleep pattern disturbances) should be discussed. The pregnant woman should be encouraged to get adequate rest and regular exercise. Preparation for labor and delivery should include several discussions on signs and symptoms indicating that labor has begun and when to go to the hospital or birthing center for delivery. Finally, signs and symptoms of possible complications (e.g., vaginal bleeding, abdominal cramping, severe headache) should be described, and the mother-to-be should know when to call her physician or clinic and when to seek emergency care.

PRENATAL SCREENING FOR GENETIC DISORDERS

One of the objectives of *Healthy People 2000* discusses the importance of offering screening and counseling for prenatal detection of fetal abnormalities. The stated purpose of these screenings is to "allow for initiation of interventions to ameliorate the consequences of the disorders through counseling and specialized obstetric and neonatal care" (USDHHS, 1990, pp. 382–383). Table 12–5 lists some prenatal screening and diagnostic tests.

The Preventative Services Task Force has developed specific guidelines for periodic health examinations for pregnant women. These recommendations are listed in Table 12–6.

Infant Care

Caring for a newborn can be a very frightening and confusing experience for new parents. Nurses who work in community settings, such as pediatric clinics, are often in a position to teach parents about care of newborns, including feeding, bathing, cord care, stooling and voiding patterns, dressing and diapering, sleeping, and observing for problems. These issues are described briefly here.

INFANT NUTRITION

Nutrition education for new parents should begin during the prenatal period and include information on the choice of breastfeeding versus bottle feeding. Basic information on both forms of infant feeding are described here. Infant feeding is also discussed in Chapter 13.

Breastfeeding

Breastfeeding is the recommended sole form of feeding for the first 5 to 6 months and should be encouraged by all health care providers (USDHHS, 1990). Indeed, one of the objectives of *Healthy People 2000* is to encourage breastfeeding in the early postpartum period (see Table 12–1). Women most likely to breastfeed their infants are mothers who are older, well educated, relatively affluent, and/or who live in the western United States. Those least likely to breastfeed are women who are low income, African-American, younger (younger than 20 years), and/or who live in the southeastern United States (USDHHS, 1990). Several barriers to breastfeeding have been identified. One barrier is the high number of women in the workforce who must leave their infants for extended periods each day, making breastfeeding more difficult. Likewise, teenage mothers (who rarely breastfeed their infants) who continue schooling are not usually able to nurse their infants during the day. Cultural and social preferences and acceptance that bottle-feeding is the "norm" also reduce breastfeeding rates.

Health care providers should instruct all pregnant women on the benefits and advantages of breastfeeding. For example, breastfeeding is more economical and convenient and provides a number of health benefits to both mother and infant. Breast milk is the ideal food for infants, supplying all nutrient needs, and immunological enhancement is a very important benefit for the baby. Furthermore, breastfeeding has psychological benefits of enhancing bonding between the infant and mother during feeding (Wong, 1995).

However, breastfeeding should be discouraged in a few cases. Breastfeeding is contraindicated for women who use illegal drugs (e.g., cocaine, marijuana), use more than minimal amounts of alcohol, or are taking certain medications or chemotherapy. Also, women who are HIV positive should not breastfeed their babies (USDHHS, 1990).

Although breastfeeding is "natural" and relatively simple, women who plan on breastfeeding their infants initially need both instruction and support. Ideally, instruction and support begin dur-

TABLE 12–5 **Types of Prenatal Genetic Testing**

Test	Purpose	Advantages	Disadvantages	Risks
Maternal serum alpha-fetoprotein (MS-AFP)	Screening test for neural tube defects, ventral wall defects, and trisomy pregnancies (e.g., Down syndrome)	Identifies women at higher risk for further testing who would not otherwise receive it	Is not diagnostic; only indicates need for further testing False-positive and false-negative results occur	Venipuncture Minimal risk
Ultrasonography	Assesses gestational age, fetal growth, placental sufficiency Detects multiple gestation and structural anomalies Screening and diagnostic test	Detects structural anomalies and effects of intrauterine environment that may not be detected by chromosome analysis	Accuracy depends on skill of ultrasonographer, quality of equipment, and size of defect Does not detect biochemical abnormalities	Noninvasive
Amniocentesis	Chromosome analysis of fetal cells DNA analysis AFP analysis, other biochemical analyses	Diagnostic for chromosome abnormalities Provides DNA for direct and indirect testing for single-gene disorders High accuracy for detection of neural tube defects by biochemical analysis	Does not detect structural anomalies not caused by chromosome abnormalities except for neural tube or ventral wall defects Usually not performed until second trimester (14–16 weeks) Results are usually available in 2–3 weeks Relatively expensive	Invasive 0.5% risk of spontaneous abortion Nongrowth of fetal cells requires repeat procedure
Chorionic villus sampling (CVS)	Chromosome analysis of chorionic (fetal) cells DNA analysis	Diagnostic for chromosome abnormalities Provides DNA for direct and indirect testing for single-gene disorders Test is done earlier than amniocentesis (9–12 weeks); therefore results are available earlier	Diagnostic accuracy may be less because of greater risk of maternal cell contamination and false evidence of mosaicism, which may require subsequent amniocentesis	Invasive Risk of spontaneous abortion about 2% Controversial evidence of limb-reduction defects

From Wong, D. L. (1995). *Whaley & Wong's Nursing Care of Infants and Children* (5th ed.). St. Louis, MO, Mosby-Year Book.

TABLE 12–6 **Preventative Services Task Force Recommendations for Pregnant Women**

Interventions Considered and Recommended for the Periodic Health Examination

Interventions for the General Population

Screening

First visit
- Blood pressure
- Hemoglobin/hematocrit
- Hepatitis B surface antigen (HBsAg)
- RPR/VDRL
- Chlamydia screen (< 25 years)
- Rubella serology or vaccination history
- D(Rh) typing, antibody screen
- Offer CVS (< 13 weeks)* or aminocentesis (15–18 weeks)* (age ≥ 35 years)
- Offer hemoglobinopathy screening
- Assess for problem or risk drinking
- Offer HIV screening†

Follow-up visits
- Blood pressure
- Urine culture (12–16 weeks)
- Offer amniocentesis (15–18 weeks)* (age ≥ 35 years)
- Offer multiple marker testing* (15–18 weeks)
- Offer serum α-fetoprotein* (16–18 weeks)

Counseling

Tobacco cessation; effects of passive smoking
Alcohol/other drug use
Nutrition, including adequate calcium intake
Encourage breastfeeding
Lap/shoulder belts
Infant safety car seats
STD prevention: avoid high-risk sexual behavior;‡ use condoms‡

Chemoprophylaxis

Multivitamin with folic acid§

Table continued on following page

ing the prenatal period and continue throughout the time the mother nurses the baby. Table 12–7 discusses some of the information needed for women who wish to breastfeed their infants. Numerous booklets and pamphlets supporting breastfeeding and providing instruction are available and should be given to the mother-to-be during early prenatal visits. Women who desire more information or who are experiencing problems should be referred to local, regional, or national support groups or organizations for more assistance (see Table 12–17).

Bottle Feeding

If the mother chooses to bottle feed her baby, she will need information on selection of a formula and instruction on formula preparation and cleaning of equipment. Commercial infant formulas are available in "ready-to-use" cans or bottles, concentrated liquid form that is to be diluted with an equal amount of water, and powdered form that must be prepared according to the manufacturer's directions. For infants with no special nutritional requirements, modified cow's milk–based formulas (e.g., Enfamil, Similac, SMA) may be used. These are available both fortified with iron and without extra iron. Soy protein formulas (e.g., Prosobee, Isomil, Nursoy) are used for infants who are sensitive to milk protein or are lactose intolerant. Hydrolysate formulas (e.g., Portagen, Ross Carbohydrate Free, Alimentum) are available for infants with malabsorption syndromes or milk allergy. Other special formulas are available for children who have special nutritional needs (e.g., to reduce sodium intake or to increase calories, protein, fat, or calcium) and for infants with phenylketonuria (Wong, 1995).

In addition to selection of formula, parents who

TABLE 12–6 **Preventative Services Task Force Recommendations for Pregnant Women** *Continued*

Interventions for High-Risk Populations

Population	*Potential Interventions* (See Detailed High-Risk [HR] Definitions‖)
High-risk sexual behavior	Screen for chlamydia (first visit) (HR1), gonorrhea (first visit) (HR2), HIV (first visit) (HR3); HbsAg (third trimester) (HR4); RPR/VDRL (third trimester) (HR5)
Blood transfusion 1978–1985	HIV screen (first visit) (HR3)
Injection drug use	HIV screen (HR3); HBsAg (third trimester) (HR4); advice to reduce infection risk (HR6)
Unsensitized D-negative women	D(Rh) antibody testing (24–28 weeks) (HR7)
Risk factors for Down syndrome	Offer CVS* (first trimester), amniocentesis* (15–18 weeks) (HR8)
Prior pregnancy with neural tube defect	Folic acid 4.0 mg,§ offer amniocentesis* (15–18 weeks) (HR9)

From U.S. Department of Health and Human Services/U.S. Preventive Services Task Force. (1996). *Guide to Clinical Preventive Services* (2nd ed). *Washington DC: Government Printing Office.*

*Women with access to counseling and follow-up services, reliable standardized laboratories, skilled high-resolution ultrasound, and, for those receiving serum marker testing, amniocentesis capabilities.

†Universal screening is recommended for areas (states, counties, or cities) with an increased prevalence of HIV infection among pregnant women. In low-prevalence areas, the choice between universal and targeted screening may depend on other considerations.

‡The ability of clinician counseling to influence this behavior is unproven.

§Beginning at least 1 month before conception and continuing through the first trimester.

‖**HR1** = Women with history of STD or new or multiple sex partners. Clinicians should also consider local epidemiology. Chlamydia screen should be repeated in third trimester if at continued risk. **HR2** = Women under age 25 with two or more sex partners in the past year, or whose sex partner has multiple sexual contacts; women who exchange sex for money or drugs; and women with a history of repeated episodes of gonorrhea. Clinicians should also consider local epidemiology. Gonorrhea screen should be repeated in the third trimester if at continued risk. **HR3** = In areas where universal screening is not performed due to low prevalence of HIV infection, pregnant women with the following individual risk factors should be screened: past or present injection drug use; women who exchange sex for money or drugs; injection drug-using, bisexual, or HIV-positive sex partner currently or in the past; blood transfusion during 1978–1985; persons seeking treatment for STDs. **HR4** = Women who are initially HBsAg negative who are at high risk due to injection drug use, suspected exposure to hepatitis B during pregnancy, multiple sex partners. **HR5** = Women who exchange sex for money or drugs, women with other STDs (including HIV), and sexual contacts of persons with active syphilis. Clinicians should also consider local epidemiology. **HR6** = Women who continue to inject drugs. **HR7** = Unsensitized D-negative women. **HR8** = Prior pregnancy affected by Down syndrome, advanced maternal age ($\geq$ 35 years), known carriage of chromosome rearrangement. **HR9** = Women with previous pregnancy affected by neural tube defect.

CVS = chorionic villus sampling; HIV = human immunodeficiency virus; RPR/VDRL = rapid plasma reagin/Venereal Disease Research Laboratory; STD = sexually transmitted disease.

choose to bottle feed their infants need instruction on formula preparation, washing the bottles, and techniques for feeding. Table 12–8 outlines information for parents who bottle feed their infants.

SLEEPING

The positioning of infants for sleep is very important, as sleeping in a prone position has been associated with sudden infant death syndrome. In 1992, the American Academy of Pediatrics recommended that almost all infants up to 6 months of age sleep on their sides or backs (exceptions are infants with gastroesophageal reflux, premature infants with respiratory distress, and some infants with upper airway problems) (Wong, 1995). Placing the infant on a firm mattress, rather than on a pillow or soft bedding, is also suggested.

TABLE 12–7 **Teaching Guidelines for Breastfeeding**

1. Wash hands. Wash nipples with warm water, no soap.
2. There are three basic positions:
   a. The *cradle position* is achieved by cradling the infant in one arm, head resting in the bend of the elbows. The infant's lower arm is tucked out of the way, and the infant's mouth is close to the breast. The mother can be sitting up in bed with pillows supporting the back or sitting in a chair.
   b. The *lying down position* is attained by having the mother lie on her side in bed with the infant lying on his or her side also.
   c. A pillow is needed to be successful with the *football hold*. The mother is seated in a chair and a pillow placed next to her on the nursing side. The pillow supports the elbow and the infant's buttocks, and should bring the infant's head up to the level of the breast.
3. Stroke the infant's cheek with the nipple.
4. The infant's mouth should be opened wide, as with a yawn, and should cover the entire areola or a large amount of the areola. If necessary, apply pressure to the infant's chin with your index finger to open the infant's mouth more widely. The breast needs to be placed far back into the infant's mouth to drain the breast adequately. Your hand position is important: Hold your hand in a "C" position around your breast with the thumb on top behind the areola and the fingers against the chest wall, and supporting the underside of the breast.
5. Both breasts are used: The first breast for about 10 minutes, the other breast for about 6 minutes. At the next feeding, the infant starts to feed on the breast used to finish the preceding feeding.
6. Retract breast tissue from the infant's nose during sucking. Break suction by placing a finger in corner of infant's mouth.
7. The neonate is nursed shortly after birth and approximately every 2–3 hours thereafter.
8. Infants should be burped after each breast and at the end of the feeding.
9. Nipples often become tender during the first week of nursing but should not become sore. Soreness and prolonged feedings are most often the result of a baby who is not latched onto the breast properly.

From Ashwill, J. W. and Droske, S. C. (1997). *Nursing Care of Children: Principles and Practice*. Philadelphia, W. B. Saunders.

Widespread adherence to these recommendations has resulted in a reported 30% decrease in sudden infant death syndrome during the past few years. All parents should be informed of these recommendations and taught to position infants on their sides or back, rather than prone, and to avoid overly soft bedding.

Choice of the infant's bed or crib is also very important to ensure safety. Federal regulations require that there should be no more than 2⅜ inches between the slats on infant beds, and no slats should be missing. Mattresses and bumper pads should fit snugly against the slats, so that the infant cannot fall between the mattress and the side of the bed. The crib should not be placed near a window where cords for blinds or drapes may be reached by the child and so the bed is free of drafts. Finally, plastic bags or plastic covering should not be used as mattress protectors. If a mattress protector is desired, parents should purchase zip-on covers specifically designed for crib mattresses (Jackson and Saunders, 1994).

BATHING AND CORD CARE

Care of the umbilical cord frequently concerns new parents. In anticipation of these concerns, parents should be taught that the umbilical stump will deteriorate in 5 to 10 days, and the cord base will heal completely about 2 weeks later. Care of the cord usually includes instruction on application of alcohol to the umbilical area two to three times per day to help it dry. Also, diapers should be folded away from the cord to prevent rubbing and to expose the cord to air (Delahoussaye, 1994). Sponge bathing the newborn is recommend until the cord falls off. Table 12–9 describes this process.

After the cord area has healed, tub baths are

TABLE 12–8 **Teaching Guidelines for Bottle Feeding**

Supplies

- Six bottles and 12 nipples. The type does not matter, but all should be the same to avoid frustrating the infant.
- Bottle brush (used to reach all crevices).
- Dishwasher basket (for securing the pieces in the dishwasher).

Preparation

- Use commercial formula rather than cow's, goat's, or soy milk. These types of milk lack the nutrients necessary for growth.
- Do not use "raw" or unpasteurized milk. This type of milk contains bacteria that can make the infant ill.
- Tap water does not need to be boiled before it is mixed with formula. Boiling can concentrate the minerals that are found in the water supply.
- If well water is used to mix formula, it should be checked for safety before use.
- Formula does not need to be sterilized. It is sterilized during the manufacturing process. It needs to be refrigerated.
- It is not necessary to heat bottles before feeding them to the infant.
- Bottles should never be heated in a microwave oven. Hot spots can occur in the formula and cause burns. Heating also changes the nutritional composition of the formula.

Feeding

- Hold the infant close, with the head elevated.
- A quivering motion during sucking indicates that the nipple has collapsed. Remove the bottle from the infant's mouth to break the vacuum.
- Low flow despite vigorous sucking indicates that the nipple opening is clogged or the screw cap is too tight. Loosen the cap and see if the flow improves. If not, inspect the nipple opening.
- Do not "prop" the bottle or put the infant to bed with a bottle in his or her mouth. Bottle propping prevents close contact and increases chances of aspiration and middle ear infections. These practices also allow sugar to accumulate around the teeth and may lead to milk bottle caries.

Storing Infant Formula

- Unopened formula should be stored in a cool, dry place and used before the expiration date printed on the can.
- Refrigerate opened cans of formula. If unrefrigerated formula is not used within 2 hours, discard it.
- Opened cans of formula (ready-to-feed or concentrate) should be used within 24 hours.
- Do not save the remainder of a bottle for later. Formula becomes contaminated with bacteria from the infant's mouth, and using it later could lead to illness.
- Formula should not be frozen.

From Ashwill, J. W. and Droske, S. C. (1997). *Nursing Care of Children: Principles and Practice*. Philadelphia, W. B. Saunders; data from Heslin, J. A. (1988). *No-Nonsense Nutrition for Your Baby's First Year.* Englewood Cliffs, NJ; Prentice-Hall; and Heslin, J. (1992). If you bottlefeed. *American Baby, 54* (5), B10–B14.

allowed. A sink or a special infant tub should be used to bathe newborns. As with the sponge bath, the bath should begin with clear water on the eye and face and progress from head to toe, finishing with the diaper area. Care should be taken to ensure that the temperature of the bath water is neither too hot nor too cold. Two or three inches of water is sufficient, and parents should be admonished to *never* leave the baby alone in the bath to prevent drowning.

DRESSING AND DIAPERING

A number of factors, such as cost, convenience, skin care, infection control, and environmental concerns, influence the parent's choice of cloth versus disposable diapers. Wong (1995) reports that "in general, home-laundered diapers are the least expensive when home labor cost is not included. Once home labor cost is included, the price difference between disposable diapers, diaper service reusable diapers and home-laundered diapers is quite small, although paper diapers tend to cost the most" (p. 314).

Diapers should be the appropriate size and positioned to fit snugly but not tightly. Soiled diapers should be changed immediately to avoid prolonged exposure of the diaper area to stools. Wet diapers should be changed frequently to minimize exposure to dampness. The genitalia, buttocks,

TABLE 12–9 **Bathing a Newborn**

- Parents should be taught to assemble all necessary items prior to beginning the bath (e.g., soap, shampoo, washcloth, towel).
- The infants eyes are washed with a washcloth and clear water from the inner to outer corner, using a different part of the washcloth for each eye.
- The face, including the nose and ears, are then washed with clear water.
- The scalp and hair is cleansed with water or shampooed with mild shampoo and rinsed with warm water. The hair is then towel dried.
- The shirt can then be removed, and the folds of the neck, the arms, axillae, chest, back, and abdomen may be washed with mild soap, then rinsed and dried. Careful attention should be made to keep the cord area dry.
- The upper part of the baby can be wrapped in the towel to prevent chilling, and the legs and feet are unwrapped and washed with mild soap and water and dried thoroughly.
- The genitalia and buttocks are washed last. The female genitalia are cleansed from front to back to avoid contamination of the urethra and vagina with fecal material. The scrotum and the penis in the boy are washed with soap and water. The foreskin on uncircumcised boys does not need to be retracted. If the male infant is circumcised, the penis should also be washed gently with soap and water and dried. Observation for signs of infection is important.
- Unscented lotions, vitamin A and D ointment, and petroleum jelly may be used to help prevent or heal skin irritations.
- Powders and oils are not recommended, as oils may clog the pores, and powders may be inhaled by the neonate, causing respiratory problems

Data from Sherwen, L. N., Scoloveno, M. A. and Weingarten, C. T. (1995). *Nursing Care of the Childbearing Family* (2nd ed.). Norwalk, CT, Appleton & Lange.

and anal area should be washed after each diaper change to prevent skin irritation.

Clothing should be appropriate for the temperature of the room or outdoors, as warranted. During cold weather, it is important to dress and wrap the baby appropriately to maintain body temperature. A bonnet, hat, or other head covering should be used when taking the infant outside during cold weather. Overdressing during warm temperatures and underdressing during cold weather can cause discomfort.

Whenever possible, a newborn's clothing should be laundered separately from the rest of the family. A mild detergent should be used, and the clothing, linens, and diapers should be double rinsed to remove all soap residue (Sherwen et al., 1995).

STOOLING AND VOIDING PATTERNS

Parents should be taught about the progression of the infant's first stools from meconium to "normal." Most normal-term infants pass meconium within 12 to 24 hours of birth (Perry, 1995). Meconium is composed of amniotic fluid, intestinal secretions, shed mucosal cells, and possibly blood and is greenish-black, viscous, and odorless. Transitional stools usually begin by the third day and are greenish-brown to yellowish-brown and are thinner and less sticky than meconium. Transitional stools last 2 to 3 days, and milk stools usually appear by 4 to 5 days. In breast-fed infants, stools are yellow to golden and pasty in consistency and smell somewhat like sour milk. The stools of formula-fed infants are pale yellow to light brown, are firmer in consistency, and have a more offensive odor (Wong, 1995).

Frequency of bowel movements for newborns varies from one with each feeding to one every 3 to 4 days. In general, the number of stools decreases in the first 2 weeks from five to six daily to one or two per day (Perry, 1995). Most newborn infants void during the first few hours of life, and neonates may void up to 20 times per day (Sherwen et al., 1995).

OBSERVING FOR COMPLICATIONS

New parents should be taught to observe their babies for relatively common problems that may arise, how to manage these problems, and when to contact their pediatrician or pediatric NP. Examples of relatively common concerns include hyperbilirubinemia, problems with temperature regulation (particularly in infants with LBW), and concerns over respiratory patterns. Parents should also be instructed on possible signs of infection (e.g., increased temperature, decreased feeding, lethargy, inconsolable crying) and taught how to take the baby's temperature.

Infertility

Infertility refers to the inability to conceive after 1 year of regular sexual intercourse without contraception (Quinn and Lowdermilk, 1995; Sherwen et al., 1995). Approximately 2.4 million married couples, or 8 to 15% of married couples, experience problems with conception (Quinn and Lowdermilk, 1995; Sherwen et al., 1995; USDHHS, 1990).

Factors related to the female partner account for 40 to 50% of infertility problems, and factors related to the male account for about 30%; a combination of factors of both partners accounts for another 20 to 30% (Sherwen et al., 1995). In women, the most common causes of infertility are problems in ovulation, blocked or scarred fallopian tubes, and endometriosis. Delay of childbirth until after the optimal age for fertility has also been identified as contributing to problems with conception.

In men, abnormal or too few sperm is the most frequent cause of infertility (USDHHS, 1990). Factors that contribute to problems with sperm and thus male infertility include underlying disease processes, trauma, poor nutrition, prolonged exposure to high temperature in the scrotal area (e.g., associated with wearing tight briefs, use of hot tubs), and varicocele (Quinn and Lowdermilk, 1995).

Complications (e.g., pelvic inflammatory disease) of sexually transmitted diseases—primarily gonorrhea and chlamydia—contribute to about 20% of cases of infertility. Other factors that may affect fertility of U. S. residents include previous abortion, the use of IUDs, stress, and exposure to environmental factors (e.g., radiation, pollution, and toxic chemicals) (USDHHS, 1990).

The process of trying to discover the cause of infertility can be expensive, painful, embarrassing, and emotionally draining. To diagnose infertility, both partners must undergo testing, including complete health history and physical examination. A detailed sexual history of both partners is also necessary. Based on information from the histories and physical examination, one or more diagnostic tests may be performed. Table 12–10 lists some tests that may be conducted to diagnose the cause of infertility.

Following identification of the reason for infertility, the couple is counseled on treatment options. Treatment of infertility can be *very* expensive, and outcomes are far from certain.

If the problem is related to ovulation, medications such as clomiphene citrate (Clomid) may be given to increase or regulate ovulation. Endometriosis may be treated medically, through use of hormones, or, in more severe cases, surgical repair of the uterus or fallopian tubes (Sherwen et al., 1995).

Similarly, treatment of male infertility may involve use of drug therapy and lifestyle changes (e.g., improved nutrition, wearing boxer shorts, no hot baths or hot tubs, stopping smoking). Surgery may be required if a varicocele is detected.

If initial therapies are unsuccessful, a number of other options are available for infertile couples. Again, the possible treatments depend on the identified cause of the problem. For example, if the cervical mucous is not supportive of sperm, artificial insemination with the partner's sperm is an option. Artificial insemination with donor sperm is an option if the male's sperm are insufficient in number or motility.

"Assisted reproductive technology" refers to a number of therapies that have been developed to treat infertility. Some of the available options cited by Quinn and Lowdermilk (1995) and Sherwen et al. (1995) include

- In vitro fertilization (IVF; "test tube" fertilization)—the woman's eggs are laparoscopically collected from her ovaries and fertilized in the laboratory, then transferred back to her uterus after normal embryo development has begun. Success rate is about 20%.
- Gamete intrafallopian transfer (GIFT)—the eggs are harvested from the ovary and placed in a catheter with washed, motile sperm and immediately transferred into the end of the fallopian tube(s). Fertilization occurs in the

TABLE 12–10 **Tests for Impaired Fertility**

Test/Examination	Timing (Menstrual Cycle Days)	Rationale
Hysterosalpingogram	7–10	Late follicular, early proliferative phase will not disrupt a fertilized ovum; may open uterine tubes before time of ovulation
Postcoital (Huhner test)	Peak cervical mucus flow*	Ovulatory late proliferative phase—look for normal motile sperm in cervical mucus
Sperm immobilization antigen-antibody reaction		Immunological test to determine sperm and cervical mucus interaction
Assessment of cervical mucus		Cervical mucus should have low viscosity, high spinnbarkheit
Ultrasound observation of follicular collapse	Ovulation	Collapsed follicle is seen after ovulation
Serum assay of plasma progesterone	20–25	Midluteal midsecretory phase—check adequacy of corpus luteal production of progesterone
Basal body temperature (BBT)		Elevation occurs in response to progesterone
Endometrial biopsy	26–27	Late luteal, late secretory phase—check endometrial response to progesterone and adequacy of luteal phase

*Exogenous estrogen may be given to induce mucus flow if spontaneous and reasonably regular ovulation does not occur.

From Quinn, E. B. and Lowdermilk, D. L. (1995). Common reproductive concerns. In I. M. Bobak, D. L. Lowdermilk, and M. D. Jensen (Eds.). *Maternity Nursing* (4th ed.). St. Louis, MO, Mosby-Year Book.

fallopian tube rather than in the laboratory. Success rates are 20 to 30%.

- Zygote intrafallopian transfer—a combination of IVF and GIFT in which the ova are fertilized in the laboratory and then transferred to the fallopian tube for development and transport to the uterus. Success rates are comparable with those of GIFT and IVF.
- Donor ovum transfer—ova from a donor are fertilized in the laboratory by the male partner's sperm and then transferred into the recipient's uterus, which has been hormonally prepared with estrogen and progesterone therapy.
- Donor embryo (embryo adoption)—a donated embryo is transferred to the uterus of an infertile women at the appropriate time (normal or induced) of the menstrual cycle.
- Gestational carrier (embryo host)—the infertile couple undergoes IVF, but the embryo(s) are transferred to another woman's uterus (the carrier) who will carry the baby to term. The carrier does not provide ova.

Nurses who work with couples experiencing problems with fertility should be prepared to discuss their options. Information on these options and resources for referral should be made available.

Teenage Pregnancy

"Pregnancy and childbearing rates for teenagers remain high in the United States despite well-documented associated adverse health, social and economic consequences for many of these teenagers and their children" (CDC, 1995, p. 677). In the United States, teenage pregnancy is one of the most serious, complicated, and far reaching of all public health problems. The statistics are astonishing. Consider the following (CDC, 1995;

USDHHS, 1990; USDHHS/ODPHP, 1994; USDHHS/Office of Population Affairs, 1994):

- The United States has the highest rate of teenage pregnancy among developed countries
- Each year, approximately 11% of teenage girls (more than 1 million girls) 15 to 19 years of age become pregnant, and more than 500,000 give birth
- By age 18, 24% of teenage girls have become pregnant at least once
- Ninety-five percent of teenage pregnancies are unintended
- Almost 70% of all births to teenagers and more than 92% of births to African-American teenagers are to unmarried girls
- Approximately 75% of teenagers report that they use no contraception or use contraception inconsistently
- Forty-three percent of pregnancies among young women 15 to 17 years of age end in abortion

Although teenage pregnancy is a widespread problem, the rates are geographically and ethnically unequal. Teenage pregnancy rates vary markedly across the country and by racial and ethnic groups. Table 12–11 lists the states with the highest and lowest birth rates for teenagers.

CONSEQUENCES

Teenage pregnancy is associated with a number of serious problems. Teenage mothers are more likely to experience complications of pregnancy (largely because of delayed or no prenatal care, poor nutrition, and other lifestyle factors). They are more likely to experience maternal complications, including pregnancy-induced hypertension, toxemia, anemia, nutritional deficiencies, and urinary tract infections. They are more prone to deliver prematurely, experience rapid or prolonged labor, and have fetal and maternal infections. Infants born to teenage mothers are more likely to have LBW and suffer associated problems (e.g., respiratory problems, neurological defects) and are more likely to be stillborn (Maurer, 1995a).

Probably the most significant factor, however, is the socioeconomic impact of teenage pregnancy. Indeed, "teenage pregnancy is viewed as the hub of the poverty cycle in the United States, because teenage mothers are likely to rear children who repeat the cycle" (Maurer, 1995a, p. 581). Many pregnant girls and teenage mothers fail to complete high school. This, in turn, is associated with unemployment and underemployment, resulting in living below the poverty level and reliance on welfare programs.

CONTRIBUTING FACTORS

Higher teenage pregnancy rates are directly tied to reports that teenagers are becoming sexually active at younger ages. In 1970, 28.6% of adolescent women (15–19 years) were sexually active. By 1988, the rate of sexually active adolescent females had increased to 51.5% (USDHHS/Office of Population Affairs, 1994).

Factors contributing to early engagement in sexual activity include peer pressure; sexually explicit media (e.g., television, movies, music, music videos, information on the Internet); need for love, acceptance, and approval; increased acceptance of unmarried mothers; and present, rather than future, orientation (Aretakis, 1996; Maurer, 1995a).

COUNSELING TEENAGERS ON ISSUES OF SEXUALITY

The benefits of practicing sexual abstinence should be stressed by health care providers to all teenagers. Providing information on reasons to avoid initiation of sexual intercourse and how to say "no" have been shown to be helpful. A number of resources provide materials on sexuality issues for adolescents that are available for health care providers and educators who work with teenagers. Several are listed in Table 12–17 at the end of this chapter. To assist nurses working with teenagers, Table 12–12 presents guidelines for counseling to prevent pregnancy in adolescents suggested by the Preventive Services Task Force (USDHHS/ODPHP, 1994), and Figure 12–1 shows an example of some of the materials avail-

TABLE 12–11 **States (and Washington, D. C.) with Highest and Lowest Birth Rates for 15- to 19-Year-Old Teenagers by Race and Hispanic Ethnicity—1992 (per 1,000 women)**

	Race		Ethnicity		
State	***White***	***Black***	***Hispanic***	***Non-Hispanic***	**Total**
District of Columbia	26.4	130.8	*	115.1	116.1
Mississippi	57.2	116.1	*	84.6	84.2
Arizona	79.9	112.0	135.4	62.0	81.7
New Mexico	79.5	75.6	102.5	61.2	80.3
Texas	75.1	113.4	112.2	61.5	78.9
Louisiana	51.3	118.4	22.5	77.8	76.5
Arkansas	62.8	122.0	*	75.3	75.5
Georgia	54.9	115.2	97.0	74.1	74.5
California	79.3	94.6	123.5	46.6	74.0
Alabama	55.2	108.9	65.6	72.6	72.5
Nebraska	35.8	125.6	99.8	38.9	41.1
Iowa	38.4	137.7	89.1	39.9	40.8
Maine	39.9	*	*	39.8	39.8
Connecticut	32.4	94.5	139.4	28.2	39.4
New Jersey	26.1	103.2	78.1	33.3	39.2
Massachusetts	33.1	97.0	128.1	30.5	38.0
North Dakota	30.6	*	*	36.5	37.3
Minnesota	29.5	162.6	110.0	34.6	36.0
Vermont	35.6	*	*	35.8	35.6
New Hampshire	31.1	*	†	†	31.3

*Birth rate is not shown for groups with < 20 births or < 1,000 women.
†Birth rate could not be calculated because the state did not provide birth data by ethnicity.
Data from Centers for Disease Control. (1995). State-specific pregnancy and birth rates among teenagers—United States, 1991–1992. *Morbidity and Mortality Weekly Report, 44* (37), 677–683.

able to help reduce teenagers' engaging in sexual intercourse.

In addition to these guidelines, nurses who care for sexually active and pregnant teenagers should be aware of their state's laws regarding "age of consent" for engaging in sexual activity and statutory rape. Although there is no firm consensus on how and when to notify child protective services or other authorities, agencies that work with sexually active and pregnant minors should have or should develop policies describing circumstances under which to notify authorities and the process that is involved. For example, in some states, girls younger than 15 years cannot *legally* consent to sex, and adults who engage in sexual intercourse with these teenagers are subject to prosecution. Other states base "age of consent" on age differences between the girl and her partner; e.g., the older partner cannot be more than 3 years older than the younger one. Thus, it may be legally permissible for a 15-year-old girl to have intercourse with a 17-year-old boy but not with a 24-year-old man. Finally, the nurse should always consider the possibility of sexual child abuse and assess appropriately—particularly when caring for younger girls.

PRENATAL CARE

For all of the reasons cited, pregnant teenagers need early and comprehensive prenatal care, and case management is preferred. It is particularly important that teenagers be counseled on good

TABLE 12–12 **Counseling Guidelines to Prevent Adolescent Pregnancy**

1. All adolescents should be asked about their sexual experiences and use of contraceptives. The clinician should maintain a nonjudgmental, empathetic manner and should be willing to answer questions and provide contraceptive advice or refer to another clinician for prescriptions, as appropriate. Information should include consequences of pregnancy and STDs and effective methods to prevent them.
2. State laws vary regarding minimum age for consenting to treatment and receiving contraceptives for minors. Clinicians should familiarize themselves with the laws in their state regarding these issues. Adolescents should be informed about issues of confidentiality regarding pregnancy prevention, STD testing, and treatment, as directed by state regulations and agency policy.
3. Parents should be counseled about the emerging sexuality in teenagers' lives and options for contraception. Clinicians should encourage effective communication between adolescents and their families regarding responsible sexual behavior.
4. Adolescents who are sexually abstinent should be supported in remaining abstinent and should be counseled in methods to resist unwelcome or coercive sexual relationships.
5. Within the parameters set by the state and the agency, adolescents who are sexually active should be assisted in choosing an effective, appropriate method of contraception. Considerations include their personal preferences and motivation, religious beliefs, cultural norms, and relationship with their partner(s). The most popular contraceptive methods among adolescents are birth control pills and condoms; implants or injectable contraceptives may be appropriate choices for teens. Diaphragms, cervical caps, and periodic abstinence are difficult for teens to use effectively, and IUDs are not recommended for adolescents.
6. All sexually active adolescents should be taught that hormonal contraception (e.g., pills, injections, implants) *DO NOT* protect against STDs and HIV. The use of condoms, *in addition to* these contraceptives, should be encouraged to *reduce* STDs in sexually active individuals. It should be stressed that condoms are *NOT* 100% effective.
7. Adolescents of both genders should be encouraged to talk frankly with their partners about STDs, HIV, and use of contraceptives. Assertiveness with partners about the use of contraception and protective measures against STDs should be supported. *IT SHOULD BE STRESSED THAT SAYING "NO" IS EVERY PERSON'S RIGHT.*
8. Boys should be provided with as much counseling as girls about contraception and STD prevention. Young adolescent males should be taught the benefits of abstinence, the importance of responsible sexual behavior, and the importance of condom use if engaging in sexual intercourse, at an early age.
9. Adolescents using prescribed contraceptives should be followed closely to determine proper use and to monitor for side effects.

HIV = human immunodeficiency virus; STD = sexually transmitted disease.
Adapted from U. S. Department of Health and Human Services. (1994). *Clinician's Handbook of Preventive Services.* Washington, D. C., Government Printing Office.

nutritional practices, getting plenty of rest, and recognition of signs and symptoms of complications. Pregnant teenagers should be encouraged to stay in school. Because of the extent of this problem, as described earlier, many school districts have developed special programs designed to meet the educational, developmental, maturational, and social needs of the pregnant teenager. On-site health care is frequently a component of school programs. Additionally, many programs offer childbirth education, parenting classes, and after-delivery child care.

POSTDELIVERY NEEDS

After delivery, teenagers need ongoing social support and encouragement to complete their education. Financial assistance is also frequently a need, and nurses who practice in community-based settings should know how to refer new mothers to obtain social services such as Aid to Families with Dependent Children, WIC, and food stamps.

Finally, *all* pregnant teenagers should be counseled regarding sexual activity and contraception choices following delivery. Somewhat surprisingly, repeat pregnancy is frequently a problem. Maurer (1995a) reports that "fifteen percent of teenagers are pregnant again within 1 year and 30% are pregnant again by the end of 2 years" (p. 600). All teenagers who have experienced one pregnancy should be emphatically encouraged to avoid another pregnancy and supported in their contraceptive choices.

Women's Health Care

In addition to health needs related to childbearing and family planning, there are a number of health promotion and illness prevention issues that should be addressed by health care professionals who care for women of all ages in community settings. Discussed here are screening recommendations for breast cancer and diseases of the reproductive organs, prevention of osteoporosis, and prevention and identification of and interventions for domestic violence.

SCREENING RECOMMENDATIONS FOR BREAST CANCER

Breast cancer is the most common cancer among women in the United States and the second leading cause of cancer deaths in women (USDHHS/OHPDP, 1994). Risk factors for breast cancer are age over 50, personal or family history (e.g., mother, sister), first pregnancy after 30 years of age, having had no children, menarche before age 12, menopause after age 50, postmenopausal obesity, high socioeconomic status, and a personal history of ovarian or endometrial cancer (USDHHS/ODPHP, 1994). Mortality from breast cancer is strongly influenced by its stage at detection; therefore, early detection is critical to promoting a good outcome. Breast self-examination (BSE), examination by a trained clinician, and mammography are the most commonly used tools to screen women for breast cancer.

Most authorities agree that all women should be taught how to perform BSE and encouraged to practice BSE monthly, about 1 week after the end of the menstrual period. In addition, all women 20 to 39 years of age should have a breast examination performed by a health professional *at least* every 3 years and every year beginning at age 40.

The American Cancer Society and other groups have excellent teaching materials, educational pamphlets and reminders that are available to help instruct women on performing BSE. Nurses who care for women in community settings are in an excellent position to teach this important skill and should provide literature and other materials to help instruct their clients.

Mammography is the most effective means of early detection for breast cancer (USDHHS/ODPHP, 1994). There is some debate on the benefit of routinely screening women younger than 50, but most authorities agree that potential benefits are much greater than any potential harm from routine screening of younger women. In general, mammography screening recommendation are as follow (USDHHS/OHPDP, 1994):

- Women 40 to 49 years of age should have screening mammograms every 1 to 2 years
- Women 50 years or older should have screening mammograms every year
- High-risk women (women with a family history of premenopausally diagnosed breast cancer in a first-degree relative) should have mammograms beginning at 35 years of age
- Any palpable breast lump, even if not detected on a mammogram, should be carefully evaluated

When breast cancer is suspected, a surgical biopsy or needle biopsy is performed. If the lump is confirmed as breast cancer, treatment is typically a combination of surgery (e.g., lumpectomy, simple mastectomy, modified radical mastectomy) and radiation and/or chemotherapy or hormone therapy. All treatment options should be discussed thoroughly with the client, including potential outcomes, side effects, benefits, and negative consequences. Again, the nurse should assist in informed decision-making by providing literature on breast cancer and referral to organizations and agencies (e.g., American Cancer Society, Reach for Recovery) that provide information on the treatment of breast cancer.

Teen Talk

Many Teens Are Saying "NO"

DON'T BE FOOLED into thinking most teenagers are having sex. **THEY AREN'T!!** There's a lot to know before you say "yes" to having sex.

WHAT SHOULD I KNOW ABOUT MY BODY?

During the teen years, you may be strongly attracted to another person. Your body may send you messages that make you want to get closer to that person. But...

You may not know that:

Over one million *teens become pregnant each year.*

Young girls *have more problems during pregnancy.*

Babies *of young, teen mothers are more likely to be born with serious health problems.*

Sexually transmitted diseases (STDs) *are at epidemic levels. You may have heard of herpes, syphilis, gonorrhea, chlamydia, and AIDS.*

Some STDs are incurable. *They may cause pain, sterility, or sometimes even death.*

Face it! Sex for teens is pretty risky!

WHAT SHOULD I KNOW ABOUT MY FEELINGS?

Sexual feelings can be pretty strong! So think before you act. Think about your future. Think about the consequences. **Think about yourself!** Ask yourself, "Am I ready to have sex now?"

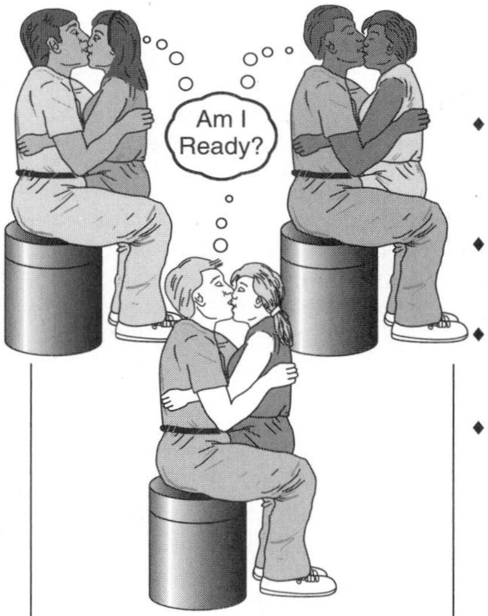

SOME QUESTIONS TO ASK YOURSELF

There's a lot to know before making your decision about whether or not to say "yes" to having sex. Here's a checklist to help you decide:

	YES	NO
♦ Is having sex in agreement with my own moral values?	❑	❑
♦ Would my parents approve of my having sex now?	❑	❑
♦ If I have a child, am I responsible enough to provide for its emotional and financial support?	❑	❑
♦ If the relationship breaks up, will I be glad I had sex with this person?	❑	❑
♦ Am I sure no one is pushing me into having sex?	❑	❑
♦ Does my partner want to have sex now?	❑	❑
♦ Am I absolutely sure my partner is not infected with an STD including AIDS?	❑	❑

If any of your answers to these questions is **"NO,"** then you'd better **WAIT.**

FIGURE 12–1 "Teen Talk." (From U. S. Department of Health and Human Services/Office of Population Affairs. [1995]. *Teen Talk*. Bethesda, MD, U. S. Department of Health and Human Services/Office of Population Affairs Clearinghouse).

SHOULD I HAVE SEX NOW OR SHOULD I WAIT?

It's true some teens decide to go ahead. But the results of your decision will fall on you.

Ask yourself these questions before making up your mind:

- Can I take full responsibility for my actions?
- Am I willing to risk STDs, including AIDS, pregnancy, and/or sterility?
- Can I handle being a single parent or placing my child up for adoption?
- Am I ready and able to support a child on my own?
- Can I handle the guilt and conflict I may feel?
- Will my decision hurt others—my parents, my friends?

DECISIONS ABOUT SEX MAY BE THE MOST IMPORTANT DECISIONS YOU'LL EVER MAKE. SO, THINK BEFORE YOU ACT.

WHAT SHOULD I KNOW IF I DECIDE NOT TO HAVE SEX?

A lot of teens decide not to have sex. Many teens are worried about hurting the other person's feeling.
BUT it's not so hard to say "NO" and still remain friends. For example, you might say:

- "I like you a lot, but I'm just not ready to have sex."
- "I don't believe in having sex before marriage. I want to wait."
- "I enjoy being with you, but I don't think I'm old enough to have sex."
- "I don't feel like I have to give you a reason for not having sex. It's just my decision."

ALSO, there are different ways to show affection for another person without having sexual intercourse.

Try to avoid situations where sexual feelings become strong. "Stopping" is much harder then. Talk about your feelings and what seems right for you.

If you and your partner can't agree, then maybe you need to find someone else whose beliefs are closer to your own.

WHAT SHOULD I KNOW ABOUT PRESSURE?

It comes from everywhere . . . advertising, friends, movies, television, shows, songs, and books.

BE POPULAR
BE PART OF THE IN-CROWD
BE A MAN/BE A WOMAN
EVERYBODY'S DOING IT
SEX IS FUN
IF IT FEELS GOOD, DO IT

BUT stop and think. Will having sex really make you more popular, more mature, or more desirable? Probably not. In fact, having sex may even cause your partner to lose interest. The one sure thing about having sex is that you may be in for problems you don't know how to handle.

WHAT SHOULD I KNOW ABOUT BOY/GIRL RELATIONSHIPS?

They're great . . . but good relationships don't develop overnight. They take time. Sex is not what makes a relationship work.
Watch out for **lines** like, **"If you care about me, you'll have sex with me."**

- You don't have to have sex with someone to prove you like or love them.
- Sex should never be used to pay someone back for something . . . all you have to say is "Thank you."
- Sharing thoughts, beliefs, feelings, and most of all, mutual respect is what makes a relationship strong.
- Saying "No" can be the best way to say "I love you."

WHERE CAN I GET INFORMATION THAT WILL HELP ME?

If you want further information or help, talk to someone who cares about you. Ask your parents, an older brother or sister, other family members, or an adult you feel will listen and give you good advice. There are people and organizations in your community who want to help —your family doctor; your priest, minister, or rabbi; your school nurse or counselor; or local health care providers.

FIGURE 12–1 *Continued*

SCREENING RECOMMENDATIONS FOR CANCERS OF THE FEMALE REPRODUCTIVE TRACT

Cancers of the cervix, ovary, and endometrium are relatively common and are successfully treatable if caught early. Screening recommendations for each are described briefly here.

Cancer of the endometrium is the most common gynecological malignancy and the fourth most common malignancy in women (after breast, colorectal, and lung cancer) (Fowler and Twiggs, 1994). Endometrial cancer most often occurs in postmenopausal women, and the average age at diagnosis is 58 years. Risk factors include nulliparity, late menopause, early menarche, obesity, a family history of breast cancer, higher socioeconomic status, pelvic irradiation, and endometrial hyperplasia (Fowler and Twiggs, 1994; Jones and Trabeaux, 1996). Abnormal vaginal bleeding and an enlarged uterus are the most common symptoms of endometrial cancer. If postmenopausal bleeding occurs, an endometrial biopsy is usually performed.

Total abdominal hysterectomy and bilateral salpingo-oophorectomy is the treatment of choice for cases of endometrial cancer. If staging determines metastases, radiation and/or chemotherapy or hormone therapy may be considered (Fowler and Twiggs, 1994).

Cancer of the cervix is one of the most common cancers in women but is highly treatable if caught early (USDHHS, 1990). Risk factors for cervical cancer include early age at first intercourse, having had multiple sexual partners, a positive test for the human papillomavirus, a history of exposure to diethylstilbestrol, and smoking (Sherwen et al., 1995). Cervical carcinoma in situ is most commonly seen in women between 20 and 30 years of age, and invasive cervical carcinoma is most common in women 40 to 45 (Bobak et al., 1989). African-American women have dramatically higher incidences of invasive cancer than white women (USDHHS/OHPDP, 1994).

Symptoms of cervical cancer include vaginal bleeding or discharge, often associated with douching or sexual intercourse. The widespread use of the Pap test for early detection of cervical cancer has contributed greatly to the decline in deaths from cervical cancer. Recommendations for routine Pap testing are as follow:

- Sexually active women 18 years of age or older should have annual Pap tests
- After a woman has had three or more consecutive "normal" examinations, the Pap test may be performed at the discretion of the physician and the patient but not less frequently than every 3 years (USDHHS/OHPDP, 1994)

Results of Pap tests are described as (Quinn, 1995)

- "Within normal limits"—minimal inflammation; no malignant cells
- "Inflammatory atypia"—mild atypical inflammation
- Cervical intraepithelial neoplasia (CIN) "grade 1"—(mild dysplasia, abnormal nucleus, normal cytoplasm)
- "CIN grade II" (moderate dysplasia, abnormal nucleus, minimal cytoplasm abnormalities)
- "CIN grade III" (abnormal chromosome and cytoplasm, abnormal cells predominate, many undifferentiated cells, severe dysplasia)

For cervical changes and abnormal Pap results, one of several diagnostic examinations and treatment options may be chosen. Colposcopy and directed cervical biopsies, cone biopsy (by cold knife, laser, or loop excision), endocervical curettage, and/or loop electrosurgical procedure may be performed (Dambro, 1996). Following treatment, Pap tests every 4 months for the first year and every 6 months thereafter are recommended.

If invasive cervical cancer is detected, a total abdominal hysterectomy is usually performed. Additional therapy (e.g., radiation and/or chemotherapy) may be recommended for advanced disease (Dambro, 1996).

Cancer of the ovary is quite rare (affecting 1 out of 70, or 1.4%, of women); however, it is the most deadly of the cancers of the reproductive organs (American Cancer Society, 1995). The high death rate is largely attributable to delay in diagnosis, as ovarian cancer rarely produces symptoms until it reaches advanced stages. Risk factors for ovarian cancer include family history; nulliparity;

older age at the first pregnancy; fewer pregnancies; and a personal history of breast, endometrial, or colorectal cancer (USDHHS/OHPDP, 1994). The pelvic examination is the most common screening examination for ovarian cancer. Treatment is usually a combination of surgery and radiation and/or chemotherapy.

PREVENTION OF OSTEOPOROSIS

Osteoporosis is a very common skeletal disease characterized by decreased bone mass, which leads to increased skeletal fragility and subsequent tendency to fracture. Osteoporosis affects about 24 million U. S. residents, including an estimated 50% of women older than 45 years and 90% of women older than 75 (USDHHS, 1990). Of those individuals, over half have fractures related to osteoporosis. Indeed, each year approximately 1.5 million fractures in the United States are related to osteoporosis (Jones and Trabeaux, 1996). The most common sites of atraumatic fractures are the vertebral column, upper femur, distal radius, and proximal humerus. The most serious fractures are hip fractures, which affect about 250,000 U. S. residents each year (USDHHS, 1990). It is estimated that about 33% of women and 17% of men experience a hip fracture by the time they reach 90 years of age (USDHHS, 1990). As the population of the United States ages, the incidence of osteoporosis-related fractures is expected to increase.

Risk factors for osteoporosis include age, family history, diet (inadequate calcium and vitamin D and excessive protein and phosphate), decreased activity, sedentary lifestyle, use of alcohol and caffeine, smoking, some medications (corticosteroids, excess thyroid replacement, long-term heparin therapy, chemotherapy, and anticonvulsants), and radiation therapy (Dambro, 1996; USDHHS/ODPHP, 1994). At greatest risk for osteoporosis-related fractures are women who are older, white, and slender and who have had a bilateral oophorectomy or early menopause. In addition to increased risk of fractures, osteoporosis is associated with both acute and chronic back pain, kyphosis, and loss of height.

Postmenopausal estrogen replacement has proven effective in reducing osteoporosis-related fractures. In addition, estrogen replacement helps decrease vasomotor symptoms associated with menopause (e.g., hot flashes) and may improve genitourinary symptoms (urgency, incontinence, frequency, and vaginal dryness) and reduce cardiovascular mortality in postmenopausal women (USDHHS, 1990; USDHHS/OHPDP, 1994). There is significant concern, however, regarding possible complications and side effects associated with hormone replacement therapy. Estrogen replacement therapy is strongly associated with increased risk of endometrial cancer, and the use of estrogen and progestin combinations may increase the risk of breast cancer. Table 12–13 presents guidelines for counseling women on the benefits and risks of hormone replacement therapy.

Other preventative measures to reduce osteoporosis include increased calcium intake (1,500 mg/day), adequate vitamin D intake (400–800 IU/day), and avoiding excess meat and phosphoric acid–containing beverages (Dambro, 1996). Premenopausal women, particularly those in high-risk groups, should be taught the benefits of calcium supplementation, with the recommended dosage being 1000 mg/day. Encouragement of weight-bearing exercise is also very important.

Domestic Violence

Studies indicate that between 2 and 4 million women in the United States are physically abused by an intimate partner each year (Grant, 1995; USDHHS, 1990). As a result, "battering of women is the foremost cause of injury to women" . . . and "40 to 60 percent of battered women are abused during pregnancy" (Grant, 1995, p. 411). Maurer (1995b) reports that 30 to 50% of police investigations involve domestic violence, as many as 70% of emergency room assault victims are women attacked at home, and around 25% of abused women require hospitalization for their injuries.

Once the pattern of domestic violence begins in a relationship, it tends to recur and become more severe over time. Furthermore, intrafamilial homicide accounts for almost one of six homicides and

TABLE 12–13 Counseling Guidelines for Hormone Replacement Therapy

- All women should be counseled about the probable risks and benefits of hormone replacement therapy and participate with their physician in deciding whether to take preventive hormone therapy.
- Women and clinicians should consider risk factors in determining whether to institute hormone replacement therapy. Risk factors include coronary heart disease risk factors (family history, blood pressure, weight, smoking status, cholesterol), osteoporosis risk factors (race, body build, physical activity level, bone mineral density), breast cancer risk factors (personal and family history, later parity, early menarche and late menopause), patient's desire for quality-of-life benefits (e.g., decreased vasomotor and genitourinary tract symptoms), patient's tolerance of side effects (e.g., endometrial bleeding and breast tenderness), and patient's willingness to participate in follow-up monitoring (endometrial sampling and mammography)
- If hormone replacement therapy is utilized, it may be desirable to begin estrogen replacement soon after the onset of menopause. Upper age limit for estrogen replacement has not been established.
- The concurrent use of progestin or careful endometrial monitoring is recommended for women with intact uteri.
- Contraindications for estrogen replacement include unexplained vaginal bleeding, active liver disease, impaired liver function, recent vascular thrombosis, breast cancer, endometrial cancer.
- Other conditions that may be considered as contraindications include seizure disorders, hypertension, uterine leiomyoma, familial hyperlipidemia, migraines, endometriosis, gallbladder disease, and thrombophlebitis.
- For women choosing estrogen therapy, a pelvic examination should be performed at initiation of therapy and yearly thereafter. Endometrial evaluation should be accomplished for women with uteri taking only estrogen. Follow-up evaluation of any vaginal bleeding should be made.
- Breast cancer screening should be the same as for women not taking hormone replacement therapy.

Adapted from U. S. Department of Health and Human Services. (1994). *Clinician's Handbook of Preventive Services.* Washington, D. C., Government Printing Office.

is often preceded by a history of physical and emotional abuse (USDHHS, 1990). Therefore, prevention of homicide among spouses and intimates should be linked to the prevention of abuse of women.

Nurses working in community settings are often in a position to identify and intervene in cases of domestic violence. Table 12–14 describes characteristics of the abuser and the victim to assist the nurse in identifying possible victims of abuse. In addition, to help nurses identify suspected cases of domestic violence, Table 12–15 lists physical and behavioral signs and symptoms that might indicate abuse. Finally, Table 12–16 presents nursing interventions for identified and suspected cases of domestic violence.

SUMMARY

This chapter has covered a number of issues related to the unique health care needs of women. Primary and secondary prevention strategies and health education for diverse topics of family planning, prenatal care, infant care, teenage pregnancy, early detection of cancers, and prevention of osteoporosis were described. The chapter concluded with information on detection and prevention of domestic violence. For further information on any of these topics, Table 12–17 lists a number of resources. Nurses in community-based practice should maintain a list of local resources and be prepared to refer their clients as needed.

Key Points

- Nursing practice in community settings includes a number of issues pertaining to women's health, including family planning, prenatal care, infertility, general health

TABLE 12–14 **Characteristics Common to Couples in Which Abuse Occurs**

Family Characteristics

- Low socioeconomic status
- Social isolation
- History of intergenerational abuse
- High levels of family stress
- Rigid boundaries

Batterer Characteristics

- Poor impulse control; unpredictable temper
- Inability to tolerate frustration
- Need to dominate
- Emotional dependency
- Egocentric
- Low self-esteem
- Poor social skills
- Excessive jealousy and frequent accusations against mate
- Unrealistic expectations
- Externalizes blame
- Victim of child abuse
- Unemployed or underemployed
- Alcohol use may facilitate aggression; may be used as an excuse

Victim Characteristics

- Low self-esteem
- Poorly educated
- Economically and emotionally dependent
- Often married young and had children early
- Emotional acceptance of guilt
- Risk increases during pregnancy
- Gradually increased isolation from friends and family
- Constant fear
- Victim of child abuse
- Hope that "things will get better"
- History of suicide attempts

Data from Watkins, A. C. (1993). Family violence. In J. M. Swanson and M. Albrecht (Eds.). *Community Health Nursing: Promoting the Health of Aggregates*. Philadelphia, W. B. Saunders; Smith-DiJulio, K. and Holzapfel, S. K. (1994). Families in crisis: Family violence. In E. M. Varcarolis (ed.). *Foundations of Psychiatric Mental Health Nursing* (2nd ed.). Philadelphia, W. B. Saunders; Grant, C. (1995). Physical and sexual abuse. In D. Antai-Otong (Ed.). *Psychiatric Nursing: Biological and Behavioral Concepts*. Philadelphia, W. B. Saunders; Maurer, F. A. (1995). Violence: A social and family problem. In C. M. Smith and F. A. Maurer (Eds.). *Community Health Nursing: Theory and Practice*. Philadelphia, W. B. Saunders.

care (e.g., screening for reproductive diseases, breast care, prevention of osteoporosis), detection and prevention of domestic violence, and prevention and intervention in teenage pregnancy.

- More than half of all pregnancies in the United States are unintended; therefore, comprehensive family planning is an important component of health care. Family planning includes consideration of a number of factors regarding childbearing, such as abstinence from sexual activity, use of contraceptives, treatment of infertility, and preconception counseling.
- A number of methods can be used to prevent pregnancy. Contraception options include barriers (e.g., condoms, diaphragm), hormonal methods (e.g., oral contraceptives, Depo-Provera, Norplant), sterilization, natural family planning, and abstinence. Each method has positive and negative consequences and should be discussed.
- Prenatal care is important for good pregnancy outcomes. Lack of prenatal care is associated with babies with LBW, prematurity, maternal complications, and infant mortality. Removing or lessening barriers to early and comprehensive prenatal care is important in improving infant mortality rates.

TABLE 12–15 **Injuries, Signs, and Symptoms Suggestive of Domestic Violence**

In an Office or Clinic

- Presenting complaints related to chronic stress or anxiety (e.g., hyperventilation, gastrointestinal disturbances, hypertension, panic attack, headache, chest pain, choking sensation)
- Depression or stress-related conditions (e.g., insomnia, anxiety, fatigue)
- Evidence of fear, embarrassment, or humiliation
- Poor grooming or inappropriate attire
- Any suspicious physical injuries (e.g., bruises, lacerations, scars, burns, swelling, fractures, ear or eye problems secondary to injury, clumps of hair missing)
- Any evidence of physical injury during pregnancy

In an Emergency Room

- Bleeding injuries, particularly to the head and face
- Perforated eardrum, eye injuries (e.g., black eye, orbital fracture)
- Broken or fractured jaw, arms, ribs, and legs
- Internal injuries; concussion
- Severe bruising, particularly on the back, buttocks, breasts, abdomen, and upper extremities
- Genital/urinary or rectal trauma
- Strangulation marks on the neck
- Burns from cigarettes, liquids, or acids
- Evidence of psychological trauma (e.g., anxiety, panic attacks, heart palpitations)
- Suicide attempt
- Miscarriage

In Any Setting

- Reports domestic problems; reports being trapped or powerless
- History of hospitalization for traumatic injuries
- Increased anxiety in presence of spouse/partner
- Inappropriate or anxious nonverbal behavior; uncontrolled crying
- Injuries in various stages of healing
- Injuries indicating failure to seek immediate care
- Timid and evasive behavior
- Inconsistent description of the cause of the injury
- Accompanied by male partner who does not wish to leave her alone

Data from Watkins, A. C. (1993). Family violence. In J. M. Swanson and M. Albrecht (Eds.). *Community Health Nursing: Promoting the Health of Aggregates*. Philadelphia, W. B. Saunders; Smith-DiJulio, K. and Holzapfel, S. K. (1994). Families in crisis: Family violence. In E. M. Varcarolis (Ed.). *Foundations of Psychiatric Mental Health Nursing* (2nd ed.). Philadelphia, W. B. Saunders; Grant, C. (1995). Physical and sexual abuse. In D. Antai-Otong (Ed.). *Psychiatric Nursing: Biological and Behavioral Concepts*. Philadelphia, W. B. Saunders; Maurer, F. A. (1995). Violence: A social and family problem. In C. M. Smith and F. A. Maurer (Eds.). *Community Health Nursing: Theory and Practice*. Philadelphia, W. B. Saunders.

- Education regarding infant care should include infant nutrition, recommending breastfeeding. If the mother chooses to bottle feed the baby, information on formula selection and preparation and cleaning of equipment should be provided. Crib selection, sleeping position, and sleeping patterns should be discussed with parents. Basics of bathing, cord care, dressing and diapering, stooling and voiding patterns, and observing for problems or complications are also important.
- Infertility affects between 8 and 15% of married couples. Diagnosis of infertility should include testing of both partners to determine the cause of infertility. Following identification of the reason(s) for infertility, the couple will be counseled on treatment options, which may include medications, surgery, lifestyle changes, artificial insemination, and more dramatic interventions, such as variations of IVF.

TABLE 12–16 **Nursing Interventions for Victims of Domestic Violence**

1. Interview women with suspicious symptoms or injuries to confirm or refute abuse
   - Talk with the woman in a quiet, private area
   - Be professional, direct, and honest in questioning
   - Be understanding; do not express anger, shock, or disapproval
2. If abuse is confirmed, assess safety and explore the victim's options to reduce danger
   - Affirm to the woman that battering is unacceptable
   - Assess the seriousness of the circumstances
   - Assist in calling and explaining the situation to friends or family when appropriate
   - Assure the victim that disclosed information will be kept confidential to the maximal extent possible
   - Counsel the victim about the dynamics of domestic violence and provide information on potential danger to the woman and her children
3. If the woman wants to leave the situation and if no other options are feasible, provide information on shelters or safe houses
   - Obtain information (telephone numbers, criteria, and process for admittance to the shelter) in advance
   - Offer to contact the shelter and make arrangements for transportation
   - Offer to contact legal authorities to report the abuse and press charges
4. If the woman chooses to stay in the relationship, encourage and assist her to develop a "safety plan" for fast escape should violence recur
   - Include ways to identify the signs of escalation of violence and select a sign that will be a cue to leave
   - Suggest that she keep a bag packed for herself and her children (include clothing, toiletries, medications, money) and ask a friend or neighbor to store the bag
   - Save money if possible
   - Take important financial records, such as rent or mortgage receipts and/or the car title
   - Provide a list of shelters and the appropriate telephone numbers—know exactly where to go and how to get there
5. Encourage follow-up care; individual and family therapy should be encouraged, when possible

Data from Watkins, A. C. (1993). Family violence. In J. M. Swanson and M. Albrecht (Eds.). *Community Health Nursing: Promoting the Health of Aggregates*. Philadelphia, W. B. Saunders; Smith-DiJulio, K. and Holzapfel, S. K. (1994). Families in crisis: Family violence. In E. M. Varcarolis (Ed.). *Foundations of Psychiatric Mental Health Nursing* (2nd ed.). Philadelphia, W. B. Saunders; Grant, C. (1995). Physical and sexual abuse. In D. Antai-Otong (Ed.). *Psychiatric Nursing: Biological and Behavioral Concepts*. Philadelphia, W. B. Saunders; Maurer, F. A. (1995). Violence: A social and family problem. In C. M. Smith and F. A. Maurer (Eds.). *Community Health Nursing: Theory and Practice*. Philadelphia, W. B. Saunders; U. S. Department of Health and Human Services/Office of Disease Prevention and Health Promotion. (1994). *Clinician's Handbook of Preventive Services*. Washington, D. C., Government Printing Office.

- Teenage pregnancy rates in the United States remain higher than in most industrialized countries and contribute to a number of health and social problems. Teenage pregnancy is associated with complications of pregnancy (both fetal and maternal), failure of the mother to complete high school, unemployment, poverty, and reliance on government assistance.
- Health promotion and illness prevention for women should also include various screenings and health education. Routine screenings for breast cancer include monthly BSE, periodic examination by a health care provider, and routine mammography for women older than 40. Screening for cancer of the cervix

TABLE 12–17 **Selected Resources for Family Planning, Maternal/Child Health, and Women's Health**

Family Planning

National Institutes of Health
National Institute of Child Health and Human Development
9000 Rockville Pike
Building 31, Room 2A32
Bethesda, MD 20892
(301) 496-5133
Office of Population Affairs
East-West Towers
Suite 200 West
5600 Fishers Lane
Rockville, MD 20857
(301) 594-4004
Office of Population Affairs
Office of Adolescent Pregnancy Programs
Room 736E, HHH Building
200 Independence Avenue, SW
Washington, D. C. 20201
Office of Population Affairs Clearinghouse
P. O. Box 30686-0686
Bethesda, MD 20824
(301) 654-6190
The Alan Guttmacher Institute
120 Wall Street
21st Floor
New York, NY 10005
(212) 248-1111
American College of Obstetricians and Gynecologists
409 12th Street SW
Washington, D. C. 20024
(202) 863-2518
National Association of Nurse Practitioners in Reproductive Health
2401 Pennsylvania Avenue, NW
Washington, D. C. 20037-1718
(202) 466-4825
National Organization on Adolescent Pregnancy, Parenting and Prevention
4421 A East-West Highway
Bethesda, MD 20814
(301) 913-0378
American Fertility Society
1209 Montgomery Highway
Birmingham, AL 35216-2809
(205) 978-5000
Association of Reproductive Health Professionals
2401 Pennsylvania Avenue, NW
Suite 350
Washington, D. C. 20037
(202) 466-3825
National Urban League
500 East 62nd Street
New York, NY 10021
(212) 310-9000
Planned Parenthood Federation of America, Inc.
810 Seventh Avenue
New York, NY 10019
(212) 541-7800
(800) 230-PLAN
National Conference of Catholic Charities
1346 Connecticut Avenue
Washington, D. C. 20036
(202) 529-6480
(adoption and foster care services)

Maternal and Child Health

U.S. Department of Agriculture
Food and Nutrition Service
3101 Park Center Drive
Alexandria, VA 22302
(703) 305-2276
(administers WIC)
Public Health Service
National Clearinghouse for Maternal and Child Health
8201 Greensboro Drive
Suite 600
McLean, CA 22102-3810
(703) 821-8955
National Institutes of Health
National Institute of Child Health and Human Development
Office of Research Reporting
Building 31, Room 2A32
9000 Rockville Pike
Bethesda, MD 20892
(301) 496-5133

TABLE 12–17 **Selected Resources for Family Planning, Maternal/Child Health, and Women's Health** *Continued*

March of Dimes Birth Defects Foundation
1275 Mamaroneck Avenue
White Plains, NY 10605
(914) 428-7100

National Center for Education in Maternal and Child Health
2000 15th Street North
Suite 701
Arlington, VA 22201
(703) 524-7802

La Leche League
P. O. Box 1209
Franklin Park, IL 60131-8209
(312) 455-7730

National Association of Childbirth Education (NACE)
3940 Eleventh Street
Riverside, CA 92501

Women's Health

National Institutes of Health

National Cancer Institute
Cancer Information Service
Building 31, Room 10A16
9000 Rockville Pike
Bethesda, MD 20892
(800) 4-CANCER
(301) 496-5583

National Cancer Institute
Surveillance, Epidemiology and End Results (SEER) Program
Division of Cancer Prevention and Control
6130 Executive Boulevard North
Room 343
Bethesda, MD 20892
(301) 496-6616

National Arthritis and Musculoskeletal and Skin Diseases Information Clearinghouse
P. O. Box AMS
9000 Rockville Pike
Bethesda, MD 20892
(301) 495-4484

American Cancer Society
Reach for Recovery
1599 Clifton Road, NE
Atlanta, GA 30329
(800) ACS-2345

National Osteoporosis Foundation
1150 17th Street NW, Suite 500
Washington, D. C. 20036
(800) 223-9994
(202) 223-2226

Domestic Violence

National Coalition Against Domestic Violence
1500 Massachusetts Avenue, NW, Suite 35
Washington, D. C. 20005
(202) 293-8260

Shelter Aid Hotline
(800) 333-SAFE

Local Battered Women's Shelters and Crisis Hotlines

through yearly or biyearly Pap tests is important. Osteoporosis affects about half of all women older than 45 years and 90% older than 75, and many develop complications such as atraumatic fractures. Postmenopausal estrogen replacement therapy has been shown to be effective in reducing osteoporosis-related fractures, and all women should be conseled regarding estrogen therapy.

- Domestic violence is the major cause of injury to women. Nurses working in community settings are often in a position to identify and intervene in cases of domestic violence and should be aware of characteristics of the victim, the batterer, and the family; recognize injuries and signs suggestive of domestic violence; and be prepared to intervene.

Learning Activities and Application to Practice

In Class

- In groups of three or four, have students research one of the issues described in this chapter (e.g., infertility, osteoporosis, domestic violence, contraception, cancer screening). What additional information were they able to identify, and how should the information be used in providing care to women in community-based settings?
- Examine the problem of teenage pregnancy in the area. How does it compare with other areas? What efforts have been made to reduce teenage pregnancy and to minimize the long-term associated problems?

In Clinical

- If feasible, allow students to provide care in a prenatal/postpartum clinic or private practice for several days. Encourage student preparation by reviewing relevant material (e.g., nutrition, developmental milestones in pregnancy, breastfeeding) to be ready for opportunities for health promotion and education.
- Encourage students to observe contraception counseling. What issues are discussed between the counselor and the client. What factors appear to determine the woman's choice? Are all relevant factors (e.g., effectiveness of method, possible complications and side effects, cost, proper use) presented and discussed?
- Allow students to participate in screening activities for women. Opportunities include teaching BSE, assisting with Pap smears, and observing for signs of domestic violence. Record impressions in a log or diary and share with other members of the clinical group.

REFERENCES

American Cancer Society. (1995). *Cancer Facts & Figures—1995*. Atlanta, GA, American Cancer Society.

Aretakis, D. (1996). Teen pregnancy. In M. Stanhope and J. Lancaster (Eds.). *Community Health Nursing: Promoting Health of Aggregates, Families and Individuals* (4th ed). St. Louis, MO, Mosby-Year Book, pp. 665–680.

Ashwill, J. W. and Droske, S. C. (1997). *Nursing Care of Children: Principles and Practice*. Philadelphia, W. B. Saunders.

Betz, C. L., Hunsberger, M. M., and Wright, S. (1994). *Family-Centered Nursing Care of Children* (2nd ed.). Philadelphia, W. B. Saunders.

Bobak, I. M., Jensen, M. D., and Zalar, M. K. (1989). *Maternity and Gynecologic Care: The Nurse and the Family*. St. Louis, MO, C. V. Mosby-Year Book, pp. 172–204.

Boyne, L. J. (1995). Maternal and fetal nutrition. In I. M. Bobak, D. L. Lowdermilk, and M. D. Jensen (Eds.). *Maternity Nursing* (4th ed.). St. Louis, MO, Mosby-Year Book, pp. 172–204.

Brown, S. S. (1989). Drawing women into prenatal care. *Family Planning Perspectives, 21* (2), 73–78.

Centers for Disease Control. (1993). Infant mortality—United States, 1990. *Morbidity and Mortality Weekly Report, 42* (9), 161–165.

Centers for Disease Control and Prevention. (1995). State-specific pregnancy and birth rates among teenagers—United States, 1991–1992. *Morbidity and Mortality Weekly Report, 44* (37), 677–683.

Clemen-Stone, S., Eigsti, D. G., and McGuire, S. L. (1995). *Comprehensive Community Health Nursing* (4th ed.). St. Louis, MO, Mosby-Year Book.

Dambro, M. R. (1996). *Griffith's 5 Minute Clinical Consult*. Baltimore, Williams & Wilkins.

Delahoussaye, C. P. (1994). Families with neonates. In C. L. Betz, M. M. Hunsberger, and S. Wright (Eds.). *Family-*

Centered Nursing Care of Children (2nd ed.). Philadelphia, W. B. Saunders, pp. 107–141.

Fowler, J. M. and Twiggs, L. B. (1994). Endometrial cancer. In R. E. Rakel (Ed.). *Conn's Current Therapy.* Philadelphia, W. B. Saunders, pp. 1074–1077.

Goldberg, M. S. (1994). Choosing a contraceptive. *Current Issues in Women's Health* (2nd ed.). Washington, D. C., Food and Drug Administration.

Grant, C. (1995). Physical and sexual abuse. In D. Antai-Otong (Ed.). *Psychiatric Nursing: Biological and Behavioral Concepts*. Philadelphia, W. B. Saunders, pp. 407–426.

Jackson, D. B. and Saunders, R. B. (1994). *Child Health Nursing: A Comprehensive Approach to the Care of Children and Their Families*. Philadelphia, J. B. Lippincott.

Jaroff, L. (1996). Rx: "Morning after" pills. *Time, July 15,* 59.

Jonas, S. (1995). Population data for health and health care. In A. R. Kovner (Ed.). *Jonas's Health Care Delivery in the United States* (5th ed.). New York, Springer Publishing Co., pp. 55–100.

Jones, L. C. and Trabeaux, S. (1996). Women's health. In M. Stanhope and J. Lancaster (Eds.), *Community Health Nursing: Promoting Health of Aggregates, Families and Individuals* (4th ed). St. Louis, MO, Mosby-Year Book, pp. 545–564.

Kovner, A. R. (1995). *Jonas's Health Care Delivery in the United States* (5th ed.). New York, Springer Publishing Co.

Maurer, F. A. (1995a). Teenage pregnancy. In C. M. Smith and F. A. Maurer (Eds.). *Community Health Nursing: Theory and Practice*. Philadelphia, W. B. Saunders, pp. 580–611.

Maurer, F. A. (1995b). Violence: A social and family problem. In C. M. Smith and F. A. Maurer (Eds.). *Community Health Nursing: Theory and Practice.* Philadelphia, W. B. Saunders, pp. 517–547.

Perry, S. E. (1995). Nursing care of the newborn. In I. M. Bobak, D. L. Lowdermilk, and M. D. Jensen (Eds.). *Maternity Nursing* (4th ed.). St. Louis, MO, Mosby-Year Book, pp. 361–406.

Quinn, E. B. (1995). Health promotion and screening. In I. M. Bobak, D. L. Lowdermilk, and M. D. Jensen (Eds.). *Maternity Nursing* (4th ed.). St. Louis, MO, Mosby-Year Book, pp. 839–856.

Quinn, E. B. and Lowdermilk, D. L. (1995). Common reproductive concerns. In I. M. Bobak, D. L. Lowdermilk, and M. D. Jensen (Eds.). *Maternity Nursing* (4th ed). St. Louis, MO, Mosby-Year Book, pp. 857–895.

Sherwen, L. N., Scoloveno, M. A., and Weingarten, C. T. (1995). *Nursing Care of the Childbearing Family* (2nd ed.). Norwalk, CT, Appleton & Lange.

Smith-DiJulio, K. and Holzapfel, S. K. (1994). Families in crisis: Family violence. In E. M. Varcarolis (Ed.). *Foundations of Psychiatric Mental Health Nursing* (2nd ed.). Philadelphia, W. B. Saunders, pp. 254–287.

U. S. Department of Health and Human Services. (1995). *Healthy People 2000: Midcourse Review and 1995 Revisions.* Washington, D. C., Government Printing Office.

U. S. Department of Health and Human Services. (1990). *Healthy People 2000: National Health Promotion and Disease Prevention Objectives*. Washington, D. C., Government Printing Office.

U. S. Department of Health and Human Services.(1989). *Your Contraceptive Choices For Now, For Later.* Bethesda, MD, U. S. Department of Health and Human Services.

U. S. Department of Health and Human Services/Office of Disease Prevention and Health Promotion. (1994). *Clinician's Handbook of Preventive Services*. Washington, D. C., Government Printing Office.

U. S. Department of Health and Human Services/Office of Disease Prevention and Health Promotion. (1996). *Guide to Clinical Preventive Services* (2nd ed.). Washington, D. C., Government Printing Office.

U. S. Department of Health and Human Services/Office of Population Affairs. (1994). *Trends in Adolescent Pregnancy and Childbearing.* Rockville, MD, U. S. Department of Health and Human Services/Office of Population Affairs.

Watkins, A. C. (1993). Family violence. In J. M. Swanson and M. Albrecht (Eds.). *Community Health Nursing: Promoting the Health of Aggregates.* Philadelphia, W. B. Saunders, pp. 459–488.

Wong, D. L. (1995). *Whaley & Wong's Nursing Care of Infants and Children* (5th ed.). St. Louis, MO, Mosby-Year Book.

13

Health Promotion and Illness Prevention for Infants, Children, and Adolescents

Case Study

Bonnie Dalton is a Registered Nurse working in a private pediatric office in a small city. In her position, Bonnie assists the pediatrician and pediatric nurse practitioner (PNP) by taking health histories, weighing and measuring the children, performing health teaching for the children and parents, administering medications, and assisting with some diagnostic and screening procedures (e.g., strep cultures, fingersticks), as well as performing many other interventions.

Last Monday, Bonnie saw Sally Benson for her 6-month well check. Sally was brought to the clinic by her mother. Bonnie observed that Sally was appropriately dressed, smiling, and responsive. Bonnie asked Mrs. Benson to remove Sally's clothes, and while this was being completed questioned her about Sally's eating and sleeping patterns and general health. She learned that Sally is breast fed and nurses six to eight times per day. Currently, she is being given only supplemental apple juice and an occasional bottle of formula when Mrs. Benson leaves her with a babysitter. Sally sleeps 10 to 11 hours at night, occasionally waking, and naps twice daily, for 1 to 2 hours.

Bonnie weighed and measured Sally and plotted the findings on a graphic chart kept in Sally's file. She noted that Sally weighed 17 pounds and measured 27 inches—a gain of 3 pounds and an increase of 1.5 inches since her 4-month visit. According to the chart, Sally's height and weight placed her within the 75th percentile for girls of her age.

When questioned, Mrs. Benson reported that Sally always rode in her car seat, there were plugs on all electrical outlets, and harmful substances and medications were in child-proof, latched cabinets. Other safety issues discussed included smoke detectors near the bedrooms and hot water heater temperature.

Bonnie assisted the PNP with a head-to-toe physical examination and Denver II Screening Test. All findings from both the physical and developmental examinations were considered "normal" for Sally's age.

The PNP instructed Mrs. Benson on slowly adding solid foods to Sally's diet, and Bonnie gave her several pamphlets and instruction guides kept in the clinic. The nurses also discussed several other safety issues, including poison control. Mrs. Benson was counseled to buy syrup of ipecac and to keep the number of the local poison control center near her telephone.

Routine neonatal screening tests (phenylketonuria, thyroid function, hemoglobin) had been performed shortly after Sally was born, and all results were normal. She was up to date on her immunizations and was scheduled to get her third vaccinations for hepatitis B, diphtheria/tetanus/pertussis, polio, and Haemophilus influenzae *B. Mrs. Benson reported that the only problem from previous immunizations was a slight fever during the afternoon and evening of the injections, which responded to administration of acetaminophen. Mrs. Benson was counseled again concerning possible side effects of immunizations and how to manage them.*

Bonnie gave Sally the oral polio first and followed with the injections. Sally cried a little but was consoled by her mother and stopped crying quickly. Mrs. Benson was encouraged to give Sally acetaminophen this afternoon and to call the office if she developed a temperature higher than 103°F or was crying inconsolably. Finally, Mrs. Benson was instructed to bring Sally back for her next well check when she was 12 to 15 months old.

The Health of Infants, Children, and Adolescents

Preventative health care for infants and children has had a profound effect on morbidity and mortality. In 1900, 87% of infants lived to age 1 year, and only 77% survived to age 20 years. In comparison, in 1990, 99.1% of infants survived until their first birthday, and 98.2% could expect to live to age 20 (National Center for Health Statistics [NCHS], 1994). This increase has been attributed to a number of factors. Improved prenatal and intrapartum care has reduced infant mortality dramatically. Infant mortality declined from approximately 165/1,000 births in 1900 to 47/1,000 in 1940 to 29.2/1,000 in 1950 to 9.1/1,000 in 1990 (Kovner, 1995; U. S. Department of Health and Human Services [USDHHS], 1990). Additionally, clean water, improved quality and quantity of food, and immunization against communicable diseases have contributed dramatically to infants and children reaching adulthood.

CAUSES OF MORTALITY

At present, the leading causes of death for infants younger than 1 year are congenital anomalies (20.9%), sudden infant death syndrome (SIDS) (14.5%), short gestation and low birth weight (11.3%), and respiratory distress syndrome (7.0%). Perinatal complications, including maternal complications; "complications of placenta, cord and membranes;" perinatal infections; and "intrauterine hypoxia and birth asphyxia" collectively account for 10.8% of infant deaths, and 35.5% are the result of "other causes" (Centers for Disease Control [CDC], 1993).

Causes of childhood mortality change dramatically after the first year of life. The leading causes of death per 100,000 children aged 1 to 4 years are unintentional injury (17.5), congenital anomalies (5.7), malignant neoplasms (3.5), homicide (2.8), and diseases of the heart (2.2). For children 1 to 14 years of age, the leading cause of death per 100,000 is unintentional injury (10.2), followed by malignant neoplasms (3.1), congenital anomalies (1.4), homicide (1.4), and heart disease (0.8). For teenagers and young adults (15–24 years of age), rates per 100,000 are accidents (42.0), homicide (22.4), suicide (13.1), cancer (5.0), and heart disease (2.7) (NCHS, 1993).

CAUSES OF MORBIDITY

The leading causes of *acute* illness in children are respiratory conditions (primarily the common cold, influenza, and acute respiratory infections), other "infective and parasitic diseases" (e.g., viral infections, intestinal virus), acute ear infections, and injuries. The most common *chronic* conditions in children include respiratory conditions (e.g., allergic rhinitis, chronic sinusitis, asthma, chronic bronchitis) and skin conditions (primarily acne and dermatitis). Musculoskeletal conditions producing orthopedic impairment (primarily back and lower extremities) and vision, speech, and hearing impairments are identified in many children (NCHS, 1994).

Respiratory conditions contribute to the most time lost from school, accounting for more than 50% of days absent. Common childhood diseases (e.g., viral infections) are responsible for almost 22% of school absences. Other common acute complaints that cause school absenteeism include ear infections, injuries (e.g., fractures, sprains), and digestive complaints (e.g., nausea, vomiting) (NCHS, 1994).

Children younger than 5 years see physicians more than any other age group until age 65 and older, averaging 6.9 physician contacts each year. In contrast, children and adolescents 5 to 17 years have 3.5 physician contacts per year.

Major reasons for hospitalization of children include respiratory conditions (e.g., asthma, bronchitis, pneumonia), injury and poisoning, digestive disorders (e.g., gastroenteritis, diarrhea), infectious and parasitic diseases, headache and seizures, chemotherapy, and unspecified viral illnesses (Betz et al., 1994; Evans and Friedland, 1994; and NCHS, 1994).

OTHER INDICATORS OF HEALTH

To prevent, detect, and minimize disease, disability, and death in infants and children, a number of indicators of health and well-being should be assessed, and appropriate interventions should be developed and implemented when problems or potential problems are identified. Health indicators to be assessed should include growth and development, vision, and hearing. General strategies for health promotion (e.g., good nutrition, exercise and fitness, dental care) should be taught and encouraged. Finally, identified threats or risk factors, such as threats to safety or substance use (e.g., tobacco, alcohol, drugs) must be addressed.

A number of *Healthy People 2000* (USDHHS, 1990) objectives specifically target health promotion and risk reduction strategies for infants, children, and adolescents. Table 13–1 presents some of these objectives. This chapter describes recommendations for primary health care, health promotion, and illness prevention activities and interventions appropriate for nurses caring for infants, children, and adolescents in community-based settings. Identification and management of common acute and chronic illness and conditions also are described.

Special Health Programs and Services for Children

To meet health care needs of disadvantaged, underserved, and disabled children, a number of federally sponsored programs have been developed over the past 3 decades. Nurses who practice in community settings, particularly those who care for underserved children, should be aware of services provided by these programs, have an understanding of eligibility requirements, and know how to refer clients. Several of the most commonly encountered programs and services are briefly discussed here.

MEDICAID AND THE EARLY AND PERIODIC SCREENING, DIAGNOSIS, AND TREATMENT PROGRAM

Children are overrepresented among those with no health insurance or those covered by public

TABLE 13–1 *Healthy People 2000*—Examples of Health Promotion Objectives for Children

1.4—Increase to at least 75% the proportion of children and adolescents 6–17 years of age who engage in vigorous physical activity that promotes the development and maintenance of cardiorespiratory fitness 3 days per week or more for 20 mintues per occasion (baseline: 66% for youth 10–17 years of age in 1984)

2.4—Reduce growth retardation among low-income children 5 years and younger to less than 10% (baseline: up to 16% among low-income children in 1988, depending on age and race/ethnicity)

Special Population Targets

Prevalence of Short Stature	*1988 Baseline (%)*	*2000 Target (%)*
2.4a—Low-income black children <1 year of age	15	10
2.4b—Low-income Hispanic children <1 year of age	13	10
2.4c—Low-income Hispanic children 1 year of age	16	10
2.4d—Low-income Asian/Pacific Islander children 1 year of age	14	10
2.4e—Low-income Asian/Pacific Islander children 2–4 years of age	16	10

2.10—Reduce iron deficiency to less than 3% among children 1–4 years of age (baseline: 9% for chidren 1–2 years of age; 4% for children 3–4 years of age in 1980)

Special Population Targets

Iron Deficiency Prevalence	*1980 Baseline (%)*	*2000 Target (%)*
2.10a—Low-income children 1–2 years of age	21	10
2.10b—Low-income children 3–4 years of age	10	5
2.10d—Alaska Native children 1–5 years of age	22–28 (1985)	10

3.5—Reduce the initiation of cigarette smoking by children and youth so that no more than 15% have become regular cigarette smokers by age 20 years (baseline: 30% of youth had become regular cigarette smokers by 20–24 years of age in 1987)

3.8—Reduce to no more than 20% the proportion of children 6 years of age and younger who are regularly exposed to tobacco smoke at home (baseline: more than 39% in 1986)

3.26—(1995 addition) Enact in 50 states and the District of Columbia laws banning cigarette vending machines, except in places inaccessible to minors (baseline: 12 states and the District of Columbia as of January 1995)

4.5—Increase by at least 1 year the average age of first use of cigarettes, alcohol, and marijuana by adolescents 12–17 years of age (baseline: age 11.6 years for cigarettes; age 13.1 years for alcohol; and age 13.4 years for marijuana in 1988)

4.13—Provide to children in all school districts and private schools primary and secondary school educational programs on alcohol and other drugs, preferably as part of comprehensive school health education (baseline: 63% provided some instruction; 39% provided counseling; and 23% referred students for clinical assessment in 1987)

6.14—Increase to at least 75% the proportion of providers of primary care for children who include assessment of cognitive, emotional, and parent-child functioning, with appropriate counseling, referral, and follow-up, in their clinical practices (baseline data not available)

7.4—Reverse to less than 22.56 per 1,000 children the number of abused children younger than 18 years (baseline: 22.6 per 1,000 in 1986)

9.5a—Reduce drowning deaths in children 4 years of age and younger to no more than 2.3 per 100,000 people (baseline: 4.2 in 1987)

9.6a—Reduce residential fire deaths to no more than 3.3 per 100,000 children 4 years of age and younger (baseline: 4.4 in 1987)

9.8a—Reduce incidence of nonfatal poisoning among children 4 years of age and younger to no more than 520 emergency department treatments per 100,000 (baseline: 648 in 1986)

9.12—Increase use of safety belts and child safety seats to at least 85% of motor vehicle occupants (baseline: 42% in 1988)

13.2—Reduce untreated dental caries so that the proportion of children with untreated caries (in permanent or primary teeth) is no more than 20% among children 6–8 years of age and no more than 15% among adolescents 15 years of age (baseline: 27% of children 6–8 years of age in 1986; 23% of adolescents 15 years of age in 1986–1987)

TABLE 13–1 ***Healthy People 2000*****—Examples of Health Promotion Objectives for Children** *Continued*

Special Population Targets *Continued*

Untreated Dental Caries Among Children	***1986–87 Baseline (%)***	***2000 Target (%)***
13.2a—Children 6–8 years of age whose parents have less than high school education	43	30
13.2b—Native American/Alaska Native children 6–8 years of age	64	35
13.2c—Black children 6–8 years of age	38	25
13.2d—Hispanic children 6–8 years of age	36	25

17.15—Increase to at least 80% the proportion of providers of primary care for children who routinely refer or screen infants and children for impairments of vision, hearing, speech, and language and assess other developmental milestones as part of well-child care (baseline data not available)

20.9—Reduce acute middle ear infection among children 4 years of age and younger, as measured by days of restricted activity or school absenteeism, to no more than 105 days per 100 children (baseline: 135.4 days per 100 children in 1987)

21.2b—Increase to at least 80% the proportion of children 2–12 years of age who have received, as a minimum within the appropriate interval, all of the screening and immunization services and at least one of the counseling services appropriate for their age and gender as recommended by the U.S. Preventive Services Task Force (baseline data not available)

From U.S. Department of Health and Human Services (1990). *Healthy People 2000: National Health Promotion and Disease Prevention Objectives.* Washington, D.C., Government Printing Office, U.S. Department of Health and Human Services. (1995). *Healthy People 2000: Midcourse Review and 1995 Revisions,* Washington, D.C., Government Printing Office.

insurance (e.g., Medicaid). Indeed, health care is financed by public sources for 23% of all persons 18 years and younger, and almost 46% of public health care dollars cover children. An additional 15% of all children have *no* health care insurance (Evans and Friedland, 1994).

Most children without health insurance are the dependents of full-time workers whose employers provided no health insurance. Lack of health insurance has a significant effect on children's health, as they are less likely to have a usual source of care, resulting in the use of emergency rooms, hospital outpatient departments, or school health centers as the primary health care provider. As a result, children without health insurance are much less likely to receive preventative health care and are more likely to receive health care after illnesses are advanced and care is more expensive.

As discussed in Chapter 3, Medicaid is a welfare assistance health program jointly sponsored by the federal government and each state. Children with Medicaid coverage are nearly as likely as children with private health insurance to have a usual source of care. This is very important for primary prevention, health education, and early identification and treatment of medical or developmental problems.

The Early and Periodic Screening, Diagnosis, and Treatment (EPSDT) program began in 1967 to identify and treat children's health problems before they become complex and costly. EPSDT "is a comprehensive and preventive health care program for Medicaid-eligible individuals up to age 21" (USDHHS/Health Care Financing Association [HCFA], 1992, p. 7). The program services may be provided by a public health clinic, community health center, school health services, Head Start program, qualified independent practitioners, and others. Under federal guidelines, all eligible children and their families must be informed about EPSDT services and where to obtain them. Furthermore, assistance with scheduling and transportation and assistance in using health resources effectively are components of EPSDT (Evans and Friedland, 1994; USDHHS/HCFA, 1992). Table 13–2 lists EPSDT required services.

TABLE 13–2 **Required Early and Periodic Screening, Diagnosis, and Treatment**

- Screening services
  - A comprehensive health and developmental history (which includes a physical and mental health assessment)
  - A comprehensive unclothed physical examination
  - Appropriate immunizations according to age and health history
  - Laboratory tests (e.g., blood lead level, hematocrit or hemoglobin, sickle cell test, tuberculosis skin test, as appropriate)
  - Health education (including anticipatory guidance)
- Dental services
- Hearing services, including hearing aids
- Vision services, including eyeglasses
- Any other necessary health care to correct or ameliorate illnesses and conditions found in screenings

From U.S. Department of Health and Human Services/Health Care Financing Administration (1992). *EPSDT: A Guide for Educational Programs.* HCFA Pub. No. 02192. Washington, D.C., Government Printing Office.

WOMEN, INFANTS AND CHILDREN

The Special Supplemental Nutrition Program for Women, Infants and Children (WIC) provides food, nutrition counseling, and access to health services for low-income women, infants, and children. WIC is a federally funded program administered by each state. Pregnant or postpartum women, infants, and children up to age 5 who meet income guidelines and residency requirements and are determined to be at "nutritional risk" are eligible. All persons receiving Aid to Families with Dependent Children, food stamps, or Medicaid are automatically eligible.

Most WIC programs provide vouchers that participants use at authorized stores to purchase nutritious foods. The foods included are high in protein, calcium, iron, and vitamins A and C. WIC foods include iron-fortified infant formula and infant cereal, iron-fortified adult cereal, vitamin C–rich fruit or vegetable juice, eggs, milk, cheese, peanut butter, and dried beans. Special infant formulas are provided, if prescribed. Participation in WIC has been shown to be effective in increasing gestation periods, raising birth weights, and reducing infant mortality. An estimated 40% of the babies born in the United States are served by WIC (U. S. Department of Agriculture/Food and Consumer Service, 1994).

HEAD START

Head Start is a federally funded, comprehensive preschool program for children who are at risk for academic problems associated with poverty and lack of sufficient social stimulation. Head Start was begun in 1965 to incorporate health, nutrition, parent involvement, and children's learning into a comprehensive program for disadvantaged children. Low-income children 3 to 5 years of age are eligible for Head Start programs. Although programs vary by area, health care is often a component of Head Start programs.

HEALTHY START

Healthy Start is a federally funded program with the goal of reducing infant mortality. Healthy Start was instituted to ensure accessible, acceptable, prenatal care for those at risk to improve the health of mothers and babies. These objectives are accomplished through integration and coordination of health and social services and provision of education about pregnancy, childbirth, and infant care. The program began in the early 1990s by providing special grants to 15 communities in which infant mortality is particularly high (e.g., Baltimore, MD; Birmingham, AL; Cleveland, OH; and New York City). Seven more cities were added to the program in 1994.

EDUCATION FOR ALL HANDICAPPED CHILDREN ACT

In response to lack of services for handicapped children, the Education for All Handicapped Children Act (Public Law [PL] 94–142) was passed in 1975. PL 94–142 is important and encompassing, as it mandates a free public education in the least restrictive environment for all handicapped children. In essence, this law requires public school districts to provide an educational environment that can meet the demands of children with disabilities, including children with physical impairments, learning disabilities, and mental and emotional disabilities.

To encourage "early intervention," in a 1986 amendment (PL 99–457), coverage for handicapped children was ensured from birth until age 21 years. PL 94–142 and PL 99–457 are now know as the Individuals with Disabilities Education Act. Services mandated by Individuals with Disabilities Education Act include necessary physical or occupational therapy, speech therapy, transportation to and from school, and counseling or psychiatric services. Periodic health or medical procedures (e.g., intermittent catheterization, tube feeding, tracheostomy suctioning) may be provided in some areas. Mainstreaming or *normalization* (integration of special needs children with other children of the same age in a regular classroom) is encouraged whenever possible (Selekman, 1995).

Primary Health Care Recommendations: United States Preventive Services Task Force

The U. S. Preventive Services Task Force (USDHHS/Office of Disease Prevention and Health Promotion [ODPHP], 1994) has developed guidelines to direct health care services for health promotion and illness prevention for individuals in all age groups. These recommendations include frequency of visits, screenings that should be performed (e.g., history, physical examination, laboratory or diagnostic procedures), appropriate parent or patient counseling and health teaching, immunization recommendations, and specific guidelines for individuals in "high-risk categories." Table 13–3 contains the recommendations from birth to 10 years of age, and Table 13–4 contains recommendations for 11 through 24 years of age. Specific assessment tools, health teaching information, and provider guidelines that address the specific recommendations are included throughout this chapter.

SCREENING RECOMMENDATIONS AND GUIDELINES

The recommendations of the Preventive Services Task Force include screening for a number of genetic, congenital, developmental, maturational, and pathological problems and conditions. Guidelines and examples of tools and teaching tips are described briefly (USDHHS, 1997).

Infant Screenings

Although there is considerable variation between states, all states require that *all* newborns be tested for congenital diseases. Testing for hypothyroidism and phenylketonuria, for example, is required by all states, and screening for galactosemia and hemoglobinopathies (e.g., sickle cell disease, thalassemia) is required by a majority of states. Additionally, some states require newborn screening for maple syrup urine disease, congenital adrenal hyperplasia, cystic fibrosis, and other conditions (USDHHS/ODPHP, 1994). All nurses who care for newborns in community settings should know the newborn screenings required by their state.

Newborn screenings are usually accomplished by collecting drops of blood onto specifically designed filter paper. The blood spot specimens should be obtained from every neonate before discharge or transfer from the nursery, regardless of the status of the infant's feeding or age. For full-term, well infants, the specimen should be obtained as close as possible to discharge from the nursery and *no later than 7 days of age*. If the initial specimen is obtained earlier than 24 hours after birth, a second specimen should be obtained at 1 to 2 weeks of age. Premature infants, infants receiving parenteral feeding, and infants receiving treatment for illness should have a specimen obtained for screening at or near the seventh day of life if it has not been done before that time,

TABLE 13–3 Recommendations of the U.S. Preventive Services Task Force—Birth Through 10 Years of Age

Interventions considered and recommended for the periodic health examination

Leading causes of death

- Conditions originating in perinatal period
- Congenital anomalies
- Sudden infant death syndrome (SIDS)
- Unintentional injuries (non-motor vehicle)
- Motor vehicle injuries

Interventions for the General Population

Screening

Height and weight
Blood pressure
Vision screen (age 3–4 years)
Hemoglobinopathy screen (birth)*
Phenylalanine level (birth)†
T_4 and/or TSH (birth)‡

Counseling

Injury Prevention

Child safety care seats (age <5 years)
Lap-shoulder belts (age ≥5 years)
Bicycle helmet, avoid bicycling near traffic
Smoke detector, flame retardant sleepwear
Hot water heater temperature <120–130°F
Window/stair guards, pool fence
Safe storage of drugs, toxic substances, firearms, and matches
Syrup of ipecac, poison control phone number
CPR training for parents/caretakers

Diet and Exercise

Breast-feeding, iron-enriched formula and foods (infants and toddlers)
Limit fat and cholesterol, maintain caloric balance, emphasize grains, fruits, vegetables (age ≥2 years)
Regular physical activity§

Substance Use

Effects of passive smoking§
Antitobacco message§

Dental Health

Regular visits to dental care provider§
Floss, brush with fluoride toothpaste daily§
Advice about baby bottle tooth decay§

Immunizations

Diphtheria-tetanus-pertussis (DTP)||
Oral poliovirus (OPV)¶
Measles-mumps-rubella (MMR)**
H. influenzae type b (Hib) conjugate††
Hepatitis B‡‡
Varicella§§

Chemoprophylaxis

Ocular prophylaxis (birth)

regardless of feeding status (American Academy of Pediatrics/Committee on Genetics, 1992).

Nurses who work in community settings such as pediatric clinics, health maintenance organizations, and other settings are frequently in a position to perform repeat testing and to follow up on positive or inconclusive results. They may also be in a position to identify those at risk for not being screened (e.g., premature infants, infants undergoing adoption, infants born at home, children of homeless families, and infants born outside the United States) (USDHHS/ODPHP, 1994). Table 13–5 describes one technique for collection of blood samples for infant screenings. Individual states, however, may provide different guidelines for collection of samples.

All abnormal results from infant screening tests require confirmatory testing and a thorough physical examination. Counseling should be provided to all parents of children with abnormal results and should include information about the significance of the results, the need for retesting, implications for the child's health, treatment, associated symptoms and complications to watch for, and genetic counseling for future childbearing (USDHHS/ODPHP, 1994).

TABLE 13–3 **Recommendations of the U.S. Preventive Services Task Force—Birth Through 10 Years of Age** *Continued*

Interventions for High-Risk Populations

Population	*Potential Interventions (see detailed high-risk [HR] definitions)‖‖*
Preterm or low birth weight	Hemoglobin/hematocrit (HR1)
Infants of mothers at risk for human immunodeficiency virus (HIV)	HIV testing (HR2)
Low income; immigrants	Hemoglobin/hematocrit (HR1); PPD (HR3)
Tuberculosis contacts	PPD (HR3)
Native American/Alaska Native	Hemoglobin/hematocrit (HR1); PPD (HR3); hepatitis A vaccine (HR4); pneumococcal vaccine (HR5)
Travelers to developing countries	Hepatitis A vaccine (HR4)
Residents of long-term care facilities	PPD (HR3); hepatitis A vaccine (HR4); influenza vaccine (HR6)
Certain chronic medical conditions	PPD (HR3); pneumococcal vaccine (HR5); influenza vaccine (HR6)
Increased individual or community lead exposure	Blood lead level (HR7)
Inadequate water fluoridation	Daily fluoride supplement (HR8)
Family history of skin cancer; nevi; fair skin, eyes, hair	Avoid excess/midday sun, use protective clothing§ (HR9)

*Whether screening should be universal or targeted to high-risk groups will depend on the proportion of high-risk individuals in the screening area and other considerations.

†If done during first 24 hours of life, repeat by age 2 weeks.

‡Optimally between day 2 and 6, but in all cases before newborn nursery discharge.

§The ability of clinician counseling to influence the behavior is unproven.

‖2, 4, 6, and 12–18 months; once between ages 4–6 years (DTaP may be used at 15 months and older).

¶2, 4, 6–18 months; once between ages 4–6 years.

**12–15 months and 4–6 years.

††2, 4, 6 and 12–15 months; no dose needed at 6 months if PRP-OMP vaccine is used for first 2 doses.

‡‡Birth, 1 month, 6 months, or 0–2 months later, and 6–18 months. If not done in infancy; current visit, and 1 and 6 months later.

§§12–18 months; or older child without history of chickenpox or previous immunization. Include information on risk in adulthood, duration of immunity, and potential need for booster doses.

‖‖**HR1** = Infants age 6–12 months who are living in poverty, black, Native American or Alaska Native, immigrants from developing countries, preterm or low birth weight infants, or infants whose principal dietary intake is unfortified cow's milk.

HR2 = Infants born to high-risk mothers whose HIV status is unknown. Women at high risk include past or present injection drug use; persons who exchange sex for money or drugs, and their sex partners; injection drug-using, bisexual, or HIV-positive sex partners currently or in past; persons seeking treatment for sexually transmitted diseases; blood transfusion during 1978–1985.

HR3 = Persons infected with HIV, close contacts of persons with known or suspected tuberculosis, persons with medical risk factors associated with tuberculosis, immigrants from countries with high tuberculosis prevalence, medically underserved low-income populations (including homeless), residents of long-term care facilities.

HR4 = Persons ≥2 years living in or traveling to areas where the disease is endemic and where periodic outbreaks occur (e.g., countries with high or intermediate endemicity; certain Alaska Native, Pacific Island, Native American, and religious communities). Consider for institutionalized children aged ≥2 years. Clinicians should also consider local epidemiology.

HR5 = Immunocompetent persons ≥2 years with certain medical conditions, including chronic cardiac or pulmonary disease, diabetes mellitus, and anatomic asplenia. Immunocompetent persons ≥2 years living in high-risk environments or social settings (e.g., certain Native American and Alaska Native populations).

HR6 = Annual vaccination of children ≥6 months who are residents of chronic care facilities or who have chronic cardiopulmonary disorders, metabolic diseases (including diabetes mellitus), hemoglobinopathies, immunosuppression, or renal dysfunction.

HR7 = Children about age 12 months who 1) live in communities in which the prevalence of lead levels requiring individual intervention, including residential lead hazard control or chelation, is high or undefined; 2) live in or frequently visit a home built before 1950 with dilapidated paint or with recent or ongoing renovation or remodeling; 3) have close contact with a person who has an elevated lead level; 4) live near lead industry or heavy traffic; 5) live with someone whose job or hobby involves lead exposure; 6) use lead-based pottery; or 7) take traditional ethnic remedies that contain lead.

HR8 = Children living in areas with inadequate water fluoridation (<0.6 ppm).

HR9 = Persons with a family history of skin cancer, a large number of moles, atypical moles, poor tanning ability, or light skin, hair, and eye color.

From U.S. Department of Health and Human Services (USDHHS). (1997). *Guide to Clinical Preventive Services* (2nd ed.). Washington, D.C., Government Printing Office.

TABLE 13–4 **Recommendations of the U.S. Preventive Services Task Force—11–24 Years of Age**

Interventions considered and recommended for the periodic health examination

Leading causes of death

- Motor vehicle/other unintentional injuries
- Homicide
- Suicide
- Malignant neoplasms
- Heart diseases

Interventions for the General Population

Screening

Height and weight
Blood pressure*
Papanicolaou (Pap) test† (females)
Chlamydia screen‡ (females <20 years)
Rubella serology of vaccination§ (females >12 years)
Assess for problem drinking

Counseling

Injury Prevention

Lap/shoulder belts
Bicycle/motorcycle/all-terrain vehicle helmets||
Smoke detector||
Safe storage/removal of firearms*

Substance Use

Avoid tobacco use
Avoid underage drinking and illicit drug use||
Avoid alcohol/drug use while driving, swimming, boating, etc.||

Sexual Behavior

Sexually transmitted disease (STD) prevention: abstinence;|| avoid high-risk behavior;|| condoms/female barrier with spermicide||
Unintended pregnancy contraception

Diet and Exercise

Limit fat and cholesterol; maintain caloric balance; emphasize grains, fruits, vegetables
Adequate calcium intake (females)
Regular physical activity||

Dental Health

Regular visits to dental care provider||
Floss, brush with fluoride toothpaste daily||

Immunizations

Tetanus-diphtheria (Td) boosters (11–16 years)
Hepatitis B¶
MMR (11–12 years)**
Varicella (11–12 years)††
Rubella[4] (females >12 years)

Chemoprophylaxis

Multivitamin with folic acid (females planning/capable of pregnancy)

Interventions for High-Risk Populations

Population	***Potential Interventions*** (See detailed high-risk [HR] definitions)‡‡
High-risk sexual behavior	RPR/VDRL (HR1); screen for gonorrhea (female) (HR2), HIV (HR3), chlamydia (female) (HR4); hepatitis A vaccine (HR5)
Injection or street drug use	RPR/VDRL (HR1); human immunodeficiency virus (HIV) screen (HR3); hepatitis A vaccine (HR5); PPD (HR6); advice to reduce infection risk (HR7)
Tuberculosis contacts; immigrants; low income	PPD (HR6)
Native Americans/Alaska Natives	Hepatitis A vaccine (HR5); PPD (HR6); pneumococcal vaccine (HR8)
Travelers to developing countries	Hepatitis A vaccine (HR5)
Certain chronic medical conditions	PPD (HR6); pneumococcal vaccine (HR8); influenza vaccine (HR9)

TABLE 13–4 **Recommendations of the U.S. Preventive Services Task Force—11–24 Years of Age** *Continued*

Interventions for High-Risk Populations *Continued*

Population	***Potential Interventions***
Settings where adolescents and young adults congregate	Second MMR (HR10)
Susceptible to varicella, measles, mumps	Varicella vaccine (HR11); MMR (HR12)
Blood transfusion between 1978–1985	HIV screen (HR3)
Institutionalized persons; health care/laboratory workers	Hepatitis A vaccine (HR5); PPD (HR6); influenza vaccine (HR9)
Family history of skin cancer; nevi; fair skin, eyes, hair	Avoid excess/midday sun, use protective clothing‖ (HR13)
Prior pregnancy with neural tube defect	Folic acid 4.0 mg (HR14)
Inadequate water fluoridation	Daily fluoride supplement (HR15)

*Periodic blood pressure for persons aged ≥21 years.

†If sexually active at present or in the past: every ≤3 years. If sexual history is unreliable, begin Pap tests at age 18 years.

‡If sexually active.

‖The ability of clinician counseling to influence this behavior is unproven.

§Serological testing, documented vaccination history, and routine vaccination against rubella (preferably with measles, mumps, and rubella [MMR]) are equally acceptable alternatives.

¶If not previously immunized: current visit, 1 and 6 months later.

**If no previous second dose of MMR.

‡‡If susceptible to chickenpox.

‡‡**HR1** = Persons who exchange sex for money or drugs, and their sex partners; persons with other STDs (including HIV); and sexual contacts of persons with active syphilis. Clinicians should also consider local epidemiology.

HR2 = Females who have: two or more sex partners in the last year; a sex partner with multiple sexual contacts; exchanged sex for money or drugs; or a history of repeated episodes of gonorrhea. Clinicians should also consider local epidemiology.

HR3 = Males who had sex with males after 1975; past or present injection drug use; persons who exhange sex for money or drugs, and their sex partners; injection drug-using, bisexual, or HIV-positive sex partner currently or in the past; blood transfusion during 1978–1985; persons seeking treatment for STDs. Clinicians should also consider local epidemiology.

HR4 = Sexually active females with multiple risk factors including: history of prior STD; new or multiple sex partners; age under 25; nonuse or inconsistent use of barrier contraceptives; cervical ectopy. Clinicians should consider local epidemiology of the disease in identifying other high-risk groups.

HR5 = Persons living in, traveling to, or working in areas where the disease is endemic and where periodic outbreaks occur (e.g., countries with high or intermediate endemicity; certain Alaska Native, Pacific Island, Native American, and religious communities); men who have sex with men; injection or street drug users. Vaccine may be considered for institutionalized persons and workers in these institutions, military personnel, and day-care, hospital, and laboratory workers. Clinicians should also consider local epidemiology.

HR6 = HIV positive, close contacts of persons with known or suspected tuberculosis, health care workers, persons with medical risk factors associated with tuberculosis, immigrants from countries with high tuberculosis prevalence, medically underserved low-income populations (including homeless), alcoholics, injection drug users, and residents of long-term care facilities.

HR7 = Persons who continue to inject drugs.

HR8 = Immunocompetent persons with certain medical conditions, including chronic cardiac or pulmonary disease, diabetes mellitus, and anatomic asplenia. Immunocompetent persons who live in high-risk environments or social settings (e.g., certain Native American and Alaska Native populations).

HR9 = Annual vaccination of residents of chronic care facilities; persons with chronic cardiopulmonary disorders, metabolic diseases (including diabetes mellitus), hemoglobinopathies, immunosuppression, or renal dysfunction; and health care providers for high-risk patients.

HR10 = Adolescents and young adults in settings where such individuals congregate (e.g., high schools and colleges), if they have not previously received a second dose.

HR11 = Healthy persons aged ≥13 years without a history of chickenpox or previous immunization. Consider serologic testing for presumed susceptible persons aged ≥13 years.

HR12 = Persons born after 1956 who lack evidence of immunity to measles or mumps (e.g., documented receipt of live vaccine on or after the first birthday, laboratory evidence of immunity, or a history of physician-diagnosed measles or mumps).

HR13 = Persons with a family or personal history of skin cancer, a large number of moles, atypical moles, poor tanning ability, or light skin, hair, and eye color.

HR14 = Women with prior pregnancy affected by neural tube defect who are planning pregnancy.

HR15 = Persons aged <17 years living in areas with inadequate water fluoridation (<0.6 ppm).

From U.S. Department of Health and Human Services. (1997). *Guide to Clinical Preventive Services* (2nd ed.). Washington, D.C., Government Printing Office.

PPD = purified protein derivative; RPR/VDRL = rapid plasma reagin/Venereal Disease Research Laboratory

TABLE 13–5 **Blood Collection Technique for Infant Screenings**

1. The same standards and techniques for collection of blood specimens for neonatal screening should be applied for all of the congenital diseases. State screening agencies hold individual hospitals accountable for instituting policies that ensure the correct collection of filter paper blood samples.
2. Required information should be entered on the specimen collection kit with a ballpoint pen, not a soft-tip pen or typewriter.
3. Universal precautions (e.g., wearing gloves and disposal of used lancets) should be taken.
4. The source of blood must be the most lateral surface of the plantar aspect of the infant's heel. The central area of the newborn's foot (area of the arch) or fingers *must not be used.*
5. Warming the puncture site can increase blood flow. A warm, moist towel (no hotter than 108°F) may be placed on the site for 3 minutes. Also, holding the infant's leg in a position lower than the heart will increase venous pressure.
6. The infant's heel should be cleaned with 70% isopropyl alcohol. Excess alcohol should be wiped away with a dry sterile gauze or cotton ball and the heel allowed to air dry thoroughly. Failure to remove alcohol may dilute the specimen and affect test results.
7. To ensure that sufficient flow of blood is obtained, the plantar surface of the infant's heel should be punctured with a sterile lancet to a depth of 2.0–2.4 mm or with an automated lancet device. The first drop of blood should be wiped away with sterile gauze. The puncture site should not be milked or squeezed, as this may cause hemolysis and mixture of tissue fluids with the specimen.
8. Care should be taken to avoid touching the area within the printed circle on the filter paper before collection. The filter paper should be touched gently against a large drop of blood and a sufficient quantity of blood allowed to soak through to fill completely the circle on the filter paper. The paper should not be pressed against the puncture site on the heel and blood should be applied only to one side of the paper. Both sides of the filter paper should be examined to ensure that the blood has penetrated and saturated the paper. Successive drips of blood should not be layered within the circle. If blood flow diminishes so that the circle is not completely filled, the sample should be collected from a different site. The sample should be allowed to dry thoroughly before insertion into the envelope.
9. After the specimen has been collected, the foot should be elevated above the body and a sterile gauze pad or cotton ball pressed against the puncture site until the bleeding stops. It is not advisable to apply adhesive bandages over skin puncture sites in newborns.

Adapted from U.S. Department of Health and Human Services/Office of Disease Prevention and Health Promotion. (1994). *Clinician's Handbook of Preventive Services.* Washington, D.C., Government Printing Office; data from National Committee for Clinical Laboratory Standards. (1992). *Blood Collection on Filter Paper for Neonatal Screening Programs* (2nd ed.). Villanova, PA, National Committee for Clinical Laboratory Standards.

Body Measurement

Significant childhood conditions, such as growth retardation, malnutrition, eating disorders, and obesity, may be identified by regularly scheduled measurement of height and weight throughout infancy and childhood. In addition, head circumference should be measured at birth; at 2 to 4 weeks; and at 1, 2, 4, 6, 9, 12, 15, 18, and 24 months of age to identify potential abnormalities (e.g., hydrocephalus). General guidelines for body measurement suggested by the ODPHP (USDHHS/ODPHP, 1994) are described here.

Height. For children younger than 2 years, height should be obtained by measuring recumbent length. A measuring board with a stationary headboard and sliding vertical foot piece can be used. If one is not available, a stationary vertical surface (e.g., the wall bordering the examining table) and a yardstick or tape measure may be used. In general, the infant or child should lie flat against the center of the board, with the head held against the head board and the legs extended. The foot piece, tape measure, or yardstick is positioned to the child's heels, and the height should be read to the nearest quarter inch.

For children 2 years and older, standing height is measured with a stadiometer or a graduated ruler or tape attached to a wall with a flat surface placed horizontally on top of the head. The child should wear only socks or be barefoot, with the knees straight and feet flat on the floor. While the child looks straight ahead, the flat surface or moveable headboard should be placed on the top of the head, compressing the hair, and the height read and recorded. If height measuring devices attached to weight scales are used, they should be checked frequently for accuracy.

Weight. To improve accuracy, a balance-beam or electronic scale should be used to obtain weights. The scale should be checked to ensure that it reads "0" before each use and should be checked periodically. Infants and small children should be weighted wearing only a dry diaper or light underpants. If possible, the same scale should be used for each measurement.

Head Circumference. The circumference of the head should be measured by extending a measuring tape around the most prominent part of the occiput to the middle of the forehead and lightly tightening to compress the hair. Head circumference is usually read to the nearest quarter inch or centimeter. A plastic or disposable paper tape is preferable to a cloth tape, as the latter may stretch.

General Instructions. All measurements should be plotted on age- and gender-specific growth charts for comparison with reference standards. Further, measurements should be interpreted within the context of the individual child's family and growth history. For example, if the child's height is above the 90th percentile, assessment of the height of the parents for comparison is warranted. Furthermore, as discussed in Chapter 6, some variation in size occurs between different racial and ethnic groups; whites and African-Americans tend to be taller than children of Southeast Asian descent. Age- and gender-specific growth charts for height and weight and head circumference may be obtained from Ross Laboratories (call 1-800-227-5767) or Meade Johnson Nutritional Division (call [812] 429-5000 for name and number of area representative).

Developmental Screening

Monitoring the progression of infants, children, and adolescents through developmental tasks is a crucial component of comprehensive health care. Assessment of developmental level can be accomplished by using screening tools, a thorough history, physical assessment, and/or directed observation. To help nurses recognize appropriate developmental tasks, Table 13–6 is included to outline some common physical, psychosocial, and cognitive developmental tasks.

The Denver II is a revision of the classic tool—the Denver Developmental Screening Test. The Denver II is a screening tool used to assess the overall developmental status of children from birth to age 6 and to alert the health care professional to potential developmental difficulties. Areas covered in the Denver II are personal-social tasks (e.g., getting along with people and caring for personal needs), fine motor-adaptive tasks (e.g., hand-eye coordination, manipulation of small objects), language (e.g., hearing, understanding, and using language), and gross motor abilities (e.g., sitting, walking, jumping) (Frankenburg and Dodds, 1990). All persons using this test are urged to participate in a training program to learn to administer and interpret the test correctly. Additional information can be obtained from Denver Developmental Materials, Inc., P. O. Box 6919, Denver, Colorado 80206-0919; (303) 355-4729.

Vision Screening

Refractive errors (myopia, hyperopia, astigmatism) are the most common vision disorders in children, occurring in about 20%. Other visual disorders affecting 2 to 5% of all children include amblyopia ("lazy eye"), strabismus (ocular misalignment; "cross eyes"), and anisometropia (difference between the two eyes in nearsightedness, farsightedness, and astigmatism). Each of these conditions usually develops in children between infancy and 5 to 7 years of age. Congenital cataracts, congenital glaucoma, retinoblastoma, and retinopathy of prematurity are other, less commonly observed eye conditions occurring in in-

TABLE 13–6 **Developmental Tasks for Infants and Children (Includes Physical, Psychosocial, and Cognitive)**

	Age	Task
Infancy	3 months	Experiences decrease in primitive reflexes, except protective and postural reflexes
		Develops social smile (indicates development of memory traces)
	4 months	Laughs
	5 months	Birth weight doubles
		When prone, can push up on arms
		Rolls over
	6 months	Begins teething
		Sits with support
		Exhibits "stranger anxiety" (is wary of strangers and clings to mother)
	8 months	Sits alone
		Crawls
	9 months	Can use pincer grasp
		Holds own bottle
	10 months	Stands with support
	12 months	Birth weight triples
		Takes first steps alone
		Develops trust
		Speaks five words
		Claps hands; waves "bye-bye"
Toddlerhood	13 months–2.5 years	Masters walking
		Climbs stairs
		Feeds self (autonomy)
		Uses language (increases to 400 words and two- to three-word phrases)
		Masters toilet training/bowel and bladder control
		Has separation anxiety (screams when the mother leaves)
Preschool	2.5–4 years	Increases vocabulary; uses sentences
		Alternates feet on steps
		Copies circles and lines
		Builds a tower of blocks
		Begins to have concepts of causality, time, and numbers
		Develops body image
		Role plays
		Begins enculturation
		Begins development of conscience
		Has fears of loss of body integrity
School age	5–12 years	Vision matures by age 6 years
		Loses first baby tooth at age 6 years; gets all permanent teeth except final molars by age 12 years
		Develops peer relationships
		Enjoys activities/groups/teams
		Develops morality
		Has cognitive development: concepts of time/space, reversibility, conservation, parts/whole
		Can classify objects in more than one way
		Develops reading/spelling and math concepts
		Begins puberty: age 9 years for girls; age 11 years for boys
		Gains sense of industry
Adolescence	13–19+ years	Develops secondary sex characteristics
		Attains adult growth
		Adjusts to body changes
		Begins menses (girls)
		Develops abstract thought
		Develops an identity
		Fantasizes role in different situations
		Has increased heterosexual interests
		Has increased peer influences

From: J. Selekman. *Pediatric Nursing.* Springhouse, PA, Springhouse.

fancy and childhood (USDHHS, 1990; USDHHS/ODPHP, 1994).

Normal vision is important for development, and "failure to treat amblyopia, anisometropia and strabismus before school age may result in irreversible visual deficits, permanent amblyopia, loss of depth perception and binocularity, cosmetic defects and educational and occupational restrictions" (USDHHS, 1990, p. 454). Thus, early detection and treatment of vision disorders is essential for normal eye development. A careful history, thorough examination, vision testing, and referral of abnormal or asymmetrical results for further testing and treatment promotes normal vision development. Table 13–7 outlines guidelines for vision testing of infants and children.

Hearing Screening

Hearing impairment affects all aspects of an individual's life, including developmental, educational, cognitive, emotional, and social components. An estimated 1 to 2% of children in the United States have some degree of hearing impairment. Hearing loss may be congenital or acquired during infancy or childhood. Temporary hearing loss associated with otitis media is fairly common among school-aged children, occurring in 5 to 7% of all children (USDHHS, 1990). Infants at greatest risk for hearing loss include those with low birth weight; congenital infection (e.g., rubella, toxoplasmosis, syphilis, cytomegalovirus, herpes); craniofacial anomalies; hyperbilirubinemia requiring exchange transfusion; Apgar scores of 0 to 3 at 5 minutes; mechanical ventilation for cardiopulmonary disease for 2 days or more; and neonatal intracranial hemorrhage, prematurity, and hospitalization in the intensive care nursery. Indicators and risk factors for hearing loss in children younger than 2 years include parental concern that a hearing, speech, language, or developmental delay is present; bacterial meningitis; head trauma (particularly in the temporal bone area); infectious

TABLE 13–7 **Guidelines for Vision Screening in Children**

1. The child's health history should include assessment of the child and family for risk factors for vision disorders, including
   - Family history of vision or eye problems
   - History of maternal, intrapartum, or neonatal conditions that may place the child at risk for visual disorders
   - Parental concern about the child's visual function
   - Changes in school performance, such as worsening grades and other difficulties that may be related to vision problems
2. Physical examination of the eye should include inspection of the lids, lashes, tear ducts, orbit, conjunctiva, sclera, cornea, iris, pupillary responsiveness, range of motion, anterior chamber, lens, vitreous, retina, and optic nerve and vessels
3. A comprehensive eye examination should include red reflex examination, corneal light reflex test (to detect strabismus), differential occlusion test (to detect strabismus), fixation (to determine if the eyes are aligned in the same direction without deviation), cover/uncover test (to detect strabismus), and stereotesting (binocular depth perception); to test for visual acuity, the use of charts such as the Snellen Letters, Tumbling E, or Allen Figures is recommended; for children, a distance of 10 feet (using an appropriate chart) may encourage better compliance; a passing score should be given for a line on which the child gives more than 50% correct responses
4. Referral should be made for a child with any abnormalities detected by any test, a visual acuity examination showing a difference in scores of two or more lines between eyes, children younger than 5 years scoring 20/40 or worse in either eye, and children older than 5 years scoring 20/30 or worse in either eye
5. Parents and children should be counseled about eye safety and the use of protective equipment (e.g., safety lenses and frames for science laboratories, shop class, or certain sports)

Adapted from U.S. Department of Health and Human Services. *Clinician's Handbook of Preventive Services.* Washington, D.C., Government Printing Office.

diseases known to be associated with sensorineural hearing loss (e.g., mumps, measles); a neurodegenerative disorder associated with hearing loss; and/or ototoxic medications used for more than 5 days (USDHHS/ODPHP, 1994).

Prevention, early detection, and intervention, particularly in infants, is critical in reducing functional limitation and disability due to hearing impairment (USDHHS, 1990). Some congenital hearing impairments and some acquired during infancy are preventable. Hearing loss due to otitis media and other diseases can be reduced through appropriate primary care. In addition, steps to minimize or manage hearing deficits through employment of assistive devices (e.g., hearing aids and special equipment) should be instituted as soon as possible to minimize developmental delays. Table 13–8 describes guidelines for hearing screening.

Lead Screening

The threat of childhood exposure to lead was discussed in Chapter 5. A few key points are repeated here and expanded to include guidelines for screening and treatment.

High blood lead levels have been identified as a *very* serious threat to children in the United States. This condition disproportionately affects minority and poor children in inner cities, where an estimated 3 million children younger than 6 years (about 15% of all children in this age group) have blood lead levels high enough to adversely affect their intelligence, behavior, and development (CDC/National Center for Environmental Health, 1994). At greatest risk for lead poisoning are children who

1. Live in a house or regularly visit a day care center, preschool, babysitter, or other house built before 1960
2. Live in or regularly visit a house built before 1960 with recent, ongoing, or planned renovation
3. Have a brother, sister, or playmate being treated for lead poisoning
4. Live with an adult whose job, hobby, or use of ethnic remedies involves lead
5. Live near an active lead smelter, battery recycling plant, or other industry likely to release lead

General guidelines for lead screening suggested by the CDC (1991) include initiation of risk assessment and counseling from prenatal visits until

TABLE 13–8 **Guidelines for Hearing Screening**

1. The health history of each child should assess for risk factors of hearing impairment
2. Parents should be questioned about the auditory responsiveness and speech and language development of young children; any parental reports of impairment should be seriously evaluated
3. Clinicians should consider referring all infants and young children with suspected hearing difficulties to an audiologist for evaluation
4. During physical examinations, clinicians should assess the ear, head, and neck for defects; abnormalities of the ear canal (inflammation, cerumen impaction, tumors, or foreign bodies) and the tympanic membrane (perforation, retraction or evidence of effusion) should be noted and addressed
5. Beginning about age 3 years, children may be screened by pure-tone audiometry; the test should be performed in a quiet environment using earphones; each ear should be tested at 500, 1000, 2000, and 4000 Hz
6. Audiometric evidence of hearing impairment should be substantiated by repeat screening; earphones should be removed and repositioned and instructions carefully repeated to the child; referral to a qualified specialist (e.g., audiologist, otolaryngologist) is recommended if repeat examination suggests impairment
7. The audiometer should be calibrated yearly, and the operator should listen to it each day of use to detect gross abnormalities

Adapted from U.S. Department of Health and Human Services. (1994). *Clinician's Handbook of Preventive Services.* Washington, D.C., Government Printing Office.

the child is 6 years of age. Although some disagreement exists among pediatric health care authorities, in general, recommendations are that children with any risk factors listed here should be tested for lead exposure. Screening should be done at about 6 to 12 months of age and again at about 24 months. Infants at high risk should be screened initially at 6 months and every 6 months. After two consecutive measurements of under 10 μg/dL, the child should be retested in 1 year. Rescreening should occur at any time when history suggests that exposure has increased, up to about age 6 years, unless otherwise indicated (USDHHS/ODPHP, 1994).

To screen for lead, capillary specimens should be carefully collected to minimize contamination. Recommendations include washing the child's hand (or feet for infants younger than 1 year) with soap and water, then cleansing with alcohol. The first drop of blood should be wiped off with sterile gauze or a cotton ball. Elevated blood lead results (over 15 μg/dL) should be confirmed using venous blood. Table 13–9 details CDC recommendations for interpretation of blood lead levels. Finally, all families should be counseled on sources of lead exposure and how to prevent exposure. See Chapter 5 for teaching tips to avoid lead exposure.

Anemia Screening

Iron deficiency anemia is the most common nutritional disorder in the United States, affecting an estimated 16% of low-income children (Wong, 1995). In infants and children, anemia is associated with fatigue, apathy, growth and development impairment, and decreased resistance to infection. Risk of anemia is related to low socioeconomic status, consumption of cow's milk before 6 months of age, consumption of formula not fortified with iron, and low birth weight. General recommendations are that the hemoglobin or hematocrit levels be checked during infancy (6–9 months), early childhood, late childhood, and early adolescence (USDHHS/ODPHP, 1994). Table 13–10 presents standards for diagnosis of anemia in children and adolescents.

Therapeutic management of iron deficiency anemia focuses on increasing the amount of iron that the child receives. Dietary supplementation includes the use of iron-fortified formulas and cereal for infants. Oral supplements may be recommended and the child retested in 3 to 4 months if anemia is fairly significant. If anemia does not improve, intramuscular or intravenous iron may be administered. Transfusions are only indicated in severe anemia (Wong, 1995). *Prevention* of iron deficiency anemia is described later in this chapter.

HEALTH PROMOTION

Health promotion refers those activities that are related to individual lifestyle choices that can influence health. Components of health promotion for infants and children that are of particular importance to nurses who practice in community settings are physical activity and fitness, nutrition, and dental health. Basic information for assessment, health teaching, and counseling is presented here.

Nutrition

Good nutrition is essential for life, health, and well-being. Conversely, poor nutrition can be harmful, as dietary factors are associated with 5 of the 10 leading causes of death (i.e., heart disease, some types of cancer, stroke, diabetes, and atherosclerosis) (USDHHS, 1990). Malnutrition in the United States is rarely the result of a lack of a sufficient quantity of food, but is more often caused by deficiencies of certain nutrients (e.g., iron, calcium, protein, and some vitamins) and excesses of others (e.g., calories, fats, simple sugars).

According to Wong (1995), most food preferences and dietary habits are established during childhood. The importance of good nutritional habits should be taught from an early age. In general, good nutrition for children includes three healthy meals per day and two healthy snacks. Providing nutrition education for children from preschool through high school should be encouraged.

TABLE 13–9 **Centers for Disease Control and Prevention Recommendations for Follow-Up of Blood Lead Measurements**

Class	Blood Lead Concentration (μg/dL)	Action
I	≤9	Low risk: 6–35 months of age—retest at 24 months of age (when blood levels peak), if resources allow ≥36 and <72 months of age—retesting not necessary unless history suggests exposure has increased High risk: 6–35 months of age—retest every 6 months; after two subsequent consecutive measurements are <10 μg/dL, or three are <15 μg/dL, retest once a year ≥36 to 72 months of age—retest once a year until sixth birthday
IIA	10–14	Low risk: 6–35 months of age—retest every 3–4 months After two consecutive measurements are <10 μg/dL or three are <15 μg/dL, retest once a year ≥36 and <72 months of age—retesting not necessary if all previous test results are <15 μg/dL, unless history suggests exposure has increased High risk: 6–35 months of age—retest every 3–4 months After two consecutive measurements are <10 μg/dL or three are <15 μg/dL, retest once a year ≥36 and <72 months of age—retest once a year until sixth birthday
IIB	15–19	Retest every 3–4 months; the family should be given education and nutritional counseling and a detailed environmental history should be taken to identify any obvious sources or pathways of lead exposure; if venous blood level is in this range in two consecutive tests 3–4 months apart, environmental investigation and abatement should be conducted, if resources permit
III	20–44*	Retest every 3–4 months. Conduct a complete medical evaluation, including iron deficiency testing; environmental lead sources should be identified and eliminated; pharmacological treatment may be necessary
IV	45–69*	Begin medical treatment and environmental assessment and remediation within 48 hours
V	≥70*	Begin medical treatment and environmental assessment and remediation immediately

*Based on confirmatory blood lead level.

From U.S. Department of Health and Human Services. (1994). *Clinician's Handbook of Preventive Services.* Washington, D.C.; Government Printing Office; data from Centers for Disease Control. (1991). *Preventing Lead Poisoning in Young Children. A Statement by the Centers for Disease Control.* Atlanta, GA, Centers for Disease Control.

TABLE 13–10 **Hemoglobin and Hematocrit Cutpoints for Anemia in Children 1 Year of Age or Older**

Gender	Age (years)	Hemoglobin (g/dL)	Hematocrit (%)
Both	1.0–1.9	11.0	33.0
	2.0–4.9	11.2	34.0
	5.0–7.9	11.4	34.5
	8.0–11.9	11.6	35.0
Female	12.0–14.9	11.8	35.5
	15.0–17.9	12.0	36.0
	≥18	12.0	36.0
Male	12.0–14.9	12.3	37.0
	15.0–17.9	12.6	38.0
	≥18	13.6	41.0

From Centers for Disease Control. (1989). CDC criteria for anemia in children and childbearing-aged women. *Morbidity and Mortality Weekly Report, 38,* 400–404.

Infant Nutrition. As described previously, iron deficiency anemia is the most common nutritional disorder in infants and children. To prevent anemia, the American Academy of Pediatrics recommends use of breast milk or commercial infant formula for the first year of life, use of iron supplementation (e.g., iron-fortified commercial formula or iron-fortified cereal for breast-fed babies) to provide 1 mg/kg/day of iron by 4 to 6 months of age, use of iron (ferrous sulfate) drops (from 2–3 mg/kg/day to 15 mg/kg/day) to breastfed preterm infants after 2 months of age and iron-fortified infant cereal when solid foods are introduced, and limiting the amount of formula to no more than 1 L/day to encourage the intake of iron-rich solid foods (Wong, 1995).

Addition of solid foods into the infant's diet should be done gradually. Commercially prepared infant cereal (e.g., rice, barley, oatmeal) is usually introduced first. Rice cereal is often suggested because of its easy digestibility and low allergic potential (Wong, 1995). Most often, strained fruits are introduced initially, followed by vegetables and then meats. Crackers or zwieback is offered at about 6 months of age. Small amounts of raw fruits and vegetables can be added gradually. General guidelines for the addition of solid foods is another important consideration in nutrition counseling. Table 13–11 presents information on feeding during the first year that is helpful when counseling parents. Most clinics and physician's offices have pamphlets and brochures to provide parents more detailed information on these topics; these materials can be used by the nurse to supplement health teaching.

Infant nutrition is also discussed in Chapter 12. Included in that chapter are strategies to encourage breastfeeding, how to choose infant formulas, and techniques for bottle-feeding.

Nutritional Needs of Children. Adequate caloric and nutrient intake is critical for supporting growth and development of children. In general, recommended nutrition intake for children includes two to three servings (2–3 ounces) per day of meat or meat substitutes (e.g., beans, lentils), 2 to 4 cups of milk or milk equivalent servings, depending on age and size, five or more servings of vegetables and fruits (including a dark green or deep yellow vegetable for vitamin A and fruits or vegetables that contain vitamin C), and four or more servings of breads and cereals. Fats, oils, and sweets should be eaten sparingly (Murray and Zentner, 1993).

Nutritional Needs of Adolescents. In general, adolescents should consume more total nutrients than they did as young children. Accelerated physical and emotional development works to increase the metabolic rate and, as a result, nutritional needs. Maximal growth in girls takes place between ages 10 and 12 and approximately 2 years later in boys. Protein, calcium, and calorie needs

TABLE 13–11 **Feeding During the First Year**

Birth to 6 Months (Breastfeeding or Bottle Feeding)

Breastfeeding

Most desirable complete diet for first half of year*
Requires supplements of fluoride (0.25 mg), regardless of the fluoride content of the local water supply, and iron by 6 months of age
Requires supplements of vitamin D (400 units) if mother's diet is inadequate

Formula

Iron-fortified commercial formula is a complete food for the first half of the year*
Requires fluoride supplements (0.25 mg) when the concentration of fluoride in the drinking water is below 0.3 parts per million (ppm)
Evaporated milk formula requires supplements of vitamin C, iron, and fluoride (in accordance with the fluoride content of the local water supply)

6–12 Months (Solid Foods)

May begin to add solids by 5 to 6 months of age
First foods are strained, pureed, or finely mashed
Finger foods such as teething crackers, raw fruit, or vegetables can be introduced by 6–7 months
Chopped table food or commercially prepared junior foods can be started by 9–12 months
With the exception of cereal, the order of introducing foods is variable, a recommended sequence is weekly introduction of other foods, beginning with fruit, then vegetables, and then meat
As the quantity of solids increases, the amount of formula should be limited to approximately 900 mL (30 oz) daily

Method of Introduction

Introduce solids when infant is hungry
Begin spoon feeding by pushing food to back of tongue because of infant's natural tendency to thrust tongue forward
Use small spoon with straight handle; begin with 1 or 2 teaspoons of food; gradually increase to 2–3 tablespoons per feeding
Introduce one food at a time usually at intervals of 4–7 days, to identify food allergies
As the amount of solid food increases, decrease the quantity of milk to prevent overfeeding
Never introduce foods by mixing them with the formula in the bottle

Cereal

Introduce commercially prepared iron-fortified infant cereals and administer daily until 18 months
Rice cereal is usually introduced first because of its low allergenic potential
Can discontinue supplemental iron once cereal is given

Fruits and Vegetables

Applesauce, bananas, and pears are usually well tolerated
Avoid fruits and vegetables marketed in cans that are not specifically designed for infants because of variable and sometimes high lead content and addition of salt, sugar, and/or preservatives
Offer fruit juice only from a cup, not a bottle, to reduce the development of "nursing caries"

Meat, Fish, and Poultry

Avoid fatty meats
Prepare by baking, broiling, steaming, or poaching
Include organ meats such as liver, which has a high iron, vitamin A, and vitamin B complex content
If soup is given, be sure all ingredients are familiar to child's diet
Avoid commercial meat/vegetable combinations because protein is low

Eggs and Cheese

Serve egg yolk hard boiled and mashed, soft cooked, or poached
Introduce egg white in small quantities (1 t) toward end of first year to detect an allergy
Use cheese as a substitute for meat and as finger food

*Breastfeeding or commercial formula feeding for up to 12 months of age is recommended. After 1 year, whole cow's milk can be given.
From Wong, D.L. (1995). *Whaley & Wong's Nursing Care of Infants and Children* (5th ed.). St. Louis, MO, Mosby-Year Book.

are higher during this time. In the United States, adolescent girls typically begin menstruating at 12.5 years; menstruation increases the need for iron.

Meal skipping, frequent snacking, the eating of fast foods, and the drinking of soft drinks contribute to imbalances in the diet of adolescents. In general, adolescents between 12 and 18 years of age should consume four servings of dairy products (low-fat milk is preferred), two to three servings of meat and meat alternatives, four to five servings of fruits and vegetables, and 6 to 11 servings of breads and cereals. As with children, fats, oils, and sweets should be used sparingly.

Eating disorders (e.g., anorexia nervosa and bulimia) most often occur in adolescent girls. Teaching adolescents the importance of good nutrition should include discussion of the consequences of eating disorders and how to recognize them. These issues are covered in Chapter 17.

Physical Activity and Exercise

Exercise and physical activity are necessary for muscular development and refinement of coordination and balance, gaining strength, and enhancing other functions, such as circulation and elimination (Murray and Zentner, 1993). Toddlers and small children usually have an abundance of energy and rarely need encouragement to promote physical activity. Many school-aged children and adolescents, however, often need to be encouraged to exercise. Several goals of *Healthy People 2000* (USDHHS, 1990) address the importance of physical activity in children 6 years of age through adolescence. In general, all children should engage in light to moderate physical activity for at least 30 minutes each day to develop and maintain cardiorespiratory fitness and improve overall physical fitness. In addition to exercises that improve heart and lung functioning, physical activities that enhance and maintain muscular strength, muscular endurance, and flexibility are recommended.

School-based physical education programs, as well as non–school related activities such as sports (e.g., soccer, baseball, basketball, hockey) and recreational activities (e.g., skating, swimming, bicycling), can be good sources of exercise. The use of appropriate safety equipment (e.g., helmets, pad, mouth protectors), however, must be stressed. Activities that can be easily incorporated into a child's daily routine and enjoyed all year should be encouraged, as activity levels tend to decrease in the winter.

Sleep and Rest

Sleep and rest are essential to good health. Sleep needs vary dramatically with age, ranging from 20 hours or more per day for neonates to 8 hours per day for older teenagers. Table 13–12 outlines sleep and rest needs for infants, children, and adolescents.

The positioning of infants for sleep is very important, as sleeping in a prone position has been associated with SIDS. In 1992, the American Academy of Pediatrics recommended that almost all infants up to 6 months of age sleep on their sides or backs (exceptions are infants with gastroesophageal reflux, premature infants with respiratory distress, and some infants with upper airway problems) (Wong, 1995). Placing the infant on a firm mattress, rather than a pillow or soft bedding, is also suggested. Widespread adherence to these recommendations has resulted in a reported 30% decrease in SIDS during the past few years. All parents should be informed of these recommendations and taught to position infants on their sides or backs, rather than prone, and to avoid overly soft bedding.

Dental Health

Dental caries have been described as the most prevalent disease known. In recent years, however, the oral health of children has improved dramatically, largely because of community water fluoridation, use of preventive services (e.g., sealants, topical fluoride treatment), and appropriate tooth care (e.g., brushing, flossing). As a result, half of school-aged children have no decay in their permanent teeth (USDHHS, 1990). *Healthy People 2000* objectives to promote oral health include increasing the percentage of communities with

TABLE 13–12 **Sleep and Rest Needs of Infants, Children, and Adolescents**

Age Group	Hours of Daily Rest (Naps)	Nighttime Sleep
Neonates	As many as seven to eight naps per day*	6–12 hours, interrupted for feedings*
Infants	Morning nap time will shorten, then be eliminated; by 12 months, one daily nap of 1–4 hours†	9–11 hours; many babies sleep through the night by 7–8 months†
Toddlers	Daily nap—1–2 hours	10–12 hours
Younger preschoolers (3 years of age)	Daily nap—1–2 hours; nap time may diminish, but a "rest" time (1–2 hours) should be encouraged	10–12 hours
Older preschoolers (4–5 years of age)	Often will refuse to nap; afternoon "rest" times should be encouraged	10–11 hours
Younger school-aged (6–9 years)		10–11 hours
Older school-aged (10–12 years)		9–10 hours
Adolescents (13 years of age and older)	May occasionally nap or "sleep in" to "catch up" on rest needs	8–10 hours (variable)—sleep and rest needs may increase due to rapid growth and energy expenditure

*Total of 16–20 hours of sleep/day during the first few weeks.
†Total of 14–15 hours of sleep/day by 3–4 months of age.
Data from Murray, R. B. and Zenter, J. P. (1993). *Nursing Assessment and Health Promotion: Strategies Through the Life Span* (5th ed.). Norwalk, CT, Appleton & Lange; Wong, D. L. (1995). *Whaley & Wong's Nursing Care of Infants and Children.* (5th ed.). St. Louis, MO, Mosby-Year Book.

fluoridated water, encouraging the use of dental sealants, and increasing the use of topical or systemic fluorides (e.g., tooth pastes, mouth rinses, fluoride drops) (USDHHS, 1990). Prevention of baby bottle tooth decay and screening of all preschool children for tooth decay are also encouraged.

"Community water fluoridation is the single most effective and efficient means of preventing dental caries in children" . . . and . . . "widespread exposure to fluorides through drinking water and dental products appears to be the primary cause of the declining prevalence of dental caries in the school-age population" (USDHHS, 1990, p. 357). According to Ripa (1993), approximately 62% of United States residents have drinking water containing optimal levels of fluoride, with the highest levels (73%) being in the midwestern states (i.e., Minnesota, Michigan, Wisconsin, Iowa, Missouri, Illinois, Indiana, and Ohio) and the lowest (17.9%), in the pacific states (i.e., Washington, Oregon, California).

Dental care of neonates and infants may include fluoride supplementation. If the infant is fed with formula concentrate or powdered formula prepared with fluoridated water, supplements are not necessary. If the baby is breast fed or if the community does not have fluoridated water, supplemental fluoride drops should be used. It is important for parents to discontinue fluoride drops when the child is drinking fluoridated water, as excessive fluoride may be harmful to the permanent teeth, producing discoloration or defects (Jackson and Saunders, 1993). For older children, dentists often recommend using fluoride tablets, fluoride application in the dental office, or use of fluoride toothpaste or mouthwash (American Dental Association [ADA], 1992).

Dental sealants are thin plastic coatings painted on the chewing surfaces of the back teeth and are applied in the dentist's office or clinic and sometimes in schools. The process is simple, painless, and effective in preventing tooth decay. The process lasts up to 10 years and is fairly inexpensive (National Institutes of Health, 1994). All parents should be encouraged to discuss dental sealants with their child's dentist.

"Bottle mouth syndrome," or baby bottle tooth decay, occurs in older infants and toddlers who are allowed to fall asleep with a bottle of formula or milk or another sweetened fluid in their mouth. These fluids pool in the mouth, particularly around the upper front teeth. Bacteria normally present in the mouth consume the carbohydrates from the milk or juice, and as a byproduct the bacteria produce metabolic acids. These acids decalcify the tooth enamel, resulting in destruction of the tooth. All parents should be taught to prevent baby bottle tooth decay by using only plain water in naptime and bedtime bottles (ADA, 1989; Betz et al., 1994).

The primary teeth (deciduous teeth or baby teeth) begin erupting at about 6 months of age and continue until 2 years of age; they start shedding at about 6 years of age. The permanent teeth begin erupting at about 6 to 7 years of age and continue into adulthood. Figure 13–1 depicts normal tooth formation.

To promote oral health, the ADA (1992) offers the following recommendations:

- Take children to the dentist regularly, beginning at 6 months of age
- Put only water in a child's naptime or bedtime bottle
- Clean the child's mouth daily
- Begin brushing as soon as the first tooth erupts
- Ensure that children get adequate fluoride for decay-resistant teeth (this varies based on the community—consult a dentist)
- Brush and floss the child's teeth daily until the child can be taught to do it alone; then encourage the child to brush and floss

Thumb sucking or use of a pacifier generally does not cause permanent dental problems for children younger than 4 years of age. However, alignment problems in the permanent teeth may develop if thumb sucking persists beyond age 5 years. Observation of thumb sucking or use of pacifiers in small children should alert the nurse to inform the parents of potential problems. If thumb sucking persists, the child should be referred to a dentist.

Oral injuries are common during childhood. Children should be encouraged to wear mouth protectors or mouthguards when participating in activities that may involve falls, head contact, tooth clenching, or flying equipment (e.g., gymnastics, football, skateboarding, soccer, basketball). In addition to protecting teeth, mouthguards also prevent injury to lips, cheeks, and tongue (ADA, 1992). Mouth protectors are available at sporting goods stores or may be custom made by the dentist.

If a dental injury occurs, the child should be taken to the dentist immediately. If a permanent tooth is knocked out, it should be rinsed gently with cool water without removing any attached tissue and immediately reinserted into the socket. If that is not possible, the tooth should be placed in cool water or milk, and the child should see a dentist as soon as possible, bringing the tooth along.

Maturation and Puberty

Like infancy, adolescence is a period of accelerated growth and development. When caring for older children and young teenagers in community settings, nurses are frequently in a position to teach adolescents and their parents about growth and development changes associated with puberty.

Puberty is the time of physical development in which individuals develop sexual maturity. Tables 13–13 and 13–14 describe physical changes in girls and boys, respectively, during preadolescence.

In girls, puberty begins between 10 and 14 years of age; menarche marks puberty and sexual maturity. Age at menarche ranges from 10 to 16, with a mean of about 12.5 years. During puberty, the breasts enlarge, and axillary and public hair grows thicker and darker (Murray and Zentner,

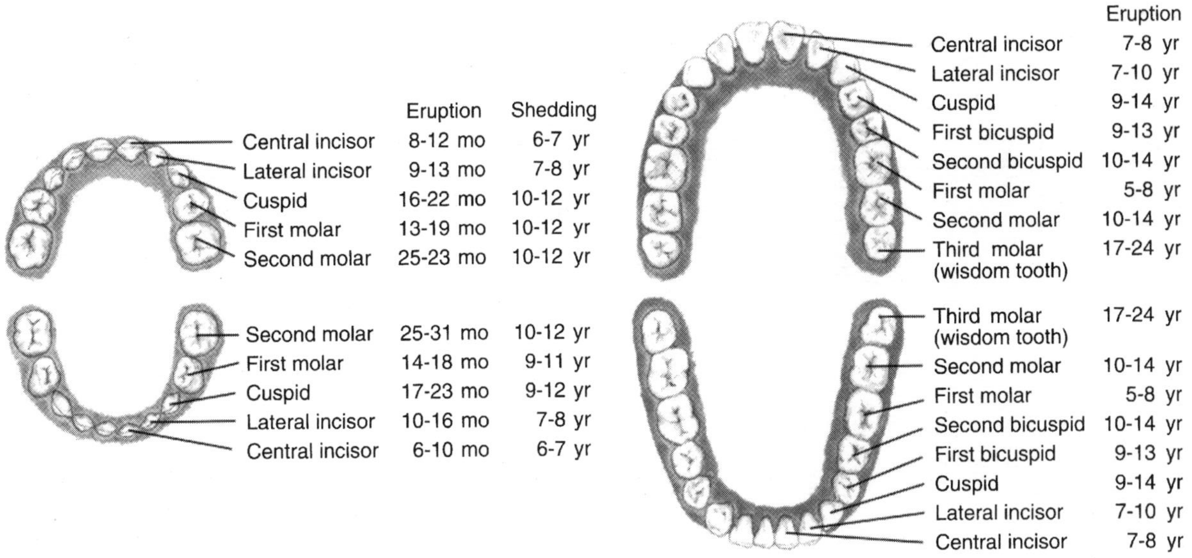

FIGURE 13–1 Normal tooth formation in the child. (From Ashwill, J. W. and Droske, S. C. [1997]. *Nursing Care of Children.* Philadelphia, W. B. Saunders, p. 244.)

TABLE 13–13 Physical Changes in Girls During Preadolescence*

- Increase in transverse diameter of the pelvis
- Broadening of hips
- Tenderness in developing breast tissue and enlargement of areolar diameter
- Axillary sweating
- Change in vaginal secretions from alkaline to acid pH
- Change in vaginal layer to thick, gray, mucoid lining
- Change in vaginal flora from mixed to Döderlein's lactic acid–producing bacilli
- Appearance of pubic hair from 8–14 years (hair first appears on labia and then spreads to mons; adult triangular distribution does not occur for approximately 2 years after initial appearance of pubic hair)

*These physical changes for girls are listed in the approximate sequence of their occurrence.

From Murray, R. B. and Zentner, J. P. (1993). *Nursing Assessment and Health Promotion: Strategies Through the Life Span* (5th ed.). Norwalk, CT, Appleton & Lange.

1993). Early instruction on menstruation should be provided.

In boys, puberty begins between 12 and 16 years. At that time, hair begins to grow at the axilla and the pubis. Also, body hair, particularly facial hair, increases, and the voice deepens. Additionally, the penis, scrotum, and testes enlarge; the scrotum reddens; and the scrotal skin changes texture. Penile development occurs between 10 and 16 years, and testicular development, between 9 and 17 years. Spermatogenesis and seminal emissions designate puberty and sexual maturity in boys. Nocturnal emissions occur approximately at age 14 (Murray and Zentner, 1993).

ILLNESS PREVENTION AND HEALTH PROTECTION

When working in community settings, nurses can dramatically affect the health of infants, children, and adolescents through measures to prevent illness and protect health and safety. Illness prevention and health protection strategies for children include prevention of communicable diseases; prevention of initiation of tobacco, alcohol, and drug use; promoting safety; and prevention and detection of child abuse. Prevention of communicable disease in children is addressed at length in Chapter 15. Interventions to improve safety; prevent alcohol, tobacco, and drug use; and detect and prevent child abuse are described here.

Prevention of Substance Use

Drugs and Alcohol. Alcohol use contributes dramatically to the three leading causes of adolescent deaths. As stated earlier, injuries are the leading cause of death in adolescents, and an estimated 40% of injury deaths in this age group are related to the use of alcohol. Alcohol use also contributes significantly to adolescent homicide and suicide (the second and third leading causes of death in this age group) (USDHHS/OHPDP, 1994).

School-based alcohol and drug education programs have been somewhat successful, as alcohol and marijuana use among adolescents (aged 12–17 years) declined between 1988 and 1992. Rates of alcohol and drug use, however, began to increase slowly beginning in 1992. To assist in reducing alcohol and drug use, health care providers are encouraged to screen and counsel

TABLE 13–14 Physical Changes in Boys During Preadolescence

- Axillary sweating
- Increased testicular sensitivity to pressure
- Increase in size of testes
- Changes in color of scrotum
- Temporary enlargement of breasts
- Increase in height and shoulder breadth
- Appearance of lightly pigmented hair at base of penis
- Increase in length and width of penis

*These physical changes for boys are listed in the approximate sequence of their occurrence.

From Murray, R. B. and Zentner, J. P. (1993). *Nursing Assessment and Health Promotion: Strategies Through the Life Span* (5th ed.). Norwalk, CT, Appleton & Lange.

adolescents for alcohol and other drug use. Components of alcohol and drug abuse counseling suggested by the USDHHS/OHPDP (1994) include the following:

- Begin education on alcohol and drug use during the preteen years. All children and adolescents should be informed of the dangers of alcohol and other drugs, emphasizing associated dangers of human immunodeficiency virus exposure and motor vehicle accidents while under the influence of alcohol and other drugs.
- Ask parents about their own use of alcohol and other drugs and whether they discuss the use of alcohol and drugs with their children. Assessment for a family history of alcoholism or drug use should be made.
- Establish a caring and confidential relationship with adolescents; however, the adolescent must be informed of the limits of confidentiality.
- As nonthreateningly as possible, question children and adolescents about drug and alcohol use in their environment (e.g., home, school, work). Suggested questions to be asked include "Do most of your friends drink alcohol or smoke marijuana at parties?" "Have you ever tried alcohol? marijuana? other drugs?" "Do your parents know that you've used ________?" "Have you ever been drunk or stoned and driven a car?"
- If alcohol or drug use is determined, assess the type of drugs used, and the quantity, frequency, and setting of use.
- Evaluate the extent to which alcohol or other drugs are affecting the adolescent's life (e.g., school performance, peer relationships, family relationships, work).
- Be aware of signs and symptoms of dependence, addiction, and withdrawal and teach them to parents and adolescents.
- Refer for evaluation and treatment if evidence of significant psychosocial impairment or physiological dependence is present. Familiarity with available treatment options in the community is essential.

Tobacco. "Use of tobacco products is the leading preventable cause of death in the United States accounting for more than 400,000 deaths each year or about one out of every five deaths" (USDHHS, 1995, p. 36). Initiation of smoking occurs almost entirely during adolescence, as surveys have indicated that 25% of those who have ever smoked started by the 6th grade, 50% by the 8th grade, 75% by the 9th grade, and 94% by the 11th grade (USDHHS, 1990). Approximately 19% of high school seniors have reported daily smoking, and in 1990, the average age of initial cigarette use was 11.5 years (USDHHS/OHPDP, 1994). Because of these statistics, reduction of the initiation of cigarette smoking by teenagers has been termed a "national priority." Strategies to prevent tobacco use among children and teenagers include enforcement of youth access laws, establishment of tobacco-free environments, and ongoing prevention programs in schools and the community.

Surveillance and enforcement of retail restriction of sale of tobacco to nonadults is essential to reduce the prevalence of smoking among teenagers (CDC, 1992a). Most states have a minimum age of 18 years for purchasing cigarettes; however, almost 58% of teenage smokers report that they usually buy their own cigarettes (CDC, 1992a). Small stores are the most commonly mentioned site for purchase of cigarettes, as almost 80% of youths 12 to 15 and 87% of youths 16 to 17 years of age reported buying cigarettes from small stores. Interestingly, vending machines were the source of cigarettes for fewer than 20% of adolescents 12 to 15 and less than 12% of older youths (CDC, 1992a).

The establishment of tobacco-free environments and tobacco use prevention education programs is an important component in decreasing the initiation of tobacco use among youth. To meet the *Healthy People 2000* (USDHHS, 1990) objectives, the Pro-Children Act of 1994 was instituted, requiring that federally funded facilities that provide services to children (e.g., schools and libraries) be smoke free (USDHHS, 1995). Increasingly, state and city ordinances and laws are being enacted that prohibit smoking in public places. These efforts should be supported by all health care workers.

Health education and counseling strategies developed by the USDHHS/ODPHP (1994) to encourage teenagers to prevent initiation of or to stop tobacco use include the following:

- Assess tobacco use in the child's household. If parents or other family members smoke, the importance of stopping should be stressed. Emphasizing the negative health consequence for the child can be effective in working with parents.
- Ask all adolescents about tobacco use. Information should be elicited in a nonthreatening manner, preferably in the absence of the parents.
- Discuss tobacco use prevention or cessation, emphasizing the unattractive cosmetic consequences (e.g., stained teeth, oral sores, bad breath), athletic consequences (e.g., decreased endurance, shortness of breath), and negative social consequences (e.g., disapproval by peers and parents). These strategies are usually more effective with children and adolescents than discussing long-term health consequences.
- Strenuously discourage the use of smokeless tobacco because of its addictive potential and associated health problems (e.g., oral cancer).
- Use other strategies that may be helpful, including age-appropriate pamphlets and other informational materials, written "contracts," and setting a "quit date."
- Support adolescents with positive feedback and suggest ways to avoid peer pressure.
- Do not recommend the use of nicotine gum and dermal patches, as they have not been adequately tested in children and adolescents.

Safety

In the United States, injuries are the leading cause of mortality in children and adolescents, accounting for about 20,000 deaths each year. Almost half (47%) of fatal accidents involve motor vehicle crashes. Homicide accounts for about 13% of injury deaths; suicide, 10%; drowning, 9.2%; fire or burns, 7.2%; and "other" (e.g., choking, falls, poisoning, sports, accidental firearms), 14% (CDC, 1990). Childhood injuries also cause an estimated 16 million emergency room visits and 600,000 hospitalizations. Interventions for childhood injury prevention are discussed in this section.

Vehicle Safety. As mentioned, motor vehicles are involved in almost half of all injury deaths and contribute to numerous hospitalizations in children and adolescents. More than 45,000 people are killed annually in motor vehicle accidents (CDC, 1990), including those who are an occupant in a vehicle and those struck while riding a bicycle or as a pedestrian. Motorcycle (11% of total), bicycle (4.5% of the total), and pedestrian (14.5% of total) casualties account for almost 30% of motor vehicle deaths each year. In children 5 to 9 years of age, pedestrian injuries were the leading cause of injury death (CDC, 1990).

Motor vehicle safety begins with the ride home from the hospital. Although some variation exists in specific regulations, all states require the use of child safety seats. General recommendations are to

- Use only car seats that meet safety standards (all car seats manufactured after 1981 meet standards)
- Install child safety seats according to manufacturer's directions, preferably in the center rear seat
- Use the child safety seat *each* time the child rides in the vehicle
- Turn the safety seat to face the rear of the vehicle until the child weighs 18 to 20 pounds and is able to sit up well
- Use a safety seat until the child weighs at least 40 pounds (some states have age as well as weight requirements)
- Secure the child in the seat according to the manufacturer's instructions
- Use a correctly secured booster seat for children up to 70 pounds
- If possible, have children sit in the rear seat of cars (particularly if the car has air bags) and use safety belts *every* time they ride
- Use safety belts for adolescents and parents

every time they operate or ride in a motor vehicle, even for short trips

Other interventions that have been suggested include adoption and enforcement of seat belt laws and ordinances, enforcement of strict penalties for operating a vehicle under the influence of drugs or alcohol, adoption and enforcement of laws and ordinances requiring motorcyclists and bicyclists to wear helmets, enforcement of speed limits, enforcement of minimum drinking age laws, and enforcement of laws and ordinances requiring child safety seat use and the extension of these laws and ordinances to cover all passengers sitting in all vehicles (CDC, 1990). Equipping vehicles with both driver and passenger airbags, improving vehicle designs to better protect both occupants (e.g., side impact protection, improved door design, roof crush resistance, and restraint system), and developing community-based pedestrian and bicycle safety programs are other safety measures.

Poisoning. Each year almost 700,000 children younger than 5 years are exposed to some type of poison, and more than 107,000 children are treated in hospital emergency rooms for poisoning. Most poisoning accidents take place in the home and involve children younger than 5 years. Any nonfood item is a potential poison, and many children die or are injured from swallowing medicines, polishes, insecticides, antifreeze, drain cleaners, and other household products (Texas Department of Health, 1990). Table 13–15 presents general guidelines to protect children against accidental poisoning, and Table 13–16 describes emergency actions for poisoning.

Head Injury. Head injuries are the most common severe disabling injuries in the United States, with an estimated half million new cases occurring annually (USDHHS, 1990). The most common causes of head injury include motor vehicle (including bicycles and motorcycles) crashes, falls, diving and other water-related accidents, and violence. Recently, efforts to prevent head injuries in children have targeted laws and ordinances requiring bicycle helmets.

Each year nearly 1,000 bicyclists are killed in the United States, and more than 550,000 persons are treated in emergency departments for bicycle-related injuries. More than 87% of bicyclist fatalities occur in males, and more than one third occur in boys between the ages of 5 and 15 years (CDC, 1995). The majority of bicycle fatalities are caused by bicyclist error (e.g., failure to yield right of way, improper crossing of an intersection or road, failure to obey traffic signs and lights), and alcohol is involved in many bicycle fatalities.

Head injury accounts for 62% of bicycle-related deaths and 67% of bicycle-related hospital admissions. Based on evidence that 74 to 85% of the risk of head injury can be reduced by the use of bicycle helmets, the CDC (1995) has recommended that state and local agencies and organizations develop programs to increase their use. These recommendations are as follow:

- Bicycle helmets should be worn by all persons (i.e., bicycle operators and passengers) at any age when bicycling
- Bicycle riders should wear helmets whenever and wherever they ride a bicycle
- Bicycle helmets should meet the standards of the American National Standards Institute, the Snell Memorial Foundation, or the American Society for Testing and Material
- To effectively increase helmet use rates, states and communities must implement programs that include legislation, education and promotion, enforcement, and program evaluation

Other measures to improve bicycle safety include education and training to improve knowledge of and adherence to traffic laws, use of appropriate clothing (light colored and marked with reflective materials) when riding at night, and bicycle maintenance. Bicycle safety programs are available in most communities. The National Highway Traffic Safety Administration or the Consumer Product Safety Commission (see Table 13–29) provides information on establishing bicycle safety programs.

Head injury is also the most commonly recorded cause of deaths for motorcycle drivers and passengers who die in crashes, and nonhelmeted riders are two and a half times more likely than helmeted riders to sustain a fatal head injury. Further, helmet use is the single most important factor in preventing death and head injuries (Advocates for Highway and Auto Safety, 1994). As of July

TABLE 13–15 **Protection of Children from Accidental Poisoning**

1. Request "safety-lock" tops on all prescription drugs
2. Keep household cleaners, bug sprays, medicines, and garage products out of reach and out of sight of children; lock them up if possible
3. Never store food and household cleaners together
4. Always store medicines in their original containers and throw out medicine when old or no longer in use; rinse out empty containers
5. Do not take medicines in front of your child because children love to imitate
6. Never call medicine"candy"
7. Read the label before taking medicine; turn on the light when giving or taking medicine
8. If you leave the room when using a medicine or a household product, take it or the child with you; a child can get into it in only a few seconds
9. Anticipate your child's curiosity and abilities; for example, if you have a crawling infant, keep household products locked up, not under the kitchen sink or on the refrigerator
10. Never put products like kerosene, gasoline, insecticides, or household cleaning agents in another container, such as a soft drink bottle, cup, or bowl
11. If you need potentially poisonous products, buy them only when needed and only enough to do the specific job
12. Always prepare and use products according to label directions
13. Place "Mr. Yuk" stickers (available from many pharmacies or health departments) on all poisons in the home if children are older than 3 years of age, and teach them that this means danger
14. Be alert for repeat poisoning; a child who has swallowed a poison is more likely to become poisoned again within a year
15. The child's life may depend on how fast you get expert emergency information and treatment—*be prepared*
    Post the poison control center number for your area near the phone; tell all babysitters it is there
    Have the following products on hand (use only on the advice of the Poison Control Center, emergency center, or a physician)
        1-ounce bottle of syrup of ipecac for each child in the house
        Epsom salt
        Activated charcoal

From Texas Department of Health. (1990). *Protect Your Child Against Accidental Poisoning.* Austin, TX, Texas Department of Health.

1994, 47 states and the District of Columbia had laws requiring that motorcycle helmets be worn by all motorcyclists or partial use laws requiring their use by persons 17 years of age and younger. Only Colorado, Illinois, and Iowa had no helmet laws. All motorcycle riders should be informed of these statistics, and helmet laws should be encouraged in those states where they do not exist and strongly enforced in all other states. Nurses and other health care providers should consistently encourage parents, adolescents, and children to use protective helmets whenever using a bicycle or motorcycle.

Fire and Burns. Fire and burns are the fifth leading cause of childhood deaths due to injury but the second leading cause of deaths due to injury in children 1 to 9 years of age (CDC/National Center for Injury Prevention and Control [NCIPC]. Ten leading causes of deaths due to injury—1991, Unpublished data, Atlanta, 1994). Indeed, 73% of burn deaths in children occurred in those younger than 9 years. Overall, 80% of deaths from fire or burns resulted from house fires, 9% from electrical burns, and 2% from scalding (CDC, 1990).

According to the USDHHS (1990), those who live in substandard housing without smoke detectors are at the highest risk for fire death. Improved public awareness of home fire safety, including use of functional smoke detectors in all sleeping areas and establishment of home evacuation plans,

TABLE 13–16 **Emergency Action for Poisoning**

Swallowed Medicine

1. *Call the poison control center*—if not available, call 911; do not give anything to drink by mouth until you call; *do not wait for symptoms to develop*
2. If emergency personnel tell you to make the child vomit, give 1 T of syrup of ipecac; keep the child moving; if the child does not vomit within 15 minutes, give a second tablespoon; do *not* give a third
3. If you go to an emergency treatment center, take the medicine container

Swallowed Chemical or Household Products

1. If child is conscious, *immediately* give one or two glasses of milk (give water if milk not available)
2. *Call the poison control center*—if not available, call 911
3. *Do **not** make the child vomit for acid, alkali, or petroleum poisoning!*

Inhaled Poison

1. Immediately get the child to fresh air; avoid breathing fumes; open doors and windows wide
2. If victim is not breathing, start artificial respiration
3. Call 911

Poison on the Skin

1. Remove contaminated clothing, and flood skin with water for 10 minutes
2. Wash gently with soap and water; rinse
3. Call the Poison Control Center

Poison in the Eye

1. Flood the eye with lukewarm (not hot) water, poured from a large glass held 2–3 inches from the eye
2. Repeat for 15 minutes
3. Have the child blink as much as possible while flooding the eye; do not force the eyelid open
4. Call a physician or the Poison Control Center

From Texas Department of Health. (1990). *Protect Your Child Against Accidental Poisoning.* Austin, TX, Texas Department of Health.

can help reduce home fire deaths and disabilities. The most common sources of fire and burns, as well as safety instructions on how to reduce or eliminate the risk, are included in Table 13–17.

Many fire death and injuries are caused by smoke and gases, as the victims inhale smoke that occurs ahead of the flames. Early warning and having an escape plan can dramatically diminish injury and death. General recommendations for fire safety from the U. S. Consumer Products Safety Commission (1994) include the following:

- Read the manufacturer's instructions on installation and location of fire detectors. Install smoke detectors on each floor of the house, near all sleeping areas, and in the kitchen.
- Follow the manufacturer's instructions for cleaning and maintenance; replace the battery annually or when a "chirping" sound is heard.
- Develop an escape plan and an alternate escape plan for the family, and practice the escape routes periodically. The escape plan should include choosing a place outside the house where the family will meet to be sure that everyone got out safely.
- Ensure that there are at least two exits from each part of the house.

Finally, it is important to note that many infants and small children are burned each year by scalding water. To prevent scalding, parents are encouraged to reduce the temperature of hot water heat-

TABLE 13–17 **Home Fire Safety**

Potential Source of Fire	Potential Safety Threats	Recommendations
Wood stoves	Improper installation/construction; creosote buildup in chimney or stovepipe; proximity to combustibles (e.g., curtains, chairs, firewood); improper use of fuel	Do not use wood-burning stoves and fireplaces unless they are properly installed and meet building codes; have chimney inspected and cleaned by a professional chimney sweep; inspect and clean stovepipes according to manufacturer's recommendations; keep all combustibles at least 3 feet away from the stove; use only proper fuels in the stove or fireplace—never burn trash or use gasoline or other flammable liquid to start fires
Space heaters (e.g., kerosene, gas, electric)	Inappropriate ventilation; improper installation; improper lighting of gas or kerosene heaters; proximity to combustible materials (e.g., bedding, furniture, drapes); use of extension cord (for electric heaters); leaving the heater unattended	**Kerosene heaters—**never use gasoline in a kerosene heater; place heater so it will not be knocked over; use only 1-K kerosene; never fill the heater while it is operating, and always refuel the heater outdoors; keep the room ventilated (keep door open or the window ajar); keep flammable liquids and fabrics away from the heater; if a flare-up occurs, activate the manual shut-off switch and call the fire department—do not try to move the heater or try to smother the flames with a rug or blanket; **gas space heaters—**follow the manufacturer's instructions regarding where and how to use heaters; do not use unvented heaters in small enclosed areas; follow the manufacturer's instructions for lighting the pilot; light matches before turning on the gas to prevent gas buildup; do not operate a vented-style heater unvented; **electric heaters—**operate heater away from combustible materials; avoid using extension cord; never place heaters on cabinets, tables or furniture
Cooking equipment	Storage of combustible items above the stove; loose-fitting sleeves that could catch fire while cooking; leaving the stove unattended when in use	Never store pot holders, plastic utensils, towels, or other flammable materials on or near the stove; roll up or fasten long loose sleeves while cooking; keep constant vigilance over any cooking
Cigarette lighters and matches	Leaving cigarette lighters and matches where children may reach them; allowing children to "play with" matches and lighters	Keep lighters and matches out of sight and out of reach of children; never allow a child to play with a lighter or think of it as a toy; always check to see that cigarettes are extinguished before emptying ashtrays
Materials that burn (e.g., mattresses/bedding, wearing apparel, flammable liquids)	Smoking on upholstered furniture or in bed; heaters, ash trays, and other fire sources located near bedding; children's sleepwear and other clothing that is not flame resistant; improperly stored flammable liquids	*Do not smoke in bed*; locate heaters 3 feet from the bed; always check furniture where smokers have been sitting for improperly discarded smoking materials or ashes; do not place or leave ashtrays on the arms of chairs; look for fabrics that resist burning (e.g., polyester, nylon, wool, and silk)—cotton, cotton/polyester blends, rayon, and acrylic burn rapidly and easier to ignite; consider purchasing garments that are easily removed; purchase flame-resistant sleepwear, and follow manufacturer's care and cleaning instructions; store and use flammable liquids (gasoline, paint thinner) carefully; store outside the house

*Adapted from U. S. Consumer Product Safety Commission. (1994). *Your Home Fire Safety Checklist.* Washington, D. C., Government Printing Office.

ers to 120 to 130°F. Always test bath water to ensure that it is comfortably warm and not hot.

Drowning. Drowning is the third leading cause of deaths due to injury in children 1 to 4 years and the fourth for children 5 to 14 years. In Arizona, California, and Florida, drowning was the leading cause of fatal injury for children younger than 4 years (CDC/NCIPC, Unpublished data, Atlanta, 1994). Those at highest risk for drowning are men and boys, children younger than 5 years, African-Americans, and Native Americans. The highest drowning rates are among children 4 years and younger and males 15 to 19 years of age. The drowning rate for African-American children (4.5/100,000) is almost twice that for white children (2.6/100,000). For adolescents, drownings are most often associated with water activities (e.g., boating, skiing). Alcohol is a factor in an estimated 40 to 50% of adolescent drownings (CDC, 1990; USDHHS/ODPHP, 1994).

As many as 90% of drownings occur in residential swimming pools. Fencing of all pools, use of pool alarms and pool covers, and safety regulations can prevent pool drowning by preschool children and should be encouraged. Counseling of parents should include admonishment to *never* leave infants, toddlers, and small children in or near the bathtub, wading pool, or swimming pool without supervision.

To prevent deaths in adolescents, all states have laws prohibiting operating a boat under the influence of alcohol or drugs. Enforcement of these laws, as well as increasing public awareness of safe operating practices and discouraging alcohol use, can be helpful (USDHHS/ODPHP, 1994).

Violent Behavior. "The United States ranks first among industrialized nations in violent death rates, and deaths caused by violent and unintentional misuse of firearms exceed in number the combined total of the next 17 nations" (USDHHS, 1990, p. 226). Furthermore, "violence is a major health and social problem affecting children and adolescents in the U. S." (USDHHS/ODPHP, 1994, p. 1125). Homicide is the 11th leading cause of death in the United States and the leading cause of deaths in African-Americans 15 to 24 years of age (USDHHS, 1990). In 1991, almost 8,200 homicide deaths in individuals 15 to 24 years of age and almost 400 homicides in children 10 to 14 years of age occurred (CDC/NCIPC, Unpublished data, 1994).

Firearms, particularly handguns, have been implicated in an alarming number of homicides and suicides. According to the CDC/NCIPC (Unpublished data, 1994), statistics for 1991 showed that more than 36,500 deaths were attributed to guns (18,500 suicide and 18,000 homicide). Additionally, in that year almost 12,300 suicides and 8,500 homicides termed "nonfirearm," totaling 57,200 violent deaths, occurred. In comparison, during 1991, motor vehicle deaths totaled 43,500 (CDC/NCIPC, Unpublished data, 1994), deaths from breast cancer were approximately 46,000 (American Cancer Society, 1995), and 32,000 deaths were attributed to acquired immunodeficiency syndrome (CDC/NCIPC, 1993). Firearms accounted for 75% of the suicide/homicide deaths for the 15- to 24-year-old age group and 66% of deaths in those 10 to 14 years of age. Basic education and counseling of parents for prevention of violent behavior and firearm safety are described in Table 13–18.

Homicide is the 11th leading cause of death in the United States, most often affecting men, teenagers, and minority groups members—particularly African-Americans and Hispanics. To assist in the detection and prevention of violence, Table 13–19 lists sociological, developmental, and familial risk factors, and Table 13–20 outlines ways to prevent youth violence.

Other Safety Hazards. There are a number of additional threats to safety of infants, children, and adolescents. These include participation in hazardous sports and recreational activities, choking or aspiration, suffocation, and other concerns.

To prevent injuries from sports and recreational activities, all children should be taught to wear appropriate protective gear *at all times* when participating. For example, batting helmets, catcher's gear, and protective gear for all participants and athletic supporters and protective "cups" for all boys should be required when playing baseball; helmets, wrist guards, knee pads, and elbow pads should be worn for in-line skating and skateboarding; and hockey and football players should wear the full complement of pads, helmets, and

TABLE 13–18 **Counseling Strategies for Prevention of Gun-Related Injuries and Violent Behaviors**

1. Every child and family should be assessed for the potential for injury from violence; areas to assess include
   Is there a history of violent injury to the child or other family members?
   Is there a history of alcohol or other drug abuse by the child or the other family members?
   Are there guns or other weapons in the home?
   Is violent injury a prevalent problem in the community?
2. All parents should be advised about the danger of keeping a gun in the home; basic rules of safety include
   Never keep a loaded gun in the house or car
   Keep guns and ammunition locked in separate places
   Always treat a gun as if it were loaded and ready to fire
   Never allow children access to guns
   Have a gunsmith check antique and souvenir guns to ensure that they are not loaded and fix them so they cannot be fired
3. Parents should be advised to inquire about the availability of guns in places where their children spend time, such as at friends' houses, schools, and recreational facilities; parents should be encouraged to take an active role in limiting the availability of guns in their children's environment
4. When treating patients with injuries that have been or may have been caused by violence, ask questions about the cause of the injury; if the injury has been caused by violence, attempt to determine if the conflict has been settled or may lead to further violence; questions to be addressed might include
   Has the argument been settled?
   Do you have a place to go if this is not settled?
   Are you safe?
   Is there anyone who can help settle the argument?
5. Despite the desirability of maintaining confidentiality, it may be necessary to consult with parents, police, and other authorities to protect the safety of children and adolescents involved in potentially violent situations
6. Parents and children should be given the facts about violence through a variety of media in classes, offices, or clinics; posters, videotapes, lectures, and brochures may be helpful
7. Children and adolescents should be encouraged to discuss how they deal with anger and to develop positive ways to manage anger and arguments; one suggested strategy for anger management reported by Berger (1994) is termed CALM:
   C—Cool down and count to 10; consider the cause and consequences
   A—Accept responsibility for your actions and reactions
   L—Listen to all sides and talk it over
   M—Move away and move on to something else

Adapted from U. S. Department of Health and Human Services/Office of Disease Prevention and Health Promotion. (1994). Counseling: Violent behavior and firearms. In *Clinician's Handbook of Preventive Services.* Washington, D. C., Government Printing Office, pp. 126–128; data from American Academy of Pediatrics/Center to Prevent Handgun Violence. (1992). *Rx for Safety: Preventing Firearms Injuries Among Children and Adolescents.* Washington, D. C., Center to Prevent Handgun Violence; American Academy of Pediatrics/Committee on Injury Control for Children and Youth. (1987). *Injury Control for Children and Youth.* Elk Grove Village, IL, American Academy of Pediatrics; Violence Prevention Project. (1992). *Identification and Prevention of Youth Violence: A Protocol of Health Care Providers.* Boston, Violence Prevention Project.

mouthguards whenever they play. Parents should be counseled to ensure that children are properly supervised when engaging in activities that are associated with injury risk. Finally, many organized athletic organizations require a yearly physical examination by a health care professional prior to participation. A physical examination may identify undetected problems that might threaten health (e.g., asthma, heart problems, musculoskeletal problems).

Each year, many children suffer serious injury or death through inappropriate use of objects or

TABLE 13–19 **Factors Associated with Risk of Violence**

Sociological

Low socioeconomic status
Involvement with gangs
Drug dealing
Access to guns
Media exposure to violence
Community exposure to violence

Developmental/Psychological

Alcohol or drug abuse
Rigid sex role expectations
Peer pressure, especially for adolescents
Poor impulse control
History of mental health problems
High individual stress level
Manual laborer, unemployed, or employed part time
Younger than 30 years

Family

History of intergenerational abuse
Social isolation
Parents verbally threaten children
High levels of family stress
Two or more children

From Maurer, F. A. (1995). Violence: A social and family problem. In C. M. Smith and F. A. Mauer (Eds.). *Community Health Nursing: Theory and Practice.* Philadelphia, W. B. Saunders, pp. 517–547.

toys (e.g., beanbags, plastic bags, balloons), misuse of equipment (e.g., highchairs, baby walkers), and lack of close supervision or precautions (e.g., leaving the side rail down on the crib, giving a toddler food that might cause choking, not covering electric outlets). Table 13–21 presents general guidelines for child safety that are an essential component of health teaching for all parents.

Child Abuse: Detection and Prevention

Child abuse and neglect refers to "any physical or mental injury, sexual abuse or exploitation, negligent treatment or maltreatment of a child by a person who is responsible for the child's welfare, under circumstances which indicate the child's health or welfare is harmed or threatened" (USDHHS, 1990, p. 232). Incidence of child abuse appears to be rising. Estimates of the number of children who suffer abuse and neglect range from 1.6 to 2.7 million each year, and these numbers appear to be increasing. Child abuse results in an estimated 1,100 deaths each year—about half from physical abuse and half from neglect.

TABLE 13–20 **Activities to Prevent Youth Violence**

Education

Adult mentoring
Conflict resolution
Training in social skills
Firearm safety
Parenting centers
Peer education
Public information and education campaigns

Legal/Regulatory Change

Regulate the use of and access to weapons
- Weaponless schools
- Control of concealed weapons
- Restrictive licensing
- Appropriate sale of guns

Regulate the use of and access to alcohol
- Appropriate sale of alcohol
- Prohibition or control of alcohol sales at events
- Training of servers

Other types of regulation
- Appropriate punishment in schools
- Dress codes

Environmental Modifications

Modify the social environment
- Home visitation
- Preschool programs, such as Head Start
- Therapeutic activities
- Recreational activities
- Work/academic experiences

Modify the physical environment
- Make risk areas visible
- Increase use of an area
- Limit building entrances and exits
- Create sense of ownership

From Centers for Disease Control/National Center for Injury Prevention and Control. (1993). *The Prevention of Youth Violence: A Framework for Community Action.* Atlanta, GA, Centers for Disease Control.

TABLE 13–21 **Child Safety Home Checklist**

Safety: Fire, Electrical, Burns

- ☐ Guards in front of or around any heating appliance, fireplace, or furnace (including floor furnace)*
- ☐ Electrical wires hidden or out of reach*
- ☐ No frayed or broken wires; no overloaded sockets
- ☐ Plastic guards or caps over electrical outlets, furniture in front of outlets*
- ☐ Hanging tablecloths out of reach, away from open fires*
- ☐ Smoke detectors tested and operating properly
- ☐ Kitchen matches stored out of child's reach*
- ☐ Large, deep ashtrays throughout house (if used)
- ☐ Small stoves, heaters, and other hot objects (e.g., cigarettes, candles, coffee pots, slow cookers) placed where they cannot be tipped over or reached by children
- ☐ Hot water heater set at 49°C (120°F) or lower
- ☐ Pot handles turned toward back of stove, center of table
- ☐ No loose clothing worn near stove
- ☐ No cooking or eating hot foods or liquids with child standing nearby or sitting in lap
- ☐ All small appliances, such as iron, turned off, disconnected, and placed out of reach when not in use
- ☐ Cool, not hot, mist vaporizer used
- ☐ Fire extinguisher available on each floor and checked periodically
- ☐ Electrical fuse box and gas outlet accessible
- ☐ Family escape plan in case of a fire practiced periodically; fire escape ladder available on upper-level floors
- ☐ Telephone number of fire or rescue squad and address of home with nearest cross-street posted near phone

Safety: Suffocation and Aspiration

- ☐ Small objects stored out of reach*
- ☐ Toys inspected for small removable parts or long strings*
- ☐ Hanging crib toys and mobiles placed out of reach
- ☐ Plastic bags stored away from young child's reach, large plastic garment bags discarded after tying in knots*
- ☐ Mattress or pillow not covered with plastic or in manner accessible to child*
- ☐ Crib design according to federal regulations with snug-fitting mattress*†
- ☐ Crib positioned away from other furniture or windows*
- ☐ Portable playpen gates up at all times while in use*
- ☐ Accordion-style gates not used*
- ☐ Bathroom doors kept closed, and toilet seats down*
- ☐ Faucets turned off firmly*
- ☐ Pool fenced with locked gate
- ☐ Proper safety equipment at poolside
- ☐ Electric garage door openers stored safely, and garage door adjusted to rise when door strikes object
- ☐ Doors of ovens, trunks, dishwashers, refrigerators, and front-loading clothes washers and dryers kept closed*
- ☐ Unused appliance, such as a refrigerator, securely closed with lock or doors removed*
- ☐ Food served in small noncylindric pieces*
- ☐ Toy chests without lids or with lids that securely lock in open position*

Safety: Suffocation and Aspiration *Continued*

- ☐ Buckets and wading pools kept empty when not in use*
- ☐ Clothesline above head level
- ☐ At least one member of household trained in basic life support (cardiopulmonary resuscitation) including first aid for choking‡

Safety: Poisoning

- ☐ Toxic substances, including batteries, placed on a high shelf, preferably in locked cabinet
- ☐ Toxic plants hung or placed out of reach*
- ☐ Excess quantities of cleaning fluid, paints, pesticides, drugs, and other toxic substances not stored in home
- ☐ Used containers of poisonous substances discarded where child cannot obtain access
- ☐ Telephone number of local poison control center and address of home with nearest cross-street posted near phone
- ☐ Syrup of ipecac in home containing two doses per child
- ☐ Medicines clearly labeled in childproof containers and stored out of reach
- ☐ Household cleaners, disinfectants, and insecticides kept in their original containers, separate from food and out of reach
- ☐ Smoking in areas away from children

Safety: Falls

- ☐ Nonskid mats, strips, or surfaces in tubes and showers
- ☐ Exits, halls, and passageways in rooms kept clear of toys, furniture, boxes, or other items that could be obstructive
- ☐ Stairs and halls well lighted, with switches at both top and bottom
- ☐ Sturdy handrails for all steps and stairways
- ☐ Nothing stored on stairways
- ☐ Treads, risers, and carpeting in good repair
- ☐ Glass doors and walls marked with decals
- ☐ Safety glass used in doors, windows, and walls
- ☐ Gates on top and bottom of staircases and elevated areas, such as porch, fire escape*
- ☐ Guardrails on upstairs windows with locks that limit height of window opening and access to areas such as fire escape*
- ☐ Crib side rails raised to full height; mattress lowered as child grows*
- ☐ Restraints used in high chairs, walkers, or other baby furniture; preferably walkers not used*
- ☐ Scatter rugs secured in place or used with nonskid back
- ☐ Walks, patios, and driveways in good repair

Safety: Bodily Injury

- ☐ Knives, power tools, and unloaded firearms stored safely or placed in locked cabinet
- ☐ Garden tools returned to storage racks after use
- ☐ Pets properly restrained and immunized for rabies
- ☐ Swings, slides, and other outdoor play equipment kept in safe condition
- ☐ Yard free of broken glass, nail-studded boards, other litter
- ☐ Cement birdbaths placed where young child cannot tip them over*

From Wong, D. L. (1995). *Whaley & Wong's Nursing Care of Infants and Children* (5th ed.). St. Louis, MO, Mosby-Year Book.

*Safety measures are specific for homes with young children. All safety measures should be implemented in homes where children reside and visit frequently, such as those of grandparents or babysitters.

†Federal regulations are available from U. S. Consumer Product Safety Commission; (800) 638-CPSC.

‡Home care instructions for infant cardiopulmonry resuscitation and infant/child choking are available in *Wong and Whaley's Clinical Manual of Pediatric Nursing*.

Although child abuse and neglect cases cross all age, race, education, and socioeconomic lines, "statistics of *reported* cases show individuals who are poor, young, black and who have little education are more frequent abusers" (Maurer, 1995, p. 523). It is important to realize that *reported* data may be biased, and observation for and reporting of suspected cases should consider suspicious cases from any social class, race, or age.

Nurses who practice in community settings are sometimes in a position to recognize and intervene in cases of suspected child abuse. To assist in recognizing individuals at risk to be abusive parents, Table 13–22 lists characteristics of abusive parents, and Table 13–23 details physical and behavioral indicators of child abuse and neglect.

Child abuse and neglect are crimes in all 50 states, and nurses have a legal responsibility to report suspected or actual cases of child abuse. Most institutions providing care to children have a written policy regarding reporting of suspected child abuse. These policies need to be reviewed periodically. Table 13–24 outlines standard procedure for notification and investigations of child abuse and neglect cases. Finally, to assist in the reduction of family violence, Table 13–25 de-

TABLE 13–22 **Characteristics and Behaviors of Abusive Parents**

Characteristics

At or below poverty level
History of abuse or neglect as a child
Poor parenting skills
Poor coping skills
Involved in a crisis situation (e.g., unemployment, divorce, financial difficulties)
Does not understand normal growth and development patterns
Unrealistic expectations of their child's behavior
Looking to child for satisfaction of needs of love, support, and reassurance
Poor impulse control
Low tolerance for frustration
Poor or inadequate role models
Socially isolated from support systems
Women more frequently physically abuse children
Men more frequently sexually abuse children
Stepfathers are five to eight times more likely to engage in sexual abuse of their children than birth fathers

Behaviors

Frequent use of harsh punishment
Projection of blame onto the child
History of drug or alcohol abuse
Delay getting medical attention for child
Respond inappropriately to child during treatment (e.g., ignore, show no concern or overinvolved with attention)
Use different facilities for treatment of child
Blame siblings, babysitters, or others without substantiation or place blame on child's clumsiness
Tell contradictory stories to explain injury
Vague about cause of the injury

Data from Watkins, A. C. (1997). Violence in the community. In J. M. Swanson and M. A. Nies (Eds.). *Community Health Nursing: Promoting the Health of Aggregates.* (2nd ed.). Philadelphia, W. B. Saunders; Smith-DiJulio, K. and Holzapfel, S. K. (1994). Families in crisis: Family violence. In E. M. Varcarolis (Ed.). *Foundations of Psychiatric Mental Health Nursing* (2nd ed.). Philadelphia, W. B. Saunders; Grant, C. (1995). Physical and sexual abuse. In D. Antai-Otong (Ed.). *Psychiatric Nursing: Biological and Behavioral Concepts.* Philadelphia, W. B. Saunders, pp. 407–426; Maurer, F. A. (1995). Violence: A social and family problem. In C. M. Smith and F. A. Maurer (Eds.). *Community Health Nursing: Theory and Practice.* Philadelphia, W. B. Saunders, pp. 517–547.

TABLE 13–23 **Physical and Behavioral Indicators of Child Abuse and Neglect**

Physical Indicators	Behavioral Indicators
Physical Abuse	
The skin is the largest and most frequently injured organ system; it may show Unexplained bruises and welts in various stages of healing that may form patterns Unexplained burns by cigars or cigarettes of immersion burns (e.g., socklike, glovelike, or on buttocks or genitalia) Rope burns Unexplained lacerations or abrasions Skeletal injuries Unexplained fractures in various stages of healing; multiple or spiral fractures Unexplained injuries to mouth, lips, gums, eyes, or external genitalia	Wary of adult contacts Apprehensive when other children cry Constantly on the alert for danger Extremes of behavior; aggressiveness or passive and withdrawn Frightened of parents Afraid to go home Reports injury by parents
Physical Neglect	
Hunger Poor hygiene Poorly or inappropriately dressed Lack of supervision for prolonged periods Lack of medical or dental care Constant fatigue, listlessness, or falling asleep in class	Begs or steals food Alone at inappropriate times or for prolonged periods Delinquent Steals Early arrival and late departure from school Reports no caretaker
Sexual Abuse	
Difficulty in walking or sitting Torn, stained, or bloody underwear Genital pain or itching Bruises or bleeding from the external genitalia, vaginal, or anal areas Venereal disease, especially in preteens Drug and alcohol abuse Developmental delays Teen pregnancy	Negative self-esteem Inability to trust and function in intimate relationships Cognitive and motor dysfunctions Deficits in personal and social skills Bizarre, sophisticated, or unusual sexual behavior or knowledge Delinquent or runs away Suicide ideation Reports sexual assault
Emotional Maltreatment	
Failure to thrive Lags in physical development Speech disorders Developmental delays	Behavior extremes from passivity to aggression Habit and conduct disorders (e.g., sucking and biting to antisocial behavior and destructiveness) Neurotic traits Attempted suicide

From Watkins, A. C. (1997). Violence in the home. In J. M. Swanson and M. A. Nies (Eds.). *Community Health Nursing: Promoting the Health of Aggregates.* (2nd ed.). Philadelphia, W. B. Saunders, pp. 576–598.

scribes prevention strategies for individuals, families, and communities.

Nursing Care for Common Health Problems

Nurses who care for infants and children in community settings should be aware of common illnesses and conditions. Table 13–26 describes some of the more frequently encountered acute and episodic illnesses and chronic conditions in infants and children, including prevention strategies, identification, and treatment.

SUMMARY

Nurses who practice in community settings are uniquely able to affect the health and well-being of children through appropriate assessment, counseling, health teaching, and providing other interventions as needed. Early detection of congenital, developmental, or acquired health problems and referral for treatment can dramatically influence the child's health and development. Preventive measures, such as encouraging appropriate, consistent use of safety devices (e.g., car seats, helmets, smoke detectors) and advance preparation (e.g., keeping poisons and matches away from children, having ipecac available), can be life saving. Furthermore, establishing healthy habits (e.g., good nutrition, dental hygiene, regular exercise) and failure to establish poor habits (e.g., smoking, drug and alcohol use) while in childhood can improve the quality and length of the individual's life.

This chapter has presented a great deal of information regarding health promotion and illness prevention for infants, children, and adolescents.

TABLE 13–24 **Typical Procedure for Notification and Investigation of Child Abuse and Neglect Cases**

Actions Taken by Community Health Nurse

Identify suspected case abuse/neglect
Verbally report to
1. Child protection agency
   or
2. Local law enforcement

Send written report to child protection agency within 48 hours of initiating complaint and send a copy to the state's attorney's office

Actions Taken by Designated Child Protection Agency

Prompt investigation within 24 hours if abuse, usually longer—perhaps as much as 5 days—if neglect
Completed investigation within 10 days and report of findings to state's attorney's office
Dispensation of case
1. No evidence found
2. Inconclusive, file kept open
3. Evidence exists, action taken

Possible actions include
1. Mandated supervision in home
2. Conditions imposed on parents to continue custody (e.g., attend parenting classes, drug rehabilitation)
3. Temporary removal of children to foster care or other relatives' homes
4. Permanent removal of child from home
5. Court action to cease parental rights to clear for adoption

From Maurer, F. A. (1995). Violence: A social and family problem. In C. M. Smith and F. A. Maurer (Eds.). *Community Health Nursing: Theory and Practice.* Philadelphia; W. B. Saunders, pp. 517–547.

There are many agencies and organizations that assist in providing care and information to promote the health of children. Table 13–27 presents a list of some of these resources.

Text continued on page 406

TABLE 13–25 **Components of a Comprehensive Program to Reduce Family Violence of Individuals, Families and the Community**

Individuals	Family	Community
Primary Prevention—Goal: Promotion of Family Wellness		
Birth control services for sexually active teens Family life education in schools, churches, and community centers Child care education for teenagers who babysit Preventive mental services for adults and children Training for professionals in early detection of violence	Parenting classes in hospitals, schools, and other community agencies Provision of bonding opportunities for new parents Social services for families Referral of at-risk families to community health nurses for follow-up services	Community education concerning family violence Development of community services such as crisis lines, respite placement for children, respite care for families with dependent elderly members, homemaker education, and evaluation
Secondary Prevention—Goal: Diagnosis of and Service for Families in Stress		
Nursing assessment for evidence of family violence in all health care settings Shelter or foster home placement for victims Social services for individuals or families Referral to community health agencies	Referral to self-help groups	Trauma center with 24-hour reporting, 24-hour response, 24-hour case intake, coordination with legal and medical authorities, coordination with voluntary agencies that have services, coordination with social services department responsible for provision of services Multidisciplinary committees to review cases and make recommendations for treatment Public authority involvement, police, district attorney, courts
Tertiary Prevention—Goal: Reeducation and Rehabilitation of Violent Families		
Professional counseling services for individuals and families	Parenting reeducation—formal training in child rearing	Foster homes Self-help groups Public authority involvement Follow-up care for known cases

From Watkins, A. C. (1997). Violence in the home. In J. M. Swanson and M. A. Nies (Eds.). *Community Health Nursing Promoting the Health of Aggregates.* (2nd ed.). Philadelphia, W. B. Saunders, pp. 576–598.

TABLE 13–26 Common Health Problems in Infants and Children

Disease/ Condition	Definition/Etiology	Prevention Strategies	Signs and Symptoms/ Complications	Management/Treatment
Acute Respiratory/Ear, Nose, and Throat Conditions				
Viral infection (e.g., cold, influenza)	*Cold:* caused by up to 200 virus strains. Incubation 1–7 days (usually 2–3 days). Children have 6–10 colds/year, decreasing with age.	Avoid exposure. Wash hands carefully; avoid touching nose or eyes with contaminated fingers. Influenza may be prevented or lessened with vaccination. Those in high-risk groups should be immunized yearly. Amantidine and rimantadine may be used prophylactically in high-risk groups and during epidemics of influenza A.	*Cold:* nasal stuffiness, sneezing, scratchy throat, coughing, malaise, headache, slight fever. *Influenza:* Sudden onset of moderate to high fever (102°F or higher), chills, headache, anorexia, malaise, muscle aches, cough, runny nose, sore throat, cervical lymphadenopathy, hoarseness, possible abdominal pain, vomiting, nausea, diarrhea. *Complications:* otitis media, pneumonia, bronchitis, sinusitis are most common.	*Medications:* analgesics and antipyretics (avoid aspirin), decongestants, antitussives. *Symptom management:* bed rest, oral hydration. Observe for complications.
Bacterial pharyngitis (e.g., strep throat, tonsillitis)	*Strep throat:* caused by group A beta-hemolytic streptococci bacteria. Greatest incidence in children 5–18 years of age.	Avoid contact with respiratory secretions. Children should not return to school until after 24 hours of antibiotic therapy.	Sore throat, reddened throat, enlarged tonsils, soft palate petechia, cervical adenopathy, fever (moderate to high), anorexia, chills, malaise, headache. Abdominal pain and vomiting may occur. *Complications:* Scarlet fever (red, papular rash beginning in the axilla and chest, spreading to the abdomen and extremities). *Progressive complications:* rheumatic fever, glomerulonephritis, myocarditis.	Throat culture for suspected infection. For streptococcal pharyngitis, a 10-day course of penicillin is the standard. Erythromycin or cephalexin may be used for penicillin-allergic children. Teach parents the importance of completing the 10-day course of therapy. Monitor for complications.
Otitis media	Inflammation of the middle ear, usually bacterial. Almost 93% of children have one or more cases of otitis media by age 7 years; 36% of children have six or more cases of otitis. Peak incidence is at 6–12 months; declines after age 7 years.	*Risk factors:* upper respiratory infection, smoking in household, family history of middle ear infections.	Ear pain, decreased hearing, may have accompanying nasal discharge and cough, fever. Infants—irritability, may have slight fever. Otoscopic examination reveals decreased eardrum mobility, bulging eardrum redness. *Complications:* perforation of eardrum, hearing loss, scarring of eardrum, mastoiditis.	*Medications:* Amoxicillin, cephalosporin. Antihistamines and decongestants may be used, but not always effective. Referral for tympanostomy tubes and adenoidectomy for multiple infections, middle ear fluid that persists for 4–6 months, and/or hearing loss.

Respiratory infections: bronchitis and pneumonia	Inflammation and infection of the respiratory tract, usually as a secondary infection. May be caused by a virus or bacteria. *Viral pneumonia:* most common cause of lower respiratory tract infections in young children and often follows an upper respiratory infection. About 90% of pneumonia in children is viral. *Bacterial pneumonia:* usually caused by pneumonocci, streptococci and staphylococci.	Monitor colds and influenza for complications and secondary infection.	Coughing—may be dry and hacking; nonproductive cough is common in bronchitis. Fever (may be mild to severe); chills, dyspnea, pulmonary rales and rhonchi, altered breath sounds, pleurisy, friction rub, headache. Tachypnea, malaise, wheezing.	*Medications:* antibiotics for bacterial bronchitis or pneumonia. Analgesics, antipyretics, cough suppressant.
Chronic Respiratory Diseases				
Asthma	Reversible airway disease characterized by bronchial construction, mucosal edema, and increased mucus production.	Avoidance of triggers: allergens (e.g., pollens, molds, dust mites, animal dander), smoke and other pollutants, viral infections. Use of medications to prevent inflammation and exacerbation.	Abnormal pulmonary function tests, wheezing, cough, prolonged expiration, hyperresonance, decreased breath sounds, nocturnal dyspnea, cyanosis, use of accessory respiratory muscles.	*Medication:* steroids, beta-agonists, anticholinergics, theophylline; monitoring of peak expiratory flow rates (PEFR); identify and eliminate irritants.
Vaccine-Preventable Diseases				
Measles (rubeola)	Highly contagious, acute viral infection; incubation 8–12 days postexposure. Contagious from 1–2 days before symptoms to 4 days after onset of rash.	Vaccine preventable. Post-exposure prophylaxis— vaccine is protective if given within 72 hours postexposure; immune globulin prevents/modifies illness if given within 6 days postexposure.	*Prodromal phase:* fever and cold-like symptoms, conjunctivitis, photophobia, nasal congestion, cough, Koplik spots (small white spots circumscribed in red, opposite lower molars). *Acute phase:* rash begins as fever peaks; dark red, maculopapular rash begins behind ears and at hairline and spreads from head to feet and lasts 10–15 days. Rash turns brown and scaly after 5–6 days. *Complications:* otitis media, bronchitis, and pneumonia are most common.	Bed rest, antitussives, antipyretics (avoid aspirin). *Notify Health Department.*
Mumps	Acute viral infection presenting with unilateral or bilateral parotitis. Incubation period 14–24 days. 85% of cases occur before age 15 years.	Vaccine preventable.	Parotid pain and swelling in one or both glands. Swelling peaks in 1–3 days and lasts 3–7 days. Mild to moderate fever.	Analgesics for pain (avoid aspirin). Liquid or soft diet, warm or cold compresses for swelling. *Complications:* orchitis or epididymitis are fairly common in postpubertal boys. Less common: meningoencephalitis, nephritis, pancreatitis, and oophoritis.

Table continued on following page

TABLE 13–26 Common Health Problems in Infants and Children *Continued*

Disease/ Condition	Definition/Etiology	Prevention Strategies	Signs and Symptoms/ Complications	Management/Treatment
Vaccine-Preventable Diseases *Continued*				
Chicken pox	Highly contagious infection caused by the varicella zoster virus. Most commonly affects children age 5–9 years of age but can develop in any age. Incubation period: 13–17 days postexposure.	Vaccine preventable. Postexposure varicella zoster immune globulin may be given to high-risk children. Avoidance of exposure (communicability—1 day before eruption of lesions until all vesicles have crusted).	*Prodromal stage:* slight fever, malaise, mild headache, and anorexia for first 24 hours. Rash begins on the trunk, spreads to face and then extremities. Lesions may develop on oral and vaginal mucous membranes. Lesions begin as macules and rapidly progress to papule, then vesicle, and present in varying degrees at one time.	Isolate child in home until vesicles have dried (usually 1 week after onset); decrease itching with antipruritic agents (e.g., calamine lotion), antihistamines and oatmeal baths. Use mild antipyretics for fever but *avoid aspirin.*
Genitourinary Conditions				
Urinary tract infection (UTI)	Inflammation or infection of the urethra, bladder, or kidney. In neonates, UTIs are more common in boys; by 4 months, they are *much* more common in girls, and this continues throughout childhood. *Escherichia coli* causes 75–90% of UTIs in children.	Good toileting hygiene (e.g., teaching girls to wipe from front to back); encourage frequent emptying of bladder; use cotton underpants. Avoid bubble baths.	Urinary urgency and frequency, burning, lower abdominal pain and cramping, hematuria, foul-smelling urine, fever. High fever and flank pain may indicate kidney infection. Recurrent infections may indicate renal anomalies, and referral for diagnostic evaluation is very important.	*Medications:* antibiotics based on culture/ sensitivity. A 7- to 10-day course of trimethoprim-sulfamethoxazole (TMP/ SMZ) or amoxicillin is usually given. Stress the importance of completing all medications.
Enuresis	Nocturnal enuresis is involuntary urination during sleep more than once a month in girls over 5 years and boys over 6 years of age. Enuresis affects about 10% of children (40% of 3 year olds, 10% of six year olds, and 3% of 12 year olds), with boys more commonly affected than girls.	More common if one or both parents report being enuretic as a child. Associated with reduced bladder capacity and/or frequent uninhibited bladder contractions.	Inability to keep from urinating while asleep at least once per month. Some children may be withdrawn and shy.	Encourage daytime fluids and less frequent urination to increase bladder size. Discourage any fluids 2 hours before bedtime; void just before bedtime; protect bed by having the child wear extra-thick underwear (not diaper), and put a towel under the child; encourage the child to get up to urinate during the night, but parents should not awaken the child to urinate; do not punish the child for wet night; praise dry nights. Bed-wetting alarms may help. *Medications:* Imipramine may be used. Intranasally administered desmopressin helps reduce nighttime production of urine and assists about 70% of children. Relapse is common after medications are discontinued. Emotional support of the child and parents is important.

Gastrointestinal Problems

Colic	Excessive crying seen in young infants who are otherwise well. Believed to be caused by paroxysmal abdominal cramping. Colic affects 10–25% of infants age 3 weeks to 3 months.	Milk allergy may contribute to some cases.	Inconsolable crying, often more than 3 hours per day; fist clenching, arching back, and drawing up of legs; excessive flatus.	Use of a pacifier, gentle rhythmic motions (e.g., rocking, car rides), music. Usually subsides by 3 months of age. Changing the baby's formula from a cow's milk formula or removing dairy products from the diet of lactating mothers may help in some cases. Give smaller, frequent feedings; burp during and after feedings; and place infant upright after feeding; place prone over a warm towel, hot water bottle, recovered heating pad. Emotional support and respite care for the primary caregiver is very important.
Gastroenteritis/stomach "flu"	In the United States, most cases of nausea, vomiting, and diarrhea are caused by viruses (rotavirus, parvovirus, adenovirus, and coronavirus). Symptoms usually occur 1–2 days after exposure.	Good handwashing, avoidance of exposure.	Nausea, vomiting, diarrhea, abdominal pain and distention, anorexia, malaise. Usually self-limiting, lasting 1–3 days. Dehydration in infants and small children may occur rapidly, however, and parents need to observe for fever, increasing thirst; decreasing urine production, sunken eyes or fontanel, diminished skin turgor, lethargy, cool extremities.	Replacement of fluids and electrolytes by encouraging consumption of clear liquids, such as uncaffeinated beverages, broth, flavored gelatin, water, or rehydration fluids (e.g., Pedialyte, Gatorade). As nausea and diarrhea decrease, slowly add mild foods, such as saltines, dry toast, rice, baked potato; avoid dairy products, most fruits, vegetables, meats. Hospitalization for intravenous rehydration may be necessary in severe cases.
Appendicitis	Acute inflammation of the vermiform appendix. Affects about 7% of all persons; children, adolescents, and young adults (10–30 years of age) are most commonly infected, although may affect person of any age.	Familial tendency is possible. High-fiber diets may help prevent appendicitis.	Constant abdominal pain—initially periumbilical then right-lower quadrant; guarding of the abdomen; anorexia; nausea; vomiting; slight fever. Leukocytosis (10,000 to 18,000/mm^3); ultrasound usually reveals appendix inflammation. *Complications:* perforation with abscess, peritonitis, bowel obstruction, gangrene.	*Surgery:* Emergency appendectomy. If uncomplicated, broad-spectrum antibiotic given postoperatively.

Table continued on following page

TABLE 13–26 **Common Health Problems in Infants and Children** *Continued*

Disease/ Condition	Definition/Etiology	Prevention Strategies	Signs and Symptoms/ Complications	Management/Treatment
Gastrointestinal Problems *Continued*				
Hepatitis A	Hepatitis A (infectious hepatitis) is the most common form of acute viral hepatitis. The virus is spread directly through the fecal-oral route directly or indirectly through ingestion of contaminated food or water. The highest incidence occurs among preschool- and school-aged children. Incubation is approximately 4 weeks.	Vaccine is available. Immune globulin for postexposure (given 1–2 weeks after exposure prevents illness in 80–90% of individuals). Proper handwashing.	Usually rapid onset of fever, malaise, nausea, anorexia, jaundice, dark urine, abdominal pain. *Complications:* rare.	*Supportive/symptomatic care:* Children should not return to school until jaundice has resolved and serum enzyme levels are no more than twice normal. Household contacts should be given immune globulin.
Pinworms (*Enterobius vermicularis*)	The most common helminthic infection in the United States, infecting about one third of all U. S. children at any one time. Predominant age is 5–14 years, with girls being more frequently infected than boys. More common in warm climates and crowded living conditions.	Prevention of reinfection includes treating all family members with two doses of medication 2 weeks apart. Washing all sleeping garments and bed linen in hot water and vacuuming around the beds may be helpful. Careful, thorough handwashing after toileting and before eating and daily showering may also help.	Intense perianal itching, particularly nocturnal, poor sleep, restlessness, enuresis, and distractibility.	*Tape test:* to diagnose, parents press transparent tape firmly against the child's perianal area as soon as the child awakens in the morning. The tape is placed in a container and taken to a clinic for microscopic examination. *Medication:* Mebendazole (Vermox) is used to treat all family members (not recommended for children <2 years or pregnant women).
Infectious diarrhea	Diarrhea and related symptoms are frequently caused by bacteria or parasites, in addition to viral gastrointestinal conditions described above. Bacteria include *E. coli, Staphylococcus, Salmonella* species, *Shigella* species, *Campylobacter jejuni, Vibrio cholerae,* and *Yersinia enterocolitica*. Parasitic organisms include *Giardia* species, *Cryptosporidium* species.	Etiology is typically contaminated food or water. Symptoms usually occur within a few hours of exposure. See Chapter 5 for information on food preparation and clean water. Good handwashing (particularly following toileting and changing diapers) is essential.	Symptoms vary somewhat based on causative organism. Severe, watery diarrhea; abdominal cramps; nausea; vomiting; headache; anorexia; malaise. Stools may contain blood or mucus. With *Giardia* species, pale, greasy stools; fatigue; and weight loss are seen. Observe for signs and symptoms of dehydration (see above).	*Medication:* antibiotics appropriate for the organism. Symptomatic treatment (see above).
Constipation	Stool is passed infrequently or consists of hard, small masses. Etiology is usually dietary, such as too much milk or insufficient fluids or bulk-forming foods. More common in boys 1–5 years of age, although not uncommon in infants.	Good dietary practices, including recommended servings of fruits, vegetables and grain products. Prunes or prune juice may help infants and small children who have hard stools. Encourage drinking noncaffeinated, noncarbonated fluid and good elimination patterns.	Infrequent, hard stools, pain or difficulty during defecation. Chronic constipation may be caused by underlying conditions (e.g., anorectal malformation, Hirschsprung's disease, endocrine disorder or side effect of medication [e.g., iron]). Referral for evaluation may be indicated.	Occasional constipation in infants may be treated with glycerin suppositories, but caution parents not to overuse. Stool softener, such as docusate sodium (Colace), may be prescribed. Laxatives and cathartics are generally not recommended. Promote good toileting and dietary changes.

Dermatologic Disorders

Diaper dermatitis	Caused by irritation in the diaper area.	Change diapers frequently; use of ointments and exposing the diaper area to air periodically may help prevent. Wash cloth diapers in mild soap and rinse thoroughly. Avoid commercial wipes.	Redness and irritation in the diaper area.	
Impetigo	A superficial skin infection usually caused by *Staphylococcus aureus* or *Group A streptococci.* Most common bacterial skin infection in children. Predominate age, 2–5 years. Most often occurring in hot, humid climates.	Good hygiene. Discourage children from scratching scabs or insect bites. Keep fingernails short and clean.	Begins as an erythematous papule, which progresses to a vesicle and crusts over. Pustules most frequently occur on face (around mouth or nose) or at a site of skin breakage (scratch or insect bite). Often multiple sites or satellite lesions occur. May be a complication of scabies, chicken pox, pediculosis, or eczema.	*Medication:* Erythromycin, cephalosporins, topical antibiotic ointments. Encourage cleanliness; wash areas two or three times per day with diluted antibacterial soap; wash linens and clothing separately from other family members' (this may need to be done daily until lesions have resolved). Exclude from school or day care until after antibiotics have been administered for 24 hours. Monitor for signs of spread.
Pediculosis	Infestation of lice—*Pediculus humanus captitis* (head lice) is the most common type of lice found in children. Whites, Asians, Hispanics and Native Americans are most commonly affected, and girls are more commonly infected than boys.	Lice are transmitted by close personal contact. Encourage children to avoid sharing objects such as combs, brushes, hats and clothing with other children. May also be transmitted through bed linen and upholstered chairs.	Nits (egg cases) are white spheres on the hair shaft. Nits are found most often on the back of head and neck and behind the ears and are "glued" to the shaft and thus cannot be moved (distinguishing them from dandruff). Adult lice are small black specks that move and jump on the scalp and hair. Itching is very common. Eyelashes may be involved.	*Medication:* Lindane (Kwell) or permethrin (Nix) shampoo. Treat the entire family. After treatment, remove nits with a nit comb. Wash all linens, brushes, combs, and hats in hot water. (Infants and pregnant women should not use Lindane.) Exclude from school or day care until treated.
Scabies	Skin infestation by the mite *Sarcoptes scabiei.* Most common in children and young adults.	Good general hygiene.	Generalized itching, which is often worse at night. Burrows are commonly found in finger webs, wrists, hands, feet, penis, scrotum, buttocks, and waistline. Vesicle and pustules may be evident if infection occurs.	*Medication:* Permethrin (Elimite cream), Lindane (Kwell), or Crotamiton (Eurax) cream or lotions are applied into the skin from the head to the soles of the feet and left on for 8–14 hours, then thoroughly washed off. A second application 48 hours later is usually recommended. Treat all intimate contacts and family members. Wash clothing, bed linen, and towels.

Table continued on following page

TABLE 13–26 **Common Health Problems in Infants and Children** *Continued*

Disease/ Condition	Definition/Etiology	Prevention Strategies	Signs and Symptoms/ Complications	Management/Treatment
Dermatologic Disorders *Continued*				
Ringworm (fungal infections of the skin)	Refers to several related fungi infections. Commonly infected are the scalp *(Tinea capitis)*, body *(Tinea pedis)*, and groin (*Tinea cruris*—jock itch)	Associated with confined living quarters, poor hygiene. May become epidemic in schools and day care centers. Good personal hygiene, avoidance of sharing clothing, shoes, brushes, combs can stop spread. Identification and treatment of infected individuals and household pets are important.	Although some variation occurs depending on site. Lesions usually appear as round patches of scale that spread. Itching is very common.	*Medications:* Topical administration of anti-fungal agents. Encourage good hygienic practices.
Acne	*The* most common skin disorder. An inflammatory disorder of the sebaceous glands resulting in progression of comedones (whiteheads, blackheads), to papules, inflammatory pustules. Scarring occasionally occurs. Acne most commonly affects adolescents during early to later puberty.	Diet probably has little effect on acne. Good nutrition and adequate sleep and exercise are beneficial.	Presence of comedones (whiteheads and blackheads). Inflammatory lesions, including papules, pustules, and nodules occur. Most often affected are the face, upper chest, and upper back.	*Medications:* Topical medications such as benzoyl peroxide and topical erythromycin are helpful for milder cases. Low-dose oral tetracycline, erythromycin, and oral contraceptives can be effective in more severe acne. Isotretinoin (Accutane) may also help. Good skin care should include daily washing with a mild soap.

Data from Dambro, M.R. (1996). *Griffith's 5 Minute Clinical Consult.* Baltimore: Williams & Williams; Jackson, D. B. and Saunders, R. B. (1994). *Child Health Nursing: A Comprehensive Approach to the Care of Children and Their Families.* Philadelphia; J. B. Lippincott; Betz, C. L., Hunsberger, M. M., and Wright, S. (1994). *Family-Centered Nursing Care of Children* (2nd ed.). Philadelphia; W. B. Saunders.

TABLE 13–27 **Resources for Infants and Children**

Governmental Programs

Healthy Start
U. S. Department of Health and Human Services/
Public Health Service
Health Resources and Services Administration
Maternal and Child Health Bureau
Division of Healthy Start
5600 Fishers Lane, Room 11A-05
Rockville, MD 20857
(301) 443-8427

U. S. Department of Health and Human Services
Health Care Financing Administration
Medicaid Bureau

Supplemental Nutrition Program for Women, Infants and Children (WIC)
United States Department of Agriculture
Food and Consumer Service
Public Information
3101 Park Center Drive
Alexandria, VA 22302
(703) 305-2286

National Maternal and Child Health Clearinghouse
38th and R Streets, NW
Washington, D. C. 20057
(202) 625-8410

Association of Maternal and Child Health Programs
2001 L Street, NW, Suite 308
Washington, D. C. 20036
(202) 775-0436

Safety

National SAFE KIDS Campaign
111 Michigan Avenue, NW
Washington, D. C. 20010
(202) 884-4993

National Highway Traffic Safety Administration
Safety Countermeasures Division
NTSs-23
400 7th Street, SW
Washington, D. C. 20590
(202) 366-2121
(202) 366-2683

Children's Safety Network
38th and R Streets, NW
Washington, D. C. 20057
(202) 625-8400

Consumer Product Safety Commission
Washington, D. C. 20207
(800) 638-2772

Injury and Violence

Kempe National Center for the Prevention and Treatment of Child Abuse and Neglect
1205 Oneida Street
Denver, CO 80220
(303) 321-3963

Children's Safety Network
Adolescent Violence Prevention Resource Center
Education Development Center, Inc.
55 Chapel Street
Newton, MA 02158
(617) 969-7100 (ext. 2374)

Children's Defense Fund
122 C. Street NW, Suite 400
Washington, D. C. 20015
(202) 628-8787

Parents Anonymous
(800) 421-0353

National Abuse Hotline
(800) 422-4453

Dental Care

American Dental Association
211 East Chicago Avenue
Chicago, IL 60611

American Association of Public Health Dentistry
10619 Jousting Lane
Richmond, VA 23235

National Institute of Dental Research
National Institutes of Health
P. O. Box 54793
Washington, D. C. 20032

Miscellaneous

Easter Seal Society for Crippled Children and Adults
70 East Lake Street
Chicago, IL 60601
(800) 221-6827

March of Dimes Birth Defects Foundation
1275 Mamaroneck Avenue
White Plains, NY 10605
(914) 428-7100

Mothers Against Drunk Driving
511 East John Carpenter Freeway
Suite 700
Irving, TX 75062
(214) 744-MADD
(800) GET-MADD

Students Against Driving Drunk
P. O. Box 800
Marlboro, MA 01752
(508) 481-3568

Key Points

- The leading causes of mortality for infants are congenital anomalies, SIDS, low birth weight, and respiratory distress syndrome. After 1 year of age and through adolescence, the leading causes of death are unintentional injury, cancer, homicide, and heart disease. In teenagers, suicide is added to the list.
- The leading causes of acute illness in children are respiratory conditions (e.g., cold, influenza, and respiratory infection), other infections (e.g., viral infections, intestinal virus), acute ear infection, and injuries. Major chronic conditions are respiratory conditions (e.g., allergic rhinitis, asthma, chronic bronchitis); skin conditions (e.g., acne, dermatitis), musculoskeletal conditions; and vision, speech, and hearing impairment.
- There are a number of federal- and state-sponsored health programs and services for disadvantaged, underserved, and disabled children. These include Medicaid EPSDT, WIC; Head Start, Healthy Start, and PL 94-142 (education for All Handicapped Children Act).
- The Preventive Services Task Force has issued screening guidelines for infants and children to test for genetic, congenital, developmental, and pathological problems and conditions. These include routine infant screenings (e.g., testing of newborns for phenylketonuria, congenital hypothyroidism), body measurement (height, weight, and head circumference), developmental screening, vision screening, hearing screening, lead screening, and screening for anemia.
- Health promotion activities for infants, children, and adolescents include nutrition education and counseling on nutrition, physical activity and exercise, sleep and rest patterns, dental health, and maturation and puberty.
- Illness prevention should include information on prevention of substance (drugs and alcohol) use and abuse, prevention of use of tobacco products, and safety issues (e.g., vehicle safety, poisoning, head injury prevention, drowning prevention, and prevention of fire and burns).
- Detection and prevention of child abuse is very important in community-based nursing practice, and nurses should be informed regarding patterns of abuse and how to identify suspected abuse and how and when to intervene.

Learning Activities and Application to Practice

In class

- Invite a guest speaker from the local agency responsible for child protection services. Have the speaker discuss signs and symptoms that might indicate child abuse and how and when to refer suspected cases. Encourage a discussion of the legal and ethical requirements of health care professionals in addressing child abuse.

- Discuss the Preventive Services Task Force recommendations for infants, preschool children, school-aged children, and adolescents) (see Tables 13–3 and 13–4). Are these guidelines followed by most practitioners? Why or why not?

In clinical

- Allow students to observe and assist in completion of an EPSDT screening.
- Allow students to collect blood samples for routine infant screenings. Ensure that agency protocols are carefully followed.
- Assign students to complete developmental screening, such as the Denver II, on two or three children of differing ages. Share results with the clinical group.
- In groups of three or four, have students develop and present a health education program on one of the topics included in the chapter. For example, groups might teach parents of preadolescents about maturational changes, or parents of infants about how to protect children from poisoning or about infant nutrition needs.
- Complete a "child safety home checklist" for a family encountered during clinical or a neighbor or friend. Share findings and suggestions or recommendations for change with the clinical group.

REFERENCES

Advocates for Highway and Auto Safety. (1994). *Motorcycle Helmet Laws: Questions & Answers.* Washington, D. C., Advocates for Highway and Auto Safety.

American Academy of Pediatrics/Committee on Genetics. (1992). Issues in newborn screening. *Pediatrics, 89,* 345–349.

American Cancer Society. (1995). *Cancer Facts & Figures —1995.* Atlanta, GA, American Cancer Society.

American Dental Association. (1989). *Baby Bottle Tooth Decay.* Chicago, American Dental Association.

American Dental Association. (1992). *Your Child's Teeth.* Chicago, American Dental Association.

Berger, E. (1994). Violence prevention in the schools—programs that work. *TBI Challenge!, 2* (3), 43.

Betz, C. L., Hunsberger, M. M., and Wright, S. (1994). *Family-Centered Nursing Care of Children* (2nd ed.). Philadelphia, W. B. Saunders.

Centers for Disease Control. (1989). Criteria for anemia in children and childbearing-aged women. *Morbidity and Mortality Weekly Report, 38,* 400–404.

Centers for Disease Control. (1990). Fatal injuries to children—United States, *Morbidity and Mortality Weekly Report, 39,* 442–445.

Centers for Disease Control. (1991). *Preventing Lead Poisoning in Young Children: A Statement by the Centers for Disease Control.* Atlanta, Centers for Disease Control.

Centers for Disease Control. (1992a). Accessibility of cigarettes to youths aged 12–17 years—United States, 1989. *Morbidity and Mortality Weekly Report, 41* (27), 485–488.

Centers for Disease Control. (1993). Infant mortality-United States, 1991. *Morbidity and Mortality Weekly Report, 42* (48), 926–930.

Centers for Disease Control. (1992b). Selected tobacco-use behaviors and dietary patterns among high school students—United States, 1991. *Morbidity and Mortality Weekly Report, 41* (24), 417–421.

Centers for Disease Control/National Center for Injury Prevention and Control. (1993). *The Prevention of Youth Violence: A Framework for Community Action.* Atlanta, Centers for Disease Control and Prevention/National Center for Injury Prevention and Control.

Centers for Disease Control and Prevention/National Center for Environmental Health. (1994). *Childhood Lead Poisoning Prevention Program.* Atlanta, U. S. Department of Health and Human Services/Centers for Disease Control.

Centers for Disease Control and Prevention. (1995). Injury-control recommendations: Bicycle helmets. *Morbidity and Mortality Weekly Report, 44* (RR-1).

Dambro, M. R. (1996). *Griffith's 5 Minute Clinical Consult.* Baltimore, Williams & Wilkins.

Evans, A. and Friedland, R. B. (1994). *Financing and Delivery of Health Care for Children.* Washington, D. C., National Academy of Social Insurance.

Frankenburg, W. K. and Dodds, J. B. (1990). *DENVER II: Training Manual.* Denver, Denver Developmental Materials, Inc.

Grant, C. (1995). Physical and sexual abuse. In D. Antai-Otong (Ed.). *Psychiatric Nursing: Biological and Behavioral Concepts.* Philadelphia, W. B. Saunders, pp. 407–426.

Jackson, D. B. and Saunders, R. B. (1993). *Child Health Nursing: A Comprehensive Approach to the Care of Children and Their Families*. Philadelphia, J. B. Lippincott.

Kovner, A. R. (1995). *Jonas's Health Care Delivery in the United States* (5th ed.). New York, Springer Publishing Co.

Maurer, F. A. (1995). Violence: A social and family problem. In C. M. Smith and F. A. Maurer (Eds.). *Community Health Nursing: Theory and Practice*. Philadelphia, W. B. Saunders, pp. 517–547.

Murray, R. B. and Zentner, J. P. (1993). *Nursing Assessment and Health Promotion: Strategies Through the Life Span* (5th ed.). Norwalk, CT, Appleton & Lange.

National Center for Health Statistics. (1994). *Advance Data from the National Ambulatory Medical Care Survey: 1992 Summary*. DHHS Publication No. (PHS) 94–1250. Hyattsville, MD, National Center for Health Statistics.

National Center for Health Statistics. (1993). Advance report of final mortality statistics, 1991. *Monthly Vital Statistics Report, 42* (Suppl 21), 21. DHHS Publication No. (PHS) 93–1120.

National Center for Health Statistics. (1994). *Vital Statistics of the United States, 1990*. DHHS Publication No. (PHS) 94–1104. Washington, D. C., Public Health Service.

National Institutes of Health. (1994). *Seal out Dental Decay*. NIH Publication No. 94–489. Washington, D. C., National Institutes of Health.

Ripa, L. W. (1993). A half-century of community water fluoridation in the United States: Review and commentary. *Journal of Public Health Dentistry, 53* (1), 17–44.

Selekman, J. (1995). Children in the community. In C. Smith and F. A. Maurer (Eds.). *Community Health Nursing: Theory and Practice*. Philadelphia, W. B. Saunders, pp. 693–718.

Selekman, J. (1993). *Pediatric Nursing*. Springhouse, PA, Springhouse.

Smith-DiJulio, K. and Holzapfel, S. K. (1994). Families in crisis: Family violence. In E. M. Varcarolis (Ed.). *Foundations of Psychiatric Mental Health Nursing* (2nd ed.). Philadelphia, W. B. Saunders.

Texas Department of Health. (1990). Protect your child against accidental poisoning. Austin, TX, Texas Department of Health.

U. S. Consumer Product Safety Commission. (1994). *Your Home Fire Safety Checklist*. Washington, D. C., Government Printing Office.

U. S. Department of Agriculture/Food and Consumer Service. (1994). *Special Supplemental Nutrition Program for Women Infants and Children*. Alexandria, VA, U. S. Department of Agriculture/Food and Consumer Service.

U. S. Department of Health and Human Services. (1990). *Healthy People 2000: National Health Promotion and Disease Prevention Objectives*. Washington, D. C., Government Printing Office.

U. S. Department of Health and Human Services. (1995). *Healthy People 2000: Midcourse Review and 1995 Revisions*. Washington, D. C., Government Printing Office.

U. S. Department of Health and Human Services/Health Care Financing Administration. (1992). *EPSDT: A Guide for Educational Programs*. HCFA Pub. No. 02192. Washington, D. C., Government Printing Office.

U. S. Department of Health and Human Services/Office of Disease Prevention and Health Promotion. (1994). *Clinician's Handbook of Preventive Services*. Washington, D. C., Government Printing Office.

U. S. Department of Health and Human Services/Office of Disease Prevention and Health Promotion. (1997). *Guide to Clinical Preventive Services* (2nd ed.). Washington D. C., Government Printing Office.

Watkins, A. C. (1997). Violence in the community. In J. M. Swanson and M. A. Nies (Eds.). *Community Health Nursing: Promoting the Health of Aggregates* (2nd ed.). Philadelphia, W. B. Saunders, pp. 576–589.

Wong, D. L. (1995). *Whaley & Wong's Nursing Care of Infants and Children* (5th ed.). St. Louis, MO, Mosby-Year Book.

14

Health Promotion and Illness Prevention for Elders in the Community

Case Study *Frank Fox is a Registered Nurse (RN) working in a senior health clinic in a small city. The clinic provides comprehensive, integrated, and systematic care for individuals aged 65 years and older. In addition to three RNs, the clinic employs two physicians, two nurse practitioners, a dietitian, a pharmacist who specializes in geriatrics, laboratory and radiology technicians, and a social worker. Services are individualized, and clients are seen in the clinic, at home, or in the hospital, as warranted.*

On Friday, Frank saw Mr. Peterson, a 75-year-old retired postal worker, for his annual physical examination. Mr. Peterson lives with his wife in a small house not far from the clinic. Five years earlier, Mr. Peterson had a mild heart attack and was hospitalized for 1 week. He has been hospitalized on two other occasions: 10 years ago for a cholecystectomy and last year for prostate surgery. He takes daily medication for hypertension, a multivitamin, and 325 mg of aspirin. He has occasional bouts of constipation that, he states, are relieved with over-the-counter laxatives. Mr. Peterson has no physical limitations, drives without difficulty, and wears glasses.

Physical findings showed that his weight was unchanged from 1 year ago, blood pressure was 142/88, pulse rate was 76 beats per minute and regular, and respiration rate was 20 breaths per minute. In accordance with guidelines from the U. S. Preventive Services Task Force, Mr. Peterson was given a complete physical examination, including a complete blood count with a blood lipid profile, an electrocardiogram (ECG), and test for fecal occult blood. Mr. Peterson reported no problems with depression, and because his mental and cognitive states were appropriate, formal assessments were not performed. According to clinic records, Mr. Peterson had received a pneumococcal immunization 3 years earlier. Because it was the beginning of the influenza season, he was offered an opportunity to be immunized and he agreed.

Physical examination revealed a relatively healthy older adult. Blood pressure appeared controlled, the ECG showed no new changes, and digital rectal findings were negative. The eye examination, however, showed some degree of cataract formation, and Mr. Peterson was referred to an ophthalmologist. In addition, several small lesions were detected on his hands and face, and he was referred to a dermatologist for evaluation.

Health teaching performed by Frank and other members of the clinic staff focused on diet and physical activity, prevention of falls, signs and symptoms of heart attack, and warning signs of cancer. Before Mr. Peterson left, Frank gave him a flu shot, informing him that the results of the blood tests would be available early the next week and that he would call with the results.

In 1900, people over 65 years of age constituted 4% of the population. By 1988, that proportion increased to 12.4%; by 2000 it is projected to reach 13%; and by the year 2030, it may reach 22%. The most rapid population increase over the next decade is expected to be among those over age 85 years (USDHHS, 1990). Seeking to improve the health and limiting disabilities of older Americans are key components of *Healthy People 2000*. Table 14–1 presents examples of related objectives.

Because of the complex and unique health needs of the aging population, as well as the anticipated growth in this aggregate and the resulting impact on the health care delivery system, all nurses should be knowledgeable about health care needs of elders. To offer a better understanding of this population, Table 14–2 presents some "fast facts" about older Americans.

According to Evashwick (1993), of persons age 65 and older, 80% have at least one chronic health problem, and most have multiple problems (p. 180). Arthritis and other orthopedic impairments, hypertension, hearing loss, heart conditions, and cataracts and other visual impairments are the most common chronic conditions among older adults. The extent of chronic conditions associated with aging is illustrated in Table 14–3. These conditions, in turn, are often accompanied by functional disabilities.

Improving functional independence through prevention or control of chronic illnesses, such as heart disease, cancer, stroke, chronic obstructive pulmonary disease, arthritis, and osteoporosis, as well as conditions associated with aging (i.e., vision and hearing impairments, incontinence and dementia), is a goal for all older adults. Promoting regular, moderate physical activity (e.g., walking, gardening, swimming) can help control or limit chronic conditions. Enhanced clinical services directed at prevention of illnesses, such as immunization against pneumonia and influenza, and screening for cancer and heart disease can help prevent serious conditions and may provide early diagnosis and referral for prompt treatment when they are detected. In addition, enhanced primary care can assist in the management of chronic problems such as hypertension, arthritis, and diabetes. Improving social networks can promote independence and reduce social isolation, thereby decreasing depression, nutritional deficits, and other related conditions associated with aging.

Nurses practicing in community settings frequently have an opportunity to work with older people and their families and to address these and related issues. This chapter describes tools for assessment of older adults, materials for health education, and resources for organizations that work with the elderly.

Assessment of Older Adults

The Standards of Gerontological Nursing Practice require regular assessment "in a comprehensive, accurate and systematic manner" (American Nurses' Association, 1987). A comprehensive assessment should include gathering information on the individual's physical health, health history,

TABLE 14–1 ***Healthy People 2000:* Examples of Objectives for Older Adults**

9.4 Reduce deaths from falls and fall-related injuries to no more than 2.3 per 100,000. (Age-adjusted baseline: 2.7 per 100,000 in 1987)

Special Population Targets

Deaths from Falls and Fall-Related Injuries (per 100,000)	***1987 Baseline***	***2000 Target***
9.4a People aged 65–84 years	18	14.4
9.4b People aged 85+ years	131.2	105.0

9.7 Reduce hip fractures among people aged 65 years and older so that hospitalizations for this condition are no more than 607 per 100,000 people. (Baseline: 714 per 100,000 in 1988)

17.1 Increase years of healthy life to at least 65 years. (Baseline: an estimated 62 years in 1980)

Special Population Targets

Years of Healthy Life	***1987 Baseline***	***2000 Target***
17.1a Blacks	56	60
17.1b Hispanics	62	65
17.1c People aged 65+ (years of healthy life remaining at age 65)	12	14

17.3 Reduce to no more than 90 per 1,000 people the proportion of all people aged 65 years and older who have difficulty in performing two or more personal care activities, thereby preserving independence. (Baseline: 111 per 1,000 in 1984–1985)

17.6a Reduce significant hearing impairment among people aged 45 years and older to a prevalence of no more than 180 per 1,000. (Baseline: average of 203 per 1,000 during 1986–1988)

17.7a Reduce significant visual impairment among people aged 65 years and older to a prevalence of no more than 70 per 1,000. (Baseline: average of 87.1 per 1,000 during 1986–1988)

17.17 Increase to at least 60% the proportion of providers of primary care for older adults who routinely evaluate people aged 65 years and older for urinary incontinence and impairments of vision, hearing, cognition and functional status. (Baseline data not available)

17.18 Increase to at least 90% the proportion of perimenopausal women who have been counseled about the benefits and risks of estrogen replacement therapy (combined with progestin, when appropriate) for prevention of osteoporosis. (Baseline data not available)

21.2f Increase to at least 40% the proportion of adults aged 65 years and older who have received, as a minimum within the appropriate interval, all of the screening and immunization services and at least one of the counseling services appropriate for their age and gender as recommended by the U. S. Preventive Services Task Force. (Baseline data not available)

Modified from U. S. Department of Health and Human Services (USDHHS). (1990). *Healthy People 2000: National Health Promotion and Disease Prevention Objectives.* Washington, D. C.: Government Printing Office.

functional ability, cognitive and mental state, and nutritional status. Consistent with use of the nursing process in other areas, interventions should be based on assessment findings and anticipated or potential threats to health and well-being of the patient.

GENERAL ASSESSMENT

A thorough health history is necessary to learn as much about the client as possible to discover issues and problems that might need attention and to assign priority. Most agencies have health his-

TABLE 14–2 **Facts About the Elderly**

Life Expectancy and Population Trends

- The "life expectancy at birth" for Americans is almost 75 years (white men, 72.3; white women, 78.9; nonwhite men, 64.9; nonwhite women, 73.4).
- Persons 65 years of age can expect to live for more than 16 more years.
- Persons aged 85+ years, America's "oldest old," increased almost 38% and constitute the most rapidly growing segment of the population.
- By 2040, the United States may have more people aged 65 and older than persons younger than 20 years of age.

Living Patterns

- Most men aged 65+ years live with their wives (75%).
- Most women aged 65+ years are widows (48.7%); an additional 39.9% live with their husbands.
- Less than 5% of the older population is institutionalized at any given time; however, about one in four older adults will spend some time in a nursing home during the last years of their lives.
- California, New York, Florida, Pennsylvania, and Texas have the greatest *numbers* of older adults. Florida, Pennsylvania, Iowa, and Rhode Island have the greatest *percentages* of older adults, and populations are rising most dramatically in Nevada, Alaska, Hawaii, and Arizona.
- More than 66% of the elderly live in a family setting; about 31% live alone.

Retirement and Income

- Around two thirds of American workers retire before age 65 and spend more than 20% of their lives in retirement.
- Social Security benefits are the major source of income for the elderly, providing more than half of the monthly income for the majority of recipients.

Health and Health Care

- The leading causes of death for persons aged 65 years and older are (in order): heart disease, cancer, cerebrovascular accident, chronic obstructive pulmonary disease, pneumonia/influenza, diabetes, and accidents.
- Elderly persons use 32% of all prescription medications.
- Adults over 65 years of age average almost nine visits to a physician annually.
- Medicare is the major source of payment for health care of the elderly and pays approximately 93% of hospital costs for this population.

Data from Eliopoulos, C. (1993). *Gerontological Nursing* (3rd ed.). Philadelphia, J. B. Lippincott; Roen, O. T. (1993). Senior health. In J. M. Swanson and M. Albrecht (Eds.). *Community Health Nursing: Promoting the Health of Aggregates.* Philadelphia, W. B. Saunders; Lashley, M. E. (1995). Elderly persons in the community. In C. M. Smith and F. A. Maurer (Eds.). *Community Health Nursing: Theory and Practice.* Philadelphia, W. B. Saunders; U. S. Department of Commerce (USDOC). (1990). *Statistical Abstract of the U. S.* (110th ed.). Washington, D. C., Bureau of the Census; and American Association of Retired Persons. (1993). *Profile of Older Americans 1993.* Washington, D. C., *American Association of Retired Persons.*

tory tools and assessment guides available for collecting this information. Minimal information should include (Luggen, 1996)

- Biographical data (name age, date of birth, sex, race)
- Informant identification (self, relative, friend)
- Chief complaint (reason the patient is seeking help)
- History of present illness (onset, location, and severity of symptoms; treatment or control methods; precipitating factors; associated symptoms)
- Past history (allergies, drug reactions, past illnesses, hospitalizations, current prescription and over-the-counter medications)
- Family history (diseases, particularly heart disease, diabetes, tuberculosis, hypertension, arthritis, and cancer, in near relatives—parents, siblings, children)

TABLE 14–3 **Most Prevalent Chronic Conditions Among Older Americans: Prevalence per 1,000 People**

Conditon	Age 65–74 Years	Age 75+ Years
Arthritis/gout	477	562
Hypertension	361	352
Heart conditions (incuding ischemic heart disease and heart rhythm disorders)	272	404
Hearing impairment	257	415
Orthopedic impairment	162	222
Cataracts	126	226
Chronic sinusitis	158	160
Diabetes	114	105
Visual impairment	71	112
Tinnitus	85	96

From National Center for Health Statistics (1994). Current Estimates from the National Health Interview Survey, 1992. *Vital and Health Statistics, Series 10,* Washington, D. C., Government Printing Office, p. 189.

- Psychosocial history (marital status; occupation; retirement history; current life situation; nutritional history; alcohol, smoking, or drug use; immunization history; education; leisure and exercise activities)
- Review of symptoms (history of concerns, symptoms or illnesses, such as cardiovascular system [palpitations, murmur, hypertension], gastrointestinal system [nausea, abdominal pain, hemorrhoids], neurological problems [headache, syncope, seizures], and psychiatric problems [depression, memory loss, insomnia])
- Functional capacity (*activities of daily living* [ADL], such as bathing, toileting, feeding) and *instrumental activities of daily living* [IADL], such as driving, using the telephone, preparing meals)

The Comprehensive Older Person's Evaluation (COPE) is an example of a tool that elicits essential information from patients regarding a number of areas, including cognition, social support, financial status, psychological health, and physical health. Use of a tool of this type can be valuable in ensuring that all factors that affect health are addressed. The COPE instrument is presented in Figure 14–1.

PHYSICAL CHANGES

The process of aging results in a number of physical changes that contribute to development of chronic illnesses and conditions. To illustrate the "expected" differences, illnesses, and problems commonly found with aging, Table 14–4 lists normal physical changes and related health implications. Nurses who frequently care for older adults in community settings should be aware of these changes to recognize expected findings and to assist in detection of unusual or abnormal findings. In addition, Table 14–5 presents some of the most common health problems encountered in older people, including etiology, symptoms, risk factors, identification, and clinical management.

NUTRITION

When assessing nutritional status in older people, the nurse must recognize physical changes and other factors that can influence dietary intake. Table 14–6 describes some factors and potential clinical manifestations. Nurses who routinely work with older patients should assess for signs of nutritional deficiencies and develop interventions that will minimize or eliminate them.

Interventions for nutritional deficits might include referral to a variety of providers or community resources that address the identified problem. For example, the nurse might obtain a referral for Meals on Wheels if the patient is not able to cook or might obtain assistance for dental care or dentures for patients with missing teeth. Nutrition education is vitally important, and the nurse might suggest the use of dietary supplements and tips on how to manage constipation.

Promoting Functional Independence

Functional independence refers to the extent to which the individual (in this case, the older pa-

Text continued on page 429

COMPREHENSIVE OLDER PERSONS' EVALUATION (COPE)

PROVIDER NAME (PRINT): ______________________ DATE OF VISIT: ____________
CHIEF COMPLAINT: ________________________________

Today I will ask you about your overall health and function and will be using a questionnaire to help me obtain this information. The first few questions are to check your memory.
PRELIMINARY COGNITION QUESTIONNAIRE: RECORD IF ANSWER IS CORRECT WITH (+). IF ANSWER IS INCORRECT WITH (−). RECORD TOTAL NUMBER OF ERRORS.

(+, −)

A. What is the date today? ____
B. What day of the week is it? ____
C. What is the name of this place? ____
D. What is your telephone number? (RECORD ANSWER) ______________ ____
IF SUBJECT DOES NOT HAVE PHONE, ASK: What is your street address? ______________ ____
E. How old are you? (RECORD ANSWER) ______________ ____
F. When were you born? (RECORD ANSWER FROM RECORDS IF PATIENT CANNOT ANSWER) ______________ ____
G. Who is the President of the United States now? ____
H. Who was the President just before him? ____
I. What was your mother's maiden name? ____
J. Subtract 3 from 20 and keep subtracting from each new number you get, all the way down ____

(CORRECT: 17, 14, 11, 8, 5, 2)
TOTAL ERRORS____

IF MORE THAN 4 ERRORS, ASK K. IF MORE THAN 6 ERRORS, COMPLETE QUESTIONNAIRE FROM INFORMANT.

K. Do you think you would benefit from a legal guardian, someone who would be responsible for your legal and financial matters?
4. Yes 2. Have functioning legal guardian (DESCRIBE: ______________)
3. Have legal guardian 1. No

DEMOGRAPHIC SECTION

1. PATIENT'S RACE OR ETHNIC BACKGROUND (RECORD) ______________
2. PATIENT'S GENDER (CIRCLE) Male Female
3. How far did you go in school?
6. 0–8 years 4. High school complete 2. Four year degree
5. High school incomplete 3. College or technical school 1. Post-graduate education

SOCIAL SUPPORT SECTION: Now there are a few questions about your family and friends.

4. Are you now married, widowed, separated, or divorced, or have you never been married?
1. Now Married 2. Widowed 3. Separated 4. Divorced 5. Never Married
5. Who lives with you? (CIRCLE ALL RESPONSES)
1. Spouse 4. Live alone
2. Other relative or friend (SPECIFY: ______________) 5. Nursing home
3. Group living situation (non-health)
6. Have you talked to any friends or relatives by phone during the last week? 1. Yes 2. No
7. Are you satisfied by seeing your relatives and friends as often as you want to, or are you somewhat dissatisfied about how little you see them? 1. Satisfied (SKIP TO #8) 2. Dissatisfied (ASK A)
A. Do you feel you would like to be involved in a Senior Citizens Center for social events, or perhaps meals? 3. Yes 2. Am Involved (DESCRIBE: ______________) 1. No

Figure 14–1

8. Is there someone who would take care of you for as long as you needed if you were sick or disabled?
    1. Yes (SKIP TO C) 2. No (ASK A)
    A. Is there someone who would take care of you for a short time? 1. Yes (SKIP TO C) 2. No (ASK B)
    B. Is there someone who could help you now and then? 1. Yes (ASK C) 2. No (ASK C)
    C. Whom would we call in case of an emergency? (RECORD NAME AND TELEPHONE) ____________

____

FINANCIAL SECTION: The next few questions are about your finances and any problems you might have.
9. Do you own, or are you buying, your own home? 1. Yes (SKIP TO #10) 2. No (ASK A)
    A. Do you feel you need assistance with housing?
        3. Yes (DESCRIBE: ____________)
        2. Have subsidized or other housing assistance
        1. No
10. Are you covered by private medical insurance, Medicare, Medicaid, or some disability plan? (CIRCLE ALL THAT APPLY)
    1. Private insurance (SPECIFY BELOW AND SKIP TO #11) ____________
    2. Medicare 3. Medicaid
    4. Disability (SPECIFY: ____________) (ASK A)
    5. None 6. Other (SPECIFY: ____________)
    A. Do you feel you need additional assistance with your medical bills? 2. Yes 1. No
11. Which of these statements best describes your financial situation?
    3. My expenses are so heavy that I cannot meet my bills (ASK A)
    2. My expenses make it difficult to meet my bills (ASK A)
    1. My bills are no problem to me (SKIP TO #12)
    A. Do you feel you need financial assistance such as (CIRCLE ALL THAT APPLY)
        1. Food stamps 3. Assistance in paying your heating or electical bills
        2. Social Security or disability payments 4. Other financial assistance? (DESCRIBE: ____________)

PSYCHOLOGICAL HEALTH SECTION: The next few questions are about how you feel about your life in general. There are no right or wrong answers, only what best applies to you. *Please answer yes or no* to each question.
12. Is your daily life full of things that keep you interested? 1. Yes 2. No
13. Have you, at times, very much wanted to leave home? 2. Yes 1. No
14. Does it seem that no one understands you? 2. Yes 1. No
15. Are you happy most of the time? 1. Yes 2. No
16. Do you feel weak all over much of the time? 2. Yes 1. No
17. Is your sleep fitful and disturbed? 2. Yes 1. No
18. Taking everything into consideration, how would you describe your satisfaction with your life in general at the present time—good, fair, or poor? 1. Good 2. Fair 3. Poor
19. Do you feel you now need help with your mental health; for example, a counselor or psychiatrist?
    3. Yes 2. Have (SPECIFY: ____________) 1. No

PHYSICAL HEALTH SECTION: The next questions are about your health.
20. During the past month (30 days), how many days were you so sick that you couldn't do your usual activities, such as working around the house or visiting with friends? TOTAL NUMBER OF DAYS: ____________
21. Relative to other people your age, how would you rate your overall health at the present time; excellent, good, fair, poor, or very poor?
    1. Excellent (SKIP to #22) 3. Good (ASK A) 5. Poor (ASK A)
    2. Very Good (SKIP TO #22) 4. Fair (ASK A)
    A. Do you feel you need additional medical services such as a doctor, nurse, visiting nurse, or physical therapy? (CIRCLE ALL THAT APPLY)
        1. Doctor 2. Nurse 3. Visiting nurse 4. Physical therapy 5. None
22. Do you use an aid for walking, such as a wheelchair, walker, cane, or anything else? (CIRCLE AID USUALLY USED) 5. Wheelchair 4. Walker 3. Cane 2. Other (SPECIFY): ____________ 5. None
23. How much do your health troubles stand in the way of your doing things you want to do; not at all, a little, or a great deal?
    1. Not at all (SKIP TO #24) 2. A Little (ASK A) 3. A great deal (ASK A)
    A. Do you think you need assistance to do your daily activities; for example, do you need a live-in aide or choreworker?
        1. Live-in aide 3. Have aide, choreworker or other assistance (DESCRIBE: ____________)
        2. Chore worker 4. None needed

Figure 14–1 *Continued*

24. Have you had, or do you currently have, any of the following health problems? (IF YES, PLACE AN "X" IN APPROPRIATE BOX AND DESCRIBE [MEDICAL RECORD INFORMATION MAY BE USED TO HELP COMPLETE THIS SECTION.])

	HX	CURRENT	DESCRIBE
a. Arthritis or rheumatism?			
b. Lung or breathing problem?			
c. Hypertension?			
d. Heart trouble?			
e. Phlebitis or poor circulation problems in arms or legs?			
f. Diabetes or low blood sugar?			
g. Digestive ulcers?			
h. Other digestive problem?			
i. Cancer?			
j. Anemia?			
k. Effects of stroke?			
l. Other neurological problem? (SPECIFY): ______			
m. Thyroid or other glandular problem? (SPECIFY): ______			
n. Skin disorders such as pressure sores, leg ulcers, burns?			
o. Speech problem?			
p. Hearing problem?			
q. Vision or eye problem?			
r. Kidney or bladder problems, or incontinence?			
s. A problem of falls?			
t. Problem with eating or your weight? (SPECIFY): ______			
u. Problem with depression or your nerves? (SPECIFY): ______			
v. Problem with your behavior? (SPECIFY): ______			
w. Problem with your sexual activity?			
x. Problem with alcohol?			
y. Problem with pain?			
z. Other health problems? (SPECIFY): ______			

Figure 14–1 *Continued*

25. What medications are you currently taking, or have been taking, in the last month? (May I see your medication bottles?) (IF PATIENT CANNOT LIST, ASK CATEGORIES A–R AND NOTE DOSAGE AND SCHEDULE, OR OBTAIN INFORMATION FROM MEDICAL OR PHARMACY RECORDS AND VERIFY ACCURACY WITH THE PATIENT.)

	Rx (DOSAGE AND SCHEDULE)
a. Arthritis medication	
b. Pain medication	
c. Blood pressure medication	
d. Water pills or pills for fluid	
e. Medication for your heart	
f. Medication for your lungs	
g. Blood thinners	
h. Medication for your circulation	
i. Insulin or diabetes medication	
j. Seizure medication	
k. Thyroid pills	
l. Steroids	
m. Hormones	
n. Antibiotics	
o. Medicine for nerves or depression	
p. Prescription sleeping pills	
q. Other prescription drugs	
r. Other non-prescription drugs	

26. Many people have problems remembering to take their medications, especially ones they need to take on a regular basis. How often do you forget to take your medications? Would you say you forget often, sometimes, rarely, or never? 4. Often 3. Sometimes 2. Rarely 1. Never

ACTIVITIES OF DAILY LIVING: The next set of questions ask whether you would need help with any of the following activities of daily living.

27. I would like to know whether you can do these activities without any help at all, or if you need assistance to do them. Do you need help to: (IF YES, DESCRIBE, INCLUDING PATIENT NEEDS)

	Yes	No	DESCRIBE (INCLUDE NEEDS)
a. Use the telephone?			
b. Get to places out of walking distance? (Use transportation?)			
c. Shop for clothes and food?			
d. Do your housework?			
e. Handle your money?			
f. Feed yourself?			
g. Dress and undress yourself?			
h. Take care of your appearance?			
i. Get in and out of bed?			
j. Take a bath or shower?			
k. Prepare your meals?			
l. Have any problem getting to the bathroom on time?			

28. During the past six months, have you had any help with such things as shopping, housework, bathing, dressing, and getting around?
    2. Yes (SPECIFY: ________________________________)
    1. No

Figure 14–1 *Continued*

TABLE 14–4 Normal Physical Assessment Findings

Cardiovascular Changes	
Cardiac output	Heart loses elasticity. Therefore heart contractility decreases in response to increased demands
Arterial circulation	Decreased vessel compliance with increased peripheral resistance to blood flow occurs with general or localized arteriosclerosis
Venous circulation	Does not exhibit change with aging in the absence of disease
Blood pressure	Significant increase in the systolic, slight increase in the diastolic, increase in peripheral resistance and pulse pressure
Heart	Dislocation of the apex is due to kyphoscoliosis, therefore diagnostic significance of location is lost
	Premature beats increase, but are rarely clinically important
Murmurs	Over half the aged have diastolic murmurs, the most common are heard at the base of the heart due to sclerotic changes on the aortic valves
Peripheral pulses	Easily palpated because of increased arterial wall narrowing and loss of connective tissue; vessels feel more tortuous and rigid
	Pedal pulses may be weaker due to arteriosclerotic changes; lower extremities are colder, especially at night; feet and hands may be cold and have mottled color
Heart rate	No changes with age at normal rest
Respiratory Changes	
Pulmonary blood flow and diffusion	Decreased blood flow to the pulmonary circulation: decreased diffusion
Anatomic structure	Increased anterior-posterior diameter
Respiratory accessory muscles	Degeneration and decreased strength; increased rigidity of chest wall
	Muscle atrophy of pharynx and larynx
Internal pulmonic structure	Decreased pulmonary elasticity creates senile emphysema
	Shorter breaths taken with decreased maximum breathing capacity, vital capacity, residual volume, and functional capacity
	Airway resistance increases: there is less ventilation at the bases of the lung and more at the apex
Integumentary Changes	
Texture	Skin loses elasticity: wrinkles, folding, sagging, dryness
Color	Spotty pigmentation in areas exposed to sun; face paler, even in the absence of anemia
Temperature	Extremities cooler; perspiration decreases
Fat distribution	Less on extremities, more on trunk
Hair color	Dull gray, white, yellow, or yellow-green
Hair distribution	Thins on scalp, axilla, pubic area, upper and lower extremities; facial hair decreases in men, women may develop chin and upper lip hair
Nails	Decreased growth rate

TABLE 14–4 **Normal Physical Assessment Findings** *Continued*

Genitourinary and Reproductive Changes	
Renal blood flow	Due to decreased cardiac output, reduction in filtration rate and renal efficiency; subsequent loss of protein from kidneys may occur
Micturition	In men frequency may increase due to prostatic enlargement In women decrease in perineal muscle tone leads to urgency and stress incontinence Nocturia increases for both men and women Polyuria may be diabetes-related Decreased volume of urine may relate to decrease in intake, but evaluation is needed
Incontinence	Occurrence increases with age, specifically in those with organic brain disease
Male reproduction	
Testosterone production	Decreases; phases of intercourse slower, refractory time lengthens
Frequency of intercourse	Changes in libido and sexual satisfaction should not occur, but frequency may decline to one or two times weekly
Testes	Decreased size; sperm count decreases, and the viscosity of seminal fluid diminishes
Female reproduction	
Estrogen	Production decreases with menopause
Breasts	Diminished breast tissue
Uterus	Decreased size, mucous secretions cease; uterine prolapse may occur due to muscle weakness
Vagina	Epithelial lining atrophies, canal narrows and shortens
Vaginal secretions	Become more alkaline as glycogen content increases and acidity declines
Gastrointestinal Changes	
Mastication	Impaired due to partial or total loss of teeth, malocclusive bite, and ill-fitting dentures
Swallowing and carbohydrate digestion	Swallowing more difficult as salivary secretions diminish Reduced ptyalin production impairs starch digestion
Esophagus	Decreased esophageal peristalsis Increased incidence of hiatus hernia with accompanying gaseous distention
Digestive enzymes	Decreased production of hydrochloric acid, pepsin, and pancreatic enzymes
Fat absorption	Delayed, affecting the rate of fat-soluble vitamins A, D, E, and K absorption
Intestinal peristalsis	Reduced gastrointestinal motility Constipation due to decreased motility and roughage
Musculoskeletal Changes	
Muscle strength and function	Decrease with loss of muscle mass, bony prominences normal in aged since muscle mass decreased
Bone structure	Normal demineralization, more porous Shortening of the trunk due to intervertebral space narrowing
Joints	Become less mobile; tightening and fixation occur Activity may maintain function longer Posture changes are normal; some kyphosis Range of motion limited
Anatomic size and height	Total decrease in size as loss of body protein and body water occur in proportion to decrease in basal metabolic rate Body fat increases, diminishes in arms and legs, increases in trunk Height may decrease 1 to 4 inches from young adulthood

Table continued on following page

TABLE 14–4 **Normal Physical Assessment Findings** *Continued*

Nervous System Changes	
Response to stimuli	All voluntary or automatic reflexes are slowed Decreased ability to respond to multiple stimuli
Sleep patterns	Stage IV sleep reduced in comparison to younger adulthood, frequency of spontaneous awakening increases The elderly stay in bed longer but get less sleep; insomnia is a problem, which should be evaluated
Reflexes	Deep tendon reflexes remain responsive in the healthy aged
Ambulation	Kinesthetic sense less efficient, may demonstrate an extrapyramidal Parkinson-like gait Basal ganglions of the nervous system are affected by the vascular changes and decreased oxygen supply
Voice	Range, duration, and intensity of voice diminish; may become higher pitched and monotonous
Sensory Changes	
Vision	
Peripheral vision	Decrease
Lens accommodation	Decreases, requires corrective lenses
Ciliary body	Atrophy in accommodation of lens focus
Iris	Development of arcus senilis
Choroid	Structure shows atrophy around disc
Lens	May develop opacity, cataract formation; more light is needed to see
Color	Fades or disappears
Macula	Degeneration occurs
Conjunctiva	Thins and looks yellow
Tearing	Decreases; increased irritation and infection
Pupil	May be different in size
Cornea	Presence of arcus senilis
Retina	Vascular changes can be observed
Stimuli threshold	Threshold for light touch and pain increases Ischemic paresthesias in the extremities are common
Hearing	High-frequency tones are less perceptible, hence language understanding is greatly impaired; promotes confusion and seems to create increased rigidity in thought processes
Gustatory	Acuity decreases as taste buds atrophy; may increase the amount of seasoning on food

From Ebersole, P., and Hess, P. (1985). *Toward Healthy Aging.* St. Louis, C. V. Mosby, pp. 184–186. Data from Malasonnos, L., et al. (1981). *Health Assessment* (2nd ed.). St. Louis, C. V. Mosby; Blake, D. (1979). Physiology and Aging Seminar for Nurses. Napa, CA, May 1979; and Wardell, S. (1979). *Acute Interventions: Nursing Process Throughout the Life Span.* Reston, VA, Reston Publishing Co.

TABLE 14–5 **Common Health Problems in Later Maturity**

Disease/Condition	Definition/Etiology	Risk Factors	Signs/Symptoms	Management/ Treatment
Cardiovascular System				
Coronary artery disease (CAD); angina	Progressive obstruction of blood flow through one or more coronary arteries caused by a build-up of plaque (cholesterol and lipids) on interior artery walls	Age (increases with age), gender, race and genetic inheritance, elevated serum lipids, hypertension, smoking, obesity, diabetes, stress, sedentary lifestyle	Substernal chest pain that may radiate to the left arm, neck, jaw, or shoulder; tachycardia or bradycardia; apprehension; dyspnea; diaphoresis; nausea and vomiting; syncope; fatigue	Dependent on degree of damage and physical findings *Diagnosis:* history and physical, chest x-ray, electrocardiogram, serum enzyme levels, serum lipids, stress test, echocardiogram *Medication:* nitroglycerin (sublingual, patches or ointment), beta-blocking agents, calcium channel blockers, antithrombotic therapy *Surgery:* coronary artery angioplasty or coronary artery bypass graft when indicated
Congestive heart failure (CHF)	Condition of altered cardiac function in which there is not enough cardiac output to meet demands of tissue metabolism	Age, hypertension, arteriosclerosis, CAD, other heart and lung conditions (arrhythmia, pneumonia, mitral stenosis, endocarditis)	Rales (crackles), difficulty breathing, tachypnea, confusion, insomnia, agitation, depression, nausea, anorexia, dyspnea, orthopnea, weight gain, bilateral ankle edema	*Medication:* digitalis, diuretics *Other interventions:* reduction in sodium intake, bed rest
Arrhythmias	Cardiac conduction irregularities characterized by chaotic electrical activity	Age, hypertension, CAD, valvular heart disease, CHF, diabetes pulmonary embolus, hyperthyroidism	Irregular pulse, tachycardia, palpitations, lightheadedness, fatigue, dyspnea, syncope, angina	Avoidance of risk (ethanol, caffeine, nicotine), management of underlying disease, prevention of complications (embolus) *Medication:* control ventricular rate (beta blockers, calcium channel blockers, cardiac glycosides), anticoagulants *Surgery:* surgical or invasive methods when appropriate (pacemaker implantation, implantable defibrillator)

Table continued on following page

TABLE 14–5 **Common Health Problems in Later Maturity** *Continued*

Disease/Condition	Definition/Etiology	Risk Factors	Signs/Symptoms	Management/ Treatment
Cardiovascular System *Continued*				
Peripheral vascular disease (atherosclerotic occlusive disease)	Obstruction or narrowing of the arteries causing interruption of blood flow to extremities (most commonly to feet and legs)	Complication of atherosclerosis, smoking, hyperlipidemia, diabetes, hypertension, and physical stress	Intermittent claudication, diminished or absent pulses, affected limb is cold, pale	Smoking cessation, foot and limb care, exercise program, weight control, cholesterol management, management of diabetes *Surgery:* bypass surgery, angioplasty, stent placement, amputation if necessary
Respiratory System				
Chronic obstructive pulmonary disease (COPD)	Consists of chronic bronchitis (increased mucus production and recurrent cough), emphysema (destruction of interalveolar septa)	Cigarette smoking, passive smoking, aging, air pollution, occupational exposure, severe viral pneumonia early in life	*Chronic bronchitis:* cough, sputum production, frequent infections, dyspnea, cyanosis, wheezing, diminished breath sounds *Emphysema:* minimal cough, scant sputum, dyspnea, weight loss, occasional infections, barrel chest, use of accessory muscles of respiration, pursed-lip breathing, diminished breath sounds	Smoking cessation, aggressive treatment of infections, treat reversible bronchospasm, pulmonary rehabilitation, avoidance of cold weather *Medication:* anticholinergics, theophylline, corticosteroids, bronchodilators, expectorants; supplemental oxygen when necessary
Asthma	Reversible airway disease characterized by bronchial constriction, mucosal edema, and increased mucus production	Allergic factors (pollens, molds, dust mites, animal dander), smoke and other pollutants, viral infections, exercise, family history	Abnormal pulmonary function tests, wheezing, cough, prolonged expiration, hyperresonance, decreased breath sounds, nocturnal dyspnea, cyanosis, use of accessory respiratory muscles	*Medication:* steroids, beta-agonists, anticholinergics, theophylline; monitoring of peak expiratory flow rate (PEFR); identify and eliminate irritants
Pneumonia	Acute inflammation of the lungs caused by bacterial, viral, fungal, chemical, or mechanical agents; most commonly caused by viral or bacterial infection in adults	Age, viral infection, alcoholism, immunosuppression, smoking, COPD, diabetes, malnutrition, general anesthesia, malignancy, mechanical ventilation, altered level of consciousness	Cough, fever, chest pain, chills, dark, thick or bloody sputum, anorexia, anxiety, chest dull to percussion, crackles (rales), cyanosis, diminished breath sounds, dyspnea, pleuritic pain, rhonchi, tachypnea, tachycardia, weakness	*Medication:* antibiotic therapy; bed rest; in severe cases, oxygen therapy, mechanical ventilation, chest physiotherapy when necessary

TABLE 14–5 **Common Health Problems in Later Maturity** *Continued*

Disease/Condition	Definition/Etiology	Risk Factors	Signs/Symptoms	Management/ Treatment
***Respiratory System** Continued*				
Tuberculosis (TB)	Caused by infection with *Mycobacterium tuberculosis;* causative organism may invade any organ but usually develops in the lungs	Human immunodeficiency virus (HIV) infection, homelessness, institutionalization (i.e., correctional or other facility), chronic conditions such as diabetes, renal failure, malnutrition, close and prolonged exposure to an infected individual	Productive cough, hemoptysis, fever, night sweats, weight loss, pleuritic pain, fatigue	*Medication:* based on diagnostic testing; prophylaxis with isoniazid (INH) for positive purified protein derivative (PPD) skin test for 9 months; for active disease, three anti-TB drugs for 6–12 months; careful monitoring of patient and condition to ensure compliance with medication regimen
Musculoskeletal System				
Osteoporosis	Progressive bone loss predisposing to atraumatic fractures, particularly of the vertebra, upper femur, distal radius, humerus, and ribs; in women, may be due to excessive and prolonged acceleration of bone resorption following menopausal loss of estrogen secretion	Gender (more common in women), age, family history, inadequate calcium and vitamin D intake, sedentary lifestyle, alcohol use, caffeine, smoking, steroid use, chemotherapy, radiation therapy	Acute or chronic back pain, kyphosis, scoliosis, atraumatic fractures, loss of height, absence of peripheral bone deformities	Weight reduction if appropriate; increase calcium intake to 1500 mg/day; avoid excess phosphate or protein intake; encourage ambulation and exercise; avoid exercises that increase compression and mechanical stress on spine *Medication:* hormone replacement therapy (estrogen/progesterone), synthetic calcitonins
Osteoarthritis	Degeneration of articular cartilage and hypertrophy of bone; leading cause of disability in elderly affecting between 33 and 90% of those over age 65; caused by biomechanical, biochemical, inflammatory, immunological factors	Age, obesity, prolonged occupational or sports stress, injury	Slowly developing joint pain, pain following use of joint, stiffness (particularly in the morning), joint enlargement, decreased range of motion, possibly joint tenderness, local pain, and stiffness	Weight reduction, fitness program, heat, physical therapy, protection of joints *Medication:* nonsteroidal anti-inflammatory agents, corticosteroids *Surgery:* may be indicated with advanced disease (joint replacement, debridement, osteotomy)

Table continued on following page

TABLE 14–5 **Common Health Problems in Later Maturity** *Continued*

Disease/Condition	Definition/Etiology	Risk Factors	Signs/Symptoms	Management/ Treatment
Genitourinary Tract				
Prostate conditions	Benign prostatic hyperplasia (BPH) is the benign growth of the prostate, which may result in bladder outlet obstruction; possibly arises from hormonal alterations associated with aging	Gender (male), age, family history	*Obstructive symptoms:* decrease in force of urine stream, hesitancy, postvoid dribbling, incomplete bladder emptying, overflow incontinence, urinary retention, inability to voluntarily stop stream *Irritative symptoms:* frequency, nocturia, urgency, urge incontinence *Other symptoms:* hematuria, distended bladder, enlarged prostate, renal failure due to obstruction	*Medication:* alpha-adrenergic antagonist, hormonal agents *Surgery:* transurethral resection of prostate (TURP), open prostatectomy, other procedures
Incontinence	See Tables 14–11 and 14–12			
Gastrointestinal Tract				
Periodontal disease (gingivitis)	Degeneration of tissues supporting the teeth; more than 80% of older adults have moderate periodontal disease, and 50% of adults over age 65 have lost some teeth from tooth decay or peridontal disease	Malnutrition, aging, inadequate plaque removal, diabetes, poor dental hygiene, faulty dental restoration (irritation by faulty bridges or partial dentures)	Mouth odor, gum swelling, redness, and bleeding, loose teeth, tooth loss	Removal of irritating factors (plaque, faulty dentures), promoting good oral hygiene, regular dental check-ups, smoking cessation *Medication:* antibiotic therapy sometimes indicated in severe cases
Diverticulitis (diverticular disease)	*Diverticulum* of colon: herniation of colon mucosa through the muscular layer; more common in sigmoid and distal colons *Diverticulitis:* an abscess or inflammation initiated by the rupture of a mucosal abscess; incidence increases with age; present in 40–50% of older population (aged 60–80 years)	Low-fiber diet, defects in colon wall strength, age (over age 40 years), low-residue diet, family history	*Diverticulosis:* 10–25% of individuals with diverticula have symptoms, pain, diarrhea, constipation, a palpable mass in the left iliac fossa; abdomen may be distended; no signs of peritoneal inflammation *Diverticulitis:* pain (acute, localized in left lower quadrant), fever, anorexia, nausea, vomiting, constipation or diarrhea, rebound tenderness, guarding, palpable mass, abdomen distended and tympanic, bowel sounds depressed	Nothing by mouth (NPO) status during acute diverticulitis; all patients with diverticula should increase dietary fiber intake *Medication:* oral treatment with antibiotics, analgesics *Surgery:* colon resection when indicated

TABLE 14–5 **Common Health Problems in Later Maturity** *Continued*

Disease/Condition	Definition/Etiology	Risk Factors	Signs/Symptoms	Management/ Treatment
Gastrointestinal Tract *Continued*				
Constipation	Decrease in frequency from usual bowel elimination pattern or difficulty in defecating	More common with age, sedentary lifestyle, electrolyte abnormalities, concomitant illness, inadequate fluid intake, inadequate fiber or bulk, side effects of drugs, chronic abuse of laxatives; psychiatric, cultural, emotional and environmental factors	Less frequency of bowel movements than the patient perceives as "normal" (typically 3–5 times/week), change in baseline defecating pattern; smaller stools than normal, impaction of stool, difficulty expelling feces from the rectum, painful evacuation, sensation of incomplete emptying of bowel, abdominal fullness	Encourage measures to improve bowel habits, routine time for toileting, avoid straining, respond to urge to defecate, daily physical exercise, increase fluid intake, increase dietary fiber *Medication:* bulk-forming agents (Metamucil, Citrucel), laxatives, stool softeners, lubricants (mineral oil), suppositories, cathartics, enemas
Endocrine System				
Diabetes	Non–insulin-dependent diabetes (NIDDM) (type II diabetes) accounts for 70–80% of all cases; hyperglycemia and glucose intolerance due to defects in insulin secretion and peripheral insulin action; almost 50% of elderly may have glucose intolerance	Family history, obesity, age	Polyuria, polydipsia, and polyphagia (however, classical symptom triad may be absent in NIDDM); weight loss; constipation; numbness and tingling in peripheral extremities; diminished peripheral pulses; headache; weakness; fatigue; frequent infections; abnormal plasma glucose levels	Combination of diet management (increased complex carbohydrate intake; decreased fat intake; avoidance of alcohol); weight loss when appropriate; regular exercise; home monitoring of blood or urine glucose; careful instruction on self-monitoring for, and management of, complications. *Medication:* oral hypoglycemic agents or insulin when necessary if conservative measures fail to control glucose levels

Table continued on following page

TABLE 14–5 **Common Health Problems in Later Maturity** *Continued*

Disease/Condition	Definition/Etiology	Risk Factors	Signs/Symptoms	Management/ Treatment
Neurological System				
Alzheimer's disease (see text and Tables 14–10 and 14–11)	Degenerative organic mental disorder characterized by progressive brain deterioration and dementia; usually occurs at age 65 years and older; cause unknown, although there is a genetic predisposition (50% of all patients have a positive family history); other theories include excessive amounts of an amyloid protein (beta-amyloid peptide), which is destructive to brain tissue; a virus; exposure to metals (particularly aluminum and mercury); an autoimmune disorder; and acceleration in aging	Family history, age, head trauma, low education level, Down syndrome	Progressive cognitive impairment lasting 3–20 years; three stages: early, middle, late *Early* (2–4 years): recent memory loss, forgets routine tasks, is distractible, forgets names or events, gets lost in familiar surrounding, has difficulty telling time and making decisions, is easily angered and aware of losses. *Middle* (2–5 years): patient has increased memory loss, may not recognize friends and family; wanders, confabulates; is preoccupied with thoughts; is immodest; undergoes gait changes; experiences bowel and bladder incontinence; has decreased ability to understand and express language; has flat affect, has hallucinations and delusions; becomes suspicious *Late* (1–3 years): inability to perform activities of daily living, little response to stimuli, loss of body weight, seizures, loss of bodily functions	Combination of improvement of cognitive function by slowing disease progression, managing or preventing behavior disturbances, and providing support and guidance to caregivers *Medication:* Tacrine HCl (Cognex) is only drug approved to treat Alzheimer's disease; other medications (e.g., neuroleptics, tricyclic antidepressants, anticonvulsants) are used to manage symptoms

TABLE 14–5 **Common Health Problems in Later Maturity** *Continued*

Disease/Condition	Definition/Etiology	Risk Factors	Signs/Symptoms	Management/ Treatment
Neurological System *Continued*				
Parkinson's disease	Neurodegenerative disorder of extrapyramidal system; characterized by a combination of tremor at rest, rigidity, and bradykinesia; cause not known, although probably the result of exposure to a toxic or infectious agent, or loss of dopamine neurons	Age; slightly more common in males	Rhythmic tremors of fingers, feet, lips, and head, with progressive rigidity of facial and trunk muscles; characteristic sign is shuffling gait while patient is leaning forward at the trunk	Maintain activity to highest degree possible, use cane for walking, avoid tension and frustration, minimize emotional upsets. Physical and occupational therapy may be indicated *Medication:* levodopa, dopamine agonists, monoamine oxidase (MAO) inhibitors, anticholinergics.
Cerebrovascular accidents (CVAs)	Sudden onset of a focal neurological deficit resulting from infarction or hemorrhage within the brain. CVAs are the second leading cause of death of people over 72 years of age.	Age, arteriosclerosis, hypertension, smoking, diabetes, family history	Symptoms depend on site of CVA *Carotid (hemispheric):* hemiplegia, hemianesthesia, aphasia, visual field defects, headache, seizure, amnesia, confusion *Vertebrobasilar (brainstem or cerebellar):* diplopia, vertigo, ataxia, facial paresis, dysphagia, dysarthria, impaired level of consciousness, behavioral changes	Maintain oxygenation; monitor cardiac rhythm; control hypertension; promote physical therapy, occupational therapy, and speech therapy when indicated *Medication:* antithrombotic measures (heparin, Coumadin, aspirin) *Surgery:* carotid endarterectomy when indicated
Sensory Disorders				
Cataract	Clouding or opacity of lens; may be congenital, related to metabolic or systemic conditions, or traumatically induced; most commonly associated with aging ("senile" cataract)	Aging; exposure to ultraviolet B rays	Blurred vision, problems with visual acuity in bright light or at night, falls, or accidents; lens opacity on eye examination; pupil may appear cloudy-white	*Surgery:* removal of cataract if visual impairment produces symptoms that interfere with lifestyle or occupation or pose risk of injury; in most cases, the cataract is replaced by a plastic intraocular lens

Table continued on following page

TABLE 14–5 **Common Health Problems in Later Maturity** *Continued*

Disease/Condition	Definition/Etiology	Risk Factors	Signs/Symptoms	Management/ Treatment
Sensory Disorders *Continued*				
Glaucoma	Damage to optic nerve and loss of visual field and visual acuity associated with high intraocular pressure *Acute* (closed-angle) (~10% of cases) *Chronic* (open-angle) (~90% of cases)	*Acute:* small cornea, Native Alaskan/Inuit ancestry, hyperopia, use of antidepressants or anticholinergics, cataract *Chronic:* positive family history, diabetes, African-American	*Acute:* severe eye pain, blurred vision, halos around lights, nausea and vomiting, elevated intraocular pressure *Chronic:* None until advanced, then gradual loss of peripheral vision, headaches, misty vision	*Acute:* medical emergency *Medication:* carbonic anhydrase inhibitors, hyperosmotic agents (e.g., mannitol) to lower pressure *Surgery:* peripheral iridectomy or iridotomy if glaucoma not managed through medication *Chronic: Medication:* used singly or in combination include topical beta-adrenergic blockers, carbonic anhydrase inhibitors, cholinergic agents *Surgery:* may be necessary if medical management is not successful
Hearing loss	Hearing loss may be complete or partial; may be classified as conductive or sensorineural *Conductive:* cerumen impaction, perforation of tympanic membrane, serous otitis media, damage to ossicles, thickening of the tympanic membrane, growth of skin into middle ear *Sensorineural:* noise induced (most common cause of hearing loss), acoustic tumor, Ménière's disease, heredity, congenital, viral, medication toxicity, or presbycusis (related to aging)	Eustacian tube obstruction, exposure to loud noise levels for extended periods of time; ototoxic medications; heredity; aging	Difficulty hearing (may be gradual or sudden); other symptoms include tinnitus, dizziness, pain and blockage; otoscopy may reveal abnormalities; audiometry tests for pure tone and/or impedance (middle ear pressure) may indicate loss	*Conductive:* cerumen impaction—remove with suction and irrigation or use of a wire curet; serous otitis: decongestants; surgery if hearing loss persists; other conditions: tympanic membrane, perforation, damaged ossicles and thickening of eardrum may need surgical correction *Sensorineural:* Depending on etiology, patient may require surgical correction (tympanoplasty, stapedectomy) or use of assistive devices (hearing aids, telephone enhancement aids)

TABLE 14–5 **Common Health Problems in Later Maturity** *Continued*

Disease/Condition	Definition/Etiology	Risk Factors	Signs/Symptoms	Management/ Treatment
Mental Health				
Depression	Clinical syndrome characterized by lowered mood, difficulty thinking, and somatic changes precipitated by feelings of loss (incidence higher in women) or guilt; between 10 and 65% of elderly may suffer from depression; it may be biochemical, genetic, or a deficiency in neurotransmitters, or situational (highest rate in persons with physical ailments)	Prior episode or diagnosis of depression, history of suicide attempt, lack of social support, stressful life events, gender, family history, substance abuse, alcoholism, chronic disease, chronic pain, retirement, age	Patient reports depressive feelings, poor appetite, sleep disorder (insomnia or hypersomnia), fatigue, restlessness, irritability, withdrawal, lack of interest or lack of desire to seek pleasure, poor self-image, poor memory, inability to make decisions, suicidal thoughts *Note:* in elderly, disorientation, memory loss, and distractibility may be signs of depression rather than dementia	Counseling or psychotherapy, often combined with antidepressants; in extreme cases, electroconvulsive therapy may be beneficial

Data from Dambro, M. R. (1996). *Griffith's 5-Minute Clinical Consult.* Baltimore: Williams & Williams; Luggen, A. S. (1996). *Core Curriculum for Gerontological Nursing.* St. Louis, Mosby-Year Book; Murray R., Zentner, J., Pinnell, N. (1993). Assessment and health promotion for the person in later maturity. In R. B. Murray and J. P. Zentner (Eds.). *Nursing Assessment and Health Promotion: Strategies Through the Life Span* (5th ed.). Norwalk, CT, Appleton & Lange; Eliopoulos, C. (1993). *Gerontological Nursing* (3rd ed.). Philadelphia, J. B. Lippincott.

tient) is able to complete "normal" and "instrumental" activities of daily living without assistance from others. Activities of daily living generally include bathing, dressing, eating, getting in and out of bed and chairs, walking, going outside, and toileting. The ability to perform necessary functions of life, such as taking transportation, preparing meals, shopping, and using the telephone, are examples of instrumental activities of daily living. Managing money as well as accomplishing routine housework is another example.

In older adults, functional impairment can be caused by cognitive, physical, social, and/or psychological disorders. According to Evashwick (1993), between 14 and 50% of older patients need help with one or more activities of daily living, with the percentage increasing markedly with age from 15% for ages 65 to 69 years to 50% for those over age 85 years. In addition, some 20% of those aged 65 to 69 years need assistance with at least one instrumental activity of daily living; similarly, the percentage increases with age, to approximately 55% by age 85 years.

Several objectives of *Healthy People 2000* address screening and referral of all elderly patients for threats to functional independence. Areas specifically targeted are presented in Table 14–1, and include

- Hearing impairment
- Impaired vision
- Cognitive deficits
- Urinary incontinence
- Decreased functional status

It is essential that all nurses working with older populations recognize potential threats and limita-

TABLE 14–6 **Factors That May Affect Nutrition in Later Maturity**

Factor and Process	Effect	Clinical Manifestation
Ingestion		
Loss of teeth; poor dentures; atrophy of jaws	Improper mastication; deletion of important foods from diet	Irritable bowel syndrome; constipation; malnutrition
Dietary habits	Overeating; eccentric diets	Obesity; malnutrition
Psychologic losses and changes; changes in social environment; lack of socialization	Poor appetite	Anorexia; weight loss
Reduced income; difficulty with food preparation and ingestion	Excessive ingestion of carbohydrates	Obesity; malnutrition
Decreased fluid intake	Dry feces	Impacted stools
Digestion and Absorption		
Decreased secretion of hydrochloric acid and digestive enzymes	Interference with digestion	Dietary deficiencies
Hepatic and biliary insufficiency	Poor absorption of fats	Fat-soluble vitamin deficiency; flatulence
Atrophy of intestinal mucosa and musculature	Poor absorption; slower movement of food through intestine	Vitamin and mineral deficiencies; constipation
Decreased secretion of intestinal mucus	Decreased lubrication of intestine	Constipation
Metabolism		
Impaired glucose metabolism and use	Diabetic-like response to glucose excesses	Hyperglycemia; hypoglycemia
Decrease in renal function	Inability to excrete excess alkali	Alkalosis
Impaired response to salt restriction	Salt depletion	Low-salt syndrome
Decline in basal metabolic rate	Lower caloric requirements but same amount of food eaten	Obesity
Changes in iron and calcium (phosphorus, magnesium) metabolism	Iron deficiency; increased requirements for calcium	Anemia; demineralization of bone; osteoporosis
Changes in vitamin metabolism	Deficiency in vitamins K and C especially	Peripheral neuropathy, sensorimotor changes; easy bruising and bleeding tendencies

From Murray, R., Zentner, J., and Pinnell, N. (1993). Assessment and health promotion for the person in later maturity. In R. B. Murray and J. P. Zentner (Eds.). *Nursing Assessment and Health Promotion: Strategies Through the Life Span* (5th ed.). Norwalk, CT, Appleton & Lange, pp 542–603.

tions to functional independence and associated health problems. Tools, health information, and teaching tips to prevent or manage threats to functional independence are described next.

HEARING DEFICITS

According to the National Center for Health Statistics (1994), more than 25% of individuals aged 65 years and over and more than 40% of those over age 75 years have some degree of hearing impairment. A a result of embarrassment or frustration, hearing loss in the elderly can contribute to social isolation, depression, and exacerbation of coexisting psychiatric problems. Hearing loss may be the result of cerumen impaction, calcification of the ossicles, or loss of nerve cells in the eighth cranial nerve (Murray et al., 1993).

All older adults should be questioned about signs of hearing loss. If hearing loss is suspected or confirmed following questioning, the nurse should perform pure-tone testing using an audiometer (USDHHS/ODPHP, 1994).

Patients with evidence of hearing loss should be referred to a specialist, since medical or surgical treatment may improve or restore hearing function. Hearing aids, when appropriate, are prescribed by specialists. Nurses in community settings, however, may be in a position to assist the patient in exploring resources to help obtain a hearing aid and to instruct in its proper use and maintenance. Finally, for health care providers working with older patients who are hearing-impaired, Table 14–7 contains guidelines that should assist communication.

VISION DEFICITS

Vision loss in adults is common, and the prevalence increases with age. It is estimated that more than 90% of older people require the use of corrective lenses (USDHHS/ODPHP, 1994); further, approximately 25% of all older people have significant visual deficits, and approximately 50% of all individuals identified as legally blind are 65 years of age or older (Eliopoulos, 1993). Cataracts, glaucoma, macular degeneration, and diabetic retinopathy often cause visual problems in the elderly. Loss of vision, in turn, may result in trauma from falls, automobile crashes, and other injuries and may significantly affect quality of life (USDHHS/ODPHP, 1994). Because most vision problems can be successfully managed through medical or surgical treatment or use of corrective lenses, early detection and prompt treatment are very important.

A comprehensive eye examination, including screening for visual acuity and glaucoma, should be performed yearly for individuals aged 65 years and over. Use of a standard Snellen wall chart or a tumbling "E" chart at 20 feet is used for basic screening. The patient should wear corrective lenses, if prescribed, during screening.

To determine the impact of visual impairment, the nurse should question the patient regarding limitations to normal and instrumental activities of daily living associated with poor vision. For example, the nurse might ask, "Does your vision make it difficult for you to feed yourself, read medication labels, groom yourself, handle money, or find your way around places outside of your home?" Determining whether the patient is using visual assistance devices, such as glasses, contact lenses, magnifying lenses, or large print books, can be beneficial in recognizing the degree of adaptation. After a complete assessment, the nurse should refer patients with significant changes in visual acuity or visual acuity of 20/40 or less with corrective lenses to an eye care specialist for further evaluation (USDHHS/ODPHP, 1994, p. 238).

In addition to identifying patients with visual difficulties and referring them for follow-up treatment, the nurse may be able to help the patient obtain needed treatment, visual aids (magnifying lenses, portable lights, large print books), or corrective lenses. Table 14–8 outlines tips for working with individuals who are significantly visually impaired or blind.

COGNITIVE IMPAIRMENT

Some degree of cognitive impairment is common among older individuals and often increases with age. An estimated 5 to 10% of individuals older

TABLE 14–7 **Guidelines for Communicating With the Hearing-Impaired Person**

- When you meet a person who seems inattentive or slow to understand you, consider the possibility that hearing, rather than manners or intellect, may be at fault. Some hard-of-hearing persons refuse to wear a hearing aid. Others wear aids so inconspicuous or clearly camouflaged that you may not spot them at first glance. Others cannot be helped by a hearing aid.
- Remember the hard-of-hearing may depend to a considerable extent on reading your lips. They do this even though they may be wearing a hearing aid, for no hearing aid can completely restore hearing. You can help by trying *always to speak in a good light* and by facing the person and the light as you speak.
- When in a group that includes a hard-of-hearing person, try to carry on your conversation with others in such a way that he or she can watch your lips. Never take advantage of the disability by carrying on a private conversation in his or her presence in low tones that cannot be heard.
- Speak distinctly but naturally. Shouting does not clarify speech sounds, and mouthing or exaggerating your words or speaking at a snail's pace makes you harder to understand. On the other hand, try not to speak too rapidly.
- Do not start to speak to a hard-of-hearing person abruptly. Attract his or her attention first by facing the person and looking straight into the eyes. If necessary, touch the hand or shoulder lightly. Help him or her grasp what you are talking about right away by starting with a key word or phrase, for example, "Let's plan our weekend now," "Speaking of teenagers. . . ." *If he or she does not understand you, do not repeat the same words.* Substitute synonyms: "It's time to make plans for Saturday," and so on.
- If the person to whom you are speaking has one "good" ear, always stand or sit on that side when you address him or her. Do not be afraid to ask a person with an obvious hearing loss whether he or she has a good ear and, if so, which one it is. The person will be grateful that you care enough to find out.
- Facial expressions are important clues to meaning. Remember that an affectionate or amused tone of voice may be lost on a hard-of-hearing person.
- In conversation with a person who is especially hard-of-hearing, do not be afraid occasionally to jot down key words on paper. If he or she is really having difficulty in understanding you, the person will be grateful for the courtesy.
- Many hard-of-hearing persons, especially teenagers, who hate to be different are unduly sensitive about their disability and will pretend to understand you even when they do not. When you detect this situation, tactfully repeat your meaning in different words until it gets across.
- Teach the family to avoid use of candles. Electric light will give the person a better chance to join the conversation because he or she can see the lips during conversation. Similarly, in choosing a restaurant or night club, remember that *dim lighting may make lipreading difficult.*
- Teach family members that they do not have to exclude the hard-of-hearing person from all forms of entertainment involving speech or music. Concerts and operas may present problems, but movies, plays, ballets, and dances are often just as enjoyable to people with a hearing loss as to those with normal hearing. (Even profoundly deaf persons can usually feel rhythm, and many are good and eager dancers.) For children, magic shows, pantomimes, and the circus are good choices.
- When sending a telegram to someone who does not hear well, instruct the telegraph company to deliver your message, not telephone it.
- The speech of a person who has been hard-of-hearing for years may be difficult to understand since natural pitch and inflection are the result of imitating the speech of others. To catch such a person's meaning more easily, watch the face while he or she talks.
- Do not say such things as "Why don't you get a hearing aid?" or "Why don't you see a specialist?" to a person who is hard-of-hearing. Chances are he or she has already explored these possibilities, and there is no need to emphasize the disability.
- *Use common sense* and tact in determining which of these suggestions apply to the particular hard-of-hearing person you meet. Some persons with only a slight loss might feel embarrassed by any special attention you pay them. Others whose loss is greater will be profoundly grateful for it.

From Murray, R., Zentner, J., and Pinnell, N. (1993). Assessment and health promotion for the person in later maturity. In R. B. Murray and J. P. Zentner (Eds.). *Nursing Assessment and Health Promotion: Strategies Through the Life Span* (5th ed.). Norwalk, CT, Appleton & Lange, pp 542–603.

TABLE 14–8 Guidelines for Helping the Blind Person

- Talk to the blind person in a normal tone of voice. The fact that he or she cannot see is no indication that hearing is impaired.
- Be natural when talking with a blind person.
- Accept the normal things that a blind person might do such as consulting the watch for the correct time, dialing a telephone, or writing his or her name in longhand without calling attention to them.
- When you offer assistance to a blind person, do so directly. Ask, "May I be of help?" Speak in a normal, friendly tone.
- In guiding a blind person, permit him or her to take your arm. Never grab the blind person's arm, for he or she cannot anticipate your movements.
- In walking with a blind person, proceed at a normal pace. You may hesitate slightly before stepping up or down.
- Be explicit in giving verbal directions to a blind person.
- There is no need to avoid the use of the word *see* when talking with a blind person.
- When assisting a blind person to a chair, simply place his or her hand on the back or arm of the chair. This is enough to give location.
- When leaving the blind person abruptly after conversing with him or her in a crowd or where there is a noise that may obstruct hearing, quietly advise that you are leaving so that he or she will not be embarrassed by talking when no one is listening.
- Never leave a blind person in an open area. Instead, lead him or her to the side of a room, to a chair, or some landmark from which he or she can obtain direction.
- A half-open door is one of the most dangerous obstacles that blind people encounter.
- When serving food to a blind person who is eating without a sighted companion, offer to read the menu, including the price of each item. As you place each item on the table, call attention to food placement by using the numbers of an imaginary clock. ("The green beans are at 2 o'clock.") If he or she wants you to cut up the food, he or she will tell you.
- Be sure to tell a blind person who the other guests are so that he or she may know of their presence.

From Murray, R., Zentner, J., and Pinnell, N. (1993). Assessment and health promotion for the person in later maturity. In. R. B. Murray and J. P. Zentner (Eds.). *Nursing Assessment and Health Promotion: Strategies Through the Life Span* (5th ed.). Norwalk, CT, Appleton & Lange, pp. 542–603.

than 65 years of age and almost 50% of those over 85 years of age experience some degree of mental impairment (USDHHS/ODPHP, 1994). Alzheimer's disease, vascular infarctions, and pharmaceuticals are frequently implicated as inducing cognitive changes.

Screening for cognitive function should include orientation, short-term memory, receptive and expressive language ability, attention, and visual-spatial ability. Use of a short screening instrument, such as the Mini-Mental State Examination (Table 14–9) may be helpful in eliciting important information quickly. If cognitive impairment is noted, consultation with family members and referral to a specialist may be indicated.

In regard to care of individuals with cognitive impairments, Alzheimer's disease is of particular concern for nurses who routinely work with the elderly. According to Selkoe (1992), Alzheimer's disease accounts for almost 56% of causes of dementia in older adults, followed by stroke (14.5%), multiple causes (12.2%), Parkinson's disease (7.7%), and other causes (9.9%).

Alzheimer's disease is a degenerative mental disorder characterized by progressive brain deterioration, resulting in impaired memory and in thought and behavioral changes (see Table 14–5 for a review of risk factors, manifestations, and clinical management). Table 14–10 lists current statistics and should be helpful to nurses who work with older people to understand the scope and significance of the problem. Table 14–11 presents management guidelines for afflicted patients and their caregivers.

INCONTINENCE

Incontinence (the involuntary loss of urine) is a significant cause of disability and dependency in older adults. An estimated 15 to 30% of noninstitutionalized elderly persons experience urinary incontinence, which contributes to social isolation, embarrassment, feelings of loss of control, and low self-esteem (Lashley, 1995). Despite its prevalence, urinary incontinence is widely underdiagnosed and underreported. Reasons cited include lack of education about the condition on the part of health care providers and shame or embar-

TABLE 14–9 **Mini-Mental State Examination**

Patient ______________ Examiner ______________ Date ______________

Maximum Score	*Score*	
		Orientation
5	( )	What is the (year) (season) (date) (day) (month)?
5	( )	Where are we: (state) (county) (town) (hospital) (floor)
		Registration
3	( )	Name three objects: 1 second to say each. Then ask the patient all three after you have said them. Give 1 point for each correct answer. Then repeat them until he or she learns all three. Count trials and record. Trials ______
		Attention and Calculation
5	( )	Serial 7's. 1 point for each correct. Stop after five answers. Alternatively spell "world" backwards.
		Recall
3	( )	Ask for the three objects repeated above. Give 1 point for each correct.
		Language
9	( )	Name a pencil, and watch (2 points) Repeat the following: "No ifs, ands, or buts." (1 point) Follow a three-stage command: "Take a paper in your right hand, fold it in half, and put it on the floor." (3 points) Read and obey the following: *Close Your Eyes* (1 point) Write a sentence (1 point) Copy design (1 point)
______		***Total Score***
		ASSESS level of consciousness along a continuum ______ Alert Drowsy Stupor Coma

rassment on the part of these individuals (USDHHS/AHCPR, 1992).

According to the Urinary Incontinence Guideline Panel, treatment can improve or cure most patients (USDHHS/AHCPR, 1992, p. xi). Following an intensive study, this panel recommended a "vigorous" information campaign targeting the public and health professionals about the problem, including effects, causes, and treatment options.

To comply with their recommendations as well as to meet objectives of *Healthy People 2000*, health care providers should routinely ask older patients about problems with bladder control using an open-ended question, such as "Do you have trouble with your bladder?" or "Do you have trouble holding your urine (water)?" If urinary continence is identified by questioning, detection of an odor, visualization of wetness, or patient complaint, and if it represents a problem for the patient or caregiver, further evaluation is needed.

Several types of urinary continence have been identified (Table 14–12). The basic evaluation should include a thorough history, physical examination, and urinalysis. General guidelines for evaluation are listed in Table 14–13.

Treatment options include a variety of behavior techniques, pharmacologic therapy, surgery, or a

TABLE 14–9 **Mini-Mental State Examination** *Continued*

Instructions for Administration of Mini-Mental State Examination

Orientation

(1) Ask for the date. Then ask specifically for parts omitted, e.g., "Can you also tell me what season it is?" One point for each correct.

(2) Ask in turn "Can you tell me the name of this hospital?" (town, country, etc.). One point for each correct.

Registration

Ask the patient if you may test his or her memory. Then say the names of three unrelated objects, clearly and slowly, about 1 second for each. After you have said all three, ask him or her to repeat them. This first repetition determines his or her score (0–3), but keep saying them until he or she can repeat all three, up to six trials. If he or she does not eventually learn all three, recall cannot be meaningfully tested.

Attention and Calculation

Ask the patient to begin with 100 and count backwards by 7. Stop after five subtractions (93, 86, 79, 72, 65). Score the total number of correct answers.

If the patient cannot or will not perform this task, ask him or her to spell the word "world" backwards. The score is the number of letters in correct order, e.g., dlrow = 5, dlorw = 3.

Recall

Ask the patient if he or she can recall the three words you previously asked him or her to remember. Score 0–3.

Language

Naming: Show the patient a wrist watch and ask him or her what it is. Repeat for pencil. Score 0–2.

Repetition: Ask the patient to repeat the sentence after you. Allow only one trial. Score 0 or 1.

Three-stage command: Give the patient a piece of plain blank paper and repeat the command. Score 1 point for each part correctly executed.

Reading: On a blank piece of paper print the sentence "Close your eyes," in letters large enough for the patient to see clearly. Ask him or her to read it and do what it says. Score 1 point only if he or she actually closes his or her eyes.

Writing: Give the patient a blank piece of paper and ask him or her to write a sentence for you. Do not dictate a sentence; it is to be written spontaneously. It must contain a subject and verb and be sensible. Correct grammar and punctuation are not necessary.

Copying: On a clean piece of paper, draw intersecting pentagons, each side about 1 inch, and ask him or her to copy it exactly as it is. All 10 angles must be present, and 2 must intersect to score 1 point. Tremor and rotation are ignored.

Estimate the patient's level of sensorium along a continuum, from alert on the left to coma on the right.

From Folstein, M. J., Folstein, S. E., and McHugh, P. R. (1975). "Mini-Mental State": A practical method for grading the cognitive state of patients for the clinician. *Journal of Psychiatric Research* 12:189–198. Reprinted with permission of Elsevier Science, Ltd., Pergamon Imprint.

combination of these (Table 14–14). According to an expert panel, "surgery should be the last resort and should be performed only after a precise, focused assessment including estimation of surgical risk, objective confirmation of the diagnosis and its severity, correlation of anatomic and physiologic findings with the surgical plan, and an estimation of the impact of the proposed surgery on the patient's quality of life" (USDHHS/AHCPR, 1992, p. 47).

Health Promotion and Illness Prevention

Although health promotion and illness prevention interventions for older adults can be very beneficial in reducing death and disability and in improving quality of life, the health care system has not systematically encouraged or provided preventive health services for this population. Most older

TABLE 14–10 **Alzheimer's Disease: Statistics**

- Approximately 4 million Americans have Alzheimer's disease, and 14 million Americans will have it by the year 2050 unless a cure or prevention is found.
- Alzheimer's disease is the fourth leading cause of death among adults.
- One in 10 persons over age 65 and nearly half of those over 85 have Alzheimer's disease.
- A person with Alzheimer's disease can live 3 to 20 years after the onset of symptoms.
- More than 70% of people with Alzheimer's disease live at home with care provided by family and friends.
- Half of all nursing home patients have Alzheimer's disease or a related disorder. The average cost for a patient's care in a nursing home is $42,000/year.
- Alzheimer's disease is the third most expensive disease in the United States after heart disease and cancer.
- Alzheimer's disease cost United States citizens approximately $80 to $100 billion a year. Neither Medicare nor private health insurance covers the long-term care most patients need.

Modified from Alzheimer's Disease Association. (1994). *Alzheimer's Disease Statistics.* Chicago, Alzheimer's Disease Association.

adults seek out medical care only in response to illness and are unlikely to see health care providers when they have no symptoms. Thus, they rely on health care professionals to recommend preventive tests and screenings. Because older patients may be unaware of activities that would improve their health and well-being, it is incumbent on providers in a variety of community settings to seek opportunities to provide health teaching, perform screenings, and encourage other preventive services.

PREVENTIVE SERVICES GUIDELINES

Priority Area "21" of *Healthy People 2000* specifically addresses "clinical preventive services" and encourages providers to improve access to primary care, to work to remove barriers to preventive care, and to provide patients with prescribed screening, counseling, and immunization services. The recommendations for screening and counseling for older adults from the U. S. Preventive Services Task Force are presented in Table 14–15.

TABLE 14–11 **Intervention Guidelines for Alzheimer's Disease**

Direct goals toward helping the client experience the highest possible physical, emotional, intellectual, and social functions for as long as possible.

Client and caregiver education should focus on

- Manifestations of the disease
  - Stages and progression of the disease (what to expect)
  - Pharmacologic management (provide information on clinical drug trials)
- Behavioral management
  - Provision of a consistent routine
  - Avoid chemical or physical restraints
- Communication strategies
  - Simple commands and directions
- Monitoring for acute illnesses and effects of medications

Caregiver and client counseling and referral should include

- Locating community resources
- Legal/financial issues
  - Durable power of attorney
  - Conservatorship or guardianship
  - Establishment of trusts
  - Advance directives and living will
- Financial assistance
  - Medicare
  - Medicaid
  - Long-term care insurance
  - Social Security Disability Insurance
  - Supplemental Security Income (SSI)
- Long-term care options (i.e., home care, respite care, nursing homes, Alzheimer's disease units)
- Family and social support
- Management of stress and lifestyle changes

Data from Lukacs, K. (1996). Neurological/Alzheimer's disease. In A. S. Luggen (Ed.). *Core Curriculum for Gerontological Nursing.* St. Louis, Mosby-Year Book, pp. 564–580; and American Association of Retired Persons. (1993). *Coping & Caring: Living with Alzheimer's Disease.* Washington, D. C., American Association of Retired Persons.

TABLE 14–12 **Common Types and Causes of Urinary Incontinence in Adults**

Transient Urge Incontinence
Delirium (confusional state)
Infection
Atrophic urethritis or vaginitis
Pharmaceuticals (sedatives, diuretics, anticholinergic agents, calcium channel blockers)
Psychological factors (depression)
Excessive urine production
Restricted mobility
Stool impaction

Stress Incontinence (involuntary loss of urine during coughing, sneezing, laughing, or other physical activities)
Hypermobility of the urethra
Displacement of the urethra and bladder neck during exertion
Congenital sphincter weakness
Acquired sphincter weakness (following prostatectomy, trauma, radiation)

Overflow Incontinence (involuntary loss of urine associated with overdistention of the bladder)
Underactive or acontractile bladder musculature (due to medication, fecal impaction, or neurologic conditions, such as spinal cord injury)
Urethral obstruction (prostatic hyperplasia or prostatic carcinoma in men; severe pelvic prolapse in women)

From U. S. Department of Health and Human Services/Agency for Health Care Policy and Research (USDHHS/AHCPR). (1992). *Urinary Incontinence in Adults: Clinical Practice Guideline.* AHCPR Pub. No. 92—0038. Rockville, MD, Agency for Health Care Policy and Research.

Health care providers who routinely work with older patients should be familiar with these guidelines and should be prepared to perform the suggested assessments, laboratory tests, counseling, and immunizations as appropriate. Health professionals or specialists for referral should be determined in advance, and mechanisms for timely, systematic, and streamlined care by specialists through interagency and interdisciplinary collaboration and communication should be strongly encouraged.

IMMUNIZATION RECOMMENDATIONS

Although primary prevention through immunization against a variety of illnesses is strongly encouraged (if not mandated) for children, immunization recommendations for older adults are often overlooked. Deaths due to vaccine-preventable diseases are common in older people. Approximately 80 to 90% of influenza deaths occur in individuals 65 years of age or older, particularly older adults with underlying health problems, such as pulmonary or cardiovascular disorders (USDHHS/ODPHP, 1994).

Improving the immunization status of Americans over age 65 years is one of the goals of *Healthy People 2000* (see Table 14–1). The Immunization Practices Advisory Committee recommends that all older adults should have completed a primary series of diphtheria and tetanus toxoids (Centers for Disease Control, 1991). In addition, a single dose of pneumococcal polysaccharide vaccine and annual vaccination against influenza should be strongly encouraged for all adults over age 65, particularly those with pre-existing chronic health conditions.

Table 14–16 contains immunization recommendations for adults by age groups.

Safety Concerns for Older Adults

Several objectives from *Healthy People 2000* concerning older Americans relate to safety. The document specifically addresses injuries from falls and poisoning caused by drug interactions and/or inadvertent overdosing. Additionally, encouraging health care providers to identify, treat, and refer victims of elder abuse is discussed as a component of the objectives to decrease violent and abusive behaviors.

FALLS

Falls are the leading cause of death from injury for people aged 65 and older and are particularly

TABLE 14–13 **Basic Evaluation for Urinary Incontinence**

History of Urinary Incontinence

Duration and characteristics of urinary incontinence (stress, urge, dribbling, etc.)
Frequency, timing, and amount of continent and incontinent voids
Precipitants and associate symptoms of incontinence (situational antecedents, cough, surgery, injury, medications, etc.)
Other lower urinary tract symptoms (nocturia, dysuria, straining, hematuria, perineal or suprapubic pain, frequency, urgency)
Fluid intake pattern
Alteration in bowel habit or sexual function
Previous treatment for urinary incontinence and its effect
Use of pads, briefs, or other protective devices

Physical Examination

Abdominal examination to detect masses, fullness, or tenderness
Genital examination in men to detect abnormalities of the foreskin, glans, penis, and perineal skin
Pelvic examination in women to assess perineal skin condition, genital atropy, pelvic prolapse, pelvic mass, perivaginal muscle tone, or other abnormality
Rectal examination to test for perineal sensation, sphincter tone, fecal impaction, rectal mass, and estimation of residual urine and to evaluate the consistency, size, and contour of the prostate in males
General examination to detect conditions that may contribute to nocturia; detect neurologic abnormalities or other potentially contributing conditions (multiple sclerosis, stroke, cognition)

Urinalysis

Basic test to detect associated or contributing conditions (hematuria, infection, glycosuria, proteinuria)
Culture and sensitivity if bacteria and/or white blood cells are present

From U. S. Department of Health and Human Services/Agency for Health Care Policy and Research (USDHHS/AHCPR). (1992). *Urinary Incontinence in Adults: Clinical Practice Guideline.* AHCPR Pub. No. 92—0038. Rockville, MD, Agency for Health Care Policy and Research.

common among those over age 85 (USDHHS, 1990, p. 276). Falls and fall-related injuries are of special concern in older adults because of the severity of injuries combined with longer recovery periods and resultant threats to long-term health and functioning. In addition to the immediate pain and disability caused by the injury, falls are associated with loss of confidence in ability to function independently, restriction of physical and social activities, increased dependence, and increased need for long-term care.

About one third of all elderly people have reported a fall during the previous 12 months (Eliopoulos, 1993; Stone and Chenitz, 1991). Although most falls do not result in serious injury, between 5 and 15% of those individuals who fall sustain fractures or other significant injuries. Fracture of the hip, femur, humerus, wrist, and ribs are the most common severe injuries from falls.

Nurses working with older adults in any setting should be aware of risk factors for falls and should direct interventions accordingly. Table 14–17 details factors that contribute to falls, and Table 14–18 presents guidelines to prevent falls.

COMPLIANCE WITH MEDICATION

Another threat to the safety of older people is the use and misuse of medications. An estimated 5 to 30% of geriatric hospital admissions are associated with inappropriate drug administration (Eliopoulos, 1993). Nurses who work with older patients should be aware of factors that contribute to medication noncompliance, should anticipate and recognize actual and potential problems, and should be prepared to intervene. To improve medication safety for older adults, nurses may refer to

Text continued on page 444

TABLE 14–14 Treatment of Urinary Incontinence

Behavioral and Related Techniques

- Bladder training (retraining): combines education, scheduled voiding, and positive reinforcement
- Habit training (timed voiding): teaches scheduled, planned voiding at regular intervals
- Prompted voiding: teaches the individual to discriminate his or her incontinence status and request toileting assistance from caregivers and is particularly useful for dependent or cognitively impaired nursing home patients
- Pelvic muscle exercises (Kegel exercises): indicated for women with stress incontinence and for men following prostatic surgery. Strengthens voluntary periurethral and pelvic muscles to improve urethral resistance. Consists of alternating contracting and relaxing the perivaginal muscles for 10 seconds followed by a 10-second relaxation period. Repeat 30–80 times a day for at least 6 weeks.
- Biofeedback: uses electronic or mechanical instruments to relay information through auditory or visual displays to teach individuals to change physiologic responses that mediate bladder control.
- Vaginal cone retention: used as an adjunct to pelvic muscle training in premenopausal women.
- Electrical stimulation: primarily for neurologically impaired person. Involves stimulating the pelvic viscera, pelvic muscles or their nerve supplies thus modifying bladder sensation and/or induce bladder contraction.

Pharmacologic Treatment of Incontinence

Stress Incontinence

- Alpha-adrenergic agonists: used to increase bladder outlet resistance
- Estrogen supplementation: restores urethral mucosal tone, increases vascularity and alpha-adrenergic responsiveness of the urethral muscle in postmenopausal women
- Combined alpha-adrenergic agonist and estrogen supplementation

Urge Incontinence

- Anticholinergic agents: block contraction of the normal bladder
- Combined anticholinergic and smooth muscle relaxants
- Combined anticholinergic and calcium channel blockers
- Tricyclic agents
- Smooth muscle relaxant
- Other drugs may also be used

Surgical Treatment—Dependent on etiology of urinary incontinence

Bladder Neck or Urethral Obstruction

- Women: caused by prior surgery or severe pelvic prolapse (severe cyctocele, enterocele, uterine prolapse)—surgical treatment urethrolysis
- Men: caused by benign prostatic hyperplasia, urethral stricture or prostate cancer; surgical treatment is transurethral prostatectomy

Involuntary Bladder Contractions

- Augmentation cystoplasty

Intrinsic Sphincter Deficiency (Males) (due to congenital anomaly [myelomeningocele or epispadias] or acquired after prostatectomy or radiation therapy)

- Periurethral bulking injections
- Placement of an artificial sphincter

Intrinsic Sphincter Deficiency (Females)

- Artificial urinary sphincter
- Sling operation

Stress Incontinence

- Anterior vaginal repair
- Retropubic suspension
- Needle suspension

Other Measures for Management of Incontinence

- Intermittent self-catheterization
- Indwelling catheters
- Suprapubic catheters
- External collection catheters
- Penile clamps
- Pessaries
- Absorbent pads or garments

Modified from U. S. Department of Health and Human Services/Agency for Health Care Policy and Research (USDHHS/AHCPR). (1992). *Urinary Incontinence in Adults: Clinical Practice Guideline.* AHCPR Pub. No. 92—0038. Rockville, MD, Agency for Health Care Policy and Research.

TABLE 14–15 **Recommendations of the U.S. Preventive Services Task Force: Ages 65 and Older**

Interventions Considered and Recommended for the Periodic Health Examination

Leading Causes of Death
- Heart diseases
- Malignant neoplasms (lung, colorectal, breast)
- Cerebrovascular disease
- Chronic obstructive pulmonary disease
- Pneumonia and influenza

Interventions for the General Population

Screening
- Blood pressure
- Height and weight
- Fecal occult blood test* and/or sigmoidoscopy
- Mammogram ± clinical breast exam† (women ≤69 years)
- Papanicolaou (Pap) test (women)†
- Vision screening
- Assess for hearing impairment
- Assess for problem drinking

Counseling

Substance Use
- Tobacco cessation
- Avoid alcohol/drug use while driving, swimming, boating, etc.§

Diet and Exercise
- Limit fat and cholesterol; maintain caloric balance; emphasize grains, fruits, vegetables
- Adequate calcium intake (women)
- Regular physical activity§

Injury Prevention
- Lap/shoulder belts
- Motorcycle and bicycle helmets§
- Fall prevention§
- Safe storage/removal of firearms§
- Smoke detector§
- Set hot water heater to <120–130°F§
- CPR training for household members

Dental Health
- Regular visits to dental care provider§
- Floss, brush with fluoride toothpaste daily§

Sexual Behavior
- STD prevention: avoid high-risk sexual behavior;§ use condoms§

Immunizations
- Pneumococcal vaccine
- Influenza*
- Tetanus-diphtheria (Td) boosters

Chemoprophylaxis
- Discuss hormone prophylaxis (women)

Interventions for High-Risk Populations

Population	***Potential Interventions*** (See detailed high-risk definitions)
Institutionalized persons	PPD (HR1); hepatitis A vaccine (HR2); amantadine/rimantadine (HR4)
Chronic medical conditions; TB contacts; low income; immigrants; alcoholics	PPD (HR1)
Persons ≥75 years or ≥70 years with risk factors for falls	Fall prevention intervention (HR5)
Cardiovascular disease risk factors	Consider cholesterol screening (HR5)
Family history of skin cancer; nevi; fair skin, eyes, hair	Avoid excess/midday sun, use protective clothing* (HR7)
Native Americans/Alaska Natives	PPD (HR1); hepatitis A vaccine (HR2)
Travelers to developing countries	Hepatitis A vaccine (HR2); hepatitis B vaccine (HR8)
Blood product recipients	HIV screen (HR3); hepatitis B vaccine (HR8)
High-risk sexual behavior	Hepatitis A vaccine (HR2); HIV screen (HR3); hepatitis B vaccine (HR8); RPR/VDRL (HR9)
Injection or street drug use	PPD (HR1); hepatitis A vaccine (HR2); HIV screen (HR3); hepatitis B vaccine (HR8); RPR/VDRL (HR9); advice to reduce infection risk (HR10)

TABLE 14–15 Recommendations of the U.S. Preventive Services Task Force: Ages 65 and Older *Continued*

Health care/laboratory workers	PPD (HR1); hepatitis A vaccine (HR2); amantadine/rimantadine (HR4); hepatitis B vaccine (HR8)
Persons susceptible to varicella	Varicella vaccine (HR11)

HR1 = HIV positive, close contacts of persons with known or suspected TB, health care workers, persons with medical risk factors associated with TB, immigrants from countries with high TB prevalence, medically underserved low-income populations (including homeless), alcoholics, injection drug users, and residents of long-term care facilities.

HR2 = Persons living in, traveling to, or working in areas where the disease is endemic and where periodic outbreaks occur (e.g., countries with high or intermediate endemicity; certain Alaska Native, Pacific Island, Native American, and religious communities); men who have sex with men; injection or street drug users. Consider for institutionalized persons and workers in these institutions, and day care, hospital, and laboratory workers. Clinicians should also consider local epidemiology.

HR3 = Men who had sex with men after 1975; past or present injection drug use; persons who exchange sex for money or drugs, and their sex partners; injection drug-using, bisexual, or HIV-positive sex partner currently or in the past; blood transfusion during 1978–1985; persons seeking treatment for STDs. Clinicians should also consider local epidemiology.

HR4 = Consider for persons who have not received influenza vaccine or are vaccinated late; when the vaccine may be ineffective owing to major antigenic changes in the virus; for unvaccinated persons who provide home care for high-risk persons; to supplement protection provided by vaccine in persons who are expected to have a poor antibody response; and for high-risk persons in whom the vaccine is contraindicated.

HR5 = Persons aged 75 years and older; or aged 70–74 with one or more additional risk factors including use of certain psychoactive and cardiac medications (e.g., benzodiazepines, antihypertensives); use of ≥4 prescription medications; impaired cognition, strength, balance, or gait. Intensive individualized home-based multifactorial fall prevention intervention is recommended in settings where adequate resources are available to deliver such services.

HR6 = Although evidence is insufficient to recommend routine screening in elderly persons, clinicians should consider cholesterol screening on a case-by-case basis for persons aged 65–75 with additional risk factors (e.g., smoking, diabetes, or hypertension).

HR7 = Persons with a family or personal history of skin cancer, a large number of moles, atypical moles, poor tanning ability, or light skin, hair, and eye color.

HR8 = Blood product recipients (including hemodialysis patients), persons with frequent occupational exposure to blood or blood products, men who have sex with men, injection drug users and their sex partners, persons with multiple recent sex partners, persons with other STDs (including HIV), travelers to countries with endemic hepatitis B.

HR9 = Persons who exchange sex for money or drugs and their sex partners; persons with other STDs (including HIV); and sexual contacts of persons with active syphilis. Clinicians should also consider local epidemiology.

HR10 = Persons who continue to inject drugs.

HR11 = Healthy adults without a history of chickenpox or previous immunization. Consider serologic testing for presumed susceptible adults.

*Annually.

†Mammogram every 1–2 years, or mammogram every 1–2 years with annual clinical breast examination.

‡All women who are or have been sexually active and who have a cervix: every 3 years or less. Consider discontinuation of testing after age 65 years if previous regular screening with consistently normal results.

§The ability of clinician counseling to influence this behavior is unproven.

CPR = cardiopulmonary resuscitation; HIV = human immunodeficiency virus; PPD = purified protein derivative; RPR = rapid plasma reagin (test); STD = sexually transmitted disease; TB = tuberculosis; VDRL = Venereal Disease Research Laboratory.

Modified from Department of Health and Human Services (USDHHS). Guide to Clinical Preventive Services (2nd ed.). Washington, D. C., Government Printing Office.

TABLE 14–16 **Vaccines Recommended for Adults, by Age Groups, United States***

Age Group (Years)	Vaccine/Toxoid					
	Td†	*Measles*	*Mumps*	*Rubella*	*Influenza*	*Pneumococcal Polysaccharide*
18–24	X	X	X	X		
25–64	X	X‡	X‡	X		
≥65	X				X	X

*Refer also to sections in text on specific vaccines or toxoids for indications, contraindications, precautions, dosages, side effects, adverse reactions, and special considerations.

†Td = Tetanus and diphtheria toxoids, adsorbed (for adult use), which is a combined preparation containing <2 flocculation units of diphtheria toxoid.

‡Indicated for persons born after 1956.

From Centers for Disease Control (CDC). (1991). Update on adult immunization: Recommendations of the Immunization Practices Advisory Committee (ACIP). *Morbidity and Mortality Weekly Report 40* (RR-12).

TABLE 14–17 **Contributing Factors for Falls in Elders**

Intrinsic Factors

Age-related changes in vision, posture, and gait
Poor judgment
Emotional/mental state: agitated, depressed, pressured, rushed, distracted, confused, fearful, and anxious
Weakness/deconditioning
Fear of incontinence
Denial of illness, weakness, and dependence
Pain
Podiatric conditions such as ingrown toenails, corns, bunions
Adjusting to new environment: recent move, recent admission, transfer
Multiple diagnoses: conditions affecting stability, mobility, and cognitive function
Drugs: prescribed/over-the-counter/self-prescribed; alcohol, sedatives/hypnotics, tricyclic antidepressants, antihypertensive agents, analgesics, and diuretics

Extrinsic Factors

Lighting: dark, too dim, glare, shadows
Walking surfaces: uneven, wet and slippery, patterned floor
Stairs: inadequate handrails, edges not clearly defined, poor step design
Furniture: too low, too soft, tips easily, on wheels
Bathroom: slippery tub or shower, lack of grab rails for toilet or tub
Shoes/slippers: too loose, badly worn heels, soles too slick
Clothing: too long, loose, and flowing
Equipment: worn out or broken, improper use of equipment, use of restraints and siderails

From Stone, J. T., and Chenitz, W. C. (1991). The problem of falls. In Chenitz, W. C., Stone, J. T., and Salisbury, S. A. (Eds.). *Clinical Gerontological Nursing: A Guide to Advanced Practice.* Philadelphia, W. B. Saunders, pp. 291–308.

TABLE 14–18 **Guidelines for Prevention of Falls in the Home**

Lights and Lighting

1. Eyes tire quickly in improper lighting. Illuminate reading material or the object worked on. Illuminate steps, entranceways, and rooms before entering. Use 70- or 100-watt bulbs, not 60-watt bulbs.
2. Avoid glaring light caused by highly polished floors or large expanses of uncovered glass. Use sunglasses to avoid the glare of highway driving, but use light tints or photoray lenses.
3. Allow more time to adjust to changes in light levels. When going from a dark to a light room or vice versa, allow a minute or two for the eyes to accommodate to the change in light before proceeding.
4. Dirty glasses or outgrown prescription lenses inhibit vision. Keep glasses clean. Have regular eye examinations to identify changes and to get new glasses when needed. If possible, do not use bifocals when walking because you cannot see the ground clearly.
5. Ability to see up, down, and sideways decreases with age. Observe the "lay of the land"; learn to look ahead at the ground to spot and avoid hazards such as cracks in the sidewalks. Use canes, walking sticks, and walkers that are prescribed.
6. At night, keep a nightlight on in your bedroom and bathroom. When getting out of bed at night, put the light on and wait a minute or two for the eyes to adjust before getting up. Have a telephone in the bedroom so you don't have to get out of bed to answer the phone. Before you go out in the evening or late afternoon, turn a light on for your return.

Activity

1. Get up from a chair slowly.
2. When getting out of bed, sit up, then wait a minute or two. Move to the side of the bed and wait another minute. Rise after you have sat for a few minutes.
3. If you are dizzy, sit down immediately. Sit on a step or a chair, or ease yourself to the sidewalk if you are outdoors.
4. Avoid tipping the head backward (extending the neck). Activities to avoid that extend the neck are washing windows, hanging clothes, and getting things from high shelves.
5. Use shelves at eye level. Avoid rapid turning of the head.
6. If weather is rainy and windy, avoid going out.
7. Use alcohol and tranquilizers with caution.
8. Exercise programs keep bodies limber. Consult your physician and then enroll in a senior exercise program.
9. Shoes and slippers should be flat and rubber-soled. Avoid clothing such as long robes and loose-fitting garments that may catch on furniture or door knobs.

Around the House

1. Avoid scatter rugs and small bathroom mats that can slide. Repair loose, torn, wrinkled, or worn carpet.
2. Avoid slick, high polish on floors.
3. Put things in easy reach, and avoid reaching to high shelves.
4. Use nonskid treads on stairs and nonskid mats in tub.
5. May wish to install a grab rail in the bath, shower, and also by the toilet.
6. Install handrails on both sides of the stairs. Paint stair edge in bright contrasting color.
7. Remove door thresholds.
8. Remove low-lying objects, such as coffee tables and extension cords.
9. Wipe up spills immediately.
10. Watch for pets underfoot and scattered pet food.
11. Check for even, nonglare lighting in every room, with easily accessible light switches.
12. Avoid floor coverings with complex patterns.
13. Avoid clutter in living areas.
14. Select furniture that provides stability and support, such as chairs with arms.
15. Check walking aids routinely, such as rubber tips on canes and screws on walkers.

From Chenitz, W. C., Kussman, H. L., and Stone, J. T. (1991). Preventing falls. In W. C. Chenitz, J. T., Stone, and S. A. Salisbury (Eds.). *Clinical Gerontological Nursing: A Guide to Advanced Practice.* Philadelphia, W. B. Saunders, pp. 309–328.

Table 14–19 for factors that contribute to medication misuse. Table 14–20 should be helpful for planning interventions to prevent and manage noncompliance.

Polypharmacy refers to the prescribing of multiple drugs for a patient, and it is a fairly common practice that affects older people. Both prescription and nonprescription medications contribute to problems encountered in polypharmacy. To avoid problems associated with medication, the nurse should

Table 14–19 Factors That Interfere With Medication Regimen Compliance in Elders

- Physiologic changes associated with aging affecting absorption, metabolism, and excretion of drugs
- Lack of knowledge or information about the reason for taking the medication and the prescribed regimen; stopping the medication when symptoms subside
- Inaccessibility to pharmacy services
- Problems with self-administration, such as failure to take the medication as prescribed, inability to open drug containers, forgetfulness, vision problems
- Multiple prescriptions or related medications for the same condition from different providers
- Lack of financial resources to purchase necessary medications (medications are not covered by Medicare)
- Complexity of drug regimens and volume of drugs needed
- Desire to avoid unpleasant side effects
- Fear of drug dependency
- Failure to discard discontinued or outdated medications
- Sharing of prescription medications with spouse or others
- Failure to report self-medication with over-the-counter drugs
- Interactions between different medications

Data from Graves, M. (1988). Drug use and abuse. In M. O. Hogstel (Ed.). *Nursing Care of the Older Adult* (2nd ed.). New York, John Wiley and Sons; Eliopoulos, C. (1993). *Gerontological Nursing* (3rd ed.). Philadelphia, J. B. Lippincott, pp. 271–276; and Lashley, M. E. (1995). Elderly persons in the community. In C. M. Smith and F. A. Maurer (Eds.). *Community Health Nursing: Theory and Practice.* Philadelphia, W. B. Saunders, pp. 719–746.

- Help the patient make and maintain a list of *all* prescription and over-the-counter medications, including purpose, dosage, frequencies, dates of use, and side effects
- Simplify the medication regimen as much as possible
- Ensure that the patient brings all medications when seeing a practitioner
- Evaluate potential medication interactions whenever a new medication is prescribed
- Inform the patient about possible side effects and symptoms of toxicity and explain what to do in the event of an occurrence
- Use a medication box that can be filled weekly and distribute the medications based on the day (e.g., Sunday through Saturday) and time of day (morning, noon, evening, before bed)

ELDER ABUSE

Elder abuse refers to neglect, physical injury, or exploitation that results in harm to an older adult. As a result of widespread underreporting, the incidence of elder abuse is difficult to determine. One source estimates that at least 5% of older Americans are victims of abuse and neglect each year (Eliopoulos, 1993). According to another source, between 700,000 and 1.5 million cases of elder abuse occur each year in the United States (Maurer, 1995). Elder abuse can take on a number of forms. The most common types of elder abuse are listed in Table 14–21.

It is estimated that only 8 to 25% of cases of elder abuse are reported. Clark (1995) cites the following reasons for failure to report abuse:

- Reluctance of older people to admit that their child or loved one might abuse them
- Love for abuser
- Dependence on the abuser
- Fear of further injury
- Inability to report the abuse

Further, health care providers may neglect to report elder abuse, often because of failure to recognize the problem, ignorance of their legal respon-

TABLE 14–20 **Barriers to Compliance and Interventions to Prevent and Treat Noncompliance in Elderly Clients**

Barrier to Compliance	Nursing Intervention
Patient Related	
Impaired vision	Ask pharmacist to use large type on labels. Affix label on central axis. Use color-coding system.
Impaired hearing	Get patient's attention before speaking. Speak clearly and slowly. Do not shout.
Impaired dexterity	Use nonchildproof medication container.
Memory loss	Write out medication schedule. Use compliance aids (medication boxes, medication calendars). Involve caregiver.
Social isolation	Suggest volunteer home visitor or telephone program.
Drug Therapy Related	
Complex drug regimen	Work with physician and pharmacist to simplify schedule. Use compliance aids.
Cost of drugs	Suggest generic drugs. Discourage use of unnecessary nonprescription drugs. Suggest nondrug alternatives.
Health Professional Related	
Inadequate knowledge about drug use	Provide specific detailed oral and written information about the drug regimen.
Diffidence of patient toward health professionals	Ask about patient's previous experience with health professionals. Allow time for questions and concerns.

From Hashizume, S. (1991). Home health care. In W. C. Chenitz, J. T. Stone, and S. A. Salisbury (Eds.). *Clinical Gerontological Nursing: A Guide to Advanced Practice.* Philadelphia, W. B. Saunders, pp. 557–576.

sibilities to report suspected cases, and failure to adequately assess at-risk situations (Maurer, 1995).

In most cases, the abuser is a caregiver, either a close family member or provider in a nursing home. Among family members, the spouse is most often the abuser (65% of cases), followed by children (25 to 30% of cases). Risk factors common to victims of elder abuse include

- The victim's dependency on the caregiver (physical, emotional, or financial)
- Confusion
- Incontinence
- Frailty
- Illness
- Mental disabilities

Characteristics of the abuser (Maurer, 1995) include

- A previous history of violence
- Being overwhelmed by the burden of providing care
- Feelings of frustration and resentment

Whenever working with older people in community or long-term settings, nurses should be aware of indicators of possible elder abuse and should direct interventions accordingly. Indicators may include (Campbell and Landenburger, 1996; Maurer, 1995)

- Unexplained or repeated injury
- Discrepancies between injury and explanation

TABLE 14–21 **Types of Elder Abuse**

Type of Abuse	Example
Physical	Beating, slapping, rape and sexual molestation, murder
Confinement	Use of physical restraints; use of chemical restraints (sedatives); confinement to bed
Psychological or Emotional	Verbal assault; isolation; exclusion; threats of abuse or abandonment; insults; humiliation; intimidation
Financial or Material	Taking resources and possessions without consent; forcing or coercing elders to sign over properties and possessions
Neglect	Withholding food, adequate clothing, shelter, health care, or medications; deprivation of dentures or eyeglasses; failure to assist with activities of daily living; abandonment; neglect may be passive or active

Data from Kirkham, A. K. (1988). Crime and abuse. In Hogstel, M. O. (Ed.). *Nursing Care of the Older Adult* (2nd ed.). New York, John Wiley and Sons, pp. 457–476; and Watkins, A. C. (1993). Family violence. In J. Swanson and M. Albrecht (Eds.). *Community Health Nursing: Promoting the Health of Aggregates.* Philadelphia, W. B. Saunders, pp. 459–486.

- Inappropriate use of medication (overuse or underuse)
- Fear of the caregiver
- Untreated wounds (decubitus ulcers)
- Evidence of poor care (an unclean or malnourished patient)
- Withdrawal and passivity
- Failure to seek appropriate medical care
- Contractures resulting from immobility or restraints
- Unwillingness or inability of caregiver to meet the patient's needs
- An unsafe home situation

In all states, nurses and other health care professionals have a legal responsibility to report suspected cases of elder abuse. Typically, the nurse would report possible cases to the adult protective services department of the area social services agency. According to Maurer (1995), the state intervenes only in extreme cases.

Usually, interventions are directed at recognizing and reducing risks. Referral to appropriate community agencies can assist in alleviating some of the stress in caregivers and thereby reducing the possibility of neglect and abuse. Respite care providers and adult day care centers can be used to allow the caregiver an opportunity to have time away from constant duty while providing supervision for the patient. Meals on Wheels can assist in providing nutritious meals for individuals and senior citizens centers, and state or local offices on aging can provide information and resources for older patients and their caregivers.

OLDER ADULTS AS VICTIMS OF CRIME

As a result of physical, financial, and environmental factors, older people are vulnerable to becoming victims of a variety of crimes. Such crimes include burglary, assault, robbery, purse snatching, pickpocketing or mugging, and fraudulent schemes. In many communities, efforts have been made to help older people avoid becoming victims of crime. For example, to combat mugging or purse snatching, many banks encourage direct deposit of Social Security payments and some communities provide escort services for older people.

Unfortunately, the areas of fraud and "con games" directed at the elderly have been somewhat overlooked. Table 14–22 describes common "scams," often directed at older citizens.

TABLE 14–22 **Fraud: Elders as Victims**

Health-Related Fraud

- Hearing aids. Disreputable hearing aid dealers pose as audiologists offering "free" hearing test and "one-day only specials." Note: Hearing aids can be sold only with a prescription.
- Mail order health care or laboratory tests. The user is promised medical care or laboratory screening for conditions, such as acquired immunodeficiency syndrome (AIDS), high cholesterol level, cancer, through the mail.
- Medical products. The individual is urged to buy health products or "cures" through the mail.
- Health quackery. The individual is urged to undergo questionable "treatment" from a variety of providers. At risk are individuals with conditions such as cancer, obesity, alcoholism, and arthritis.
- Health insurance policy schemes. The individual is required to overpay for Medigap coverage or buy multiple policies, or the person might receive a "bill" for medical insurance that he or she has not purchased.

Home Repair and Sales Schemes

- Home repair "contractors" "working in the neighborhood" offer to repair, inspect, or remodel the home or exterminate pests. Often the work and expense are unnecessary.
- Home inspectors say they must inspect plumbing, furnace, or wiring. Once inside, they may rob the homeowner, insist that something needs repair, or charge excessively for the job.
- Salesperson offers to describe only (not sell) a product if the respondent will sign a paper proving the salesperson did it. The individual may have agreed to purchase a product or service unknowingly, or the salesperson might be using this tactic as a ruse for entry.

Real Estate Schemes

- The individual is promised cheap land or retirement and recreational facilities at a wonderful site. The land may not exist.

Obituary Watchers

- A new widow or widower is sent false bills or merchandise supposedly ordered but not paid for by the deceased.
- "Funeral vultures" are disreputable funeral directors who contact the grieving individual and promote costly or "discount" funerals.

Contest Winners

- The individual is told that he or she has won a vacation, automobile, or other prize but must send a specified amount of money for postage or registration to collect.
- Someone offers to sell a winning lottery ticket that he or she is not able to collect for a number of reasons. The "winning ticket" is phony.
- Using a "pigeon drop," the fraudulent person offers to share "found" money if the individual will put up some money to show "good faith."

Credit or Phone Card Fraud

- A salesperson asks for credit or phone card number to send a product, verify insurance, or check for unauthorized charges. The number is then used to charge against the account.

Request for "Help" Resulting in Theft

- Someone asks for help because a spouse or child is sick, the person has run out of gas, or needs money.
- A woman, child, or nonthreatening individual knocks on door and asks for entrance to use the phone.

Data from Marklein, M. (1991). Con games proliferate: New threats haunt city folk. *AARP Bulletin 32*(2), 1, 16–17; and Kirkham, A. K. (1988). Crime and abuse. In M. O. Hogstel (Ed.). *Nursing Care of the Older Adult* (2nd ed.). New York, John Wiley and Sons, pp. 457–476.

Care Assistance for Older Adults

Only about 5% of older Americans reside in institutional settings (e.g., nursing homes) (Birchfield, 1996; Clemen-Stone et al., 1995). The remainder live in their own homes, typically with their spouse or alone. If individuals have health problems or need assistance with normal or instrumental activities of daily living, they may reside with someone who can assist them, usually a child, sibling, or other relative.

Whether the person lives at home or with someone else, many times assistance from an external organization or agency can be beneficial, even if not necessary. This assistance might be temporary (e.g., home health care following hip replacement

TABLE 14–23 **Long-Term and Short-Term Care Providers and Facilities for Older Adults**

Setting/Provider	Caregivers	Services
Home	Informal caregivers (spouses, children, neighbors)	Variable, depending on needs of the elder—assist with activities of daily living, health care, meals
Home health agencies	Professional and paraprofessionals (nurses, therapists, aides)	Intermittent skilled nursing; various therapies; assistance with activities of daily living, shopping, transportation, chores
Nursing homes (skilled nursing facilities and intermediate care facilities)	Professional and paraprofessionals (nurses, therapists, aides)	Skilled nursing; monitoring; various therapies; assistance with activities of daily living, supervision as needed.
Community-based services	Professional and volunteer staff	Preventive health care; on-site and delivered meals; legal and tax services; transportation; recreation
Adult day care	Professional, paraprofessional and volunteer	Temporary care for elders who live at home with family or friends but need supervision and assistance during the workday
Respite care	Professional, paraprofessional and volunteer (friend/family)	Temporary care (few hours, day, week) for disabled or frail older person for the purpose of relieving the family or principal care provider
Housing services (retirement communities, assisted living board and care, halfway houses, congregate living)	Professional, paraprofessional	Services variable, based on individual need and functional ability; include room, meals, assistance with activities of daily living, medication management, some protective oversight

Data from Evashwick, C. J. (1993). The continuum of long-term care. In S. J. Williams and P. R. Torrens (Eds.). *Introduction to Health Services* (4th ed). Albany, NY, Delmar Publishers; Eliopoulos C. (1993). *Gerontological Nursing* (3rd ed). Philadelphia, J. B. Lippincott; and Richardson, H. (1995). Long-term care. In A. R. Kovner (Ed.). *Jonas's Health Care Delivery in the United States* (5th ed.). New York, Springer Publishing Co., pp. 194–231.

TABLE 14–24 **Resources for Elders**

General Aging

U. S. Department of Health and Human Services
Administration on Aging
330 Independence Ave. S.W.
Washington, D. C. 20201
(202) 619-0724

Eldercare Locator (Community Assistance for Seniors)
(800) 677-1116

National Institutes of Health
National Institute on Aging
9000 Rockville Pike
Bethesda, MD 20892-0001
(301) 496-4000

Social Security Administration*
Public Inquiries
6401 Security Building
Baltimore, MD 21235
(410) 965-7700

Social Issues

American Association of Retired Persons (AARP)†
601 E. St. N.W.
Washington, D. C. 20049
(202) 434-2277

Gray Panthers
P.O. Box 21477
Washington, D. C. 20009
(202) 466-3132

Hearing Loss/Vision Impairment

National Institute of Neurological and Communication Disorders
Bethesda, MD 20014
(202) 496-4000

American Speech and Hearing Association
10801 Rockville Pike
Rockville, MD 20852-3279
(301) 897-5700

National Eye Care Project
(800) 222-EYES (3937)

Lions Club
(800) 747-4448

Heart Disease

American Heart Association
7272 Greenville Ave.
Dallas, TX 75231
(214) 373-6300

Cancer

American Cancer Society
1599 Clifton Rd. N.E.
Atlanta, GA 30329
(404) 320-3333

Alzheimer's Disease

Alzheimer's Association
919 Michigan Ave., 10th Floor
Chicago, IL 60611
(312) 335-8700
(800) 272-3900

Alzheimer's Disease Education and Referral Center
P.O. Box 8250
Silver Spring, MD 20907-8250
(800) 438-4380

Parkinson's Disease

American Parkinson's Disease Association
116 John St.
New York, NY 10038
(212) 732-9550

Arthritis

Arthritis Foundation
1330 West Peachtree Street
Atlanta, GA 30309
(404) 872-7100

Arthritis Information Clearinghouse
P.O. Box 34427
Bethesda, MD 20034
(301) 881-9411

*Local or regional offices available.
†Call for listings of state offices.

TABLE 14–25 **Functions of the Gerontological Nurse**

Guide persons of all ages toward a healthy aging process
Eliminate ageism
Respect the rights of older adults and ensure that others do the same
Oversee and promote the quality of service delivery
Notice and reduce risks to health and well-being
Teach and support caregivers
Open channels for facing developmental tasks
Listen and support
Offer optimism and hope
Generate, support, implement, and participate in research
Implement restorative and rehabilitative measures
Coordinate services
Assess, plan, implement, and evaluate care in an individualized manner
Link services with needs

Nurture future gerontological nurses for advancement of the specialty
Understand the unique assets of each older individual
Recognize and encourage the appropriate management of ethical concerns
Support and comfort through the dying process
Educate to promote self-care and independence

From Eliopoulos, C. (1993). *Gerontological Nursing* (3rd ed). Philadelphia, J. B. Lippincott.

surgery) or more permanent (e.g., adult day care for a frail individual who lives with an adult child who is employed). Table 14–23 describes several types of community-based providers and agencies that assist in caring for older adults.

Referrals for assistance or services can be one of the most important interventions for nurses who work with older patients. Table 14–24 provides a collection of resources that can be used as a starting point for nurses in community settings. Each nurse, however, should assemble a list of local providers and services for quick referral for these individuals and their caregivers. For example, the nurse should have readily available the phone numbers for Meals on Wheels, a nearby respite care provider or adult day care center, and organizations that provide financial assistance to older people.

SUMMARY

The number and proportion of Americans over 65 years of age are growing at an astonishing rate. As a result, the United States needs many more health care professionals, particularly nurses, educationally prepared to work with older adults. As the vast amount of health care for the elderly is provided in community settings, nurses should be trained and equipped to manage care appropriately, focusing special attention on health promotion and illness prevention and recognizing the unique needs of this population. Table 14–25 creatively describes the multiple roles and functions of the gerontological nurse.

Key Points

- Because *22% of Americans will be over age 65 by the year 2030,* improving the health and limiting disabilities in older adults is essential.
- *Assessment* of older adults should be comprehensive and should include evaluation of physical health, health history, functional ability, cognitive and mental state, and nutritional status.
- *Functional independence* refers to the extent to which an indiviudal is able to perform *activities of daily living* (ADL) and *instrumental activities of daily living* (IADL) without assistance from others.
- To *promote* functional independence, the nurse should identify and manage potential threats and limitations and associated health problems. Areas of assessment and intervention include hearing deficits, vision deficits, congnitive impairment, and urinary incontinence.
- *Health promotion and illness prevention guidelines* adopted by the U.S. Preventive Services Task Force include recommendations on immunization, addressing safety concerns (falls and medication compliance), and assessment and intervention in elder abuse.
- *Common health problems* in older adults include cardiovascular conditions (coronary artery disease, congestive heart failure, peripheral vascular disease), respiratory diseases (chronic obstructive pulmonary disease, asthma), musculoskeletal problems (osteoporosis, arthritis), genitourinary conditions (prostate enlargement, incontinence), gastrointestinal problems, endocrine disorders (diabetes), neurological conditions (Alzheimer's disease, cerebrovascular accidents), sensory disorders (cataract, hearing impairment), and mental health problems (depression).
- *Care assistance arrangements* for older adults include nursing homes, home health agencies, adult day care providers, and respite care providers.

Learning Activities and Application to Practice

In Class

- Discuss *Healthy People 2000* objectives that address older adults. What progress has been made in achieving the objectives? Outline strategies and interventions that nurse can implement to contribute to achieving the objectives.
- Discuss recommendations of the Preventive Services Task Force for older adults (see Table 14–15). Are recommendations followed by primary care providers? Why or why not?
- Invite a guest speaker from area Adult Protective Services to discuss the problem of elder abuse. Ask the speaker to include discussion of types of elder abuse, when elder abuse might be suspected, the risk factors for elder abuse, and what to do if elder abuse is suspected (process for referral).

In Clinical

- In groups of two or three, have students visit providers of assistive care for elders (i.e., assign one group to visit a local adult day care center; another can visit a nursing home or retirement center). Have students note which services are provided and who is the provider. What activities are available? How are services funded? Share findings with the group.
- Have each student complete the Comprehensive Older Person's Evaluation (COPE) on one patient being cared for in clinical practice. Use the questionnaire to develop a preventive plan of care for that patient.
- In a log or diary, have each student record the chronic conditions identified in clinical practice. What percentage of elders encountered have more than one chronic condition? What are common combinations (e.g., chronic obstructive pulmonary disease and asthma, diabetes, peripheral vascular disease, coronary artery disease)? Share observations with members of the group.
- Assess the home of an older patient for threats to safety, particularly falls. Develop a plan or strategy to reduce identified threats.

REFERENCES

Alzheimer's Disease Association. (1994). *Alzheimer's Disease Statistics*. Chicago, Alzheimer's Disease Association.

American Association of Retired Persons. (1993). *Profile of Older Americans 1993*. Washington, D. C.: American Association of Retired Persons.

American Association of Retired Persons. (1993). *Coping & Caring: Living with Alzheimer's Disease*. Washington, D. C., American Association of Retired Persons.

American Nurses' Association. (1987). *Standards and Scope of Gerontological Nursing Practice*. Kansas City, MO, American Nurses' Association.

Birchfield, P. C. (1996). Elder health. In M. Stanhope and J. Lancaster (Eds.). *Community Health Nursing: Promoting Health of Aggregates, Families and Individuals* (4th ed.). St. Louis, Mosby–Year Book, pp. 581–600.

Campbell, J. and Landenburger, K. (1996). Violence and human abuse. In M. Stanhope and J. Lancaster (Eds.). *Community Health Nursing: Promoting Health of Aggregates, Families and Individuals* (4th ed). St. Louis, Mosby–Year Book.

Centers for Disease Control (CDC). (1991). Update on adult immunization: Recommendations of the Immunization Practices Advisory Committee (ACIP). *Morbidity and Mortality Weekly Report 40* (RR-12).

Chenitz, W. C., Kussman, H. L., and Stone, J. T. (1991). Preventing falls. In W. C. Chenitz, J. T. Stone, and S. A. Salisbury (Eds.). *Clinical Gerontological Nursing: A Guide to Advanced Practice*. Philadelphia, W. B. Saunders, pp. 309–328.

Clark, M. J. (1995). *Nursing in the Community* (2nd ed.). Norwalk, CT, Appleton & Lange.

Clemen-Stone, S., Eigsti, D. G., and McGuire, S. L. (1995). *Comprehensive Community Health Nursing* (4th ed). St. Louis, Mosby–Year Book.

Dambro, M. R. (1996). *Griffith's 5-Minute Clinical Consult*. Baltimore, Williams & Williams.

Ebersole, P. and Hess, P. (1985). *Toward Healthy Aging*. St. Louis, C. V. Mosby.

Eliopoulos, C. (1993). *Gerontological Nursing* (3rd ed). Philadelphia, J. B. Lippincott.

Evashwick, C. J. (1993). The continuum of long-term care. In S. J. Williams and P. R. Torrens (Eds.). *Introduction to Health Services* (4th ed). Albany, NY, Delmar Publishers, pp. 177–218.

Folstein, M. F., Folstein, S. E., and McHugh, P. R. (1975). "Mini-Mental State": A practical method for grading the cognitive state of patients for the clinician. *Journal of Psychiatric Research, 12,* 189–198.

Graves, M. (1988). Drug use and abuse. In M. O. Hogstel (Ed.). *Nursing Care of the Older Adult* (2nd ed). New York, John Wiley and Sons, pp. 261–276.

Hashizume, S. (1991). Home health care. In W. C. Chenitz, J. T. Stone, and S. A. Salisbury (Eds.). *Clinical Gerontological Nursing: A Guide to Advanced Practice.* Philadelphia, W. B. Saunders, pp. 557–576.

Kirkham, A. K. (1988). Crime and abuse. In M. O. Hogstel (Ed.). *Nursing Care of the Older Adult* (2nd ed). New York, John Wiley and Sons, pp. 457–476.

Lashley, M. E. (1995). Elderly persons in the community. In C. M. Smith and F. A. Maurer (Eds.). *Community Health Nursing: Theory and Practice*. Philadelphia, W. B. Saunders, pp 719–746.

Luggen, A. S. (1996). Aging process. In A. S. Luggen (Ed.). *Core Curriculum for Gerontological Nursing*. St. Louis, Mosby-Year Book, pp. 35–43.

Lukacs, K. (1996). Neurological/Alzheimer's disease. In A. S. Luggen (Ed.). *Core Curriculum for Gerontological Nursing*. St. Louis, Mosby–Year Book, pp. 564–580.

Marklein, M. (1991). Con games proliferate: New threats haunt city folk. *AARP Bulletin, 32*(2), 1, 16–17.

Maurer, F. A. (1995). Violence: A social and family problem. In C. M. Smith and F. A. Maurer (Eds.). *Community Health Nursing: Theory and Practice*. Philadelphia, W. B. Saunders, pp. 517–547.

Murray, R., Zentner, J., and Pinnell, N. (1993). Assessment and health promotion for the person in later maturity. In R. B. Murray and J. P. Zentner (Eds.). *Nursing Assessment and Health Promotion: Strategies Through the Life Span* (5th ed.). Norwalk, CT, Appleton & Lange, pp. 542–603.

National Center for Health Statistics. (January 1994). Current Estimates from the National Health Interview Survey, 1992. *Vital and Health Statistics, Series 10,* p. 189. Washington, D. C.

Richardson, H. (1995). Long-term care. In A. R. Kovner (Ed.). *Jonas's Health Care Delivery in the United States* (5th ed.). New York, Springer Publishing Co., pp. 194–231.

Roen, O. T. (1993). Senior health. In J. M. Swanson and M. Albrecht (Eds.). *Community Health Nursing: Promoting the Health of Aggregates*. Philadelphia, W. B. Saunders, pp. 329–368.

Selkoe, D. J. (1992). Aging brain, aging mind. *Scientific American, 267*(3), 134–142.

Stone, J. T. and Chenitz, W. C. (1991). The problem of falls. In W. C. Chenitz, J. T. Stone, and S. A. Salisbury (Eds.). *Clinical Gerontological Nursing: A Guide to Advanced Practice*. Philadelphia, W. B. Saunders, pp. 291–308.

U. S. Department of Commerce (USDOC). (1990). *Statistical Abstract of the U. S.* (110th ed.). Washington D. C., Bureau of the Census.

U. S. Department of Health and Human Services (USDHHS). (1990). *Healthy People 2000: National Health Promotion and Disease Prevention Objectives. Summary Report*. Washington, D. C., Government Printing Office.

U.S. Department of Health and Human Services/Agency for Health Care Policy and Research (USDHHS/AHCPR). (1992). *Urinary Incontinence in Adults: Clinical Practice Guideline*. AHCPR Pub. No. 92–0038. Rockville, MD, Agency for Health Care Policy and Research.

U. S. Department of Health and Human Services/Office of Disease Prevention and Health Promotion (USDHHS/ODPHP). (1994). *Clinician's Handbook of Preventive Services*. Washington, D. C., Government Printing Office.

U. S. Department of Health and Human Services/Office of Disease Prevention and Health Promotion. (1996). *Guide to Clinical Preventive Services* (2nd ed.). Washington, D. C., Government Printing Office.

U.S. Department of Health and Human Services (USDHHS). (1997). *Guide to Clinical Preventive Services* (2nd ed.). Washington, D. C., Government Printing Office.

Ventry, I. M. and Weinstein, B. E. (1983). Identification of elderly people with hearing problems. *ASHA (American Speech-Language-Hearing Association),* (25), 7–42.

Watkins, A. C. (1993). Family violence. In J. Swanson and M. Albrecht (Eds.). *Community Health Nursing: Promoting the Health of Aggregates*. Philadelphia, W. B. Saunders, pp. 459–486.

UNIT

V

Nursing Care of Clients with Special Needs in Community Settings

15

Communicable Disease: Prevention and Intervention

Case Study

Mark Mitchell works as a nurse for the public health department in a mid-sized city. Mark's primary responsibility is investigation and follow-up of suspected cases of reportable diseases. One recent Monday, Mark received a call from a local pediatrician who reported a suspected case of measles in a 3-year-old boy named Patrick. To gather information about the case, Mark reviewed the child's presenting symptoms with the physician. The symptoms were a fever of over 101°F for 2 days, a mild cough, runny nose, conjunctivitis, and a red rash, which his mother reported began on his face and had progressed to his trunk. Upon prompting from Mark, the pediatrician looked inside the child's mouth and discovered small red spots with bluish-white centers on the buccal mucosa (Koplik's spots). Additionally, the pediatrician stated that according to her records, Patrick's immunization status was incomplete, as he had received only his initial diphtheria/pertussis/tetanus (DPT), Haemophilis influenzae *b (HIB), and oral polio vaccinations at her office. The mother denied that the child had received "shots" at any other clinic. The pediatrician concluded that although Patrick was quite ill, he did not need to be hospitalized, but would be treated with cough medication, antipyretics, and decongestants as an outpatient.*

Mark was aware that during the past 6 weeks, there had been 10 confirmed cases of measles in the county and about 20 others that were "suspect." Because of the presence of the disease in the area, Mark determined that with the symptoms Patrick was displaying, along with his incomplete immunization status, it was probable that Patrick was ill with measles. Mark instructed the pediatrician to obtain a sample of blood to send to the state laboratory for confirmation of the diagnosis. According to department protocols, Mark obtained the boy's name and address and made a visit to the boy's home later that day.

Patrick was the youngest of three (Joseph, 6, and Brittany, 9). While in the home, Mark questioned Patrick's parents regarding the immunization status of their other two children and reviewed their immunization records. Both children's records were complete and included two injections of measles/mumps/rubella (MMR) vaccine, as required by the state for all children in school. Both of Patrick's parents were born before 1957 and reported they had been ill with measles as children.

Next, Mark gathered as much information as the parents could provide pertaining to other children that Patrick had been around the previous 2 weeks. He discovered that Patrick had spent a few hours at a baby sitter's house on two separate days and in the church's nursery for about 3 hours the previous Sunday. Mark called the nursery director at the church. She stated there had been about 10 children in Patrick's class on Sunday and she knew of none that were sick. She agreed to call all of the parents and explain that their children had possibly been exposed to measles. Further, she would instruct them to call their pediatricians to check their children's immunization status.

The baby sitter was then called. She reported that one of the children she keeps on a sporadic basis had been very ill with a fever about 10 days previously, but she did not know what was wrong with her. Mark obtained that child's name and her parent's telephone number and address and continued the process of communicable disease surveillance.

Caring for individuals with communicable diseases was one of the earliest functions of nurses. Later, prevention of the spread of communicable diseases, through advocating of cleanliness and use of immunizations and medications, became an integral part of nursing practice. Indeed, the first intervention learned by virtually every nursing student relates to the spread of communicable diseases: "Wash your hands!" The importance of frequent and thorough hand washing is repeatedly stressed and cannot be overstated for prevention of the spread of communicable diseases.

Around 1900, communicable diseases accounted for 4 of the top 10 causes of death for Americans. At that time, pneumonia and influenza were designated collectively as the leading cause of death, followed closely by tuberculosis. Diarrhea and enteritis were collectively the third major cause of death, and diphtheria was 10th. A similar list for 1995 contains only two communicable diseases. "Pneumonia and influenza" (fifth) was the only duplication from the earlier list, and acquired immunodeficiency syndrome (AIDS) (and human immunodeficiency virus [HIV] infection), not heard of in 1900, was 10th. With these exceptions, communicable disease as a cause of *mortality* has largely been managed. In terms of *morbidity*, however, although there has been much improvement, many Americans are sickened each year by a variety of communicable diseases ranging from mild (colds or "stomach flu") to serious and life threatening (influenza or tuberculosis).

This chapter presents an overview of contemporary health problems and issues that relate to communicable disease prevention, transmission, and management. *Healthy People 2000,* the national health objectives publication introduced in Chapter 1, lists three priority areas that relate specifically to prevention and management of communicable disease. These are: HIV Infection (18), Sexually Transmitted Diseases (19), and Immunization and Infectious Diseases (20). Examples of goals from two of these priority areas (Sexually Transmitted Diseases and Immunization and Infectious Disease) are shown in Table 15–1. Goals for AIDS and HIV infection are discussed separately in Chapter 16.

Communicable Disease Transmission

Communicable diseases may be transmitted either directly, through physical contact between infected individuals, or indirectly, through a source other than another human. Direct transmission can be through physical contact including biting, kissing, and touching (e.g., for influenza, colds, strep throat) or sexual contact (e.g., for HIV, sexually transmitted diseases [STDs], hepatitis B). Indirect transmissions can be vehicle borne through "fomites" (objects that absorb and transmit infec-

TABLE 15–1 ***Healthy People 2000:* Examples of Objectives for Prevention of Communicable Disease**

19.1—Reduce gonorrhea to an incidence of no more than 225 cases per 1000,000 people. (Baseline: 300 per 100,000 in 1989)

19.3—Reduce primary and secondary syphilis to an incidence of no more than 10 cases per 1000,000 people. (Baseline: 18.1 per 100,000 in 1989)

19.7—Reduce sexually transmitted hepatitis B infection to no more than 30,500 cases. (Baseline: 58,300 cases in 1988)

19.9—Reduce the proportion of adolescents who have engaged in sexual intercourse to no more than 15% by age 15 and no more than 40% by age 17. (Baseline: 27% of girls and 33% of boys by age 15; 50% of girls and 66% of boys by age 17; reported in 1988)

19.12—Include instruction in prevention of sexually transmitted disease transmission in the curricula of all middle and secondary schools, preferably as part of quality school health education. (Baseline: 95% of schools reported offering at least one class on sexually transmitted disease as part of their standard curricula in 1988)

19.14—Increase to at least 75% the proportion of primary care and mental health care providers who provide age-appropriate counseling on the prevention of HIV and other sexually transmitted diseases. (Baseline: 10% of physicians reported that they regularly assessed the sexual behaviors of their patients in 1987)

20.1—Reduce indigenous cases of vaccine-preventable diseases as follows:

Disease	1988 Baseline	2000 Target
Diphtheria <25 years	1	0
Tetanus <25 years	3	0
Polio (wild-type virus)	0	0
Measles	3,058	0
Rubella	225	0
Congenital rubella syndrome	6	0
Mumps	4,866	500
Pertussis	3,450	1,000

20.4—Reduce tuberculosis to an incidence of no more than 3.5 cases per 100,000 people. (Baseline: 9.1 per 100,000 in 1988)

20.11—Increase immunization levels as follows:

Basic immunization series among children age 2: at least 90% (Baseline: 70–80% estimated in 1989)

Hepatitis B immunization among high-risk populations, including infants of surface antigen–positive mothers to at least 90%; occupationally exposed workers to at least 90%; IV drug users in drug treatment programs to at least 50%; and homosexual men to at least 50%. (Baseline data not available)

20.17—Increase to at least 90% the proportion of local health departments that have ongoing programs for actively identifying cases of tuberculosis and latent infection in populations at high risk for tuberculosis. (Baseline data not available)

From U.S. Department of Health and Human Services. (1990). *Healthy People 2000: National Health Promotion and Disease Prevention Objectives.* Washington, D. C., Government Printing Office.

tious material such as toys, telephones, money) or substances (food, water, blood). Communicable disease may also be transmitted indirectly through "vectors" such as animals (e.g., rabies, anthrax, toxoplasmosis) or arthropods (e.g., malaria, Lyme disease, Rocky Mountain spotted fever). Airborne transmission through dust and droplet and droplet nuclei may be either direct (spray from body fluids such as sneezing or coughing, e.g., in colds, influenza) or indirect (contaminated dusts or droplet nuclei, e.g., in legionellosis, tuberculosis) (Table 15–2). Figure 15–1 illustrates communicable disease transmission.

Efforts to prevent spread of communicable dis-

TABLE 15–2 **Types of Transmission**

Direct Transmission	Indirect Transmission
Physical contact	**Vehicle borne**
Biting	Fomites (toys)
Touching	Substances (food, blood)
Spitting	
Sexual contact	**Vector borne**
Fecal-oral	Mechanical
Anal intercourse	Biological
Oral-genital	
Airborne	**Airborne**
Dust and droplets	Dust and droplets
Droplet nuclei	Droplet nuclei

From Dash, D. (1993). Communicable disease. In J. Swanson and S. Albrecht (Eds.). *Community Health Nursing: Promoting the Health of Aggregates.* Philadelphia, W. B. Saunders.

Data from Mausner, J. S. and Kramer, S. (1985). *Epidemiology: An Introductory Text.* Philadelphia, W. B. Saunders.

eases must incorporate primary prevention strategies designed to stop transmission. Encouraging frequent hand washing, use of tissues to cover the mouth and nose when coughing or sneezing, mosquito control, rabies inoculation for all pets, and promoting sexual abstinence or appropriate use of condoms are examples of primary prevention interventions that attempt to stop the spread of communicable diseases.

Reportable Communicable Diseases

Each state has an established reporting system to monitor communicable diseases. Typically, state laws or regulations empower the state board or department of health to establish and modify reporting requirements. The individual states are then required to report selected data to the Centers for Disease Control and Prevention (CDC). Figure 15–2 illustrates this process.

According to CDC (1992, p 303), state regulations usually specify:

- The disease and conditions that must be reported
- Who is responsible for reporting
- What information is required on each case of disease reported
- How, to whom, and how quickly the information is to be reported
- Control measures to be taken for specified diseases

REPORTABLE DISEASES

Reportable diseases and those that require notification of authorities vary slightly from state to state. Table 15–3 provides a list of diseases and conditions that are required to be reported nationally and other diseases about which authorities must be notified according to individual state regulations.

WHO IS RESPONSIBLE FOR REPORTING

Although there may be differences based on state regulations, most states *require* reporting of known or suspected cases of reportable diseases by physicians, dentists, nurses, and other health professionals (medical examiners, laboratory directors, chiropractors, veterinarians) and administrators of hospitals, clinics, nursing homes, schools, and nurseries (CDC, 1992). Typically, organizations (e.g., clinics, doctor's offices, hospitals) designate one individual who is responsible for this activity and who has been trained in the process.

WHAT INFORMATION IS REQUIRED

Data to be collected vary based on the disease. Usually, case reports include the name, age, sex, race or ethnicity, date of birth, address, and telephone number of the patient and the disease, its date of onset, the attending physician, and the method of diagnosis. Some diseases (e.g., chicken-

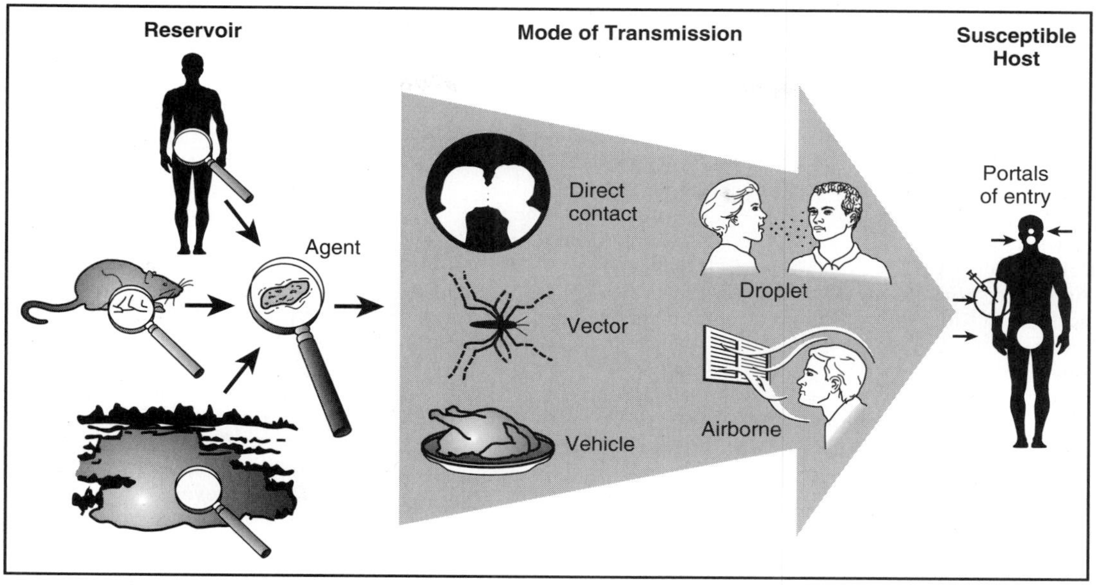

FIGURE 15–1 Chain of infection. (From Centers for Disease Control and Prevention. [1992]. *Principles of Epidemiology* (2nd ed.). Atlanta, GA, Centers for Disease Control and Prevention.)

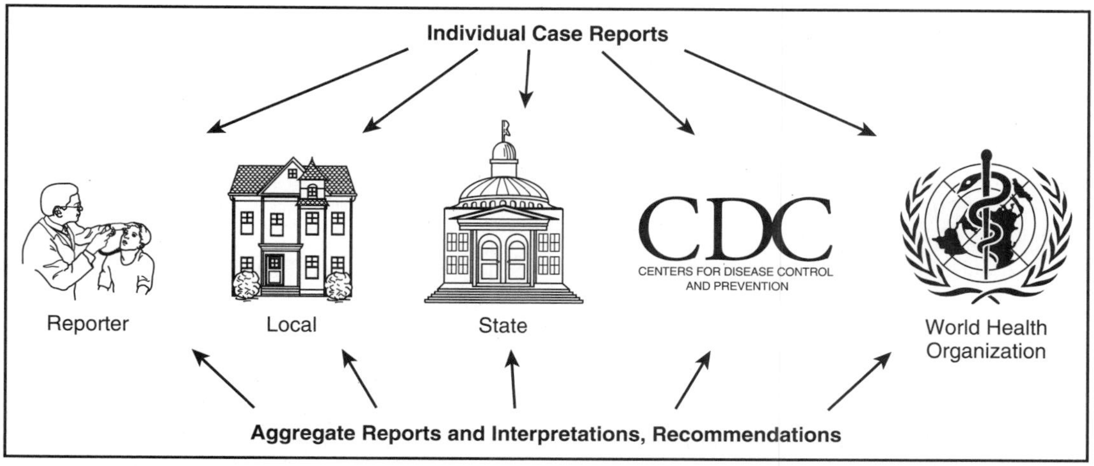

FIGURE 15–2 The reportable disease information cycle. (From Centers for Disease Control. [1992]. *Principles of Epidemiology* (2nd ed.). Atlanta, GA: Centers for Disease Control.)

TABLE 15–3 **National Notifiable Disease Surveillance System List of All Notifiable Diseases**

Surveillance Mandatory

AIDS	Hansen's disease	Rabies (animal)
Amoebiasis	Hepatitis A	Rabies (human)
Anthrax	Hepatitis B	Rheumatic fever
Aseptic meningitis	Hepatitis (non-A/non-B)	Rocky Mountain spotted fever
Botulism (infant)	Hepatitis (unspecified)	Rubella
Botulism (wound)	Legionellosis	Salmonellosis
Botulism (unspecified)	Leptospirosis	Shigellosis
Brucellosis	Lyme disease	Syphilis (all stages)
Chancroid	Lymphogranuloma venereum	Syphilis (primary and secondary)
Cholera	Malaria	Syphilis (congenital)
Diphtheria	Meningococcal infections	Toxic shock syndrome
Encephalitis (post-chickenpox)	Mumps	Trichinosis
Encephalitis (post-mumps)	Pertussis	Tuberculosis
Encepahlitis (post-other)	Plague	Tularemia
Encephalitis (primary)	Poliomyelitis (paralytic)	Typhoid fever
Gonorrhea	Psittacosis	Yellow fever
Granuloma inguinale		

Surveillance Maintained but not Mandatory

Campylobacter infection	*Listeria monocytogenes* (listeriosis)
Chlamydia trachomatis infection	Mucopurulent cervicitis
Dengue fever	Nongonococcal urethritis
Genital herpes simplex virus infection	Pelvic inflammatory disease
Genital warts	Reye's syndrome
Giardiasis	Spinal cord injury
Haemophilus influenzae (invasive disease)	Varicella
Kawasaki syndrome	All other unusual outbreaks

Data from Centers for Disease Control and Prevention. (1995c). Summary of notifiable diseases, United States: 1994. *Morbidity and Mortality Weekly Report,* 43(53), iv; and Dash, D. (1993). Communicable disease. In J. Swanson and S. Albrecht (Eds.). *Community Health Nursing: Promoting the Health of Aggregates.* Philadelphia, W. B. Saunders.

pox or influenza during an outbreak) may only be reported by number of cases.

HOW, WHEN, AND TO WHOM TO REPORT

Individual state regulations dictate the process for reporting. Some diseases, such as those that are rare, potentially very infectious, or involved in unusual outbreaks, are to be reported *immediately* by telephone. These typically include plague, rabies, measles, and poliomyelitis. Others are usually reported on a weekly basis either by telephone or by written report. Examples of illness reported weekly include: AIDS and other STDs, tuberculosis, Lyme disease, and mumps.

Most frequently, the health professional identifying a reportable disease reports to the local health department. As depicted in Figure 15–2, the local health department reports to the state health department, which then reports to the CDC.

STEPS TAKEN TO CONTROL SPREAD

States may have specific instructions to follow when certain diseases are identified. These instructions can include sending out surveillance teams to investigate and confirm reported cases; instruction on collecting of specimens; and specified control techniques such as environmental sanitation, immunization, quarantine, and education on prevention of transmission (CDC, 1992). Nurses working in public health departments, hospital infection control departments, ambulatory settings, schools, and industry should be aware of the most frequently encountered communicable diseases in their settings and learn the appropriate measures to take when a reportable disease is suspected or confirmed.

Identifying Communicable Diseases

Table 15–4 presents information on identification of some of the most common communicable diseases. Included are incubation period, mode of transmission, symptoms, and treatment. Familiarity with these illnesses will allow nurses to assist in identification, prevention, and treatment.

Incidence of Selected Reportable Diseases

Control of communicable diseases requires careful monitoring of trends and disease patterns. Table 15–5 lists several reportable diseases and the number of reported cases for selected years dating to 1945. This table graphically illustrates the effectiveness of immunization efforts in the reduction of vaccine-preventable diseases as well as trends in some communicable diseases that are interesting (fluctuation of gonorrhea, relative stability of hepatitis A), encouraging (0 cases of diphtheria in 1993), and cause for concern (increase in syphilis and tuberculosis). This table also allows insight into recent and anticipated changes in the immunization schedules (e.g., the addition of a booster for MMR following the outbreak of measles in 1989–1990 and the recent addition of immunization against chicken pox).

Vaccine-Preventable Diseases

Vaccination against communicable diseases has very dramatically affected morbidity and mortality from infectious diseases, as Table 15–5 shows. The worldwide eradication of small pox in 1980 is an example of the success that is possible through the use of global efforts to control disease through immunization. Efforts to eradicate other disease, such as measles, have been less successful to date, primarily owing to failure to appropriately immunize all those who are susceptible. Table 15–6 further illustrates the impact of routine vaccinations.

The routine immunization schedules have become very complex in recent years. Recommendations have been modified a number of times since the early 1980s with the addition of new vaccines, changes in the ages for administration, requirements for informed consent, and reporting of serious side effects. Nurses who primarily work with children in schools, clinics, and doctor's offices, and who administer immunizations, must be aware of a number of components of immunizations delivery. In addition to a basic understanding of the principles behind immunization, nurses should know the pediatric immunization schedule and standards; contraindications and precautions; requirements for parent education and consent; and the process for reporting "adverse vaccine events." Each is discussed here.

IMMUNITY

Immunity refers to protection from infectious disease. There are two basic mechanisms for acquiring immunity—active and passive.

- **Passive immunity** is protection produced by an animal or human and transferred to another human. Passive immunity often provides effective protection, but this protection wanes over time—usually a few weeks or months.
- **Active immunity** is protection that is produced by the person's own immune system.

Text continued on page 472

TABLE 15–4 Identifying Selected Communicable Infectious Diseases

Disease (Causative Agent)	Symptoms	Mode of Transmission	Complications and Community Health Concerns	Specific Treatment (If Any)
Respiratory Route				
Chickenpox (varicella-zoster virus)	Incubation period, 12–21 days. Low-grade fever, listlessness. Lesions within 2–4 days. Rash has three phases: raised spots, fluid-filled vesicles, and scabs. Rash itches and is found over entire body, including mucous membranes such as mouth.	Very contagious (person-to-person direct contact or contact with airborne droplet). Vesicles are contagious, scabs are not. Communicable 2 days before to 6 days after vesicles appear. Primarily affects children.	Grandparents and older adults should avoid caring for children because they may develop shingles.	Immunosuppressed persons should be treated with γ-globulin. Vaccine is available.
Diphtheria (*Corynebacterium diphtheriae*)	Flulike symptoms with sore throat, fever, and involvement of adenoids and larynx with potential respiratory distress. Characterized by formation of yellow-white membranes on tonsils and pharyngeal walls.	Person-to-person direct contact or contact with airborne droplet. Usually affects children under 15 years but may affect adults.	Asymptomatic carrier state possible; should be treated with antibiotics.	Antitoxin immediately on diagnosis and antibiotics (e.g., penicillin and/or erythromycin). Isolate until three negative throat cultures.
Pertussis or whooping cough (*Haemophilus pertussis* bacteria)	Incubation period, 7–10 days. Characteristic cough is nonproductive with quick expiratory phase followed by inspiratory "whoop." Pneumonia and ear infections may be present. Small scleral and conjunctival hemorrhages can occur owing to severe coughing. Convulsions may occur.	Person-to-person direct contact or droplet spread. Very contagious. Affects females more than males. Infants younger than 1 year are severely affected.	Incidence has increased in recent years because of lower immunization rates and concern about side effects of vaccine. Severity of illness and risk of death far surpass the risks from vaccination.	Antibiotics. Hospitalization with oxygen support and nasotracheal suctioning may be necessary.
German measles/rubella (rubella virus)	Incubation period, 14–21 days. Mild in adults and young children, with a macular rash on scalp, body, and limbs lasting 1–3 days. Severe in early fetal development and can result in congenital malformations and death; late fetal infection carries risk of birth defects. Conditions associated with fetal infections include low birth weight, deafness, cataracts, glaucoma, heart disease, and mental retardation.	Person-to-person direct contact or droplet spread. Communicable 4 days before to 4 days after rash appears. Highly contagious. Common in children 5 to 10 years of age.	Women of childbearing years should be immunized before pregnancy. Vaccine is live, so it must not be given to pregnant women. Reinfections can occur but are rare.	None

Measles/rubeola (rubeola virus)	Incubation period, 7–21 days. Rash, usually starting on the face and spreading to body, lasting 6 days. Koplik's spots in mouth that are bluish white and very fine. Coldlike symptoms and cough. Lasts 4–5 days.	Person-to-person direct contact with saliva or droplets. Common disease of childhood. More common in poorly immunized populations and in adolescents.	Complications are pneumonia and encephalitis. No congenital malformations, but can cause spontaneous abortion and prematurity. Children who are HIV positive and asymptomatic should be considered for the vaccine because the illness could be fatal. Persons allergic to eggs may have severe reactions to vaccine.	None
Mumps (mumps virus)	Incubation period, 14–26 days. Low-grade fever, headache, earache, pain, and swelling of parotid glands (unilateral or bilateral). Swelling lasts about a week. Early fetal infections can result in spontaneous abortion.	Person-to-person direct contact with saliva or droplets. More commonly a childhood disease. Communicable 6 days before to 9 days after swelling.	Infrequent complications are encephalitis and meningitis. Orchitis occurs in males who have reached puberty but sterility is rare. Potential for spontaneous abortion if woman is infected in early pregnancy. Persons allergic to eggs may have severe reaction to vaccine.	None
Tuberculosis (*Mycobacterium tuberculosis*)	Low-grade fever, listlessness, night sweats, respiratory congestion, cough, hemoptysis. Sites other than the lungs may be infected; if so, symptoms will be specific to the site. (Other sites include meninges, joints, bladder, and lymphatic system.)	Inhalation from droplet containing bacteria. Risk factors include poverty, poor health, and age. Very young and very old are most susceptible.	Infection with the bacteria produces disease in approximately 10% of cases in the United States. Mantoux test is used to screen for infection and disease. Incidence is on the rise owing to increased incidence in HIV patients and rise of drug-resistant strains of tuberculosis.	Multiple drug therapy with three to six drugs for 6 to 12 months for persons with the disease. Persons infected are treated prophylactically with one medication for up to 6 months. Drug-resistant individuals may need a variety and mix of drugs over time to ensure appropriate treatment.
Influenza (influenza type A or B virus, or potentially a third [type C] virus)	Respiratory symptoms such as runny nose or cough. May be accompanied by headache and fever. Sometimes may be accompanied by gastrointestinal symptoms such as nausea and vomiting.	Inhalation from droplet spread. Very infectious.	Rapid antigenic variation makes it difficult for the host to develop immune response. Influenza causes more pandemics than any other organism. Complications include pneumonia, croup, Reye's syndrome, toxic shock syndrome, myocarditis, and myocardial infarction.	None. Yearly vaccination recommended for susceptible individuals (i.e., elderly and chronically ill persons). Vaccine must be reconfigured each year to meet the specific characteristics of the current strain.

Table continued on following page

TABLE 15–4 **Identifying Selected Communicable Infectious Diseases** *Continued*

Disease (Causative Agent)	Symptoms	Mode of Transmission	Complications and Community Health Concerns	Specific Treatment (If Any)
Integumentary Route				
Pediculosis (parasitic lice)	Incubation period, 2 weeks. Lice and eggs may be present in scalp hair or pubic hair or on the body. Itching and other signs of skin irritation, such as a rash or swollen glands, may be present.	Direct contact or indirect transfer of adult lice, nits, or eggs via body contact, or contact with personal items that are infected with the parasites.	Nuisance disease; not easily transmitted from person to person.	Hair and pubic lice are treated with medicated shampoos such as Kwell in several applications. Nits (eggs) should be removed from scalp hair with a fine-toothed comb. Body lice are eliminated by dusting clothes with 1% malathion powder and washing all affected garments in very hot water.
Impetigo (group A streptococcal or staphyloccal bacteria)	Incubation period, 4–10 days. Skin blisters usually found in the corners of the mouth or near edge of nose. Blisters break and form yellow crusts that resolve with little or no scarring; blisters may be itchy, and scratching may occur. Fever, malaise, and headache may be present.	Direct contact with lesions or secretions. Very contagious. Scratching spreads the disease to other areas of the body or other persons. Communicable as long as lesions persist.	Most common in hot, humid climates. Very contagious and problematic in children. Infected children should be kept from school until completely healed.	Penicillin and/or erythromycin and topical antibiotics to treat skin eruptions.
Rabies (rabies virus)	Three phases: prodromal, neurological, and coma. Prodromal: wound heals and symptoms of minor infection are present lasting 2–10 days; these include fever, headache, chills, sore throat, and pain at site of bite. Neurological: lasts up to 7 days and includes hallucinations, stiffness, disorientation, and seizures. Coma: death may occur if treatment is not given.	Transmitted through bites from an infected animal.	Treatment is difficult, and fatality rate is high. Prevention is the main community health thrust. Domestic animals should be immunized and populations educated to avoid wild (e.g., fox, raccoon) or unknown animals.	Rabies vaccine. Hospitalization with isolation.
Scabies (parasitic mite)	Incubation period, 2–6 weeks; reinfections in 1–4 days. Skin rash, scratching may occur. Burrows on skin look like gray-white tracts; lesions may be evident around wrists and belt line.	Direct contact. Transmitted by mites that burrow under skin and lay eggs. Clothing and other personal items may hold mites or eggs. Communicable as long as eggs or mites are alive.	Concerns similar to those for pediculosis.	Hot bath, vigorous body scrub followed by application of 5% solution of benzyl benzoate or Kwell. Application should be repeated in approximately 1 week. Bedding and clothing must be thoroughly cleaned.

Gastrointestinal Route				
Candidiasis (*Candida* fungus)	Depend on site of infection. Gastrointestinal infection produces diarrhea and may be accompanied by cramping. Vaginal infections have vaginal symptoms.	Highly infectious. Found on skin and under finger- and toenails and may be passed to gastrointestinal tract by hand-to-mouth transmission. Vaginal infection common in females, easily transferred to males during sexual contact.	Infants can be infected during vaginal delivery	Multiple oral and topical drugs depending on site of infection, including nystatin, clotrimazole, and amphotericin B.
Salmonellosis (several types of *Salmonella* bacteria)	Incubation period, 6–72 hours. Sudden onset of acute gastroenteritis with abdominal cramps, diarrhea, nausea, and sometimes vomiting and dehydration. Headache and fever are present. Stools are loose for days after acute episode.	Direct via person-to-person oral-fecal contact or indirectly by ingestion of food contaminated with feces containing *Salmonella.* Communicable during entire period of infection, which may be as long as a year or more.	Infections most frequent from July to November with warm weather. Uncooked eggs and meats are major harborers of bacteria. Carriers continue to excrete organisms in stool for more than 1 year after symptoms disappear. Drug-resistant strains becoming more common.	Antibiotics for severe symptoms. Carriers treated with ampicillin.
Polio (strains of poliovirus)	Incubation period, 7–14 days or longer. Muscle weakness progressing to paralysis. May affect any muscle group, including limbs and respiratory muscles. Pain may accompany muscle weakness. There is little or no loss of sensation despite paralysis.	Direct contact of virus with mouth.	Humans are the only natural host and reservoir of the virus. Localized outbreaks in the United States are usually in unvaccinated or undervaccinated communities. Some recurring muscular weakness has been recently seen in persons who recovered from the illness years ago.	None
Shigellosis (variety of bacterial agents)	Incubation period, 1–7 days. Diarrhea, fever, and nausea. Can progress to toxemia, vomiting, and tenesmus. Blood, mucus, and pus may be found in stool.	Person-to-person by fecal-oral route or, more rarely, from contaminated water. Communicable as long as organism is present, which may be a month or more. Infants and young children are more often infected because of poor hygiene.	Most contagious condition caused by bacteria. Seasonal; more common in warm weather.	Antibiotics for severe symptoms
Intestinal parasites (roundworms and pinworms)	Abdominal pain; bloody stools or diarrhea may be present. Occasional nausea and vomiting.	Transmitted via ingestion of eggs of the worms, either directly via hands and fingernails or through food and water containing eggs.	Diagnosis of pinworms made by application of cellophane tape to anal area early in the morning to confirm eggs.	Treat with mebendazole until stools are clear of parasites.
Toxoplasmosis (protozoa)	Most persons have no symptoms or only mild symptoms, including enlarged lymph nodes, fever, night sweats, sore throat, or rash. Immunosuppressed persons, including HIV-positive individuals, may develop toxoplasmic encephalitis; hemiparesis, seizures, visual complications, mental disorientation, and listlessness. Fetal infection may result in spontaneous abortion, stillbirth, or varied complications after birth, including blindness, encephalitis, hydrocephalus, and anemia.	Contact with the protozoa via uncooked or undercooked meat or via airborne contact from the feces of cats.	Health education related to proper preparation of meats and care of cat litter is important. Toxoplasmosis screening should be done on pregnant women.	Immunosuppressed individuals are treated with a variety of drugs for up to 4–6 weeks after symptoms resolve; infected pregnant women are also treated.

Table continued on following page

TABLE 15–4 **Identifying Selected Communicable Infectious Diseases** *Continued*

Disease (Causative Agent)	Symptoms	Mode of Transmission	Complications and Community Health Concerns	Specific Treatment (If Any)
Hepatitis A (hepatitis A virus)	Incubation period, 15–30 days. Rapid onset of flulike symptoms, nausea and vomiting, abdominal cramps, jaundice; may also be asymptomatic. Long period of recovery (1–3 months).	Person-to-person by oral-fecal route. Very contagious and spreads rapidly. Also may be spread indirectly if virus is present in milk, undercooked shellfish, or contaminated water.	Common in daycare centers, homosexuals, and illicit intravenous drug users.	Immune serum globulin can be administered if exposed individuals are identified.
Serum Route				
Hepatitis B (hepatitis B virus)	Incubation period, 1–6 months. General flulike symptoms or no symptoms. Liver deterioration, if present, is noted by markedly enlarged liver, dark urine, light stool, jaundiced eyes and skin, skin eruptions. Symptoms last 4–6 weeks.	Exposure to infected blood (e.g., through sexual activity and intravenous drug paraphernalia). In health care workers, exposure to infected blood is often via accidental needle puncture.	Complications include chronic hepatitis, cirrhosis, live cancer, and death. Persons who need frequent blood transfusions are at increased risk. Health care workers are at increased risk to exposure. Chronic carriers can transmit disease to others; drug users are at risk for carrier status.	Vaccination for at-risk populations is recommended.
Human immunodeficiency virus (HIV)	Incubation period, potentially 10 years or more. Flulike symptoms may or may not be noted immediately after infection. Symptoms of immune compromise including opportunistic infections and cancers that allow for the diagnosis of AIDS (i.e., Kaposi's sarcoma, *Pneumocystis carinii* pneumonia, toxoplasmosis, candidiasis, cryptococcus, cytomegalovirus, herpes simplex, and others). Eventual outcome is death.	Exchange of secretions and semen during sexual intercourse; parenteral exposure of blood and blood products from mother to fetus; breast milk.	Testing for HIV infection is confidential. Persons positive for HIV infection may be asymptomatic for years, which is problematic because they may unknowingly engage in behavior that puts others at risk. Health teaching about safe sexual and personal habits is a concerted community health effort to control spread. HIV screening requires retesting at intervals after possible infection because the virus is not immediately detectable. There is a window period of approximately 1–12 weeks after infection when test results may be negative. People must be encouraged to retest as needed to ensure accurate testing results.	Treatment depends on specific presenting opportunistic illness or disease. Azidothymidine (AZT), didanosine (DDI), and dideoxycytidine (DDC) appear to slow the spread of the virus; AZT is particularly toxic and cannot be tolerated by many. Research continues in an attempt to find an effective treatment; at present none exists. Efforts at vaccine development continue.

Sexually Transmitted Route

Herpes (herpes simplex virus; HSV 1, oral; HSV 2, genital)	Incubation period, 2 weeks. Lesions at site of infection are fluid filled and rupture and ulcers form scabs. Lesions may or may not be painful. Virus stays dormant in body, and successive eruptions occur commonly as a result of stress or other illnesses. HSV 2 symptoms may include fever and other flulike symptoms. In women, vaginal discharge, painful intercourse, and painful urination may be present.	Direct contact with oral and genital secretions. HSV 1 and HSV 2 viruses have recently been found in genital and oral sites previously thought to be exclusive to one or the other.	Complications include increased risk of cervical cancer. Infants exposed through the birth canal may experience blindness, brain damage, or death. Recurrence in infected individuals places new sexual partners at risk. Protection of sexual partners during infectious periods should be stressed; condom use is important.	Incurable; acyclovir is given to treat existing cases and suppress recurrent episodes.
Cytomegalovirus (CMV)	Incubation period varies. If symptomatic, resembles mononucleosis; adults are mostly asymptomatic. Virus remains in body for life. Fetal infections can result in congenital anomalies, including mental retardation, deafness, jaundice, chorioretinitis, hydrocephaly, and epilepsy. Symptoms in newborns may not be immediately evident at birth but usually present during the first 6 months.	Transmitted through blood transfusions, organ transplants, breast milk, from children's urine and respiratory tract, and through sexual contact with semen and vaginal secretions.	Imunosuppressed individuals are at risk for frequent infectious episodes.	Ganciclovir is used to treat retinal CMV but is not successful against gastrointestinal, respiratory, and systemic CMV. Vaccine development is experimental and minimally useful to date.
Venereal warts (papillomavirus)	Condylomata warts, which may or may not be painful. Infants may develop respiratory symptoms.	Close contact with warts; may also be sexually transmitted. Passed to infants during passage through the birth canal.	Most serious complication is the link between the disease and malignancies of the cervix and genital tract.	Cryotherapy, laser therapy, or podophyllin in tincture of benzoin compound to remove or destroy warts.
Gonorrhea (*Neisseria gonorrhoeae*)	Incubation period, 2–30 days. Frequently asymptomatic, especially in men. Symptoms: women—pain, heavy purulent vaginal discharge, pain in the genital and pelvic area; men—discharge from penis, pain on urination, urinary frequency.	Primarily sexual contact. Can be transmitted to mucous membranes other than genitalia.	Complications include arthritis, blood, meningeal and heart infections, and sterility. In women, pelvic inflammatory disease; in men, narrowing of the urethra and swelling of the testicles. Children born during an active case may contract ophthalmia neonatorum, leading to blindness. Incidence is alarmingly high and most prevalent in young adults 15–35 years old.	One-time dose of ceftriaxone, cefixime, ciprofloxacin or ofloxacin. Antibiotics appropriate to treat for *Chlamydia* and trichomoniasis are often prescribed simultaneously. Test of cure in 4–7 days after treatment ends to ensure treatment effectiveness is especially important, because drug-resistant strains are becoming more frequent.
Chlamydia (*Chlamydia* bacteria)	Incubation period, 1–3 weeks. Symptoms consist of other infections such as nongonococcal urethritis, pelvic inflammatory disease, inflammation of cervix, and conjunctivitis. In infants, as a result of vaginal delivery: eye infections and pneumonia.	Primarily sexual contact but infections can occur in other areas of the body if contact is made with the bacteria.	Complications in women include pelvic inflammatory disease and cervical dysplasia; in men, prostatitis and epididymitis occur. Frequently occurs with other sexually transmitted diseases. This is the most frequently occurring sexually transmitted disease.	Doxycycline, azithromycin, tetracycline, or erythromycin. Test of cure in 4–7 days after treatment is completed.

Table continued on following page

TABLE 15–4 **Identifying Selected Communicable Infectious Diseases** *Continued*

Disease (Causative Agent)	Symptoms	Mode of Transmission	Complications and Community Health Concerns	Specific Treatment (If Any)
Syphilis (*Treponema pallidum*)	Incubation period, first stage, 10–90 days. Disease has three stages if left untreated. First stage: canker sore at site of infection (genital, rectum, lips); sore is usually painless. Second state: occurs 3–6 weeks later; generalized flulike symptoms and may have body rash, sores, inflamed eyes. Third stage: starts when disease becomes dormant, which may last years. Symptoms may recur, including blindness, deafness, brain damage, paralysis, heart disease, and death.	Sexual contact	Incidence is increasing, especially among young adults. Complications of untreated syphilis include blindness, deafness, brain damage, paralysis, heart disease, and death.	Large-dose intramuscular penicillin; if individual is allergic to penicillin, oral tetracycline or doxycycline is given. Patients must be rescreened at 3, 6, and 12 months because some infections are resistant to treatment. Drug-related strains are becoming problematic.
Pelvic inflammatory disease (gonorrhea, *Chlamydia*, *Trichomonas* bacteria, and other orgainsms)	Abnormal vaginal discharge, severe abdominal/pelvic pain and tenderness, painful intercourse, irregular vaginal bleeding, chills, fever, and nausea and vomiting. Can be fatal	Infections caused by sexually transmitted disease that spread to the upper genital tract of women.	Most common complication is sterility. Others include chronic abdominal pain; chronic infection of fallopian tubes, uterus, and ovaries; ectopic pregnancies.	Oral antibiotics, outpatient care; if no substantial improvement within 72 hours, hospitalization is necessary. Antibiotics should be specific for the particular organism causing the infection.
Trichomoniasis (protozoa *Trichomonas vaginalis*)	Incubation period, 1–6 weeks. Men usually asymptomatic but can have slight, clear penile discharge and itch on urination. Women have thin yellow-green-gray vaginal discharge with odor and burning, redness, itching of genitalia; may have frequency of urination.	Sexual contact with exchange of body fluids.	Sexual partners must be treated at the same time, even though men are commonly asymptomatic.	Metronidazole (flagyl, Protostat, or Metryl) given orally for 7–10 days. Vineger douche may alleviate vaginal symptoms.

From Matocha, L. K. (1995). Communicable disease. In C. M. Smith and F. A. Maurer (Eds.). *Community Health Nursing: Theory and Practice.* Philadelphia: W. B. Saunders. Compiled by Matocha, L. K. and Maurer, F. A.

TABLE 15–5 **Selected Reportable Diseases by Year**

Disease	Number of Cases								
	1945	***1950***	***1960***	***1970***	***1980***	***1985***	***1990***	***1993***	***1994***
AIDS	N/A	N/A	N/A	N/A	N/A	8,249	41,595	103,533	78,279
Diphtheria	18,675	5,796	918	435	3	3	4	0	2
Gonorrhea	287,181	286,746	258,933	600,072	1,004,029	911,419	690,169	439,675	418,068
Hepatitis A	N/A	2,820	41,666	56,797	29,078	23,266	31,441	24,238	29,796
Hepatitis B	Non-Specific			8,310	19,015	26,611	21,102	13,361	12,517
Measles	146,013	319,124	441,703	47,351	13,506	2,822	27,786	312	963
Mumps	N/A	N/A	N/A	104,953	8,576	2,982	5,292	1,692	1,537
Pertussis	133,792	120,718	14,809	4,249	1,730	3,589	4,570	6,586	4,617
Poliomyelitis	13,624	33,300	3,190	33	9	7	6	3	—
Rabies—human	43	18	2	3	2	1	1	3	6
Rubella	N/A	N/A	N/A	56,552	3,904	630	1,125	192	227
Syphilis	359,114	217,558	122,538	91,382	68,832	67,563	134,255	101,259	81,696
Tuberculosis	114,931	121,742	55,494	37,137	27,749	22,201	25,701	25,313	24,361
Varicella	N/A	N/A	N/A	N/A	190,894	178,162	173,099	134,722	151,219

From Centers for Disease Control and Prevention. (1995). Summary of notifiable diseases, United States—1994. *Morbidity and Mortality Weekly Report, 43* (53), 69–79.

TABLE 15–6 **Comparison of Maximum and Current Morbidity from Vaccine-Preventable Diseases**

Disease	Maximum Cases (n [year])	1993 Cases (n)	Change (%)
Diphtheria	206,939 (1921)	0	−100.0
Measles	894,134 (1941)	312	−99.9
Mumps	152,209 (1968)	1,692	−98.9
Pertussis	265,269 (1934)	6,586	−97.8
Polio* (paralytic)	21,269 (1952)	0	−100.0
Rubella	57,686 (1969)	192	−99.7
Congenital rubella syndrome	20,000 (1964–1965)	1	−99.3
Tetanus	601 (1948)	48	−97.3

*Due to wild poliovirus

From Centers for Disease Control and Prevention. (1995). *Epidemiology & Prevention of Vaccine-Preventable Diseases.* Atlanta, GA, Centers for Disease Control and Prevention.

This type of immunity is generally long-lasting (CDC, 1995a, p. 12).

Examples of passive immunity include transplacental transfer of immunity from a mother to her infant and injection of constituents of blood products from human donors (e.g., homologous pooled human antibody, immune globulin). Active immunity occurs following the stimulation of the body's immune system to produce antibodies and cellular immunity, often after a person has had a disease. Active immunity can also be achieved through administration of a vaccine that produces an immunological memory similar to that of the natural disease (CDC, 1995a).

Vaccines are classified as live attenuated and inactivated. Live attenuated vaccines are produced by modifying a disease-producing virus or bacterium in the laboratory. The altered vaccines allow production of an immune response as the organism replicates in the vaccinated person. Although the organisms in live attenuated vaccines replicate, they usually do not cause the disease; or if they do, the case is usually much milder than the natural disease (CDC, 1995a). Live attenuated vaccines must be handled and stored carefully, as they may be destroyed by heat and light. Examples of live attenuated vaccines include those for measles, mumps, rubella, polio, varicella, and tuberculosis (bacille Calmette-Guérin vaccine [BCG]).

Inactivated vaccines are produced by growing the organism in a culture media, then inactivating it with heat or chemicals. The organisms in inactivated vaccines do not replicate, and the vaccine's effectiveness depends on the body's immune system to develop protection following a second or third dose. Influenza, pertussis, hepatitis B, tetanus, and *Haemophilus influenzae* b (HIB) are examples of diseases that a person can be inoculated against with inactivated vaccines (CDC, 1995a). Table 15–7 lists current licensed vaccines available in the United States.

IMMUNIZATION SCHEDULE

The recommended immunization schedule for routine pediatric vaccinations has undergone several major changes over the last decade. Changes include (1) the addition of vaccination for HIB in the early 1980s; (2) the addition of an MMR booster in 1990; (3) the inclusion of vaccination against hepatitis B in 1992; and, most recently (4) proposed recommendations for the additions of vaccination against varicella and hepatitis B vaccination for adolescents. Other changes have occurred following approval of new vaccines, such as that for acellular diphtheria, pertussis, and tetanus (DPT) and a combined DPT and HIB vaccine. The current recommended schedule for pediatric immunization is presented in Table 15–8.

IMMUNIZATION STANDARDS

The Standards for Pediatric Immunization Practices were published in 1993 "to eliminate barriers and obstacles . . . that impede efficient vaccine delivery and to encourage providers to take advantage of all health-care visits as opportunities to provide vaccination" (CDC, 1993a, p 1). These standards, along with numerous programs at each local, state and federal levels of the public health system, have been quite successful in improving the rates of complete immunization for U.S. children (CDC, 1994e). The standards are outlined in Table 15–9.

CONTRAINDICATIONS AND PRECAUTIONS

Standards 6 and 7 of the Standards for Pediatric Immunizations relate to contraindications and precautions to vaccine administration. Guidelines for "true contraindications" and precautions were included with the development of the standards published by the CDC. These are given in Table 15–10. It is imperative that all nurses working in ambulatory settings who routinely administer immunizations know these contraindications and the rationales.

PARENT EDUCATION AND CONSENT

Standards 5 and 6 of the standards for pediatric immunization practices refer to parental education and providing information on the risks of vaccination. In October, 1994, the CDC instituted a re-

TABLE 15–7 **Licensed Vaccines and Toxoids Available in the United States**

Vaccine	Type	Route
Adenovirus*	Live virus	Oral
Anthrax†	Inactivated bacteria	Subcutaneous
Bacillus of Calmette and Guérin (BCG)	Live bacteria	Intradermal/percutaneous
Cholera	Inactivated bacteria	Subcutaneous or intradermal‡
Diphtheria/tetanus/pertussis (DTP)	Toxoids and inactivated whole bacteria	Intramuscular
DTP-*Haemophilus influenzae* type b conjugate (DTP–HIB)	Toxoids, inactivated whole bacteria, and bacterial polysaccharide conjugated to protein	Intramuscular
Diphtheria/tetanus/acellular pertussis (DTaP)	Toxoids and inactivated bacterial components	Intramuscular
Hepatitis B	Inactive viral antigen	Intramuscular
Haemophilus influenzae type b conjugate (HIB)§	Bacterial polysaccharide conjugated to protein	Intramuscular
Influenza	Inactivated virus or viral components	Intramuscular
Japanese encephalitis	Inactivated virus	Subcutaneous
Measles	Live virus	Subcutaneous
Measles/mumps/rubella (MMR)	Live virus	Subcutaneous
Meningococcal	Bacterial polysaccharides of serotypes A/C/Y/W-135	Subcutaneous
Mumps	Live virus	Subcutaneous
Pertussis†	Inactivated whole bacteria	Intramuscular
Plague	Inactivated bacteria	Intramuscular
Pneumococcal	Bacterial polysaccharides of 23 pneumococcal types	Intramuscular or subcutaneous
Poliovirus vaccine, inactivated (IPV)	Inactivated viruses of all three serotypes	Subcutaneous
Poliovirus vaccine, oral (OPV)	Live viruses of all three serotypes	Oral
Rabies	Inactivated virus	Intramuscular or intradermal‖
Rubella	Live virus	Subcutaneous
Tetanus	Inactivated toxin (toxoid)	Intramuscular¶
Tetanus/diphtheria (Td or DT)**	Inactivated toxins (toxoids)	Intramuscular¶
Typhoid (parenteral)	Inactivated bacteria	Subcutaneous††
(Ty21a oral)	Live bacteria	Oral
Varicella	Live virus	Subcutaneous
Yellow fever	Live virus	Subcutaneous

From Centers for Disease Control and Prevention. (1994). General recommendations on immunization. *Morbidity and Mortality Weekly Report, 43* (RR-1).

*Available only to the U.S. Armed Forces.

†Distributed by the Division of Biologic Products, Michigan Department of Public Health.

‡The intradermal dose is lower than the subcutaneous dose.

§The recommended schedule for infants depends on the vaccine manufacturer; consult the package insert and ACIP recommendations for specific products.

‖The intradermal dose of rabies vaccine, human diploid cell (HDCV), is lower than the intramuscular dose and is used only for preexposure vaccination. *Rabies vaccine, adsorbed (RVA) should not be used intradermally.*

¶Preparations with adjuvants should be administered intramuscularly.

**Td = tetanus and diphtheria toxoids for use among persons ≥7 years of age. Td contains the same amount of tetanus toxoid as DTP or DT, but contains a smaller dose of diphtheria toxoid. DT = tetanus and diphtheria toxoids for use among children <7 years of age.

††Booster doses may be administered intradermally unless vaccine that is acetone-killed and dried is used.

TABLE 15–8 Recommended Childhood Immunization Schedule, United States: 1996

	Age										
Vaccine*	Birth	1 Month	2 Months	4 Months	6 Months	12 Months	15 Months	18 Months	4–6 Years	11–12 Years	14–16 Years
Hepatitis B (Hep B-1)†‡	Hep B-1										
		Hep B-2			Hep B-3					Hep B‡	
Diphtheria, tetanus, pertussis (DTP) §			DTP	DTP	DTP	DTP§ (DTaP at 15+m)			DTP or DTaP	Td	
H. influenzae type b (Hib)‖			Hib	Hib	Hib	Hib‖					
Polio (OPV)¶			OPV¶	OPV	OPV				OPV		
Measles, mumps, rubella (MMR) **						MMR			MMR** or MMR**		
Varicella zoster virus vaccine (Var) ††						Var				Var††	

From Centers for Disease Control and Prevention. (1996). *Epidemiology & Prevention of Vaccine-Preventable Diseases.* Atlanta, GA, Centers for Disease Control and Prevention.

Approved by the Advisory Committee on Immunization Practices (ACIP), the American Academy of Pediatrics (AAP), and the American Academy of Family Physicians (AAFP).

*Vaccines are listed under the routinely recommended ages. *Solid lines* indicate range of acceptable ages for vaccination. *Broken lines* indicate catch-up vaccination: at 11–12 years of age, hepatitis B vaccine should be administered to children not previously vaccinated, and varicella zoster virus vaccine should be administered to children not previously vaccinated who lack a reliable history of chickenpox.

†*Infants born to HBsAg-negative mothers* should receive 2.5 μg of Merck vaccine (Recombivax HB) or 10 μg of SmithKline Beecham (SB) vaccine (Engerix-B). The 2nd dose should be administered ≥1 month after the 1st dose.

Infants born to HBsAg-positive mothers should receive 0.5 mL Hepatitis B Immune Globulin (HBIG) within 12 hours of birth, and either 5 μg of Merck vaccine (Recombivax HB) or 10 μg of SB vaccine (Engerix-B) at a separate site. The 2nd dose is recommended at 1–2 months of age and the 3rd dose at 6 months of age.

Infants born to mothers whose HBsAg status is unknown should receive either 5 μg of Merck vaccine (Recombivax HB) or 10 μg of SB vaccine (Engerix-B) within 12 hours of birth. The 2nd dose of vaccine is recommended at 1 month of age and the 3rd dose at 6 months of age.

‡Adolescents who have not previously received 3 doses of hepatitis B vaccine should initiate or complete the series at the 11–12 year-old visit. The 2nd dose should be administered at least 1 month after the 1st dose, and the 3rd dose should be administered at least 4 months after the 1st dose and at least 2 months after the 2nd dose.

§DTP4 may be administered at 12 months of age, if at least 6 months have elapsed since DTP3. DTaP (diphtheria and tetanus toxoids and acellular pertussis vaccine) is licensed for the 4th and/or 5th vaccine dose(s) for children aged ≥15 months and may be preferred for these doses in this age group. Td (tetanus and diphtheria toxoids, adsorbed, for adult use) is recommended at 11–12 years of age if at least 5 years have elapsed since the last dose of DTP, DTaP, or DT.

‖Three *H. influenzae* type b (Hib) conjugate vaccines are licensed for infant use. If PRP-OMP (PedvaxHIB [Merck]) is administered at 2 and 4 months of age, a dose at 6 months is not required. After completing the primary series, any Hib conjugate vaccine may be used as a booster.

¶Oral poliovirus vaccine (OPV) is recommended for routine infant vaccination. Inactivated poliovirus vaccine (IPV) is recommended for persons with a congenital or acquired immune deficiency disease or an altered immune status as a result of disease or immunosuppressive therapy, as well as their household contacts, and is an acceptable alternative for other persons. The primary 3-dose series for IPV should be given with a minimum interval of 4 weeks between the 1st and 2nd doses and 6 months between the 2nd and 3rd doses.

**The 2nd dose of MMR is routinely recommended at 4–6 years of age or at 11–12 years of age, but may be administered at any visit, provided at least 1 month has elapsed since receipt of the 1st dose.

††Varicella zoster virus vaccine (Var) can be administered to susceptible children any time after 12 months of age. Unvaccinated children who lack a reliable history of chickenpox should be vaccinated at the 11–12 year-old visit.

Immunization Protects Children

Regular checkups at your pediatrician's office or local health clinic are an important way to keep children healthy.

By making sure that your child gets immunized on time, you can provide the best available defense against many dangerous childhood diseases. Immunizations protect children against: hepatitis B, polio, measles, mumps, rubella (German measles), pertussis (whooping cough), diphtheria, tetanus (lockjaw), *Haemophilus influenzae* type b, and chickenpox. All of these immunizations need to be given before children are 2 years old in order for them to be protected during their most vulnerable period. Are your child's immunizations up-to-date?

This chart includes immunization recommendations from the American Academy of Pediatrics. Remember to keep track of your child's immunizations—it's the only way you can be sure your child is up-to-date. Also, check with your pediatrician or health clinic at each visit to find out if your child needs any booster shots or if any new vaccines have been recommended since this schedule was prepared.

If you don't have a pediatrician, call your local health department. Public health clinics usually have supplies of vaccine and may give shots free.

TABLE 15–9 **Standards for Pediatric Immunization Practices**

1. Immunization services are readily available.
2. There are no barriers or unnecessary prerequisites to the receipt of vaccines.
3. Immunization services are available free or for a minimal fee.
4. Providers utilize all clinical encounters to screen and, when indicated, vaccinate children.
5. Providers educate parents and guardians about immunization in general terms.
6. Providers question parents or guardians about contraindications and, before vaccinating a child, inform them in specific terms about the risks and benefits of the vaccinations their child is to receive.
7. Providers follow only true contraindications.
8. Providers administer simultaneously all vaccine doses for which a child is eligible at the time of each visit.
9. Providers use accurate and complete recording procedures.
10. Providers coschedule immunization appointments in conjunction with appointments for other child health services.
11. Providers report adverse events following vaccination promptly, accurately, and completely.
12. Providers operate a tracking system.
13. Providers adhere to appropriate procedures for vaccine management.
14. Providers conduct semi-annual audits to assess immunization coverage levels and to review immunization records in the patient populations they serve.
15. Providers maintain up-to-date, easily retrievable medical protocols at all locations where vaccines are administered.
16. Providers practice patient-oriented and community-based approaches.
17. Vaccines are administered by properly trained persons.
18. Providers receive ongoing education and training regarding current immunization recommendations.

From Centers for Disease Control and Prevention. (1993). *Standards for pediatric immunization practices. Morbidity and Mortality Weekly Report, 42*(RR-5), 3.

quirement that all health care providers administering any vaccine for diphtheria, tetanus, pertussis, measles, mumps, rubella, or polio provide parents with "Vaccine Information Statements" (VIS). The VIS were written to simplify explanations on the benefits and risks associated with MMR, polio, DPT and tetanus/diphtheria vaccines. Since that time, all providers are required to provide a copy of the relevant VIS each time a patient is vaccinated (CDC, 1995a). The VISs have been translated into Chinese, French, Spanish and Vietnamese and can be obtained from the CDC and the state health departments. Figure 15–3 presents the VIS for polio vaccine.

REPORTING ADVERSE VACCINE EVENTS

Standards 11 and 12 of the Pediatric Immunization Practices Standards relate to tracking and reporting "adverse events" following immunization. The Vaccine Adverse Event Reporting System (VAERS) was developed to comply with the National Childhood Vaccine Injury Act of 1986 to "provide a single system for the collection and analysis of reports on all adverse events associated with the administration of any U.S. licensed vaccine in all groups" (Chen et al., 1994, p. 542). Examples of reportable "adverse events" appear in Table 15–11. The VAERS is operated by the CDC and Food and Drug Administration, and additional information can be obtained by calling the 24-hour toll-free telephone number (1-800-822-7967).

ADULT IMMUNIZATION

In general, people are aware of pediatric immunizations, but most adults, and many health care providers, are unaware of recommended immunizations for adults. For example, the CDC reports

Text continued on page 481

TABLE 15–10 Guide to Contraindications and Precautions to Vaccinations*

True Contraindications and Precautions	Not Contraindications (vaccines may be administered)
General for all vaccines (DTP/DTaP, OPV, IPV, MMR, HIB, Hepatitis B)	
Contraindications Anaphylactic reaction to a vaccine contraindicates further doses of that vaccine Anaphylactic reaction to a vaccine constituent contraindicates the use of vaccines containing that substance Moderate or severe illnesses with or without a fever	**Not contraindications** Mild to moderate local reaction (soreness, redness, swelling) following a dose of an injectable antigen Mild acute illness with or without low-grade fever Current antimicrobial therapy Convalescent phase of illnesses Prematurity (same dosage and indications as for normal, full-term infants) Recent exposure to an infectious disease History of penicillin or other nonspecific allergies or family history of such allergies
DTP/DTaP	
Contraindications Encephalopathy within 7 days of administration of previous dose of DTP **Precautions†** Fever of ≥105°F within 48 hours after vaccination with a prior dose of DTP Collapse or shocklike state (hypotonic-hyporesponsive episode) within 48 hours of receiving a prior dose of DTP Seizures within 3 days of receiving a prior dose of DTP‡ Persistent, inconsolable crying lasting ≥3 hours within 48 hours of receiving a prior dose of DTP	**Not contraindications** Temperature of <105°F following a previous dose of DTP Family history of convulsions‡ Family history of sudden infant death syndrome Family history of an adverse event following DTP administration
OPV§	
Contraindications Infection with HIV or a household contact with HIV Known altered immunodeficiency (hematologic and solid tumors; congenital immunodeficiency; and long-term immunosuppressive therapy) Immunodeficient household contact **Precaution†** Pregnancy	**Not contraindications** Breast-feeding Current antimicrobial therapy Diarrhea
IPV	
Contraindication Anaphylactic reaction to neomycin or streptomycin **Precaution†** Pregnancy	

TABLE 15–10 **Guide to Contraindications and Precautions to Vaccinations*** *Continued*

True Contraindications and Precautions	Not Contraindications (vaccines may be administered)
MMR¶	
Contraindications	**Not contraindications**
Anaphylactic reactions to egg ingestion and to neomycin‖	Tuberculosis or positive PPD skin test
Pregnancy	Simultaneous TB skin testing¶
Known altered immunodeficiency (hematologic and solid tumors; congenital immunodeficiency; and long-term immunosuppressive therapy)	Breast-feeding
Precaution†	Pregnancy of mother of recipient
Recent immune globulin administration	Immunodeficient family member or household contact
	Infection with HIV
	Nonanaphylactic reactions to eggs or neomycin
HIB	
Contraindication	**Not a contraindication**
None identified	History of HIB disease
Hepatitis B	
Contraindication	**Not a contraindication**
Anaphylactic reaction to common baker's yeast	Pregnancy

*This information is based on the recommendations of the Advisory Committee on Immunization Practices (ACIP) and those of the Committee on Infectious Diseases (Red Book Committee) of the American Academy of Pediatrics (AAP). Sometimes these recommendations vary from those contained in the manufacturer's package inserts. For more detailed information, providers should consult the published recommendations of the ACIP, AAP, and the manufacturer's package inserts.

†The events or conditions listed as precautions, although not contraindications, should be carefully reviewed. The benefits and risks of administering a specific vaccine to an individual under the circumstances should be considered. If the risks are believed to outweigh the benefits, the vaccination should be withheld; if the benefits are believed to outweigh the risks (for example, during an outbreak or foreign travel), the vaccination should be administered. Whether and when to administer DTP to children with proven or suspected underlying neurological disorders should be decided on an individual basis. It is prudent on theoretical grounds to avoid vaccinating pregnant women. However, if immediate protection against poliomyelitis is needed, OPV is preferred, although IPV may be considered if full vaccination can be completed before the anticipated imminent exposure.

‡Acetaminophen given before administering DTP and thereafter every 4 hours for 24 hours should be considered for children with a personal or family history of convulsions in siblings or parents.

§No data exist to substantiate the theoretical risk of a suboptimal immune response from the administration of OPV and MMR within 30 days of each other.

‖Persons with a history of anaphylactic reactions following egg ingestion should be vaccinated only with caution. Protocols have been developed for vaccinating such persons and should be consulted. (J Pediatr 1983;102:196–9, J Pediatr 1988;113:504–5.)

¶Measles vaccination may temporarily suppress tuberculin reactivity. If testing can not be done the day of MMR vaccination, the test should be postponed for 4–6 weeks.

DTaP = diphtheria/tetanus/acellular pertussis; DTP = diphtheria/tetanus/pertussis; IPV = poliovirus vaccine, inactivated; OPV = poliovirus vaccine, oral.

From Centers for Disease Control and Prevention. (1994). General recommendations on immunization. *Morbidity and Mortality Weekly Report, 43*(RR-1), 24–25.

POLIO VACCINE

What you need to know before you or your child gets the vaccine

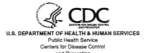

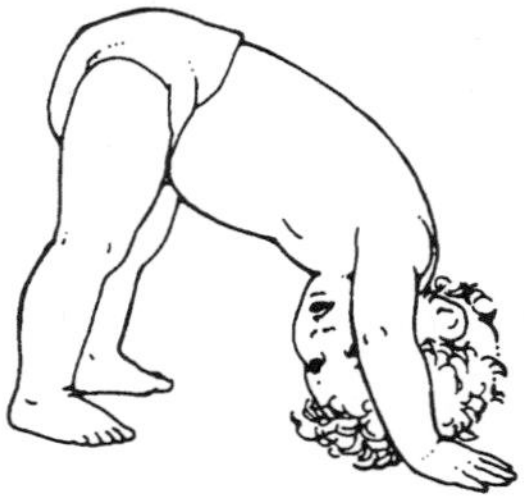

U.S. DEPARTMENT OF HEALTH & HUMAN SERVICES
Public Health Service
Centers for Disease Control and Prevention

ABOUT THE DISEASE

Polio is a serious disease. It spreads when germs pass from an infected person to the mouths of others. Polio can:

- paralyze a person (make arms and legs unable to move)
- cause death

ABOUT THE VACCINES

Benefits of the vaccines

Vaccination is the best way to protect against polio. Because most children get the polio vaccines, there are now very few cases of this disease. Before most children were vaccinated, there were thousands of cases of polio.

There are 2 kinds of polio vaccine

OPV or Oral Polio Vaccine is the one most often given to children. It is given by mouth as drops. It is easy to give and works well to stop the spread of polio.

IPV or Inactivated Polio Vaccine is given as a shot in the leg or arm.

OPV schedule

Most children should have a total of 4 OPV vaccines. They should have OPV at:

✔ 2 months of age
✔ 4 months of age
✔ 6–18 months of age
✔ 4–6 years of age

Other vaccines may be given at the same time as OPV.

Who should get OPV?

Most doctors recommend that almost all young children get OPV. But there are some cautions. Tell your doctor or nurse if the person getting the vaccine *or anyone else in close contact with the person getting the vaccine* is less able to fight serious infections because of:

- a disease she/he was born with
- treatment with drugs such as long-term steroids
- any kind of cancer
- cancer treatment with x-rays or drugs
- AIDS or HIV infection

If so, your doctor or nurse will probably give IPV instead of OPV.

If you are older than age 18 years, you usually do not need polio vaccine.

Travel
If you are traveling to a country where there is polio, you should get either OPV or IPV.

Pregnancy
If protection is needed during pregnancy, OPV or IPV can be used.

Allergy to neomycin or streptomycin
Does the person getting the vaccine have an allergy to the drugs neomycin or streptomycin? If so, she/he should get OPV, but not IPV. Ask your doctor or nurse if you are not sure.

FIGURE 15–3 Vaccination information sheet: polio vaccine. (From Centers for Disease Control and Prevention).

Tell your doctor or nurse if the person getting the vaccine:

- ever had a serious allergic reaction or other problem after getting polio vaccine
- now has moderate or severe illness

If you are not sure, ask your doctor or nurse.

What are the risks from polio vaccine?

As with any medicine, there are very small risks that serious problems, even death, could occur after getting a vaccine.

The risks from the vaccine are much smaller than the risks from the disease if people stopped using vaccine.

Almost all people who get polio vaccine have no problems from it.

Risks from OPV

Risks to the person taking OPV:
There is a very small chance of getting polio disease from the vaccine.

- about 1 case occurs for every $1\frac{1}{2}$ million first doses
- about 1 case occurs for every 30 million later doses

Risks to people who never took polio vaccine who have close contact with the person taking OPV:
After a person gets OPV, it can be found in his or her mouth and stool. If you never took polio vaccine, there is a very small chance of getting polio disease from close contact with a child who got OPV in the past 30 days. (Examples of close contact include changing diapers or kissing.)

- about 1 case occurs for every 2 million first doses
- about 1 case occurs for every 15 million later doses

Talk to your doctor or nurse about getting IPV.

Risks from IPV

This vaccine is not known to cause problems except mild soreness where the shot is given.

What to do if there is a serious reaction:

☞ Call a doctor or get the person to a doctor right away.

☞ Write down what happened and the date and time it happened.

☞ Ask your doctor, nurse, or health department to file a Vaccine Adverse Event Report form or call:
(800) 822-7967 (toll-free)

The **National Vaccine Injury Compensation Program** gives compensation (payment) to persons thought to be injured by vaccines. For details call:
(800) 338-2382 (toll-free)

If you want to learn more, ask your doctor or nurse. She/he can give you the vaccine package insert or suggest other sources of information.

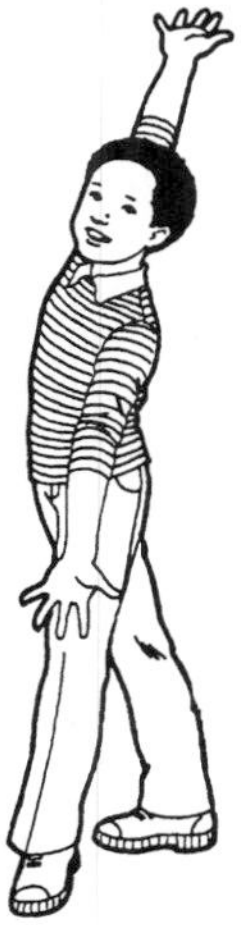

Polio 6/10/94
42 U.S.C. § 300aa-26

FIGURE 15–3 *Continued*

Figure continued on following page

Texas Department of Health
Addendum to Polio Vaccine Information Statement

Polio Vaccine

1. I agree that the person named below will get the vaccine checked below.
2. I got a copy of the Vaccine Information Statement for this vaccine.
3. I know the risks of the disease this vaccine prevents.
4. I know the benefits and risks of the vaccine.
5. I have had a chance to ask questions about the disease, the vaccine, and how the vaccine is given.
6. I know that the person named below will have a vaccine put in his or her body to prevent an infectious disease.
7. I agree that the record of giving this vaccine can be put in the Texas Department of Health immunization tracking system.
8. I agree that the record of giving this vaccine can be given to other health care providers, schools, or places that provide child care.
9. I am an adult who can legally consent for the person named below to get vaccines. I freely and voluntarily give my signed permission for this vaccine.

Vaccine to be given: ☐ OPV (Oral polio vaccine) ☐ IPV (Inactivated polio vaccine)

Information about person to receive vaccine (Please print)						
Name: Last	First	Middle Initial	Birthdate		Age	
Address: Street		City	County	State **TX**	ZIP	
Signature of person to receive vaccine or person authorized to make the request (parent or guardian): X_________ Date_____ _________ Date_____ Witness						

For Clinic/Office Use
Clinic Office Address
Date Vaccine Administered
Vaccine Manufacturer
Vaccine Lot Number
Site of Injection
Signature of Vaccine Administrator
Title of Vaccine Administrator

Texas Department of Health
C-90 (9/94)

CDC Revision (6/10/94)

FIGURE 15–3 *Continued*

TABLE 15–11 **Vaccine Injury Table**

Vaccine	Illness, Disability, Injury or Condition*	Time Period for First Symptom or Manifestation of Onset or of Significant Aggravation After Vaccine Administration
DTP; P; DT; Td; or tetanus toxoid; or in any combination with polio; or any other vaccine containing whole cell pertussis bacteria, or partial cell pertussis bacteria, or specific pertussis antigen(s)	Anaphylaxis or anaphylactic shock	24 hours
	Encephalopathy (or encephalitis)	3 days
	Shock-collapse or hypotonic or hyporesponsive collapse	3 days
	Residual seizure disorder†	3 days
Measles, mumps, rubella, or any vaccine containing any of the foregoing as a component	Anaphylaxis or anaphylactic shock	24 hours
	Encephalopathy (or encephalitis)	15 days (for mumps, rubella, measles, or any vaccine containing any of the foregoing as a component) 3 days (for DT, Td, or tetanus toxoid)
	Residual seizure disorder†	Same as for encephalopathy
Polio vaccines (other than inactivated polio vaccine)	Paralytic polio	
	In a nonimmunodeficient recipient	30 days
	In an immunodeficient recipient	6 months
	In a vaccine associated community case	Not applicable
Inactivated polio vaccine	Anaphylaxis or anaphylactic shock	24 hours

*Any acute complication or sequela (including death) of an illness, disability, injury, or condition that arose within the time period prescribed is also subject to the presumption of causation.

†Defined as follows: Patient did not suffer a seizure or convulsion unaccompanied by fever or accompanied by a fever of less than 102°F before the first seizure or convulsion after the administration of the vaccine involved and (1) in the case of measles, mumps, or rubella vaccine or any combination of such vaccines, the first seizure or convulsion occurred within 15 days after administration of the vaccine and two or more seizures or convulsions occurred within 1 year after the administration of the vaccine, which were unaccompanied by fever or accompanied by a fever of less than 102°F; and (2) in the case of any other vaccine, the first seizure or convulsion occurred within 3 days after the administration of the vaccine and two or more seizures or convulsions occurred within 1 year after the administration of the vaccine, which were unaccompanied by a fever or accompanied by a fever of less than 102°F.

From Centers for Disease Control and Prevention. (1995). *Epidemiology & Prevention of Vaccine-Preventable Diseases.* Atlanta, GA, Centers for Disease Control and Prevention.

that fewer than 28% of persons in high-risk categories have received pneumococcal polysaccharide vaccine (CDC, 1995b). Appropriately vaccinating adults should be a priority for all health care providers. The recommended vaccination schedule for adults is listed in Table 15–12. Additionally, Table 15–13 lists recommended *immunobiologicals* (vaccine, toxoid, or immune globulin) for selected individuals determined to be "at risk."

Sexually Transmitted Diseases

The number and incidence of STDs has increased dramatically over the last several decades, with almost 12 million cases occurring each year in the United States. It is of particular concern that 86% of STDs occur in people aged 15 to 29 years

TABLE 15–12 **Vaccines and Toxoids Recommended for Adults, by Age Group (United States)**

Age Group (Years)	Vaccine/Toxoid					
	*Td**	*Measles*	*Mumps*	*Rubella*	*Influenza*	*Pneumococcal Polysaccharide*
18–24	X	X	X	X		
25–64	X	X†	X†	X		
≥65	X				X	X

*Td = Tetanus and diphtheria toxoids, adsorbed (for adult use), which is a combined preparation containing <2 flocculation units of diphtheria toxoid.

†Indicated for persons born after 1956.

From Centers for Disease Control and Prevention. (1991). Update on adult immunization. *Morbidity and Mortality Weekly Report, 40*(RR-12), 56.

(USDHHS, 1994). People considered at risk for STDs and HIV infection include:

- those who are contacts of, or have a previous history of, documented STD/HIV infection
- pregnant women
- individuals who are or were recently sexually active (especially those with multiple sexual partners)
- individuals living in areas with high prevalence of HIV/STDs
- homosexual and bisexual men
- drug and alcohol abusers
- those involved in the exchange of sex for drugs or money (USDHHS, 1994)

Until as recently as the early 1980s, the only STDs (called venereal diseases at the time) commonly recognized by the public were syphilis and gonorrhea. By the 1990s, there were more than a dozen STDs. Table 15–14 lists some of the most common STDs in the United States, their incubation periods, symptoms, possible complications, and treatment information. The next sections describe primary and secondary prevention of STDs. Chapter 16 presents more detailed information on the epidemiology, prevention, and management of HIV infection and AIDS.

PRIMARY PREVENTION OF STDs

"Primary prevention of STDs is based on changing the sexual behaviors that place patients at risk" (CDC, 1993b, p. 3). Education and counseling on abstinence, high-risk behaviors, and "safer sex" strategies (e.g., the use of condoms and other barriers and spermicides) is essential in primary prevention of STDs. It is the responsibility of the health care provider to counsel and educate those at risk to change their behaviors. Generic techniques to enhance compliance through education and counseling are presented in Table 15–15. When counseling clients at risk for STDs, it is also important to use language and terminology that the patient understands and to reassure the patient that treatment will be provided regardless of ability to pay, citizenship or immigration status, language spoken, or lifestyle (CDC, 1993b).

Sexual intimacy in a mutually monogamous relationship between partners known to be disease free and sexual abstinence are the only certain ways to prevent infection. To *reduce* the possibility of exposure, "safer sex" counseling should include *correct* use of *latex* condoms (Table 15–16 includes instructions for condom use) for *each* sexual encounter; avoidance of sex with high-risk partners; avoiding anal intercourse and avoiding the use of substances that impair judgment (e.g., alcohol, cocaine, marijuana).

TABLE 15–13 **Immunobiologicals Recommended for Special Occupations, Lifestyles, Environmental Circumstances, Travel, Foreign Students, Immigrants, and Refugees (United States)**

Indication	Immunobiologic
Occupation	
Hospital, laboratory, and other health-care personnel	Hepatitis B Influenza Measles Rubella Mumps Polio
Public-safety personnel	Hepatitis B Influenza
Staff of institutions for the developmentally disabled	Hepatitis B
Veterinarians and animal handlers	Rabies Plague
Selected field workers (those who come into contact with possibly infected animals)	Plague Rabies
Selected occupations (those who work with imported animal hides, furs, wool, animal hair, and bristles)	Anthrax
Lifestyles	
Homosexual males	Hepatitis B
Intravenous drug users	Hepatitis B
Heterosexual persons with multiple sexual partners or recently acquired sexually transmitted disease	Hepatitis B
Environmental Situation	
Inmates of long-term correctional facilities	Hepatitis B
Residents of institutions for the developmentally disabled	Hepatitis B
Household contacts of HBV carriers	Hepatitis B
Homeless persons	Tetanus/diphtheria Measles Mumps Rubella Influenza Pneumococcal polysaccharide
Travel*	Measles Mumps Rubella Polio Influenza Hepatitis B Rabies Meningococcal polysaccharide Tetanus/diphtheria† Yellow fever Typhoid Cholera Plague‡ Immune globulin§
Foreign students, immigrants, and refugees	Measles Rubella Diphtheria Tetanus Mumps Hepatitis B

*Vaccines needed for travelers vary depending on individual itineraries; travelers should refer to *Health Information for International Travelers* for more detailed information.

†If not received within last 10 years.

‡In or during travel to areas with enzootic or epidemic plague in which exposure to rodents cannot be prevented.

§For hepatitis A prophylaxis.

From Centers for Disease Control. (1991). Update on adult immunization. *Morbidity and Mortality Weekly Report, 44*(RR-12), 57–58.

TABLE 15–14 Sexually Transmitted Diseases

Disease	Incubation Period	Symptoms	Treatment	Possible Complications
Chlamydia	7–14 days +	Often there are no symptoms; females have slight vaginal discharge, itching and burning of the vagina; males may have a penile discharge, burning during urination, and burning and itching at the urethral opening	Antibiotics—not penicillin	Women—pelvic inflammatory disease (PID), ectopic pregnancy, and infertility Men—prostatitis, epididymitis
Gonorrhea	2–7 days (can be longer)	Males usually have burning on urination and purulent discharge from the urethra (5–20% have no symptoms); females may have a genital discharge but most have no symptoms.	Antibiotics. Some strains have become resistant to penicillin in recent years.	Women—PID, infertility Men—narrowing of urethra, sterility Newborns—eye, nose, lung, and/or rectal infections
Herpes simplex	2–12 days	Painful blisters or sores on the genitals, rectum, or mouth that break, crust over, and heal in 2–4 weeks. The sores may reappear throughout life.	No cure at this time. Medication (acyclovir) may be given to shorten the outbreak; medications may be given to prevent bacterial infection in the open sores and to control pain	Women—possible increased risk of cervical cancer Newborns—blindness, brain damage, and/or death to baby passing through birth canal of mother with active lesions; cesarean section is indicated if mother has active lesions at the time of delivery.
HIV	Unknown, 1–3 months to 10 years	No symptoms for years; eventually, fever, weight loss, fatigue, swollen glands, and diarrhea; opportunistic infections and conditions follow.	No medical cure. AZT and other medications are being used with success.	Multiple opportunistic infections; death
Human papilloma-virus	1–20 months (average is 4 months)	Sometimes there are no symptoms. Typically, there are pink or dirty gray warts appearing on the moist areas of the genitals and anus.	Removal of the warts through freezing, laser therapy, surgical removal or application of a topical medication	Blockage of vaginal, rectal, or throat openings; cervical dysplasia; cervical cancer (possibly)

Syphilis	10 days to 3 months	Primary stage: painless chancre (sore) at site of entry; swollen glands. Secondary stage: 1 week to 6 months after chancre—may include rash, patchy hair loss, sore throat, and swollen glands.	Antibiotics	If untreated—blindness, deafness, brain damage, heart disease, death Newborns—damage to skin, eyes, teeth, and/or liver
Chancroid	3–5 days to 14 days	Single or multiple painful, necrotizing ulcers at the site of infection; swelling and pain in the regional lymph nodes. May be asymptomatic in women.	Antibiotics	Increases risk of HIV transmission; fluctuant lymphadenopathy
Hepatitis B	45–180 days; average: 60–90 days	Variable. Fatigue, weakness, anorexia, abdominal pain, muscle or joint pain, nausea and vomiting, jaundice, and dark urine.	No cure. Treatment is palliative.	Chronic hepatitis; cirrhosis; liver cancer
Tricho-moniasis	4–20 days; average: 7 days	Many women and most men have no symptoms. Women may have a white or greenish-yellow odorous discharge, vaginal itching and soreness and/or painful urination. Males may have a slight itching of the penis, painful urination and/or clear penile discharge	Oral medication (Flagyl)	None identified
Scabies	2–6 weeks in initial infection; 1–4 days after re-exposure	Small, raised, red bumps or blisters on the skin with severe itching. Generally affects webs of the fingers, elbows, underarms, external genitalia.	Over-the-counter (OTC) prescription medications. Laundering all bedding, clothing, and towels in hot water.	Secondary bacterial infection
Pediculosis pubis	3–14 days	Intense itching, blue or gray spots and insects or nits in the pubic area	OTC (NIX, RID) or prescription (lindane, Kwell) medications	None identified

Adapted from Texas Department of Health. (1992). *Educator's Guide to Sexually Transmitted Diseases* (3rd ed.). Austin, TX, Texas Department of Health; Benenson, A. S. (1990). *Control of Communicable Diseases in Man.* Washington, D. C., American Public Health Association.

TABLE 15–15 **U. S. Preventive Services Task Force's Principles of Patient Education and Counseling**

1. Develop a therapeutic alliance.
2. Counsel all patients.
3. Ensure that patients understand the relationship between behavior and health.
4. Work with patients to assess barriers to behavior change.
5. Gain commitment from patients to change.
6. Involve patients in selecting risk factors to change.
7. Use a combination of strategies.
8. Design a behavior modification plan.
9. Monitor progress through follow-up contact.
10. Involve office staff.

From U. S. Department of Health and Human Services. (1994). *Clinician's Handbook of Preventive Services.* Washington, D. C., Government Printing Office.

SECONDARY PREVENTION AND STDs

Early diagnosis and prompt, appropriate treatment are essential in stopping the spread of STDs. Treatment must include instruction on medication compliance and referral for treatment of all sex partners. In most cases, partners of patients with STDs should be examined. Resources for referral should be identified in advance, and information should be made available where STDs are most likely to be detected (e.g., drug treatment and HIV treatment centers). Table 15–24, at the conclusion of this chapter, includes sources for referral and information for STDs.

Trends in Incidence and Prevention of Selected Communicable Diseases

Nurses who work in community-based settings should continually watch for changes in rates of communicable diseases. It is particularly important to monitor trends in area populations and communities. Several diseases are discussed here because of their importance to nurses in community-based practice.

TUBERCULOSIS

After decades of decreasing incidence of tuberculosis (TB) in the United States, the number of reported cases has increased slowly but steadily since 1985. The rise in cases is attributed, in part, to opportunistic infections in those who are HIV-positive. Additionally, many new cases are identified in immigrants and those in other high-risk groups. There is cause for concern over this trend, in particular because of the emergence of multiple-drug resistant strains (USDHHS, 1994; CDC, 1990).

Persons at risk for tuberculosis include the medically underserved, particularly those of African-American, Hispanic, Asian, Native American, and Alaskan Native heritage; foreign-born individuals from high-prevalence areas (Asia, Africa, and Latin America); those in close contact with infectious TB cases; individuals with medical conditions known to increase the risk of TB (e.g., HIV, diabetes, chronic renal failure, conditions requiring prolonged corticosteroid therapy); alcoholics and intravenous drug users; and residents of high-risk environments (long-term-care facilities, correctional institutions, and mental institutions) (USDHHS, 1994). Guidelines for TB screening are as follows:

- Screening for TB should be performed on children and adults in high-risk groups.
- The Mantoux text (intradermal injection of 0.1 mL of purified protein derivative in the long axis of the forearm) should be performed whenever possible.
- The Mantoux test should be read 48 to 72 hours after placement by palpating the margin of induration and measuring and recording the diameter. Treatment is indicated if induration is greater than 5 mm to greater than 15 mm depending on exposure, age, risk factors, and presence of symptoms (see Table 15–17).
- It should be recognized that absence of a reaction does not exclude a diagnosis of TB infection, particularly when the individual has

Table 15–16 **Guidelines for Condom Use**

1. Use only *latex* (rubber) condoms.
2. Use only condoms that are not in damaged packages and are not brittle, sticky, discolored, or past expiration date.
3. Use only reservoir-tip condoms or leave 1/2 inch space at the tip of the condom to collect semen.
4. Use only water-based lubricants. Lubricants made with petroleum jelly, mineral oil, cold cream, or vegetable oils may damage the condom.
5. Spermicides, containing nonoxinol 9, inside the condom or inside the vagina may increase protection against STDs and HIV. However, if spermicides cause local irritation, they may increase the risk of HIV transmission. Spermicides do not give added protection in anal intercourse.
6. Put the condom on an erect penis and unroll slowly and completely to the base *before* the penis comes in contact with a body opening.
7. If a condom breaks, it should be replaced immediately.
8. After ejaculation, withdraw the penis while it is still erect. Hold the condom carefully against the base of the penis so that it remains in place.
9. Dispose of condoms properly. *Never* reuse condoms.
10. Remember that other contraceptives (birth control pills, depo-provera, and IUDs) cannot protect against STDs and HIV.
11. Condom failure rates are 10–15%, either as a result of product failure (breakage) or incorrect or inconsistent use.

Adapted from U. S. Department of Health and Human Services. (1994). *Clinician's Handbook of Preventive Services.* Washington, D. C., Government Printing Office; American College Health Association. (1990). *Safer Sex* [brochure]. Baltimore, MD, American College Health Association.

symptoms of active disease. Induration of less than 5 mm may occur early in the course of TB infection or in individuals with altered immune function (e.g., AIDS).

- BCG vaccination may cause false-positive Mantoux reactions, but this decreases with time and rarely causes an induration of 15 mm or greater.
- Live vaccines such as MMR and oral polio vaccine may interfere with response to the Mantoux test. TB testing may be administered either concurrently with these vaccines or 4 to 6 weeks afterwards.

Table 15–17 summarizes interpretation of Mantoux tests. Additional testing after positive Mantoux results consists of chest radiograph and sputum smear and culture, to determine if there is active disease. If the results of these tests are negative, the client is usually placed on a preventive medication regimen, typically oral isoniazid (INH) 300 mg daily for 6 to 12 months (CDC, 1994d).

For patients with active TB, as evidenced by radiographs and sputum cultures, therapy consists of administration of multiple drugs over a period of several months, depending on symptoms, exposure, pre-existing conditions, and sputum cultures. Table 15–18 depicts recommended options for treatment of active TB.

HEPATITIS B

The reported incidence of hepatitis B (HBV) decreased 59% from 1985 through 1993. This decline is largely attributed to decreases in the number of cases among homosexual men and IV drug users. These decreases are thought to result from an increase in AIDS awareness, and subsequent behavioral changes (e.g., safer sex and needle-using practices) (CDC, 1994a).

The availability of the hepatitis B vaccine and recommended use for "at risk" populations has also assisted in the decreased incidence. Identification of these individuals, and recommendation of immunization, is an important intervention for nurses who work in ambulatory settings. Those

TABLE 15–17 **Summary of Interpretation of Purified Protein Derivative (PPD)-Tuberculin Skin-Test Results**

1. An induration of $\geq$5 mm is classified as positive in:
   - persons who have HIV infection or risk factors for HIV infection but unknown HIV status
   - persons who have had recent close contact* with persons who have active TB
   - persons who have fibrotic chest radiographs (consistent with healed TB).
2. An induration of $\geq$10 mm is classified as positive in all persons who do not meet any of the criteria above but who have other risk factors for TB, including:

   High-risk groups:
   - intravenous drug users known to be HIV seronegative
   - persons who have other medical conditions that reportedly increase the risk for progressing from latent TB infection to active TB (e.g., silicosis; gastrectomy or jejuno-ileal bypass; being $\geq$10% below ideal body weight; chronic renal failure with renal dialysis; diabetes mellitus; high-dose corticosteroid or other immunosuppressive therapy; some hematological disorders, including malignancies such as leukemias and lymphomas; and other malignancies)
   - children <4 years of age.

   High-prevalence groups:
   - persons born in countries in Asia, Africa, the Caribbean, and Latin America that have high prevalence of TB
   - persons from medically underserved, low-income populations
   - residents of long-term-care facilities (e.g., correctional institutions and nursing homes)
   - persons from high-risk populations in their communities, as determined by local public health authorities.
3. An induration of $\geq$15 mm is classified as positive in persons who do not meet any of the above criteria.
4. Recent converters are defined on the basis of both size of induration and age of the person being tested:
   - $\geq$10 mm increase within a 2-year period is classified as a recent conversion for persons <35 years of age.
   - $\geq$15 mm increase within a 2-year period is classified as a recent conversion for persons $\geq$35 years of age.
5. PPD skin-test results in health-care workers (HCWs)
   - In general, the recommendations in sections 1, 2, and 3 of this table should be followed when interpreting skin-test results in HCWs. However, the prevalence of TB in the facility should be considered when choosing the appropriate cut-point for defining a positive PPD reaction. In facilities where there is essentially no risk for exposure to *Mycobacterium tuberculosis* (i.e., minimal- or very low-risk facilities), an induration $\geq$15 mm may be a suitable cut-point for HCWs who have no other risk factors. In facilities where TB patients receive care, the cut-point for HCWs with no other risk factors may be $\geq$10 mm.
   - A recent conversion in an HCW should be defined generally as a $\geq$10 mm increase in size of induration within a 2-year period. For HCWs who work in facilities where exposure to TB is very unlikely (e.g., minimal-risk facilities), an increase of $\geq$15 mm within a 2-year period may be more appropriate for defining a recent conversion because of the lower positive-predictive value of the test in such groups.

*Recent close contact implies either household or social contact or unprotected occupational exposure similar in intensity and duration to household contact.

From Centers for Disease Control and Prevention. (1994). Guidelines for preventing the transmission of *Mycobacterium tuberculosis* in health-care facilities: 1994. *Morbidity and Mortality Weekly Report, 43*(RR-13), 62–63.

TABLE 15–18 **Regimen Options for the Treatment of Tuberculosis in Children and Adults**

Option	Indication	Total Duration of Therapy	Initial Treatment Phase		Continuation Treatment Phase		Comments
			Drugs	*Interval and Duration*	*Drugs*	*Interval and Duration*	
1	Pulmonary and extrapulmonary TB in adults and children	6 months	INH RIF PZA EMB or SM	Daily for 8 weeks	INH RIF	Daily or two or three times weekly* for 16 weeks†	• EMB or SM should be continued until susceptibility to INH and RIF is demonstrated. • In areas where primary INH resistance is <4%, EMB or SM may not be necessary for patients with no individual risk factors for drug resistance.
2	Pulmonary and extrapulmonary TB in adults and children	6 months	INH RIF PZA EMB or SM	Daily for 2 weeks, then two times weekly for 6 weeks	INH RIF	Two times weekly* for 16 weeks†	• Regimen should be directly observed. • After the initial phase, EMB or SM should be continued until susceptibility to INH and RIF is demonstrated, unless drug resistance is unlikely.
3	Pulmonary and extrapulmonary TB in adults and children	6 months	INH RIF PZA EMB or SM	3 times weekly* for 6 months†			• Regimen should be directly observed. • Continue all four drugs for 6 months‡ • This regimen has been shown to be effective for INH-resistant TB.
4	Smear- and culture-negative pulmonary TB in adults	4 months	INH RIF PZA EMB or SM	Follow option 1, 2, or 3 for 8 weeks	INH RIF PZA EMB or SM	Daily or two or three times weekly* for 8 weeks	• Continue all four drugs for 4 months. • If drug resistance is unlikely (primary INH resistance <4% and patient has no individual risk factors for drug resistance), EMB or SM may not be necessary and PZA may be discontinued after 2 months.
5	Pulmonary and extrapulmonary TB in adults and children when PZA is contraindicated	9 months	INH RIF EMB or SM§	Daily for 8 weeks	INH RIF	Daily or two times weekly* for 24 weeks†	• EMB or SM should be continued until susceptibility to INH and RIF is demonstrated. • In areas where primary INH resistance is <4%, EMB or SM may not be necessary for patients with no individual risk factors for drug resistance.

EMB = ethambutol; INH = isoniazid; PZA = pyrazinamide; RIF = rifampin; SM = streptomycin.

*All regimens administered intermittently should be directly observed.

†For infants and children with miliary TB, bone and joint TB, or TB meningitis, treatment should last at least 12 months. For adults with these forms of extrapulmonary TB, response to therapy should be monitored closely. If response is slow or suboptimal, treatment may be prolonged on a case-by-case basis.

‡Some evidence suggests that SM may be discontinued after 4 months if the isolate is susceptible to all drugs.

§Avoid treating pregnant women with SM because of the risk for ototoxicity to the fetus.

Note: For all patients, if drug-susceptibility results show resistance to any of the first-line drugs, or if the patient remains symptomatic or smear- or culture-positive after 3 months, consult a TB medical expert.

From Centers for Disease Control and Prevention. (1994). Guidelines for preventing the transmission of *Mycobacterium tuberculosis* in health-care facilities: 1994. *Morbidity and Mortality Weekly Report, 43*(RR-13), 67.

identified as at risk for contracting hepatitis B include

- persons with occupational risk
- clients and staff of institutions for the developmentally disabled
- hemodialysis patients
- sexually active homosexual men
- users of illicit injectable drugs
- recipients of certain blood products
- household and sexual contacts of HBV carriers
- adoptees from countries of high HBV endemicity
- other contacts of HBV carriers
- populations with high endemicity of HBV infection in the United States (Alaskan Natives, Pacific Islanders, and refugees from HBV-endemic areas)
- sexually active heterosexual persons (particularly those requiring treatment for STDs, prostitutes, and those with a history or multiple partners)
- international travelers residing for more than 6 months in areas with high endemicity (CDC, 1990b).

Routine testing of pregnant women for hepatitis B and treatment for the infants of those who tested positive with immune globulin and vaccine was instituted in the early 1990s. As described earlier, efforts to further reduce the incidence of hepatitis B include initiation of routine immunization of all infants in 1992 and the more recent recommendation to immunize adolescents.

HEPATITIS, NON-A/NON-B

Reported cases of non-A/non-B hepatitis have steadily increased since 1990. This increase in *reported* cases is thought to be the result of the routine screening of blood for the presence of the antibody to the hepatitis C virus (available since May, 1990) rather than an actual increase in incidence of hepatitis C. Indeed, surveillance has shown a decline of 50% in the incidence of non-A/non-B hepatitis, primarily attributable to a 58% decrease in the number of reported cases among intravenous drug users (CDC, 1994a).

Identification of previously unknown and asymptomatic individuals is not uncommon in ambulatory care, however. Ongoing monitoring of reported cases and observation of the long-term effects and implications of latent disease need careful consideration.

EMERGING INFECTIONS

Emerging infectious diseases are those diseases whose incidence in humans has increased within the past two decades or threatens to increase in the near future. They may be new or previously unrecognized illnesses. Factors identified as contributing to concern over emerging infectious diseases include social and environmental changes, explosive population growth, expanding poverty, urban migration, international travel, and technology (CDC, 1994a). Table 15–19 lists several emerging infections of which nurses who work in community-based settings should be aware. All health care providers should monitor "current" concerns or trends in communicable diseases in their community to assist in identification of suspect cases, education, prevention, and early treatment, where indicated.

International Travel

International travel may greatly increase exposure to a number of communicable diseases. Jong and McMullen (1995, p. 3) state that international travelers should seek medical advice 4 to 6 weeks in advance of departure to allow "adequate time for immunizations to be scheduled, for advice and prescriptions to be given, and for specific information to be obtained when needed." Destinations will obviously dictate travel precautions with regard to health. Of particular concern are enteric diseases, malaria, rabies and other vector-borne diseases, STDs and HIV, and other illnesses, depending on destination. Individual research into

TABLE 15–19 **Emerging Infections**

NOTE: The term "emerging infectious diseases" refers to those "infectious diseases whose incidence in humans has increased within the past two decades or threatens to increase in the near future" (2). These can be new or previously unrecognized infectious diseases, reemerging diseases, or infectious diseases that have developed resistance to previously effective antimicrobial drugs.

Coccidioidomycosis

The outbreak of coccidioidomycosis in California that began in 1991 continued in 1993. From an annual average number of 428 cases reported per year in California during the period 1981–1990, 1,200 cases were reported in 1991, 4,516 in 1992, and 4,137 in 1993, 70% of which were reported from Kern County in central California. Key factors that may be associated with the ongoing outbreak include weather conditions that are conducive to the growth and spread of *Coccidioides immitis* (e.g., protracted drought followed by heavy rains), activities that disturb the soil and facilitate airborne spread of the organism, and an increasing population of persons who are susceptible to the organism because of migration from areas where coccidoidomycosis is not endemic.

Cryptosporidiosis

In spring 1993, a municipal water supply in Milwaukee, Wisconsin, contaminated with *Cryptosporidium* caused the largest recognized outbreak of waterborne illness in the history of the United States. More than 400,000 persons became ill, 4,400 of whom required hospitalization.

Escherichia coli O157:H7

In 1993, an outbreak of *E. coli* O157:H7 affected more than 500 people in four western states, resulting in 56 cases of hemolytic uremic syndrome and four deaths. Because of this outbreak, many clinical laboratories began screening stool samples for *E. coli* O157:H7, which resulted in the identification of many more cases and outbreaks. In May 1993, the Council of State and Territorial Epidemiologists (CSTE) passed a resolution recommending that *E. coli* O157:H7 infection be made reportable by all states and territories.

Group A Streptococcal Disease

During 1993, CDC surveillance for invasive group A streptococcal infections consisted of a passive nationwide surveillance system. This system operated through the collection of isolates from normally sterile sites and the collection of case reports. Although current data on incidence and trends for invasive disease, streptococcal toxic shock syndrome, and necrotizing fasciitis are not available, population-based active surveillance for these infections has begun in several geographic areas and will be expanded in 1994 as part of surveillance for emerging infectious diseases.

Hantavirus Pulmonary Syndrome

Hantavirus Pulmonary Syndrome (HPS), a newly recognized illness characterized by an influenza-like prodrome followed by the acute onset of respiratory failure, was first identified in the southwestern United States in June 1993 during the investigation of a cluster of unexplained deaths. A new hantavirus (Sin Nombre virus) and a rodent reservoir for the virus (the deer mouse *[Peromyscus maniculatus]*) were identified. As of August 31, 1994, national surveillance for HPS, initiated by CDC in coordination with CSTE, has identified 91 confirmed cases of HPS (with 48 deaths) in 20 states (case fatality rate: 53%).

Drug-Resistant Pneumococcus

The increasing incidence of drug-resistant *Streptococcus pneumoniae* (DRSP) strains in the United States has created an emerging public health challenge. CDC surveillance data from 1992 indicated that the prevalence of pneumococcal strains that are highly resistant to penicillin increased 60-fold (from 0.02% to 1.3%) when compared with the prevalence of isolates collected from 1979 through 1987. CDC, CSTE, and the infectious diseases and microbiology communities are developing recommendations for the surveillance of DRSP infections. This surveillance data will be used to determine optimal empiric treatment regimens for pneumococcal infections.

Vancomycin-Resistant Enterococci (VRE)

From 1989 through 1993, the percentage of nosocomial enterococci resistant to vancomycin reported from hospitals participating in the National Nosocomial Infections Surveillance System increased from 0.3% to 7.9%. During this period, numerous VRE outbreaks (occurring primarily among immunocompromised patients) were reported. Because of the public health importance of the emergence of VRE, CDC has published draft *Guidelines for Preventing the Spread of Vancomycin Resistance* and is conducting studies to assess the effectiveness of these guidelines in preventing disease transmission.

From Centers for Disease Control and Prevention. (1994). Summary of notifiable diseases. United States: 1993. *Morbidity and Mortality Weekly Report, 42*(53), vii–viii.

Data from Public Health Service. (1991). *Healthy People 2000: National Health Promotion and Disease Prevention Objectives—Full Report, with Commentary.* Washington, D. C., U. S. Department of Health and Human Services. Public Health Service, DHHS publication no. (PHS)191-50212; and Institute of Medicine. (1992). *Emerging Infections: Microbial Threats to Health in the United States.* Washington, D. C., National Academy Press.

specific risks and careful planning of primary and secondary prevention is vitally important.

Prior to leaving the United States, a "traveler's health history" should be completed by the traveler and carried in a safe place throughout the trip. This document should contain immunization records, list of current medications, list of medical problems, known drug allergies, blood type, name and telephone number of the regular doctor, and name and telephone number of the closest relative or friend in the United States. Tables 15–20, 15–21, and 15–22 also include important planning information for international travelers, particularly those going into areas where public health efforts are marginal, where medical care is difficult to obtain, and where certain illnesses may be endemic. Finally, Table 15–23 contains immunization recommendations for foreign travel.

SUMMARY

Primary and secondary prevention of communicable diseases is one of the most important functions of nurses who work in community-based settings. This chapter focused on several aspects of communicable disease control, including identification and reporting of suspected cases, prevention through immunization, and education and counseling efforts to reduce transmission of STDs. Encouraging monitoring of selected diseases and emerging infections as well as disease prevention during international travel concluded the discussion.

In addition to the references included at the conclusion of the chapter, Table 15–24 lists a number of resources for further information on the major topics. Each of these agencies and organizations provides literature for health care providers, and many offer educational materials for clients.

TABLE 15–20 **Pre-Travel Medical Recommendations**

1. Consult personal physician, local Public Health Department, or travel clinic about recommendations for immunizations and malaria chemoprophylaxis after selection of the travel itinerary, but preferably 4 to 6 weeks in advance of departure.
2. Prepare a Traveler's Health History and Traveler's Medical Kit.
3. Carry a telephone credit card that can be used for international telephone calls, or make sure that the friends or relatives listed in the health history would accept an international collect call in case of an emergency.
4. Make sure to have the telephone number of your personal physician, including office and after-hours numbers, and a telefax number if available. A business card attached to the Traveler's Health History is a handy way to carry this information.
5. Check medical insurance policy or health plan for coverage of illness or accidents occurring outside the United States.
6. Specifically inquire if the regular insurance policy or health plan will cover emergency medical evacuation by an air ambulance.
7. Arrange for additional medical insurance coverage or for a line of credit as necessary for a medical emergency situation.

From Jong E. C. (1995). The travel medical kit and emergency medical care abroad. In E. C. Jong and R. McMullen (Eds.). *The Travel & Tropical Medicine Manual* (2nd ed.). Philadelphia, W. B. Saunders.

TABLE 15–21 The Traveler's Personal Medical Kit

It is a wise traveler who is prepared ahead of time for unexpected emergencies that can arise. Below are listed some of the suggested items for the traveler's personal medical kit. Not all of these items are necessary or appropriate for every traveler: items should be selected based on the style of travel and destination(s).

Prescription Items

Antibiotics, General: Antibiotics may be useful for travelers at risk for skin infections, upper respiratory infections (URIs), and/or urinary tract infections (UTIs).

Skin infections:

Dicloxacillin, 250-mg capsule. Two PO q 6 h × 7 days; or
Cephalexin (or cephradine) 500-mg capsule. One PO q 6 h × 7 days
Mupirocin 2% topical antibiotic ointment. 15-g tube or 1-g foil packets. Apply to infected skin lesions three times a day.

Upper respiratory tract infections:

Erythromycin, 250-mg tablet. One PO q 6 h × 7 days; or
Trimethoprim 160-mg/sulfamethoxazole 800-mg double-strength tablet (TMP/SMX DS). One PO q 12 hr × 7 days; or
Doxycycline, 100 mg capsule. One PO q 12 hr × 7 days; or
Azithromycin, 250-mg tablet. Two PO first dose, followed by one PO q 24 h × 4 additional days.

Urinary tract infections (uncomplicated):

TMP/SMX DS tablet: One PO q 12 h × 3 days; or
Norfloxacin, 400-mg tablet: One PO q 12 h × 3 days.

Multipurpose Antibiotics: These would provide empiric coverage for skin infections, URI, and UTI. (Note that ciprofloxacin and ofloxacin are used for treatment of traveler's diarrhea as well):

Amoxicillin, 500-mg plus clavulanate, 125-mg tablet (Augmentin, 500 mg). One PO q 8 h × 3–7 days; or
Ciprofloxacin, 500-mg tablet. One PO q 12 h × 3–7 days; or
Ofloxacin, 300-mg tablet. One PO q 12 h × 3–7 days.

Allergic Reactions: (To bee, wasp, yellow jacket, or hornet stings; food, etc).

EpiPen emergency injection of epinephrine:

Use according to package directions for severe reaction to bee sting or for other allergic reaction causing shortness of breath or wheezing; or swelling of the lips, eyes, throat, or severe hives. This will give short-acting relief. As soon as the afflicted person can swallow, give them Benadryl tablets as directed below.

Benadryl (diphenhydramine), 25-mg tablet:

Take two tablets by mouth immediately, then one to two tabs q 6 h × 2 days following an allergic reaction. Use Benadryl alone for mild to moderate allergic skin reactions and itching, and take Benadryl following the use of the EpiPen.

Medrol (methylprednisolone) DosePack:

For use with severe and persistent allergic reactions or skin rashes.
Follow the instructions for the tapering dose schedule in the packet.
May be required in addition to Benadryl for severe allergic reactions.

Ventolin (albuterol) inhaler (MDI, multidose inhaler):

Use for asthma attacks or for allergic reactions that cause persistent wheezing. Two puffs 2 minutes apart, each inhaled as deeply as possible into the lungs. Do this four times a day.

Cough Suppressant: A small bottle of prescription cough syrup or a few tablets of codeine-containing medication (Tylenol #3 tablets will serve this purpose and that of medication for severe headache or pain).

Diarrhea Treatment: An antimotility drug (Lomotil or Imodium) plus an antibiotic (e.g., trimethoprim/sulfamethoxazole, ciprofloxacin, ofloxacin, tetracycline) may be prescribed for self-treatment.

High-Altitude Illness: Acetazolamide (Diamox) may be prescribed for prophylaxis of high-altitude illness for high-altitude destinations.

Jet Lag: In some cases, a short-acting sleeping medication is helpful in treating sleeping problems associated with jet lag.

Malaria Pills: As the malaria situation in many countries continues to change, malaria chemoprophylaxis changes as well. Updated information on the malaria situation for specific destination(s) needs to be carefully reviewed, and approprate medications prescribed.

Motion Sickness: Travelers who experience motion sickness may be prescribed a medication for this.

Nausea and Vomiting: Compazine (prochloperazine), 25-mg rectal suppository. This may be helpful when oral medications cannot be tolerated and an injectable antiemetic is not available.

Pain Relief: A modest supply of prescriptive pain medication may be needed for headache, toothache, or musculoskeletal injury.

Tylenol #3 (Tylenol with 30 mg codeine) tablets: one to two tablets PO q 4–6 h prn severe headache or pain; or
Dilaudid (hydromorphone), 2-mg tablets: one to two tablets PO q 4 for relief of severe pain (useful for people allergic or intolerant to codeine).

Table continued on following page

TABLE 15–21 **The Traveler's Personal Medical Kit** *Continued*

Nonprescription Items

Aspirin or Tylenol or Ibuprofen (Advil, Nuprin): For general relief of minor aches and pains or headache.
Antibiotic Ointment: (Neosporin or Bacitracin) for topical application on minor cuts and abrasions.
Antifungal Powder or Cream: For travelers prone to athletes' foot and/or other fungal skin problems.
Antifungal Vaginal Cream or Troches: For women prone to yeast vaginitis associated with changes in climate or following antibiotic use.
Decongestant Tablets (Actifed, Sudafed, Contac, etc.): For nasal congestion due to colds, allergies, or water sports.
Diarrhea Prevention: Bismuth subsalicylate (Pepto-Bismol) tablets may be taken, two tablets qid every day of the trip to prevent traveler's diarrhea.
Hydrocortisone Cream: For topical relief of itching due to insect bites or sunburn.
Laxative: For relief of "traveler's constipation" due to changes in diet and schedule. Patients with a history of this problem may need to take a fiber supplement and/or a prescription stool softener.
Oral Rehydration Salt Packets: WHO-ORS (Jianas Brothers, Kansas City, MO), IAMAT Oral Rehydration Salts; to be mixed in purified water safe for drinking for fluid replacement and rehydration during severe diarrhea.
Throat Lozenges: For relief of throat irritation due to air pollution or upper respiratory infection.

General Health and First Aid Supplies

Antiseptic Solution: Topical solution for cleansing of minor cuts and abrasions (Hibiclens).
Bandages: Band-Aids, 4 × 4-inch sterile gauze pads, 2-inch roll gauze dressing.
Elastic Bandage: For minor sprains (Ace wrap).
Eyeglasses: If corrective lenses are used, bring an extra pair of eyeglasses along.
Case (Waterproof): To hold medications and supplies.
Condoms (Latex): For prevention of sexually transmitted diseases.
Insect Repellent (with DEET): For topcal application to exposed areas of skin.
Insect Spray (with Permethrin): For application to external clothing, mosquito nets, curtains, etc.
Moleskin: For prevention of blisters on feet.
Safety Pins: The rust proof baby diaper pin types are useful for all kinds of emergency repairs, pinning room curtains shut, hanging laundry on wire hangers, etc.
Sanitary Supplies (Menstruating Women): Tampons, sanitary napkins (these may not be readily available in tropical and developing parts of the world).
Scissors: For general use (if not included in Swiss Army Knife).
Swiss Army Knife (or similar): An all-purpose gadget, especially useful if tweezers and scissors are included.
Sunglasses: With UV light protective lenses.
Sunscreen: Any brand with sun protective factor (SPF) of greater than 15.
Tape, Adhesive: For first aid wound care.
Tape, Duct: For general repairs, creating splints, etc.
Tick Pliers: For participants in outdoor activities; to remove ticks safely and completely.
Toilet Paper: Often not available in public rest facilities when one is in desperate need (buy a compact roll, available in sporting supply stores).
Towelettes (Premoistened): For cleaning hands.
Thermometer, Oral: Very important for assessment of illness while traveling.
Venom Extractor Pump: To extract venom from venomous insect stings and snake bites.
Water Disinfection Tablets
Water Disinfection Device, Portable

Dosage information applies to adults in good health without contraindications to the given drug.
Trademark names are provided for identification only and do not constitute an endorsement.
From Jong E. C. (1995). The travel medical kit and emergency medical care abroad. In E. C. Jong and R. McMullen (Eds.). *The Travel & Tropical Medicine Manual* (2nd ed.). Philadelphia, W. B. Saunders.

TABLE 15–22 Methods for Purification of Water*

Method	Brand Name	Quantity to be Added to 1 Quart or 1 Liter of Water
Iodine compound tablets*	Potable Aqua, Coughlins	Two tablets are added to water at 20°C, and the mixture is agitated every 5 minutes for a total of 30 minutes.
Chlorine solution, 2–4%	(Common laundry bleach)	Two to four drops are added to water at 20°C, and after mixing, the solution is kept for 30 minutes before drinking.
Iodine solution†	(2% tincture of iodine)	Five to ten drops of iodine are added to water at 20°C, and after mixing, the solution is kept for 30 minutes before drinking.
Heat		Water is heated to above 65°C for at least 3 minutes. (At 20,000 ft altitude or 6000 m, water boils at 70°C.)

*The methods presented here are sufficient to kill *Giardia* cysts in most situations. Heat is the best method when tested in a laboratory situation.
†Iodine-containing compounds should be used with caution during pregnancy.
From Jong E. C. (1995). The travel medical kit and emergency medical care abroad. In E. C. Jong and R. McMullen (Eds.). *The Travel & Tropical Medicine Manual* (2nd ed.). Philadelphia, W. B. Saunders.

TABLE 15–23 Immunization Recommendations for International Travel

Vaccine	Dosage (mL)	Interval
Cholera	1 dose (0.5)	Every 6 months
Hepatitis*	3 doses (1.0)	Unknown
Immune globulin†	1 dose (5.0)	Every 4–6 months
Influenza	2 doses (0.5)	First year given 4 weeks apart
	1 dose (0.5)	Every year
Japanese encephalitis	2 doses (1.0)	At 12 months; then every 4 years
Malaria‡	Prophylaxis—check for chloroquine resistance	Continuously while in endemic regions
Meningococcus A/C/Y/W-135	1 dose	Every 3 years
Plague	2 doses (0.5)	6 months apart
	1 dose (0.5)	1–2 years after second dose (above)
	1 dose (0.2)	Years of possible exposure
Rabies, human diploid cell	3 doses (1.0)	Days 0, 7, and 21 or 28
	1 dose (1.0) pending titer check	At 2-year intervals—check titer if exposure remains possible
Tuberculosis bacille Calmette-Guérin vaccine	1 dose (0.1)	Once
Typhoid	2 doses (0.5)	4 weeks apart
	1 dose (0.5)	Every 3 years
Yellow fever	1 dose (0.5)	Every 10 years

*Hepatitis vaccine can be Heptavax, Recombivax, or Engerix B.
†Immune globulin is also called γ-globulin.
‡Many different kinds of malaria prophylaxis are available for the different strains of malaria. Currently, there is no vaccine available. Check status of chloroquine resistance in area.
Data from Benenson et al. (1985). *Control of Communicable Diseases in Man* (14th ed.). Washington, D. C., American Public Health Association; Centers for Disease Control. (1988): *Health Information for International Travel.* Atlanta, Centers for Disease Control; Ghendon, Y. (1990). WHO Strategy for the global elimination of new cases of hepatitis B. *Vaccine* 8(suppl):S129–132; Sherris et al. (1986): Immunizing the world's children. *Population Rep,* L:154–192; Wolfe et al. (1989): *Health Hints for the Tropics* (10th ed.). Washington, D. C., American Society of Tropical Medicine and Hygiene.
From Dash, D. (1993). Communicable disease. In J. Swanson and S. Albrecht (Eds.). *Community Health Nursing: Promoting the Health of Aggregates.* Philadelphia, W. B. Saunders.

TABLE 15–24 **Resources for Communicable Disease Prevention**

General Information on Communicable Diseases

Centers for Disease Control and Prevention
Public Inquiries
1600 Clifton Road, NE
Mailstop A23
Atlanta, GA 30333
(404) 639-3534

National Center for Infectious Diseases
1600 Clifton Road, NE
Mailstop A23
Atlanta, GA 30333
(404) 639-3945

National Immunization Program
1600 Clifton Road, NE
Mailstop A23
Atlanta, GA 30333
(404) 639-8204

National Center for Prevention Services
1600 Clifton Road, NE
Mailstop A23
Atlanta, GA 30333
(404) 639-8008

National Institute of Allergy and Infectious Diseases (NIAID)
9000 Rockville Pike
Building 31, Room 7A-50
Bethesda, MD 20892
(301) 496-5717

Health Resources and Services Administration
National Clearinghouse for Maternal and Child Health
8201 Greensboro Drive
Suite 600
McLean, VA 22102–3810
(703) 821-8955

American Academy of Pediatrics
141 Northwest Point Boulevard
P.O. Box 927
Elk Grove Village, IL 60009
(708) 228-5005

National Foundation for Infectious Disease
4733 Bethesda Avenue, Suite 750
Bethesda, MD 20814
(301) 656-0003

Resources for Sexually Transmitted Diseases

National STD Hot Line
(800) 227-8922

American Foundation for the Prevention of Venereal Disease
799 Broadway
Suite 638
New York, NY 10003
(212) 759-2069

American Social Health Association
P. O. Box 13827
Research Triangle Park, NC 27709
(919) 361-8400
(800) 227-8922 (STD National Hotline)
(800) 342-2437 (National AIDS Hotline)
(919) 361-8488 (National Herpes Hotline)

Planned Parenthood Federation of America
810 Seventh Avenue
New York, NY 10019
(212) 541-7800
(800) 230-PLAN

Key Points

- Although there has been dramatic improvement in morbidity and mortality from communicable diseases, particularly vaccine-preventable diseases (e.g., measles, diphtheria, polio), a number of threats and risks still exist for all people from communicable illnesses (HIV, tuberculosis, influenza).
- Communicable diseases may be transmitted directly (kissing, touching, sexual contact) or indirectly (through fomites, substance, or vectors). Airborne transmission may be either direct or indirect.
- The Centers for Disease Control and Prevention and the individual state legislatures have identified "Reportable Communicable Diseases." Guidelines for reporting include who is responsible for reporting; what information is required; how, when, and to whom to report; and steps taken to control spread.
- Many communicable diseases are preventable through immunization. The recommended immunization schedule for infants and children is complex and has changed a number of times in recent years. To address potential problems with immunizations, the *Standards for Pediatric Immunization Practices* were published in 1993. The Standards outline specific information on contraindications and precautions for vaccines; parent education; consent; and reporting of adverse vaccine events.
- The number and incidence of STDs have increased dramatically over the last several decades. The most common STDs include chlamydia, gonorrhea, herpes, HIV, human papillomavirus, syphilis, and scabies.
- Nurses working in community-based settings should watch for changes in rates of communicable diseases. Diseases that should be closely monitored include tuberculosis, hepatitis B, non-A/non-B hepatitis, and "emerging infections."
- Often, nurses in community settings are asked to advise clients on issues related to international travel. Information that might be needed includes pre-travel recommendations, immunization requirements and recommendations, and tips for water purification.

Learning Activities and Application to Practice

In Class

- Discuss modes of communicable disease transmission. Identify and outline primary prevention strategies to reduce or eliminate each type of transmission.
- Invite a guest speaker from the local public health department to discuss surveillance and control of communicable diseases. Ask the speaker to include data on local and regional trends in communicable diseases and to describe the process of reporting.
- Discuss the current pediatric immunization schedule and the Standards for Pediatric Immunization Practices. Ensure that students are aware of recent changes, as well as contraindications and precautions.

In Clinical

- In a log or diary, have students compile a list of communicable illnesses encountered in the clinical setting. When possible, have students participate in the process of reporting of communicable diseases.
- Encourage students to participate in a pediatric immunization clinic or to work with nurses who routinely immunize children. If allowable, have students participate in screening children for possible contraindications, providing the required parent education and recording immunizations. Also allow students to administer the immunization according to protocol. Have them share impressions of the experience with other students.

REFERENCES

Benenson, A. S. (1990). *Control of Communicable Diseases in Man* (15th ed). Washington, D. C., American Public Health Association.

Centers for Disease Control and Prevention. (1995a). *Epidemiology & Prevention of Vaccine-Preventable Diseases.* Atlanta, GA: Centers for Disease Control and Prevention.

Centers for Disease Control and Prevention. (1995b). National Adult Immunization Awareness Week. *Morbidity and Mortality Weekly Report, 44*(40), 741–745.

Centers for Disease Control and Prevention. (1995c). Summary of notifiable diseases, United States: 1994. *Morbidity and Mortality Weekly Report, 43*(53).

Centers for Disease Control and Prevention. (1994a). Addressing emerging infectious disease threats: A prevention strategy for the United States. *Morbidity and Mortality Weekly Report, 43*(RR-5).

Centers for Disease Control and Prevention. (1994b). General recommendations on immunization. *Morbidity and Mortality Weekly Report, 43*(RR-1).

Centers for Disease Control and Prevention. (1994c). Guidelines for preventing the transmission of *Mycobacterium tuberculosis* in health-care facilities, 1994. *Morbidity and Mortality Weekly Report, 43*(RR-13).

Centers for Disease Control and Prevention. (1994d). Vaccine coverage of 2-year-old children, United States. *Morbidity and Mortality Weekly Report, 43*(39), 705–709.

Centers for Disease Control. (1993a). Standards for pediatric immunization practices. *Morbidity and Mortality Weekly Report, 42*(RR-5).

Centers for Disease Control. (1993b). 1993 Sexually transmitted diseases treatment guidelines. *Morbidity and Mortality Weekly Report, 42*(RR-14).

Centers for Disease Control. (1992). *Principles of Epidemiology* (2nd ed.). Atlanta, GA, Centers for Disease Control.

Centers for Disease Control. (1991). Update on adult immunization. *Morbidity and Mortality Weekly Report,* 40(RR-12).

Centers for Disease Control. (1990a). The use of preventive therapy for tuberculosis infection in the United States. *Morbidity and Mortality Weekly Report, 39*(RR-8).

Centers for Disease Control. (1990b). Protection against viral hepatitis: Recommendations of the Immunization Practices Advisory Committee. *Morbidity and Mortality Weekly Report, 39,* 5–22.

Chen, R. T., Rastogi, S. C., Mullen, J. R., et al. (1994). The Vaccine Adverse Event Reporting System (VAERS). *Vaccine, 12*(6), 542–550.

Dash, D. (1993). Communicable disease. In J. Swanson and S. Albrecht (Eds.). *Community Health Nursing: Promoting the Health of Aggregates.* Philadelphia, W. B. Saunders.

Jong, E. C. (1995). The travel medical kit and emergency medical care abroad. In E. C. Jong and R. McMullen (Eds.). *The Travel & Tropical Medicine Manual* (2nd ed). Philadelphia, W. B. Saunders.

Jong, E. C. and McMullen, R. (1995). Sexually transmitted disease and foreign travel. In E. C. Jong and R. McMullen (Eds.). *The Travel & Tropical Medicine Manual* (2nd ed.). Philadelphia, W. B. Saunders.

Mausner, J. S. and Kramer, S. (1985). *Epidemiology: An Introductory Text.* Philadelphia, W. B. Saunders.

Mantocha, L. K. (1995). Communicable diseases. In C. M. Smith and F. A. Maurer (Eds.). *Community Health Nursing: Theory and Practice*. Philadelphia, W. B. Saunders.

Milone-Nuzzo, P. (1995). Home health care. In C. Smith and F. A. Maurer (Eds.). *Community Health Nursing: Theory and Practice*. Philadelphia, W. B. Saunders.

Texas Department of Health. (1992). *Educator's Guide to Sexually Transmitted Diseases* (3rd ed.). Austin, TX: Texas Department of Health.

U. S. Department of Health and Human Services (USDHHS). (1994). *Clinician's Handbook of Preventive Services.* Washington, D. C., Government Printing Office. (Also marketed through the "GPO Sales Program and Federal Depository Libraries".)

U. S. Department of Health and Human Services (USDHHS). (1990). *Healthy People 2000: National Health Promotion and Disease Prevention Objectives*. Washington, D. C., Government Printing Office.

Wilson, M. E. (1995). Travel and HIV infection. In E. C. Jong and R. McMullen (Eds.). *The Travel & Tropical Medicine Manual* (2nd ed.). Philadelphia, W. B. Saunders.

16

Community-Based Nursing Care of Clients with HIV Infection and AIDS

Case Study *Amy Anderson is a Registered Nurse who works in a community-sponsored human immunodeficiency virus/acquired immunodeficiency syndrome (HIV/AIDS) clinic located in a large city. The clinic provides comprehensive services including counseling and testing, case management for those who are HIV-positive, and participation in clinical trials.*

One recent Wednesday, Amy saw several patients, for a variety of reasons. In the morning, Amy also saw Jeffrey Jackson to administer his aerosolized pentamidine treatment and to draw blood for CD4 T-cell counts. Later she saw Mark Freeman to follow-up on his treatment for tuberculosis. Later in the day, she performed pretest counseling and drew blood for testing for a young couple who were getting married; she made appointments for them to return in 2 weeks to discuss the results. In the early afternoon, she taught a nutrition class for HIV-positive individuals and their family members.

The last patient Amy saw that day was "Mary Smith," a college student 22 years of age. Ms. Smith came to the clinic to learn the results of the HIV test she had done 2 weeks ago and for post-test counseling. Ms. Smith first came to the clinic for testing because she had had unprotected sex with her former boyfriend, who reportedly used intravenous (IV) drugs, and she was concerned that she might have been exposed to HIV. In counseling Ms. Smith, Amy was happy to inform her that her HIV test results were negative at this time; but she was careful to discuss the implications of the negative results. When questioned about her past sexual history, Ms. Smith stated she had not had sex with her former boyfriend or anyone else for almost a year. Because of the length of time since her last exposure, Amy explained to Ms. Smith that it was unlikely that she needed to be retested. She was then given explicit instructions and information on how to remain HIV-negative. This information included the importance of using a Latex condom every time *she had sexual intercourse and instructions on how to use condoms correctly. Ms. Smith stated she would be* very *careful from now on and did not plan on becoming sexually involved with anyone else until she was ready for marriage.*

A June 1981 *Morbidity and Mortality Weekly Report* article described the occurrence of *Pneumocystis carinii* pneumonia (PCP) in five previously healthy, young, and sexually active homosexual men from Los Angeles. Soon afterward, cases of Kaposi's sarcoma (KS), a very rare condition, were diagnosed in young, male homosexuals in New York City. Laboratory studies revealed severe immunodeficiency in these men. During the next 12 months, the Centers for Disease Control and Prevention (CDC) investigated a growing number of cases of these and other opportunistic infections in young homosexual and bisexual men. Soon afterward, other groups, including IV drug users, Haitian immigrants, persons with hemophilia and other recipients of blood or blood components, and sexual partners and children of persons with the diseases, were found to have the same or similar problems. About the same time these conditions first appeared in the United States, a number of European countries described similar patterns of opportunistic infections affecting gay men. In central Africa, however, a somewhat different epidemic was observed. There, men and women were infected equally, leading health care professionals to determine that the virus was transmitted both heterosexually and homosexually.

In September 1982, the CDC termed the condition manifested by immunosuppression and opportunistic infections as AIDS. In 1983, it was determined that AIDS was caused by a retrovirus, later termed human immunodeficiency virus type 1 (HIV-1 or HIV). Identification of the virus subsequently led to development of a blood test for HIV antibody. This was a very important development, which allowed public health officials to identify persons infected with the virus and to screen blood and blood products to prevent transmission (Flaskerud, 1995).

Since its identification in the early 1980s, AIDS has mushroomed to epidemic levels. Table 16–1 shows approximate numbers of persons worldwide infected with HIV. The World Health Organization estimates there will be 30 to 40 million people around the world infected with HIV by the year 2000. Others experts believe the figure may be as high as 110 million (U.S. Department of Health and Human Services (USDHHS)/Agency for Health Care Policy and Research (AHCPR), 1994).

In the United States, the AIDS epidemic has had a profound effect. Through 1995, there were 513,000 reported cases of AIDS; of these infected, 62% have died (CDC, 1995a). In addition, there are an estimated 1 million people in the United States infected with HIV. Among persons 25 to 44 years of age, HIV infection is the leading cause of death in men and the third leading cause of death in women. By 2000, AIDS will be the third most common cause of death in the United States for all ages. Current studies indicate that HIV infection is present in 0.2 to 8.9% of patients visiting emergency departments and in 0.1 to 7.8% of admissions to acute care hospitals (USDHHS/AHCPR, 1994).

TABLE 16–1 **Estimated Worldwide HIV Infection by Region**

Sub-Saharan Africa	7.5 million
Americas	2 million
South and Southeast Asia	1.5 million
Western Europe	500,000
North Africa and the Middle East	75,000
Eastern Europe and Central Asia	50,000
East Asia and the Pacific	25,000
Australia	25,000

Data from Flaskerud, J. H. (1995). Overview of HIV disease and nursing. In Flaskerud, J. H., and Ungvarski, P. J. (Eds.). *HIV/AIDS: A Guide to Nursing Care* (3rd ed.). Philadelphia, W. B. Saunders. (Source: *Global AIDS News.* [1993]. 1[4].)

Economically, HIV infection costs the United States more than $10 billion annually in direct medical costs and time lost from work as well as indirect costs. Additionally, emotional and physiological pressure on individuals, families, and society at large is immense (USDHHS/AHCPR, 1994).

In response to concerns about the growing threat of HIV and AIDS, one of the "Priority Areas" of *Healthy People 2000* addresses HIV infection. Table 16–2 presents some of the objectives related to HIV infection.

The growing presence of HIV infection, therefore, necessitates that *all* health care providers be knowledgeable about HIV prevention, counseling, and treatment. This chapter presents a number of issues and concepts that are important for nurses working in community-based settings. Included are discussions of epidemiology of the disease, prevention, principles of counseling

TABLE 16–2 ***Healthy People 2000*—Examples of Objectives for Prevention of Communicable Disease**

18.1—Confine annual incidence of diagnosed AIDS cases to no more than 98,000 cases. (Baseline: An estimated 44,000 to 50,000 diagnosed cases in 1989)

Special Population Targets

Diagnosed AIDS Cases	***1989 Baseline***	***2000 Target***
18.1a Gay and bisexual men	26,000–28,000	48,000
18.1b Blacks	14,000–15,000	37,000
18.1c Hispanics	7,000–8,000	18,000

18.2—Confine the prevalence of HIV infection to no more than 800 per 100,000 people. (Baseline: An estimated 400 per 100,000 in 1989)

Special Population Targets

Estimated Prevalence of HIV Infection (per 100,000)	***1989 Baseline***	***2000 Target***
18.2a Homosexual men	2,000–42,000	20,000
18.2b Intravenous drug abusers	30,000–40,000	40,000
18.2c Women giving birth to live-born infants	150	100

18.3—Reduce the proportion of adolescents who have engaged in sexual intercourse to no more than 15 percent by age 15 and no more than 40 percent by age 17. (Baseline: 27 percent of girls and 33 percent of boys by age 15; 50 percent of girls and 66 percent of boys by age 17; reported in 1988)

18.4—Increase to at least 50 percent the proportion of sexually active, unmarried people who used a condom at last sexual intercourse. (Baseline: 19 percent of sexually active, unmarried women aged 15 through 44 reported that their partners used a condom at last sexual intercourse in 1988)

18.7—Reduce to no more than 1 per 250,000 units of blood and blood components the risk of transfusion-transmitted HIV infection. (Baseline: 1 per 40,000 to 150,000 units in 1989)

18.9—Increase to at least 75 percent the proportion of primary care and mental health care providers who provided age-appropriate counseling on the prevention of HIV and other sexually transmitted diseases. (Baseline: 10 percent of physicians reported that they regularly assessed the sexual behaviors of their patients in 1987)

18.10—Increase to at least 95 percent the proportion of schools that have age-appropriate HIV education curricula for students in 4th through 12th grade, preferably as part of quality school health education. (Baseline: 66 percent of school districts required HIV education but only 5 percent required HIV education in each year for 7th through 12th grade in 1989)

From U. S. Department of Health and Human Services (USDHHS). (1990). *Healthy People 2000: National Health Promotion and Disease Prevention Objectives.* Washington, D.C., Government Printing Office.

and testing, and basics of treatment and management.

Epidemiology

In the United States, HIV infection is predominately found in two high-risk groups, homosexual and bisexual men and intravenous drug users, although this trend has modified somewhat in the last few years. According to recent reports from the CDC, although the greatest proportion of new cases is still attributed to male-to-male sexual contact (51% of new cases), the largest increases have occurred among heterosexual men and women acquiring HIV through injecting drug use and heterosexual contact (CDC, 1995a). Females accounted for 19% of cases in 1995, the highest proportion yet reported, mostly through injecting drug use (38%) or sexual contact with a man at risk for HIV infection (38%).

AIDS/HIV affects minorities disproportionately, particularly women and children. According to the *HIV/AIDS Surveillance Report,* in 1995 for the first time the proportion of persons reported with AIDS that is black was equal to the proportion that is white (40%). Additionally, in 1995, blacks and Hispanics represented the majority of cases among men (54%) and women (76%), and the reported AIDS incidence rate per 100,000 among blacks (92.6) was six times higher than among whites (15.4) and two times higher than among Hispanics (46.2). Perhaps most disturbingly, among children with AIDS, 84% were black or Hispanic. In its report, however, the CDC notes that "measures of socioeconomic status such as education and income may more accurately predict risk of HIV than demographic factors such as race/ethnicity" (p. 5).

Geographically, rates of HIV infection are highest in the Northeast. The greatest proportionate increases in the last few years, however, have been in the South and Midwest. Incidence rates are highest in Washington D. C., Puerto Rico, New York, Florida, New Jersey, Maryland, and Connecticut. Among the most heavily affected metropolitan areas are San Francisco, West Palm Beach, Jersey City, San Juan, Baltimore, and Orlando (CDC, 1995a).

Because of the variations in the AIDS epidemic, HIV prevention and management efforts should begin at the local and regional levels. Community-based prevention programs should be based on knowledge of HIV risk behaviors in the local community, and surveillance data should be interpreted with knowledge of local practices (CDC, 1995a and USDHHS/AHCPR, 1994). To assist nurses in community settings in understanding the gender, racial/cultural, and geographic distribution of AIDS, Figures 16–1 and 16–2 present 1995 state and territory incidences rates for male and female adults, and Figure 16–3 illustrates changes in racial/ethnic distribution. Table 16–3 presents AIDS cases by age group, exposure category, and sex.

Transmission of HIV

There are several known risk factors for HIV infection. These include sharing needles or syringes to inject drugs or steroids, engaging in unprotected sex with infected individuals, being a recipient of blood or blood products between 1978 and 1985, engaging in unprotected sex with anyone in any of these categories, and having occupational exposure to blood or body fluids of infected individuals. Prevention efforts for these risk factors are discussed here.

SEXUAL EXPOSURE

About 75% of HIV infection is attributable to sexual exposure. It has been determined that certain behaviors, sexual practices, or coexisting factors increase risk of transmission.

Receptive anal intercourse is thought to be the most risky sexual practice, followed closely by insertive anal intercourse. The risk associated with vaginal intercourse is somewhat less than with anal intercourse. In vaginal intercourse, women are at higher risk than men. Transmission may occur through oral sexual practices, with oral sex on a man (with ejaculation) being the highest risk behavior, followed by oral sex on a woman and oral/anal contact (American College Health Asso-

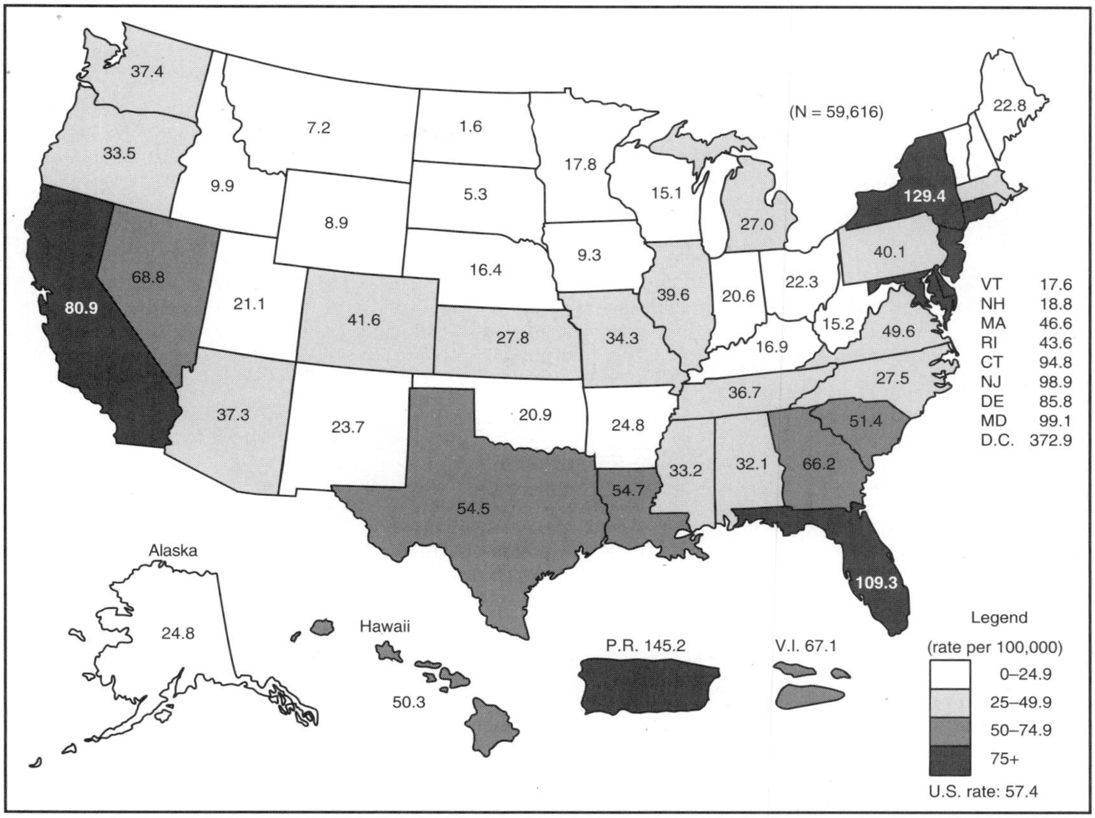

FIGURE 16–1 Male adult/adolescent AIDS annual rates per 100,000 population—1995. (From CDC. [1995]. *HIV/AIDS Surveillance Report, 1995*; 7[2], page 23).

ciation, 1990). For all sexual behaviors, coexisting conditions (i.e., open lesions on the mouth or genital area or another sexually transmitted disease) and multiple exposures or multiple partners will increase the risk.

Prevention efforts are to be stressed in the form of teaching and counseling; they should focus on promoting sexual abstinence and mutually monogamous relationships where neither partner is infected. Instructions on "safer sex," and reduction or elimination of high-risk sexual practices, should include the use of condoms *for each sexual encounter* (instructions on correct use of condoms is found in Table 15–16). In particular, it should be stressed that to reduce risk, receptive anal intercourse, rectal douching, and multiple sexual partners should be avoided.

INTRAVENOUS EXPOSURE

The spread of HIV through sharing of needles and other IV drug paraphernalia is the second most common source of transmission. More than one third of all AIDS cases are attributable to injecting drug use (USDHHS, 1994). Education and counseling efforts to prevent IV exposure should include repeated reminders *never* to share needles, syringes, or any part of the "works" with others and instruction on how to clean needles and syrin-

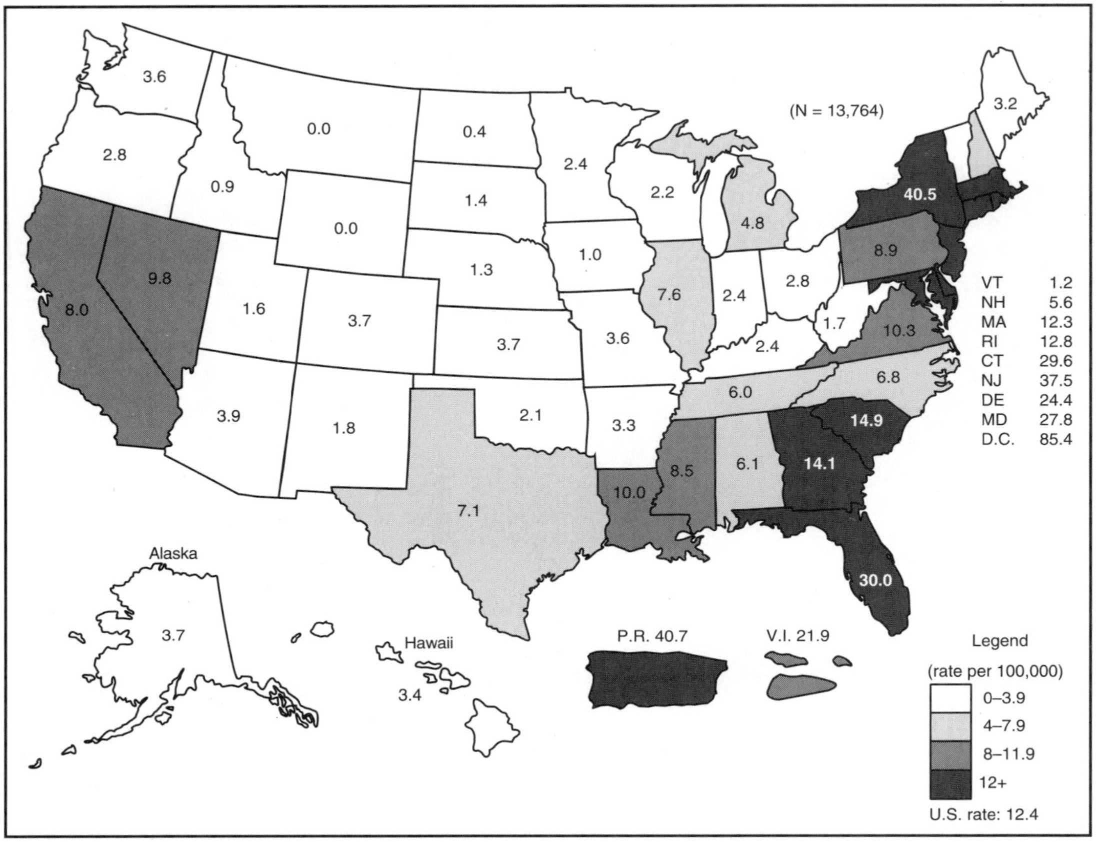

FIGURE 16–2 Female adult/adolescent AIDS annual rates per 100,000 population—1995. (From CDC. [1995]. *HIV/AIDS Surveillance Report, 1995*; 7[2], page 23).

ges with full-strength bleach. Needle exchange programs have been implemented in some areas and are reportedly successful. Referral for information, counseling, or drug treatment programs should be an integral component of HIV prevention and education. Health care providers should prepare in advance to refer IV drug users for drug treatment by maintaining a list of area programs, including the process and requirements for referral. To meet the needs of IV drug users, coordination and integration of specialized substance abuse services with the primary health care, mental health, and HIV/AIDS service systems at the state and local levels are encouraged to promote better treatment and sustained recovery of drug users and lower HIV transmission (USDHHS, 1994).

OCCUPATIONAL EXPOSURE

Primary prevention of HIV transmission for health care workers and others at risk for occupational exposure was addressed by the CDC in the development of "Universal Precautions" in 1987, which were revised in 1989. The basic premise of universal precautions is the assumption that *all* patients are potentially infected and that body fluids are assumed to be contaminated and should

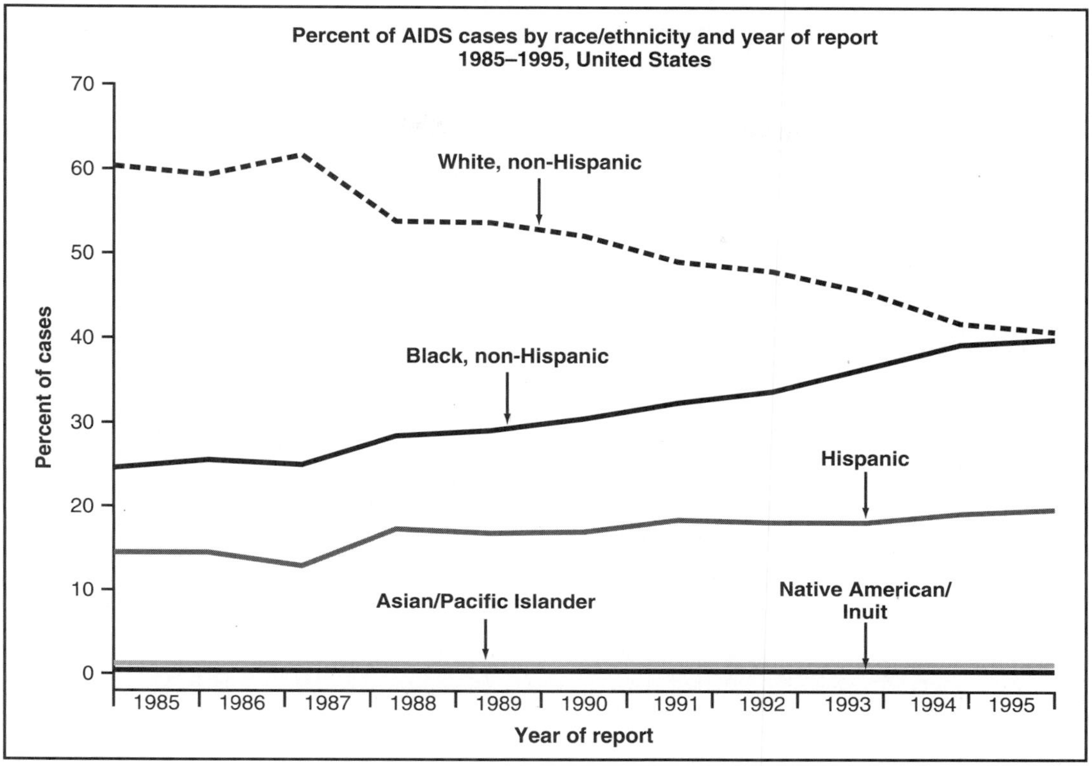

FIGURE 16–3 Percent of AIDS cases by race/ethnicity and year of report 1985–1995. (From CDC. [1995]. *HIV/AIDS Surveillance Report, 1995*; 7[2], page 23).

therefore be managed with extreme care. Perhaps due to the early directives by the CDC, awareness of modes of transmission by health care workers and efforts to minimize exposure, and prophylactic treatment for known exposures with zidovudine (ZDV), occupational exposure and resultant seroconversion to HIV has been very low. Through 1995, there have been only 39 documented cases of occupational transmission of HIV (Burnett et al., 1996). Table 16–4 outlines Principles of Universal Precautions and Table 16–5 details body fluids that require precaution to prevent transmission. Although the CDC does not formally recommend the use of ZDV for postexposure prophylaxis for known occupational exposure, it states that health care workers who are "at risk" should be informed that ZDV appears to reduce seroconversion by approximately 79% (CDC, 1995d).

EXPOSURE THROUGH CONTAMINATED BLOOD PRODUCTS

Screening of all donors to eliminate those who are at risk for HIV and hepatitis B infection has been commonplace since the middle 1980s, and testing of all blood and blood products for these viruses is now required. These measures have resulted in the dramatic decline in transfusion-related transmission of HIV, and this decline is anticipated to continue. Participation in autologous blood donation programs will prevent transmission of any bloodborne pathogens and should be encouraged whenever possible.

PERINATAL EXPOSURE

HIV can be transmitted from an infected woman to her infant during pregnancy, labor, and delivery

TABLE 16–3 **AIDS Cases by Age Group, Exposure Category, and Sex, Reported in 1994 and 1995;* and Cumulative Totals, by Age Group and Exposure Category, Through December 1995, United States**

Adult/Adolescent Exposure Category	Males 1994 No.	Males 1994 (%)	Males 1995 No.	Males 1995 (%)	Females 1994 No.	Females 1994 (%)	Females 1995 No.	Females 1995 (%)	Totals† 1994 No.	Totals† 1994 (%)	Totals† 1995 No.	Totals† 1995 (%)	Totals† Cumulative Total‡ No.	Totals† Cumulative Total‡ (%)
Men who have sex with men	35,524	(55)	30,671	(51)	—	—	—	—	35,524	(45)	30,671	(42)	259,672	(51)
Injecting drug use	16,044	(25)	14,057	(24)	5,923	(43)	5,204	(38)	21,967	(28)	19,261	(26)	128,696	(25)
Men who have sex with men and inject drugs	4,234	(7)	3,425	(6)	—	—	—	—	4,234	(5)	3,425	(5)	33,195	(7)
Hemophilia/coagulation disorder	483	(1)	423	(1)	25	(0)	22	(0)	508	(1)	445	(1)	4,107	(1)
Heterosexual contact:	3,009	(5)	2,840	(5)	5,575	(40)	5,253	(38)	8,585	(11)	8,093	(11)	40,038	(8)
Sex with injecting drug user	*963*		*928*		*2,118*		*1,921*		*3,081*		*2,849*		*18,710*	
Sex with bisexual male	—		—		*394*		*376*		*394*		*376*		*2,209*	
Sex with person with hemophilia	*2*		*12*		*56*		*50*		*58*		*62*		*330*	
Sex with transfusion recipient with HIV infection	*66*		*53*		*63*		*59*		*129*		*112*		*734*	
Sex with HIV-infected person, risk not specified	*1,978*		*1,847*		*2,944*		*2,847*		*4,923*		*4,694*		*18,055*	
Receipt of blood transfusion, blood components, or tissue§	405	(1)	366	(1)	329	(2)	298	(2)	734	(1)	664	(1)	7,433	(1)
Other/risk not reported or identified‖	5,276	(8)	7,834	(13)	2,035	(15)	2,987	(22)	7,311	(9)	10,821	(15)	33,397	(7)
Adult/adolescent subtotal	64,975	(100)	59,616	(100)	13,887	(100)	13,764	(100)	78,863	(100)	73,380	(100)	506,538	(100)

Pediatric (<13 years old) Exposure Category														
Hemophilia/coagulation disorder	14	(3)	5	(1)	—	—	—	—	14	(1)	5	(1)	227	(3)
Mother with/at risk for HIV infection:‖	463	(91)	345	(89)	494	(94)	385	(93)	957	(93)	730	(91)	6,256	(90)
Injecting drug use	*145*		*104*		*153*		*107*		*298*		*211*		*2,594*	
Sex with injecting drug user	*73*		*59*		*75*		*55*		*148*		*114*		*1,164*	
Sex with bisexual male	*10*		*6*		*9*		*4*		*19*		*10*		*128*	
Sex with person with hemophilia	*2*		—		—		*2*		*2*		*2*		*25*	
Sex with transfusion recipient with HIV infection	*3*		—		*2*		*2*		*5*		*2*		*26*	
Sex with HIV-infected person, risk not specified	*96*		*66*		*97*		*68*		*193*		*134*		*731*	
Receipt of blood transfusion, blood components, or tissue	*4*		*2*		*9*		*2*		*13*		*4*		*139*	
Has HIV infection, risk not specified	*130*		*108*		*149*		*145*		*279*		*253*		*1,449*	
Receipt of blood transfusion, blood components, or tissue§	23	(5)	17	(4)	17	(3)	9	(2)	40	(4)	26	(3)	366	(5)
Other/risk not reported or identified‖	9	(2)	20	(5)	14	(3)	19	(5)	23	(2)	39	(5)	99	(1)
Pediatric subtotal	509	(100)	387	(100)	525	(100)	413	(100)	1,034	(100)	800	(100)	6,948	(100)
Total	**65,484**		**60,003**		**14,412**		**14,177**		**79,897**		**74,180**		**513,486**	

*See Technical Notes for a discussion of the impact of the 1993 AIDS surveillance case definition for adults and adolescents (implemented January 1, 1993) on the number of cases reported annually since 1993.

†Includes 1 person whose sex is unknown.

‡Includes 9 persons known to be infected with human immunodeficiency virus type (HIV-2). See *MMWR* 1995;44:603–606.

§Thirty-three adults/adolescents and 2 children developed AIDS after receiving blood screened negative for HIV antibody. Ten additional adults developed AIDS after receiving tissue, organs, or artificial insemination from HIV-infected donors. Three of the 10 received tissue, organs, or artificial insemination from a donor who was negative for HIV antibody at the time of donation. See *N Engl J Med* 1992;326:726–732.

‖See Table 16 and Figure 7 for a discussion of the "other" exposure category. "Other" also includes 29 persons who acquired HIV infection perinatally but were diagnosed with AIDS after age 13. These 29 persons are tabulated under the adult/adolescent, not pediatric, exposure category.

From Centers for Disease Control and Prevention. (1995). *HIV/AIDS Surveillance Report, 1995* 7(2), 23.

TABLE 16–4 **Principles of Universal Precautions to Prevent Transmission of HIV and Hepatitis B Virus**

1. Assume that all patients are infectious for HIV and other bloodborne pathogens.
2. Be immunized for hepatitis B virus.
3. Wash hands frequently.
4. Use protective barriers to prevent percutaneous exposure to blood and other potentially hazardous body fluids.
5. Properly disinfect work areas, equipment, and clothing.
6. Properly dispose of contaminated waste.
7. Document exposure and report to employer, who is required to report occupational injuries to the federal government.

From Centers for Disease Control and Prevention. (1989). Guidelines for prevention of transmission of human immunodeficiency virus and hepatitis B virus to health-care and public-safety workers. *Morbidity and Mortality Weekly Report 38*(S-6).

or through breastfeeding. According to the CDC (1995e), between 1989 and 1992 approximately 7,000 HIV-infected women gave birth annually. Estimates on HIV transmission from the mother to the infant range from 13 to 40%; thus, between 1,000 and 2,000 HIV-infected infants are born each year. Urban areas, particularly in the Northeast, have the greatest incidence of perinatal infection.

Clinical trials have shown that administration of ZDV during pregnancy, labor, and delivery, as well as to the exposed newborns, reduces the risk of HIV transmission by approximately two thirds. In response to this evidence, in 1995 the U.S. Public Health Service outlined guidelines for counseling and testing of all pregnant women for HIV (CDC, 1995e).

All nurses who care for pregnant women in ambulatory care settings should be aware of these recommendations and encourage testing. Resources for referral or a plan of care for those women identified as HIV-positive should be determined in advance and should include a simple system for care, long-term management, and follow-up. Table 16–6 presents the recommendations and guidelines for counseling and testing of pregnant women.

HIV Infection

CLINICAL MANIFESTATIONS

Following initial infection by HIV, the individual may experience flulike symptoms including fever, nausea, fatigue, lymphadenopathy, headache, diarrhea, and myalgia (Casey, 1995). Following recovery of the initial infection, the HIV-positive individual will usually remain symptom-free for an extended period (median 10 years), during which HIV antibodies can be detected, and a continual decline in $CD4^+$ T-cell counts is seen. As HIV infection progresses, associated symptoms increase and progress until the individual develops full-blown AIDS. In 1993, the CDC established a system for categorization of HIV infection in adults and adolescents (13+ years) to include $CD4^+$ T-lymphocyte counts as a marker for HIV immunosuppression. The three $CD4^+$ T-lymphocyte categories are as follows:

- Category 1: $\geq$500 cell/μL
- Category 2: 200–4,999 cells/μL
- Category 3: $\leq$200 cells/μL

To simplify the classification of infection and to direct medical care for those infected, the categories or stages of infection are as follows:

- Category A—Asymptomatic HIV infection and persistent generalized lymphadenopathy, or acute (primary) HIV infection with accompanying illness
- Category B—Symptomatic conditions in an HIV-infected person with symptoms or conditions related to the infection such as bacillary angiomatosis, oral candidiasis (thrush), persistent vaginal candidiasis, cervical dysplasia/cervical carcinoma in situ, constitutional symptoms such as fever or diarrhea lasting more than 1 month, leukoplakia, herpes zoster (shingles), idiopathic thrombocytopenia purpura, listeriosis, pelvic inflammatory disease, and peripheral neuropathy

TABLE 16–5 **Body Fluids that Do and Do Not Require Universal Precautions to Prevent Transmission of HIV and Hepatitis B Virus**

Fluids that Require Precautions

Blood
Semen
Vaginal secretions
Amniotic fluid
Pericardial fluid
Peritoneal fluid
Pleural fluid
Synovial fluid
Cerebrospinal fluid
Any body fluid visibly contaminated with blood

Fluids that Do Not Require Precautions*

Feces
Nasal secretions
Sputum
Sweat
Tears
Urine
Vomitus

Other Body Fluids that May Require Precautions in Special Settings†

Human breast milk
Saliva (except in dentistry, where precautions apply due to potential for blood contamination)

*Unless they contain visible blood.
†General infection control suggests use of gloves may be appropriate, and handwashing after exposure is recommended.
From Centers for Disease Control. (1988). Update: Universal precautions for prevention of transmission of HIV, HBV and other bloodborne pathogens in health-care settings. *Morbidity and Mortality Weekly Report 37*(24), 377–388.

- Category C—HIV infection and the presence of any of the clinical conditions listed in Table 16–7

CASE DEFINITION

In 1986, the CDC published case definition guidelines for diagnoses of AIDS, and this Case Definition was revised in 1993 (CDC, 1992). Awareness of this change is important when reviewing statistical information on AIDS, as the substantial increase in the number of diagnosed cases of AIDS between 1992 and 1993 was largely due to a change in the official case definition of AIDS. Beginning in December 1992, cervical cancer, tuberculosis, recurrent pneumonia, and severely compromised immune system, as evidenced by severely decreased $CD4^+$ T-lymphocyte counts, were included in the Case Definition.

With regard to T-lymphocyte counts, the revised classification system defines AIDS cases to include "all HIV-infected persons who have <200 $CD4^+$ T-lymphocytes/microL, or a $CD4^+$ T-lymphocyte percentage of total lymphocytes of <14" (CDC, 1992, p. 1). In addition to the T-cell counts above, Table 17–7 contains the identified conditions for definitive diagnosis of AIDS in HIV-positive individuals.

Due to differences in clinical characteristics of AIDS in children, a separate classification system for identification and diagnosis of HIV infections

TABLE 16–6 **Recommendations for HIV Counseling and Testing for Pregnant Women**

HIV Counseling and Voluntary Testing of Pregnant Women and Their Infants

All pregnant women should be counseled and encouraged to be tested for HIV infection to allow them to know their infection status for their own health and then reduce the risk for perinatal HIV transmission.

HIV testing of pregnant women and their infants should be voluntary. Consent for testing should be obtained in accordance with prevailing legal requirements. Women who test positive for HIV or who refuse testing should not be denied prenatal or other health care services or reported to child protective services or discriminated against in any other way.

Health care providers should counsel and offer HIV testing to women as early in pregnancy as possible.

Uninfected pregnant women who continue to practice high-risk behaviors (e.g., injecting-drug use, unprotected sexual contact with an HIV-infected or high-risk partner) should be encouraged to avoid further exposure to HIV and retested during the third trimester of pregnancy.

Women who have not received prenatal care are at higher risk for HIV infection and should be assessed as soon as possible. For women whose HIV infection status has not been determined, HIV counseling should be provided and testing should be offered as soon as the mother's condition permits. If the mother is identified as being HIV-infected during labor and delivery, health care providers should consider offering intrapartum and neonatal ZDV.

Pregnant women should be provided access to other HIV prevention and treatment services (e.g., drug-treatment and partner-notification services) as needed.

Interpretation of HIV Test Results

HIV antibody testing should be performed, including use of an enzyme immunoassay (EIA) to test for antibody to HIV and confirmatory testing with an additional, more specific assay (e.g., Western blot technique or immunofluorescence assay).

HIV infection is defined as a repeatedly reactive EIA and a positive confirmatory supplemental test.

Pregnant women who have repeatedly reactive EIAs and indeterminate supplemental tests should be retested immediately for HIV antibody to distinguish between recent seroconversion and a negative test result. Additional tests to diagnose or exclude HIV infection may be required.

Women who have negative EIA results and those who have repeatedly reactive EIAs but negative supplemental test results should be considered uninfected.

Recommendations for HIV-Infected Pregnant Women

HIV-infected pregnant women should receive counseling, including explanation of the clinical implications of a positive HIV test result and the need for, benefit of, and means of access to HIV-related early intervention services. The risk of perinatal HIV transmission, ways to reduce the risk, and the prognosis for infants who become infected should be discussed.

HIV-infected pregnant women should be evaluated according to published recommendations to assess their need for antiretroviral therapy, antimicrobial prophylaxis, and treatment of other conditions. Evaluation of the need for psychological and social services should also be determined.

HIV-infected pregnant women should be provided information concerning ZDV therapy for reducing the risk of perinatal HIV transmission, including the potential benefit and short-term safety for ZDV, the uncertainties regarding long-term risks of such therapy, and the effectiveness in women who have different clinical characteristics than women who participated in the trials. HIV-infected pregnant women should not be coerced into making decisions about ZDV therapy, and a woman's decision not to accept treatment should not result in punitive action or denial of care. Therapy should be offered according to appropriate regimen in published recommendations.

HIV-infected pregnant women should receive information about all reproductive options, and health care providers should be supportive of any decision.

HIV-infected women should be advised against breastfeeding to reduce the risk of HIV transmission to the infant.

Positive and negative HIV test results should be available to the woman's health care provider and included on both her and her infant's confidential medical records. After obtaining consent, maternal health care providers should notify the pediatric care providers of the impending birth of an HIV-exposed child, anticipated complications, and whether ZDV should be administered after birth.

TABLE 16–6 **Recommendations for HIV Counseling and Testing for Pregnant Women** *Continued*

Recommendations for HIV-Infected Pregnant Women *Continued*

Counseling for HIV-infected pregnant women should include an assessment of the potential for negative effects resulting from HIV infection (e.g., discrimination, domestic violence, and psychological difficulties). If anticipated or identified, counseling should include information on how to minimize these consequences and assistance in identifying supportive persons or referral to appropriate psychological, social, and legal services. HIV-infected women should be informed that discrimination based on HIV status or AIDS regarding matters such as housing, employment, state programs, and public accommodations is illegal.

HIV-infected women should be encouraged to obtain HIV testing for any of their children born after they became infected or, if they do not know when they became infected, for children born after 1977.

Recommendations for Follow-Up of Infected Women and Perinatally Exposed Children

Following pregnancy, HIV-infected women should be provided ongoing HIV-related medical care, including immune function monitoring, antiretroviral therapy, and prophylaxis for and treatment of opportunistic infections and other HIV-related conditions. Gynecological care should include regular Pap smears, reproductive counseling, information on how to prevent sexual transmission of HIV, and treatment of gynecological conditions.

HIV-infected women (or the guardians of their children) should be informed of the importance of follow-up care for their children. The children should receive follow-up care to determine their infection status, initiate prophylactic therapy to prevent PCP and other prophylactic therapies, and monitor disorders in growth and development. HIV-infected children and other children living in the household with HIV-infected persons should be vaccinated according to published recommendations for altered schedules.

Referrals should be provided for medical and social services for the HIV-infected mother and the family as appropriate.

Adapted from Centers for Disease Control and Prevention. (1995). U. S. Public Health Service recommendations for HIV counseling and voluntary testing for pregnant women. *Morbidity and Mortality Weekly Report 44* (RR-7).

was deemed necessary, and in 1994 a revised system was enacted (CDC, 1994b). Table 16–8 illustrates the process of diagnosis of HIV infection in children born to HIV-infected mothers. Designated clinical categories for HIV-positive children, based on severity of symptoms and diagnosis of opportunistic infections or related conditions, are included in Table 16–9.

HIV COUNSELING AND TESTING

"Early knowledge of HIV infection allows infected individuals to seek early treatment, which has been shown to delay the onset of AIDS, and to change high-risk behavior that could contribute to disease spread. Counseling and screening are, therefore, essential strategies for preventing the spread of HIV infection and the progression of symptoms" (USDHHS, 1994, p. 214).

Programs for HIV testing and counseling must recognize the complex physical, social, psychological, and economic issues inherent with HIV infection. Because of the many issues involved, in-depth pretest and post-test counseling should be provided by trained health professionals. The issue of confidentiality is one of the most important to the individual. Agencies that provide HIV testing should have and enforce policies regarding confidentiality. Guidelines for HIV screening developed by the U.S. Public Health Service are included in Table 16–10, and important information on pretest and post-test counseling for HIV is contained in Table 16–11.

Disclosure

Individuals who have been determined to be HIV-positive should be counseled regarding disclosing

TABLE 16–7 **Conditions Included in the 1993 AIDS Surveillance Case Definition**

- Candidiasis of bronchi, trachea, or lungs
- Candidiasis, esophageal
- Cervical cancer, invasive*
- Coccidioidomycosis, disseminated or extrapulmonary
- Cryptococcosis, extrapulmonary
- Cryptosporidiosis, chronic intestinal (>1 month's duration)
- Cytomegalovirus disease (other than liver, spleen, or nodes)
- Cytomegalovirus retinitis (with loss of vision)
- Encephalopathy, HIV-related
- Herpes simplex: chronic ulcer(s) (>1 month's duration); or bronchitis, pneumonitis, or esophagitis
- Histoplasmosis, disseminated or extrapulmonary
- Isosporiasis, chronic intestinal (>1 month's duration)
- Kaposi's sarcoma
- Lymphoma, Burkitt's (or equivalent term)
- Lymphoma, immunoblastic (or equivalent term)
- Lymphoma, primary, of brain
- *Mycobacterium avium* complex or *M. kansasii,* disseminated or extrapulmonary
- *Mycobacterium tuberculosis,* any site (pulmonary* or extrapulmonary)
- *Mycobacterium,* other species or unidentified species, disseminated or extrapulmonary
- *Pneumocystis carinii* pneumonia
- Pneumonia, recurrent*
- Progressive multifocal leukoencephalopathy
- *Salmonella* septicemia, recurrent
- Toxoplasmosis of brain
- Wasting syndrome due to HIV

*Added in the 1993 expansion of the AIDS surveillance case definition.

From Centers for Disease Control. (1992). 1993 revised classification system for HIV infection and expanded surveillance case definition for AIDS among adolescents and adults. *Morbidity and Mortality Weekly Report 41* (RR-17).

their HIV status to others. They should understand that disclosure to significant others may result in increased social support and encourage others to be tested also. On the other hand, disclosure may result in housing discrimination, loss of employment or of child custody, reduction or cessation of health benefits, or rejection by friends or significant others (USDHHS/AHCPR, 1994).

In addition, health care providers should know their state's HIV reporting requirements and educate patients about them. Currently, all states and the District of Columbia require reporting of patients meeting the CDC's surveillance case definition of AIDS, and providers are responsible for giving their patients information on mandatory or voluntary HIV reporting requirements. Even in states without mandatory reporting of HIV, the provider should inform the patient that once AIDS is diagnosed, the patient must be reported to the state health department. The provider is responsible for setting procedures for reporting based on state requirements. Also, "whereas State law may require mandatory reporting of HIV status or AIDS diagnosis to public health agencies, there are no legal requirements for providers or agencies to further inform partners or others at risk" (USDHHS/AHCPR, 1994, p. 19). Table 16–12 lists each state's reporting requirements for HIV infection.

MANAGEMENT OF HIV INFECTION

The life expectancy of HIV-infected individuals has grown remarkably in the past several years.

TABLE 16–8 **Diagnosis of HIV Infection* in Children**

Diagnosis: HIV Infected

a) A child <18 months of age who is known to be HIV seropositive or born to an HIV-infected mother **and:**
- has positive results on two separate determinations (excluding cord blood) from one or more of the following HIV detection tests:
  — HIV culture,
  — HIV polymerase chain reaction,
  — HIV antigen,

or

- meets criteria for acquired immunodeficiency syndrome (AIDS) diagnosis based on the 1987 AIDS surveillance case definition.

b) A child ≥18 months of age born to an HIV-infected mother or any child infected by blood, blood products, or other known modes of transmission (e.g., sexual contact) who:
- is HIV-antibody positive by repeatedly reactive enzyme immunoassay (EIA) and confirmatory test (e.g., Western blot or immunofluorescence assay [IFA]);

or

- meets any of the criteria in a) above.

Diagnosis: Perinatally Exposed (Prefix E)

A child who does not meet the criteria above who:
- is HIV-seropositive by EIA and confirmatory test (e.g., Western blot or IFA) and is <18 months of age at the time of test;

or

- has unknown antibody status, but was born to a mother known to be infected with HIV.

Diagnosis: Seroreverter (SR)

A child who is born to an HIV-infected mother and who:
- has been documented as HIV-antibody negative (i.e., two or more negative EIA tests performed at 6–18 months of age or one negative EIA test after 18 months of age);

and

- has had no other laboratory evidence of infection (has not had two positive viral detection tests, if performed);

and

- has not had an AIDS-defining condition.

*This definition of HIV infection replaces the definition published in the 1987 AIDS surveillance case definition.

From Centers for Disease Control and Prevention. (1994). 1994 revised classification system for human immunodeficiency virus infection in children less than 13 years of age. *Morbidity and Mortality Weekly Report 43* (RR-12).

This is largely due to preventative management using antiretroviral medications and prevention of PCP and other opportunistic infections. In addition, encouragement of healthy lifestyles and aggressive treatment of medical complications have proved successful for many people. Further, ongoing research offers opportunities for HIV-positive patients to be a part of the latest treatment options through participation in clinical trials. Finally, care of AIDS patients near the end of their lives necessitates understanding of the course or progression of the illness and methods to help manage complications. Each of these areas will be discussed briefly.

Health Promotion for HIV-Infected Individuals

Health promotion for HIV-infected individuals points to encouraging a lifestyle and behaviors that prevent exposure to pathogens that might

TABLE 16–9 **Clinical Categories for Children with HIV Infection**

Category N: Not Symptomatic

Children who have no signs or symptoms considered to be the result of HIV infection or who have only one of the conditions listed in Category A.

Category A: Mildly Symptomatic

Children with two or more of the conditions listed below but none of the conditions listed in Categories B and C.

- Lymphadenopathy ($\geq$0.5 cm at more than two sites; bilateral = one site)
- Hepatomegaly
- Splenomegaly
- Dermatitis
- Parotitis
- Recurrent or persistent upper respiratory infection, sinusitis, or otitis media

Category B: Moderately Symptomatic

Children who have symptomatic conditions other than those listed for Category A or C that are attributed to HIV infection. Examples of conditions in clinical Category B include but are not limited to:

- Anemia (<8 g/dL), neutropenia (<1,000/mm^3), or thrombocytopenia (<100,000/mm^3) persisting $\geq$30 days
- Bacterial meningitis, pneumonia, or sepsis (single episode)
- Candidiasis, oropharyngeal (thrush), persisting (>2 months) in children >6 months of age
- Cardiomyopathy
- Cytomegalovirus infection, with onset before 1 month of age
- Diarrhea, recurrent or chronic
- Hepatitis
- Herpes simplex virus (HSV) stomatitis, recurrent (more than two episodes within 1 year)
- HSV bronchitis, pneumonitis, or esophagitis with onset before 1 month of age
- Herpes zoster (shingles) involving at least two distinct episodes or more than one dermatome
- Leiomyosarcoma
- Lymphoid interstitial pneumonia (LIP) or pulmonary lymphoid hyperplasia complex
- Nephropathy
- Nocardiosis
- Persistent fever (lasting >1 month)
- Toxoplasmosis, onset before 1 month of age
- Varicella, disseminated (complicated chickenpox)

Category C: Severely Symptomatic

Children who have any condition listed in the 1987 surveillance case definition for acquired immunodeficiency syndrome, with the exception of LIP.

From Centers for Disease Control and Prevention. (1994). 1994 revised classification system for human immunodeficiency virus infection in children less than 13 years of age. *Morbidity and Mortality Weekly Report 43* (RR-12).

TABLE 16–10 **Basics of HIV Screening**

1. Serologic testing for the presence of antibodies to HIV-1 is the standard method of screening for HIV disease.
2. Enzyme immunoassay (EIA) is the most widely used screening test for HIV-1 infection. Because any screening test can result in a false-positive reaction, it is necessary to validate positive results by confirmatory testing. This is usually accomplished using Western blot tests.
3. A single specimen is tested first by EIA. If the test result is positive (reactive), multiple samples from the initial specimen are retested. If at least two of three retests are reactive, the specimen is considered repeatedly reactive and must be verified with a supplemental test such as the Western blot.
4. The percentage of repeatedly reactive samples found positive with additional testing varies according to the true antibody prevalence in the tested population. Testing of the repeatedly reactive EIAs with Western blot produces predictive values nearing 100%.
5. After infection with HIV-1, antibodies to the virus develop. The interval between infection and seroconversion is called the "window period." Although there have been reports of delayed antibody response to HIV-1 infection, 95% or more of infected persons seroconvert within 6 months. Individuals whose test results are negative should be reminded that, despite their negative test results, they may be infected. They should be counseled to stop all high-risk behaviors and return for retesting in 6 months or earlier to make sure they have not converted to a positive test result. Patients who continue practicing high-risk behavior should be counseled and retested periodically.
6. HIV screening must always include pretest and post-test counseling. Individualized client-centered counseling is recommended. Specially trained clinicians or counselors should provide clients with accurate, clear, understandable information regarding HIV testing at both pretest and post-test counseling sessions.

Adapted from U. S. Department of Health and Human Services. (1994). *Clinician's Handbook of Preventive Services.* Washington, D. C., Government Printing Office.

cause symptoms as well as taking measures to enhance the body's ability to fight infection. Flaskerud (1995, pp. 36–38) describes basic health promotion strategies for HIV-infected individuals. These include the following:

Nutrition To prevent disease progression, HIV-infected individuals should be encouraged to eat a diet that consists of a variety of foods composed of 50–55% carbohydrates, 15–20% protein, and 30% or less from fat. Vitamin C and vitamin A–rich fruits and vegetables are encouraged. The addition of a multivitamin-mineral supplement containing vitamins A, B, and E, beta-carotene, zinc, selenium, and niacin may enhance immune response. However, patients should note that megadoses of vitamins and minerals might be harmful.

Exercise Regular physical exercise has been shown to be beneficial by increasing lung capacity, muscle strength, endurance, and energy. Exercise also improves sleeping, appetite, and regular bowel activity and decreases stress. An exercise program of 30–45 minutes, 4 or more days per week, is recommended.

Stress Excess stress has been associated with immunosuppression and may increase vulnerability to disease; therefore, efforts to minimize or eliminate stress should be encouraged in HIV-positive individuals. Stress reduction activities and techniques include engaging in regular exercise, ensuring adequate rest, taking part in recreational activities, and encouraging emotional expression. Joining a support group or stress reduction program may be helpful.

Recreational Drug Use The use of chemical stimulants and depressants, including tobacco, alcohol, marijuana, cocaine, and other substances, are associated with a number of physical and mental health problems. They may suppress appetite, irritate the gastrointestinal tract, inhibit food absorption, and damage the liver; therefore, they should be discouraged.

TABLE 16–11 **Pretest and Post-Test Information for HIV Testing**

Counseling should include a review of the risk factors for acquiring HIV infection along with a focused and tailored risk assessment

Counselors should review strategies for HIV prevention and assist the client in developing a plan to reduce his/her risk of HIV infection or transmission. This plan should include the following:

- Advice on abstinence, "safer sex" practices, and "safer" drug use
- Information on drug treatment programs
- Provision of condoms and bleach
- Information on pregnancy, breastfeeding, and infant immunization
- General health promotion information
- Review of potential psychological and emotional reaction to test results
- Information on medical, social, and psychiatric resources and follow-up
- Counseling

Clients should understand the difference between a positive test result for antibodies to HIV and clinical AIDS. The median duration between development of HIV antibodies and onset of clinical disease is approximately 10 years. Detection of antibodies can occur at any time between development of antibodies and clinical disease.

All clients must be informed that a negative antibody test result does not conclusively exclude the possibility of HIV infection. Typically, it takes 3 to 6 months following infection before the test (enzyme-linked immunosorbent assay) reliably detects HIV antibodies; it is important to inform the client that a false-negative test may occur during this early period.

The importance of post-test counseling should be stressed. At the completion of the initial post-test counseling session, the counselor should assess the client's need for additional sessions. Post-test counseling for persons with negative results should include the following:

- Interpretation of the test results
- Review of safer sex and drug-use practices
- Provision of condoms and bleach or information on needle-exchange programs if applicable
- Information on how to maintain a negative test-result status
- Referral for psychological, social, medical, and psychiatric services and drug rehabilitation programs as needed
- Assessment of whether further post-test counseling is needed
- Retesting every 6 to 12 months for high-risk patients, particularly if they continue to engage in high-risk behavior

Post-test counseling for persons with seropositive test results should include the following:

- Interpretation of the results (including the information that the person does not have AIDS)
- Evaluation for suicide potential
- Crisis intervention counseling as needed
- Discussion of follow-up for partners and children
- Referral to a partner notification program if needed
- Review of information on transmission, safer sex and drug-use practices
- Information on pregnancy and perinatal transmission
- Information on symptoms associated with HIV disease
- Referral to an early intervention program
- Referral to an appropriate support group
- Referral for medical follow-up
- Referral to a drug rehabilitation program if appropriate
- Information on entering clinical trials
- Referral for psychological, social, and psychiatric services as appropriate
- Discussion of potential discrimination in housing, employment, and insurance
- Assessment of whether further post-test counseling is needed

Adapted from U. S. Department of Health and Human Services. (1994). *Clinician's Handbook of Preventive Services.* Washington, D. C., Government Printing Office; Flaskerud, J. H. (1995). Health promotion and disease prevention. In Flaskerud, J. H., and Ungvarski, P. J. (Eds.). *HIV/AIDS: A Guide to Nursing Care* (3rd ed.). Philadelphia, W. B. Saunders. (Source: *Global AIDS News.* 1993. 1[4]); Centers for Disease Control. (1993). Recommendations for HIV testing services of inpatients and outpatients in acute-care hospital settings and technical guidance on HIV counseling. *Morbidity and Mortality Weekly Report 42.*

TABLE 16–12 Reporting Requirements for Human Immunodeficiency Virus (HIV) Infection

By Name	Anonymous	Not Required
Alabama	Georgia	Alaska
Arizona	Illinois*	California
Arkansas	Iowa	Connecticut
Colorado	Kansas	Delaware
Idaho	Kentucky	Florida
Indiana	Montana	Hawaii
Michigan	Maine	Louisiana
Minnesota	New Hampshire	Maryland‡
Mississippi	Oregon	Massachusetts
Missouri	Rhode Island	Nebraska
Nevada	Texas	New Mexico
New Jersey†		New York
North Carolina		Pennsylvania
North Dakota		Vermont
Ohio		Washington‡
Oklahoma		District of Columbia
South Carolina		
South Dakota		
Tennessee†		
Utah		
Virginia		
West Virginia		
Wisconsin		
Wyoming		

*With the exception of HIV-infected school-aged children, whose names must be reported confidentially to their school principals.

†Implementation date, January, 1992.

‡Requires reports of symptomatic HIV infection by name.

Note: Current as of March 1, 1993. All States require reporting of acquired immunodeficiency syndrome (AIDS) cases by name at the State/local level.

From U. S. Department of Health and Human Services/Agency for Health Care Policy and Research. (1994). *Clinical Practice Guidelines: Evaluation and Management of Early HIV Infection.* Rockville, MD.

Clinical Management of Early HIV Infection

In 1994, the Department of Health and Human Services developed clinical practice guidelines for managing HIV infection (USDHHS/AHCPR, 1994). Table 16–13 provides an overview of the guidelines for monitoring CD4 lymphocytes and initiating antiretroviral therapy and PCP prophylaxis and testing and treatment for tuberculosis. Tables 16–14, 16–15, and 16–16 contain information on antiretroviral therapy, PCP prophylaxis, and tuberculosis prevention, respectively. For more detailed information on management of HIV infection, the reader is referred to the *Clinical Practice Guidelines for Evaluation and Management of Early HIV Infection,* which is available at no charge from the National AIDS Clearinghouse (see Table 16–19).

Management of Intermediate and Advanced AIDS

The progression of HIV infection to AIDS is indicated by the development of one or more of a variety of opportunistic infections and related conditions (e.g., KS, non–Hodgkin's lymphoma, cervical dysplasia listed in the Case Definition—Table 17–7). Diagnosis and treatment of these conditions, and interventions to stop further progression of the disease, become the greatest concern as the individual progresses from HIV infection to AIDS. Table 16–17 presents some of the opportunistic infections and conditions commonly found in HIV-positive individuals and describes prevention and treatment recommendations.

AIDS Clinical Trials

An AIDS clinical trial is a study conducted to help find effective therapies to treat people infected with HIV. Controlled studies for AIDS research, or clinical trials for AIDS, have been extremely beneficial for AIDS patients. For example, during an AIDS clinical trial, it was discovered that ZDV, when given early in HIV infection, may help delay the onset of symptoms, or when given to pregnant women will help prevent transmission to the baby.

AIDS clinical trials are directed cooperatively by the National Institute of Allergy and Infectious Diseases (NIAID), the Food and Drug Administration (FDA), the National Library of Medicine, and the CDC. The NIAID is responsible for funding AIDS clinical trials and assists in enrolling patients in appropriate studies. The FDA is the agency that grants permission to pharmaceutical

TABLE 16–13 **Guidelines for Management of Early HIV Infection**

Monitoring CD4 Lymphocytes and Initiating Antiretroviral Therapy and PCP Prophylaxis

CD4 lymphocyte count is a laboratory evaluation of immune function. The HIV-positive individual's immune status should be determined as part of the initial evaluation and every 6 months if the CD4 count is greater than 600 cells/μL and every 3 months when the CD4 count is 200–600 cells, and at least every 3 months if <200.

If CD4 counts are greater than 500 cells/μL, antiretroviral therapy with zidovudine (ZDV [AZT]) should be offered to all asymptomatic HIV-infected individuals with CD4 counts less than 500 cells/μL. (Decisions regarding immediate initiation or deferral of treatment should be made jointly by the provider and patient following a discussion of risks and benefits.)

HIV-infected individuals who do not tolerate ZDV should be offered therapy with didanosine (ddI) or dideoxycytidine (ddC). Individuals whose disease progresses while receiving ZDV should be offered monotherapy with either ddI or ddC or combination therapy of ZDV with either ddI or ddC.

HIV-infected individuals receiving ZDV may benefit from a change to ddI. Combination therapy of ZDV with either ddI or ddC may provide another option. These options should be discussed with and offered to patients.

Prophylaxis for PCP should be initiated if (1) the CD4 cell count is <200 or (2) there has been a prior episode of PCP and/or (3) oral candidiasis or constitutional symptoms such as unexplained fevers are present. (Oral trimethoprim-sulfamethoxazole (TMP-SMX) is the preferred agent for PCP prophylaxis.)

Other effective prophylactic agents include aerosolized pentamidine, oral dapsone, and a combination of oral dapsone and pyrimethamine. Consider advantages and disadvantages in determining which to use.

Recommendations for Pregnant Adults and Adolescents

In HIV-infected pregnant women, CD4 counts should be determined at the time of presentation for prenatal care or at the time of delivery if the woman has received no prenatal care.

If the count is 600 cells/μL or above, it does not need to be repeated unless indicated by clinical symptoms. If the count is 200 cells/μL or less, it does not need to be repeated during the pregnancy. If the count is 200–600, it should be repeated each trimester.

Providers should inform HIV-infected pregnant women of the benefits of early ZDV therapy and potential for risk to the mother and fetus. If CD4 counts are less than 500 cells/μL, ZDV therapy should be considered.

HIV-infected pregnant women should receive PCP prophylaxis according to the same guidelines used for other adults.

Testing and Preventive Therapy for Tuberculosis Infection

The health history for all HIV-infected individuals should include assessment of previous TB infection or disease, past treatment or preventive therapy, and history of exposure; assessment of the risk for TB infection, including predisposing social conditions and suggestive symptoms (e.g., cough, hemoptysis, fever, night sweats, weight loss).

The health history for HIV-infected individuals should include an assessment of health and social conditions that may affect their ability to complete therapy (e.g., failure to keep medical appointments, alcoholism, mental illness, and substance use).

All HIV-infected individuals should be screened using purified protein derivative (PPD) during their initial evaluation. The Mantoux method, with an intradermal injection of 0.1 mL 5 tuberculin unit PPD should be used. Reactions should be assessed 48–72 hours after injection, and reactions of 5 mm or greater induration should be considered positive in persons with HIV infection.

Concurrent testing for anergy using control antigens (*Candida,* mumps, or tetanus) should be done. Any degree of induration in response to intradermal injection of these antigens constitutes a positive reaction and indicates that the individual is not anergic.

All HIV-infected individuals who are PPD-positive or anergic should receive a chest x-ray and clinical evaluation.

PPD testing should be repeated annually in persons who are not PPD-positive; retesting every 6 months is recommended for persons who reside in areas where TB prevalence is high.

All PPD-negative HIV-infected individuals who have been exposed to persons with suspected or confirmed TB should be tested with PPD and retested in 3 months.

Chest x-rays should be obtained to exclude the presence of active TB in all HIV-infected individuals who are PPD-positive or anergic or have symptoms of TB. If the chest x-ray reveals abnormality, multiple sputum smears and cultures should be performed. If sputum smears are positive the patient should be started on anti-TB therapy immediately.

Preventive therapy for TB should include isoniazid (INH) for 12 months in HIV-infected individuals who have a positive PPD but do not have active disease; preventive therapy should be considered for anergic patients who are known contacts of patients with TB and for anergic patients belonging to groups in which the prevalence of TB infection is 10% or higher (i.e., injection drug users, prisoners, homeless persons, persons living in congregate housing, migrant laborers, and persons born in countries where rates of TB are high).

HIV-infected individuals exposed to drug-resistant strains of TB should consult a pulmonary or infectious disease specialist.

From U. S. Department of Health and Human Services/Agency for Health Care Policy and Research. (1994). *Clinical Practice Guidelines: Evaluation and Management of Early HIV Infection.* Rockville, MD.

TABLE 16–14 **Drug* Dosage and Adverse Effects; Antiretroviral Therapy†**

Medication	Dosage: Adult/Tanner Stage IV and V Adolescents‡	Dosage: Infants/ Children/Tanner Stage I and II Adolescents‡	Adverse Effects§
Zidovudine (ZDV) formerly azidothymidine (AZT) Retrovir Formulation: 100 mg capsules Pediatric syrup 50 mg/5 mL	100 mg/dose administered orally every 4 hours or 5 doses given 7 days/week	180 mg/m^2 dose administered orally every 6 hours given 7 days/week	Granulocytopenia Anemia Nausea Headache Confusion Myositis Anorexia Hepatitis Seizures Nail discoloration
Didanosine (ddI) (dideoxyinosine) Videx Formulation: 25, 50, 100, 150 mg tablets Pediatric powder for oral solution 10 mg/mL	Patients under 45 kg: 100 mg/dose orally given every 12 hours 7 days/ week Patients over 45 kg: 200 mg/ dose administered orally every 12 hours given 7 days/week (Tablet should be chewed and taken on an empty stomach)	200 mg/m^2/day administered orally every 12 hours given 7 days per week	Pancreatitis, potentially fatal Peripheral neuropathy Peripheral retinal atrophy (in children only) Nausea Diarrhea Confusion Seizures
Zalcitabine (ddC) (dideoxycytidine) Formulation: 0.375 mg tablets 0.750 mg tablets Pediatric 0.1 mg/mL syrup	Patients under 45 kg: 0.375 mg/dose administered orally every 8 hours given 7 days/week Patients over 45 kg: 0.750 mg dose administered orally every 8 hours given 7 days/week	0.005–0.01 mg/kg/dose administered orally every 8 hours given 7 days/week	Aphthous ulcers Esophageal ulcers Peripheral neuropathy Stomatitis Cutaneous eruptions Thrombocytopenia Pancreatitis

*Contains only drugs discussed or recommended in the *Clinical Practice Guidelines: Evaluation and Management of Early HIV Infection.* Not all drugs or combinations of drugs used in the care of HIV-infected individuals are included.

†Dosage schedules and recommendations for use are based on review of literature or expert consensus and may not have approval of the Food and Drug Administration (FDA) for indications noted. Information included in this guideline may not represent FDA approval or FDA-approved labeling for the particular products or indications in question. Specifically, the terms "safe" and "effective" may not be synonymous with the FDA-defined legal standard for product approval.

‡For adolescents who are Tanner stage I or II, pediatric dose schedules should be followed. Adult doses should be used for adolescents who are Tanner stage IV or V. Tanner stage III adolescents should have dose individualized, recognizing that this is the stage of most rapid growth.

§For a complete list of adverse reactions to these drugs, consult the *Physicians' Desk Reference* (Medical Economics Data, Montvale, NJ, 1993) or the drug's package insert.

From U. S. Department of Health and Human Services/Agency for Health Care Policy and Research. (1994). *Clinical Practice Guidelines: Evaluation and Management of Early HIV Infection.* Rockville, MD.

TABLE 16–15 **Drug Dosage and Adverse Effects: *Pneumocystis carinii* Pneumonia Prophylaxis*†**

Medication	Dosage: Adult/Tanner Stage IV and V Adolescents‡	Dosage: Infants/Children/Tanner Stage I and II Adolescents‡	Adverse Effects§
Trimethoprim-Sulfamethoxazole (TMP-SMX) Bactrim Septra Formulations: Single-strength tablet: 80 mg TMP 400 mg SMX Double-strength tablet: 160 mg TMP 800 mg SMX Pediatric suspension: (per 5 mL) 40 mg TMP 200 mg SMX	Most commonly used regimens: one double-strength tablet taken orally three times per week on alternate days or daily 7 days per week	150 mg/m² TMP 750 mg/m² SMX Total oral daily dose given 3 times/week Can be divided into two doses or administered as a single daily dose and given on 3 consecutive or 3 alternate days per week This same oral daily dose divided into 2 doses can be given 7 days per week	Drug allergy: Skin rash Steven-Johnson syndrome Fever Arthralgia Toxic epidermal necrolysis Hematologic: Anemia Neutropenia Thrombocytopenia Gastrointestinal: Elevation of serum transaminase Nausea Vomiting Anorexia Fulminant hepatic necrosis (rare)
Pentamidine Isethionate NebuPent 300 mg The vial must be dissolved in 6 mL sterile water and used with Respirguard nebulizer	Aerosolized pentamidine (AP) (NebuPent) is given as single 300 mg (one vial) dose every 4 weeks. Nebulized dose given over 30–45 min at a flow rate of 5–9 liters/min from a 40–50 lb per square inch air or oxygen source Alternative: if a Fisons ultrasonic nebulizer is used, dose of pentamidine is 60 mg given every 2 weeks after a loading dose of five treatments given over 2 weeks	Children over 5 years can receive same inhalation dose as adults	Pulmonary: Bronchospasm with cough Pneumothorax Other: Extrapulmonary *P. carinii* infection Increased risk of environmental transmission of *M. tuberculosis*
Dapsone Formulation: 25 and 100 mg tablets	50–100 mg per day oral dose divided into two doses or administered as a single dose given 2–7 days per week	1 mg/kg administered orally as a single daily dose given 7 days per week	Hematologic: Agranulocytosis Aplastic anemia Hemolytic anemia in G6PD deficiency Methemoglobinemia Cutaneous reactions: Bullous and exfoliative dermatitis Erythema nodosum Erythema multiforme Peripheral neuropathy Gastrointestinal: Nausea Vomiting

*Contains only drugs discussed or recommended in *Clinical Practice Guidelines: Evaluation and Management of Early HIV Infection.* Not all drugs or combinations of drugs used in the care of HIV-infected individuals are included.

†Dosage schedules and recommendations for use are based on review of literature or expert consensus and may not have approval of the Food and Drug Administration (FDA) for indications noted. Information included in this guideline may not represent FDA approval or FDA-approved labeling for the particular products or indications in question. Specifically, the terms "safe" and "effective" may not be synonymous with the FDA-defined legal standard for product approval.

‡For adolescents who are Tanner stage I or II, pediatric dose schedules should be followed. Adults doses should be used for adolescents who are Tanner stage IV or V. Tanner stage III adolescents should have dose individualized, recognizing that this is the stage of most rapid growth.

§For a complete list of adverse reactions to these drugs, consult the *Physicians' Desk Reference* (Medical Economics Data, Montvale, NJ, 1993) or the drug's package insert.

From U. S. Department of Health and Human Services/Agency for Health Care Policy and Research. (1994). *Clinical Practice Guidelines: Evaluation and Management of Early HIV Infection.* Rockville, MD.

TABLE 16–16 **Drug* Dosage and Adverse Effects; Preventive Therapy (Chemoprophylaxis) for *Mycobacterium tuberculosis*†**

Medication	Dosage: Adult/Tanner Stage IV and V Adolescents‡	Dosage: Infants/Children/Tanner Stage I and II Adolescents‡	Adverse Effects§
Isoniazid INHR Nydrazid Formulation: 50 mg, 100 mg, 300 mg tablets 1 gram vial Syrup 50 mg/5mL	300 mg administered orally as a single daily dose given 7 days/week for 12 mo or 900 mg administered orally as a single daily dose given 2 days/week for 12 months	10–15 mg/kg/day (max 300 mg/day) administered orally as a single daily dose given 7 days/week for 12 months	Gastrointestinal: Hepatotoxicity (rare in children) Nausea, vomiting, anorexia Neurologic: Peripheral neuropathy Neuritis, fatigue Weakness Hematologic: Agranulocytosis Hemolytic and aplastic anemia Thrombocytopenia Eosinophilia Drug allergy: Skin rash Fever Lymphadenopathy and vasculitis (SLE-like syndrome)

*Contains only drugs discussed or recommended in the *Clinical Practice Guidelines: Evaluation and Management of Early HIV Infection.* Not all drugs or combinations of drugs used in the care of HIV-infected individuals are included.

†Dosage schedules and recommendations for use are based on review of literature or expert consensus and may not have approval of the Food and Drug Administration (FDA) for indications noted. Information included in this guideline may not represent FDA approval or FDA-approved labeling for the particular products or indications in question. Specifically, the terms "safe" and "effective" may not be synonymous with the FDA-defined legal standard for product approval.

‡For adolescents who are Tanner stage I or II, pediatric dose schedules should be followed. Adult doses should be used for adolescents who are Tanner stage IV or V. Tanner stage III adolescents should have dose individualized, recognizing that this is the stage of most rapid growth.

§For a complete list of adverse reactions to these drugs, consult the *Physicians' Desk Reference* (Medical Economics Data, Montvale, NJ, 1993) or the drug's package insert.

From U. S. Department of Health and Human Services/Agency for Health Care Policy and Research. (1994). *Clinical Practice Guidelines: Evaluation and Management of Early HIV Infection.* Rockville, MD.

companies to test experimental drugs and products in humans and that monitors the progress of the trials and reviews the results. All experimental treatments undergoing clinical testing in treating AIDS or HIV-related conditions must be approved by the FDA. The National Library of Medicine makes information available through on-line services, and the CDC operates the AIDS Clinical Trials Information Service.

Patients choose to take part in clinical trials for many reasons (e.g., live longer, feel better, or help find a cure). A trial may be designed to test a new drug or dosage of an approved drug; test drugs in combination; or test a new use of an existing drug. Types of drugs tested in clinical trials include (1) antiretroviral drugs to help prevent or delay the onset of AIDS (e.g., ZDV, foscarnet, dideoxycytidine), (2) treatments that may strengthen the im-

Text continued on page 527

TABLE 16–17 **Prevention and Management of Opportunistic Infections and Related Conditions in HIV-Infected Persons**

Disease/ Conditions	Epidemiology	Prevention	Signs/Symptoms/ Indications	Management/ Treatment
Candidiasis: **Candida albicans**	*Candida* infections occur in 75–90% of HIV patients; oropharyngeal candidiasis most frequently encountered. Vulvovaginal candidiasis is also common.	Prevention of oral *Candida* infections includes routine oral hygiene and detection of early signs/symptoms of infection.	*Thrush:* white or yellowish patches surrounded by an erythematous base on the buccal mucosa and tongue. The patches can be wiped off, leaving reddened or bleeding mucosa. *Candida leukoplakia:* White lesions on the buccal mucosa, tongue, or hard palate, which cannot be wiped off. *Vulvovaginal candidiasis:* curdlike vaginal discharge, pruritus, and erythematous vagina and labia.	*Medications: Oral or oropharyngeal*—clotrimazole (Mycelex), nystatin, ketoconazole (Nizoral), or fluconazol (Diflucan). *Vaginal*—miconazole (Monistat) cream or suppositories, clotrimazole (Mycelex, Gyne-Lotrimin) vaginal suppositories, or nystatin (Mycostatin, Nilstat) cream.
Coccidioido-mycosis	Pulmonary infection caused by a fungus found in the Southwestern United States (California, Arizona, Nevada, New Mexico, Texas, and Utah). Coccidioidomycosis may affect up to 20% of HIV-positive persons in endemic areas and can cause pulmonary infection leading to fibrosis. The infection may become extrapulmonary, involving the skin, lymph nodes, or liver.	HIV-positive persons should be counseled to avoid activities associated with increased risk of exposure to soil in endemic areas.	Symptoms are nonspecific and include malaise, fever, weight loss, cough, chest pain, chills, dyspnea, pleural friction rub, splenomegaly, and fatigue. Diagnosis is made by microscopic examination of the organism, culture, or examination of affected tissues.	*Medications:* amphotericin B, ketoconazole, fluconazole.

Cryptosporidiosis	*Cryptosporidium* is a Protozoa recently identified in humans and transmitted through human-to-human contact or via contaminated water. In the United States, approximately 15% of HIV-positive patients with diarrhea are infected with *Cryptosporidium.* In Haiti and Africa approximately 50% of AIDS patients with diarrhea are infected.	HIV-positive persons should avoid contact with human and animal feces and be taught to practice strict handwashing techniques after contact with soil or pets and to not drink water directly from lakes or rivers. Outbreaks of cryptosporidiosis have been linked to municipal water supplies. Use of filters and boiling water will reduce risk.	Severe watery diarrhea 5–14 days after exposure, abdominal pain, profound weight loss, dehydration, and electrolyte imbalance. Diagnosis is made by identification of the organism from stool specimens.	*Medications:* No effective therapy exists. Cryptosporidiosis in persons with AIDS may result in death from malabsorption, electrolyte imbalance, malnutrition, and dehydration. Therapy is directed toward symptom relief and includes fluid replacement, correction of electrolyte imbalance, analgesics, and administration of antidiarrheal agents.
Cytomegalovirus (CMV)	About 90% of HIV-positive individuals have active CMV infection during the course of their illness. CMV retinitis is seen in about 25% of patients.	Prevention efforts focus on avoidance of reinfection and early recognition of symptoms. Regular ophthalmic funduscopic examination is encouraged.	CMV occular infection may result in painless vision loss (loss of a portion of the visual field, blurred vision, or "floaters"). Pulmonary CMV is usually seen in combination with other infections PCP or *Mycobacterium avium* Complex (MAC).	*Medications:* For CMV retinitis—ganciclovir and foscarnet.
Herpes Simplex Virus: group of viruses including herpes simplex type 1 (HSV-1) (cold sores); HSV-2 (genital herpes); Varicella-zoster (VZV) (chickenpox, shingles); Epstein-Barr (infectious mononucleosis), cytomegalovirus; and others.	Common viral infection affecting 1–20% of humans at any time.	Exposure to HSV-2 should be avoided through limited sexual contact and appropriate use of condoms. For persons susceptible to VZV, zoster immune globulin should be given within 4 days of exposure to an individual infected with chickenpox or shingles. Prevention of secondary infections is important.	HSV-1 infections (oral or pharyngeal) appear as painful vesicular lesions that rapidly coalesce and rupture, producing ulcers on the lips, tongue, pharynx, or buccal mucosa. HSV-2 (genital) infection appears as small papules that become painful vesicles that ulcerate, crust over, and resolve within 3 weeks. Inguinal lymphadenopathy may be present.	*Medications:* acyclovir (Zovirax). May be given IV in severe infection and is indicated for HSV encephalitis. Topical acyclovir ointment is used to relieve symptoms of skin lesions and reduce viral shedding.
Histoplasmosis	*Histoplasma capsulatum* is a fungus found in bird and bat intestines; commonly detected in soil in central and southern states. About 2–5% of HIV-positive patients will develop histoplasmosis.	HIV-positive individuals should avoid exposure to bird and bat droppings (i.e., chicken coops, areas where birds roost, caves)	Fever, weight loss, abdominal pain, diarrhea, cough, fatigue, lymphadenopathy, hepatomegaly, splenomegaly, anemia, and leukopenia may be found.	*Medications:* intraconazole, fluconazole, or amphotericin B.

Table continued on following page

TABLE 16–17 **Prevention and Management of Opportunistic Infections and Related Conditions in HIV-Infected Persons** *Continued*

Disease/ Conditions	Epidemiology	Prevention	Signs/Symptoms/ Indications	Management/ Treatment
HIV Encephalopathy/ AIDS Dementia Complex (ADC)	ADC is a neurobehavioral deficit diagnosed in 5–15% of HIV-positive persons, and symptoms may be found in up to 70% of HIV-positive persons. Symptoms range from mild cognitive deficit to severe and fatal.	Early treatment of HIV infection with ZDV and other antiretroviral agents may help prevent ADC.	Forgetfulness, reduced ability to concentrate, slowed verbal and motor responses, loss of coordination, loss of balance, apathy, withdrawal, depression, irritability, agitation. Late stages include obvious dementia, urinary and fecal incontinence, and vegetative state.	Management of ADC may necessitate a combination of ZDV and other medications to minimize symptoms. Antipsychotic, antidepressive, or antianxiety medications may be used.
Human Papillomavirus (HPV) and Cervical Cancer	Infection with HPV is strongly correlated with cervical dysplasia and cervical cancer. Cervical dysplasia affects 20–40% of HIV-positive women.	Encourage condoms to reduce the risk of HPV transmission. HIV-positive women should have cervical Pap smears twice during the first year after diagnosis, and if the results are normal, annually thereafter. More frequent Pap smears are indicated following abnormal results.	Abnormal Pap smear, postcoital bleeding, blood-tinged vaginal discharge, irregular vaginal bleeding, foul-smelling discharge, pelvic pain, rectal bleeding, hematuria, enlarged cervix.	Colposcopic evaluation and/or cone biopsy may be indicated. For severe dysplasia and cervical cancer, laser therapy, conization, cryosurgery, electrocauterization, or hysterectomy may be performed.
Kaposi's Sarcoma (KS)	KS is a neoplasm characterized by vascular tumors of the skin. Four types: classic, non–AIDS-related KS; African KS; AIDS-related (epidemic) KS; and KS associated with immunosuppressive medications. Epidemic (AIDS-related) KS is probably attributable to a viral agent (e.g., HPV or HSV).	No preventive measures.	Widely disseminated, painless skin lesions on the face, arms, and trunk. The lesions are usually pigmented (red to blue) and palpable. Early lesions may resemble bruises. The areas can coalesce and form nodular tumors. Lesions on mucous membranes, lymph nodes, and viscera are also possible.	Treatment is determined by the extent of the disease. Radiation therapy, laser therapy, surgical excision, or cryotherapy may be used. For those with rapidly progressive disease, systemic therapy with antineoplastic drugs may be appropriate.

Non-Hodgkin's Lymphoma (NHL)	NHL most often occurs late in the course of HIV infection and affects 3+% of persons with HIV. Most cases of NHL in AIDS patients are extranodal and often involve the central nervous system, gastrointestinal tract, bone marrow, liver, jaw, rectum, orbit, lung, skin, or other area.	No preventive measures.	Most persons with NHL have nonspecific symptoms consisting of fever, night sweats, and weight loss. If lymphoma is in the central nervous system, symptoms include confusion, lethargy, and memory loss. Diagnosis is based on histological tissue examination.	Treatment includes chemotherapy and/or radiotherapy. Chemotherapy is composed of a modified, low-dose combination of antineoplastic agents.
Mycobacterium avium *Complex (MAC)*	MAC is due to an atypical mycobacterial infection acquired orally or through inhalation. Pneumonia or localized gastrointestinal tract infection may result.	The CDC recommends that HIV-positive persons with CD4 T-cell count of <100 receive prophylaxis against MAC using rifabutin.	Unexplained systemic symptoms including fever, weight loss and debilitation, chronic diarrhea, abdominal pain, anemia, malabsorption, and extrahepatic biliary obstruction. Culture of the blood, bone marrow, or lymph nodes is needed to determine MAC infection.	Treatment depends on the severity of the illness, general state of health, potential for adverse effects, or intolerance to medications and/or presence of concurrent infections. *Medications:* Treatment regimen consists of 2–6 drugs, including amikacin, clarithromycin (Biaxin), ciprofloxacin (Cipro), rifampin, rifabutin, and streptomycin.
Pneumocystis carinii *Pneumonia (PCP)*	PCP is the most common respiratory complication in HIV-positive individuals. An estimated 75% of HIV-positive individuals will develop PCP during their illness.	The CDC recommends chemoprophylaxis for CD4 T-cell counts <200; unexplained fever for 2 weeks; or a history of oral candidiasis.	Usually insidious in onset with fever, shortness of breath, cough (initially nonproductive but progressing to productive), malaise, weakness, tachypnea. Diagnosis is based on chest x-ray and cytology.	*Medications:* Pharmacologic prevention of PCP is described in Table 17–15. During an acute episode, pentamidine, trimethoprim/sulfamethoxazole (Bactrim, Septra), and/or trimetrexate glucuronate may be used.
Recurrent Bacterial Respiratory Infections/Pneumonia	Most often caused by *Streptococcus pneumoniae* or *Haemophilus influenzae*. Risk increases as CD4 T-cell count falls <200.	Immunization with polysaccharide pneumococcal vaccine is recommended as soon as possible after diagnosis with HIV. Immunization for *Haemophilus influenzae* should be considered.	Often abrupt onset: fever, productive cough. X-ray may reveal diffuse interstitial infiltrates; culture of respiratory secretions is necessary to determine treatment.	Pharmacological therapy is dependent on laboratory studies and identification of the causative organism. Oral or parenteral administration of antibiotics is necessary. Administration of fluids, antipyretic drugs, airway suction, and bronchodilators may be indicated.

Table continued on following page

TABLE 16–17 **Prevention and Management of Opportunistic Infections and Related Conditions in HIV-Infected Persons** *Continued*

Disease/ Conditions	Epidemiology	Prevention	Signs/Symptoms/ Indications	Management/ Treatment
Toxoplasmosis/ Toxoplasmic Encephalitis	*Toxoplasma gondii* is a Protozoa commonly found in humans and domestic animals, particularly cats. Almost 70% of adults in the United States are seropositive for exposure. Approximately 30–35% of HIV-positive patients will develop symptoms from toxoplasmosis, usually affecting the central nervous system.	All HIV-positive persons should be tested for immune antibody to *Toxoplasma* after diagnosis to detect latent infection. All HIV-positive persons should be counseled to minimize risk of infection through avoidance of cat litter boxes; not eating undercooked meat; washing fruits and vegetables thoroughly; and careful handwashing after contact with raw meat, soil, or cats.	Often vague and nonspecific. Headache, confusion, lethargy, delusional behavior, frank psychosis, cognitive impairment, coma, hemiparesis, aphasia, ataxia, visual field loss, and seizures may be demonstrated. Diagnosis is based on recent onset of neurological abnormality, abnormal CAT scan, and serologic evidence of *Toxoplasma* exposure.	*Medications:* pyrimethamine and sulfadiazine; trisulfapyrimidine may also be used.
Tuberculosis (TB)	HIV infection is a risk factor for development of TB, and 2–10% of HIV-positive individuals will develop TB. The majority of patients with multiple-drug-resistant TB are HIV-infected.	See Table 17–13 for prevention and diagnosis of TB in HIV-positive individuals.	May precede, coincide, or follow a diagnosis of AIDS. Fever, weight loss, night sweats, fatigue, dyspnea, hemoptysis, and chest pain. Extrapulmonary TB is not uncommon in HIV-infected persons.	See Table 17–16 for treatment of TB in HIV-positive individuals.
Wasting Syndrome	90–100% of HIV-positive persons lose weight. Criteria for diagnosis of HIV wasting syndrome include involuntary weight loss of >10% of baseline body weight plus either chronic diarrhea (at least two loose stools per day for >30 days) or chronic weakness and fever for 30 days in the absence of a concurrent illness.	Nutrition counseling and education should be provided early in the course of the illness. Strategies to maximize food intake, such as encouraging nutrient-dense foods and higher-calorie foods and beverages, increasing the number and/or size of feedings each day, and adding nutritional supplements, should be discussed.	Anorexia, diarrhea, nausea/ vomiting, oral lesions, dysphagia, taste/smell changes, medication interactions, abdominal pain, polydipsia, polyphagia, and neuropathy may contribute to weight loss.	Symptom control to manage nausea, vomiting, and diarrhea. Oral supplements such as Ensure, Sustacal, and Resource may be used. Parenteral nutrition is only used in severe cases.

Data from Centers for Disease Control and Prevention. (1995). USPHS/IDSA Guidelines for the Prevention of Opportunistic Infections in Persons Infected with Human Immunodeficiency Virus: A Summary. *Morbidity and Mortality Weekly Report 44* (RR-8); Dambro, M. R. (1996). *Griffith's 5 Minute Clinical Consult.* Baltimore, Williams & Wilkins; and Ungvarski, P. J. and Staats, J. A. (1995). Clinical manifestations of AIDS in adults. In Flaskerud, J. H. and Ungvarski, P. J. (Eds.). *HIV/AIDS: A Guide to Nursing Care* (3rd ed). Philadelphia, W. B. Saunders.

mune system (e.g., interleukin-2, interferon-alpha), or (3) treatment of AIDS-related infections and cancers (e.g., aerosol pentamidine to treat PCP, ZDV plus interferon for KS; foscarnet for cytomegalovirus infection). Almost all research studies compare a new treatment or drug with a drug already in use to see which works better. Persons are selected to become part of a clinical trial after determining if they meet the eligibility criteria (e.g., age, symptoms of HIV, results of certain laboratory tests, past treatments).

Most trials take place in large medical centers or hospitals. Occasionally private doctors and local clinics will test drugs. According to the USDHHS/NIAID (1989), benefits of being in a clinical trial include the following:

- Patients have a chance to help others.
- Trials offer access to top medical care with experts in treating HIV patients.
- Being a part of a clinical trial is seen as a positive action.
- Patients may be among the first to be helped by a new drug.
- Some medical costs (tests and drugs related to the trial) are paid by the study.

Risks of participating in a clinical trial include the following:

- The treatment may not be beneficial.
- The treatment may be harmful.
- The drug may have side effects.

Most patients are referred to clinical trials by their physician or clinic. Others may learn about trials from a support group or other source. Figure 16–4 illustrates the process of joining an AIDS clinical trial. For more information, contact the AIDS Clinical Trials Information Service (see Table 16–19).

Care of AIDS Clients Near the End of Life

At some point, virtually all AIDS patients will be described as "terminally ill." Hospice care for these clients can be very beneficial in reducing symptoms and improving quality of life.

In general, "the greater the cumulative number of opportunistic infections/illnesses, complications and/or immunological and serological markers, the more rapid the progression for HIV infection to AIDS and to decreased survival" (Kemp and Stepp, 1995, p. 17). The infections/illness most often associated with decreased survival in HIV-positive patients include oral and/or esophageal candidiasis, oral hairy leukoplakia, herpes zoster, cytomegalovirus infection, atypical mycobacteriosis complex infection, and lymphoma. In addition, symptoms associated with decreased survival include chronic diarrhea and rapid weight loss, rapid progress of the disease, hypoxemia, low body weight, progressive neurological changes (fatigue, lethargy, confusion), decreased response to therapy, and/or unexplained or severe deterioration. Table 16–18 describes symptom management in advanced and terminal-stage AIDS.

Case Management of HIV-Infected Clients

Patient-centered case management is recommended for all HIV patients to improve patient care and coordination of resources (USDHHS/AHCPR, 1994). The goals of case management are to access health and mental health care, provide or obtain social support services, and empower patients, family members, and significant others through provision of education, referral, and anticipatory guidance. Objectives of case management for HIV patients are the following:

- Assist patients, family, and significant others in achieving a coordinated set of services with client advocacy as an emphasis.
- Provide counseling on diagnosis and its implications, education about prevention and treatment, and necessary health care.
- Complete psychosocial assessments and integrate these with medical and nursing assessments.
- Develop achievable care plans, integrating psychosocial and health care goals.
- Link patients to one or more needed services.
- Support patients with follow through and continuation of services.

Referral:	Patient finds out about a study from his or her doctor or other source. The patient or doctor contacts the research staff to find out if the study might be open to the patient.	
↓		
Counseling:	Research staff explain the purpose of the trial, the risks, and what the patient will be asked to do.	
↓		
Testing:	Patient takes a number of tests, such as physical examination, blood work, biopsy, or x-ray.	
↓	*Either:*	*Or:*
Results:	Patient's test results meet the trial's needs.	Patient's test results do not meet the trial's needs.
↓	↓	↓
Outcome:	Patient signs informed consent form and enters the trial. *Or:* Patient decides not to take part.	Patient returns to private doctor or clinic for care. He or she may look for other trials.

*From U. S. Dept. of Health and Human Services/National Institute of Allergy and Infectious Diseases. (1989). *AIDS Clinical Trials: Talking it Over.*

FIGURE 16–4 Clinical Trials—Are You Eligible? (From USDHHS/National Institute of Allergy and Infectious Diseases. [1989]. *AIDS Clinical Trials: Talking it Over.*)

- Monitor and track patients to determine use, availability, and appropriateness of services.
- Reassess, together with the patient, family, and significant other, the plan and goals if the original plan is not working or cannot be achieved.
- Maintain records of unmet needs to be used in planning and advocacy efforts.
- Maintain records on each patient for evaluation of case management services. (USDHHS/AHCPR, 1994).

Typically a nurse or a social worker will serve as the case manager for HIV-positive patients. Case managers should have a knowledge of the client's disease status, knowledge of and contact with services (health care, social services, and public entitlement programs) in the community, resourcefulness in accessing services, and interpersonal skills that promote effective interaction between the client and multiple providers. Components of case management follow the nursing process and include identification of those requiring, seeking, or eligible for service; comprehensive assessment of patient needs; development of a written care plan, including setting of goals and objectives; implementation of the plan through referral, coordination, counseling, advocacy, and activities to reach the goals; ongoing monitoring and reassessment; updating as necessary, and disposition and termination (often after the death of the patient) (USDHHS/AHCPR, 1994).

International Considerations and HIV Infection

Contrary to the epidemiology of HIV infection in the United States, heterosexual transmission internationally accounts for up to 70% of HIV infections in sub-Saharan Africa and parts of the Caribbean and Asia. Similarly, in Latin America

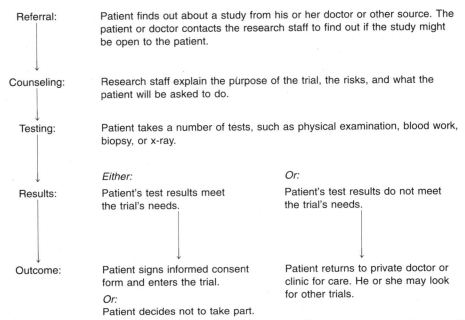

TABLE 16–18 Symptom Management in Advanced and Terminal-Stage AIDS

Pain

Principles of pain management for patients with AIDS correspond with pain management of hospice patients (see Table 9–10).

Confusion

Confusion is common in advanced AIDS and may be due to AIDS dementia complex (ADC), opportunistic infections (i.e., CMV and toxoplasmic encephalitis), side effects of medications or treatments, associated metabolic disorders, or primary neurological disease.

Treatment focuses on modification of the etiology (i.e., stop infection, change medications, manage pain). ZDT may be effective in treating ADC. If the etiology cannot be treated, symptomatic management including low-dose antipsychotic medications may be initiated. Other measures include maintenance of a familiar environment and periodic orientation to person, place, and time.

Depression and Anxiety

Depression in terminal AIDS patients is very common due to the combined effects of a fatal illness, possible family or intrapersonal conflict related to lifestyle (sexual activities or drug use), decreased social and/or financial support, and caregiver fears of infection. All patients with advanced AIDS should be regularly evaluated for depression and suicide risk.

Treatment options include psychosocial support and/or use of antidepressant medication. Support measures include reducing physical symptoms (pain), involving the patient and family in care, and giving frequent and realistic reassurance that the patient will not be alone.

Fatigue

Fatigue may be due to the HIV infection as well as to related opportunistic infections, symptoms (diarrhea, nausea), cancer, or medications. Symptomatic management of fatigue includes promoting adequate sleep, nutrition, and periodic rest. Planning of activities and rearranging the patient's environment (e.g., placing the telephone within reach) to decrease energy expenditure may help.

Fever

Fever is a common symptom in AIDS patients. Use of around-the-clock antipyretics and encouraging heat loss through using light covering may help. Maintenance of fluid and nutrition intake are important.

Dyspnea and Hypoxia

Respiratory problems are usually related to PCP and other opportunistic infections. Dyspnea may be lessened by elevating the head, using pursed-lip breathing, limiting activity, maintaining an environment that is low in humidity and cool with good ventilation, and reducing anxiety. Use of antianxiety medications and oxygen may be necessary.

Nausea and Vomiting

Nausea and vomiting may be due to an infection, treatment, or medication. To minimize nausea, increase fluids as much as can be tolerated. Using an electrolyte preparation such as Pedialyte may be helpful. Small meals should include easy-to-tolerate foods and drinks such as soft drinks, soda crackers, juices, soup, broth, or jello. Antiemetics may be used in severe cases.

Diarrhea

Most AIDS patients will experience some bouts of diarrhea, usually due to opportunistic infection or side effects of medications. Management focuses on resolving the etiology and palliative measures. Antidiarrheal medications may be used.

Wasting

Wasting may be the result of a combination of the disease process, anorexia, chronic diarrhea, chronic weakness, and fever. Treating causative infections and/or problems, increasing caloric intake, and managing symptoms may be helpful in minimizing wasting.

Dehydration

Dehydration is common in advanced disease. Symptoms include orthostatic hypotension, decreased skin turgor, dry mucous membranes, confusion, decreased urine output, and serum electrolyte changes. Hydration should be maintained with oral fluids whenever possible. Use of parenteral therapy in terminally ill patients should be discouraged.

Data from Kemp, C. and Stepp, L. (1995). Palliative care for patients with acquired immunodeficiency syndrome. *American Journal of Hospice and Palliative Care* 12 (6), 14–27.

new cases are increasingly transmitted heterosexually (Jong and McMullen, 1995).

Jong and McMullen (1995) attribute the difference in the spread of the HIV virus in the areas listed above to several factors, including high rates of prostitution, high rates of genital ulcerative disease (i.e., syphilis, chancroid, genital herpes, lymphogranuloma venereum), high rates of nonulcerative sexually transmitted diseases, cervical ectopy, lack of circumcision, inadequate or unavailable resources for disinfection and sterilization of medical equipment and supplies, and perinatal transmission. To decrease their risk of infection, travelers in areas of high endemicity (sub-Saharan Africa, Southeast Asia) are advised to do as follows:

- Abstain from casual sex while abroad.
- Select low-risk partners if they choose to engage in sex.
- Stringently avoid participation in sexual tourism.
- Use condoms purchased in the United States if possible, and use them consistently.
- Be aware that cultural biases may strongly deter the use of condoms.
- Be aware of the effects of alcohol and other mind-altering substances that might contribute to negligent behavior.
- Take along sterile syringes and needles if there is any possibility of need.
- Choose medical facilities and practitioners very carefully (Wilson, 1995; Jong and McMullen, 1995).

SUMMARY

HIV/AIDS is a major concern for all nurses. As the greatest proportion of health care for HIV-positive individuals is provided in community settings, most nurses working in clinics, home health care, hospices, and other areas should be knowledgeable about HIV/AIDS, including epidemiology, prevention, identification, and management. For further information on any of these topics as well as resources for referral, Table 16–19 lists a number of national resources. Local, regional, and state resources are available in most areas, and nurses who routinely work with HIV-positive clients should be aware of all resources in their community.

Key Points

- Acquired immunodeficiency syndrome (AIDS) was first recognized in 1982, and the causative agent (HIV-1) was identified about a year later. Today, AIDS is a pandemic, and the World Health Organization estimates that worldwide, there will be 30–40 million infected persons by the year 2000.
- In the United States there have been more than 500,000 persons diagnosed with AIDS, of which 62% have died, and there are approximately 1 million people in the United States infected with HIV. HIV infection is one of the 10 leading causes of death and is expected to be the third most common cause by 2000.
- In the United States, HIV infection is predominately found in two high-risk groups—homosexual/bisexual men and intravenous drug users. HIV infection is much more common in men, but the proportion of women is growing; females accounted for 19% of cases in 1995. It affects minorities disproportionately, particularly women and children.
- About 75% of HIV infection is attributed to sexual exposure. Prevention should focus on promoting sexual abstinence and a mutually monogamous relationship between uninfected partners. Instruction on "safer sex" and reduction or elimination of "high-risk" sexual practices should include the correct use of condoms.

TABLE 16–19 **Resources for AIDS Prevention and Treatment**

Centers for Disease Control and Prevention
Public Inquiries
1600 Clifton Road, NE
Mailstop A23
Atlanta, GA 30333
(404) 639-3534

National Center for Prevention Services
1600 Clifton Road, NE
Mailstop A23
Atlanta, GA 30333
(404) 639-8008

Resources Specifically for HIV Infection

National AIDS Program Office
Humphrey Building, Room 738-G
200 Independence Avenue SW
Washington, D. C. 20201
(202) 690-5560

CDC National AIDS Clearinghouse
P. O. Box 6003
Rockville, MD 20849-6003
(800) 458-5231 (information/publications)
(800) 342-AIDS (hotline)
(800) 344-SIDA (Publications—Spanish)
(800) HIV-0440 (AIDS Treatment Information Service)
Call the national AIDS hotline (800) 342-2437 for state hotlines

Health Resources and Services Administration
Bureau of Health Professions
5600 Fishers Lane
Parklawn Building, Room 8-101
Rockville, MD 20857
(301) 443-6864
(800) 933-3413 (HIV Telephone Consultation for Health Care Providers)

NIAID AIDS Clinical Trials
Information Service
(800) TRIALS-A
(800) 874-2572

Substance Abuse and Mental Health Services Administration
Center for Substance Abuse Prevention
National Clearinghouse for Alcohol and Drug Information
P. O. Box 2345
Rockville, MD 20847
(800) 729-6686
(301) 468-2600

American Foundation for AIDS Research
733 Third Avenue, 12th Floor
New York, NY 10017
(212) 682-7440

National Association of People Living with AIDS
1413 K Street NW
Washington, D. C. 20005
(202) 898-0435

- The spread of HIV through sharing of needles or other IV drug paraphernalia is the second most common source of transmission. To prevent IV exposure, individuals should be reminded *never* to share needles or syringes. Needle exchange programs may be successful.
- To prevent or greatly minimize occupational exposure, the CDC developed Universal Precautions in 1987. Due to the early directives by the CDC and prophylactic treatment, occupational exposure and resultant seroconversion to HIV-positive status has been very low (39 cases through 1995).
- Screening of all donors of blood and blood products has resulted in the dramatic decline in transfusion-related transmission of HIV.
- Between 13 and 40% of HIV-infected pregnant women will transmit HIV infection to their infant perinatally. The prophylactic administration of zidovudine (AZT/ZDV) during pregnancy, labor, and delivery reduces the risk of HIV transmission by approximately two thirds. As a result, the Public Health Service has recommended testing of all pregnant women for HIV.

- Beginning in 1993, the CDC began categorization of HIV infection to include $CD4^+$ T-lymphocyte counts as a marker for immunosuppression. The case definition for diagnosis states that all HIV-infected persons who have less than 200 $CD4^+$ T-lymphocytes/μL and one of the identified conditions has AIDS.
- Management of HIV-infected individuals includes efforts to promote health through encouraging a lifestyle and behaviors that prevent exposure to pathogens that might cause symptoms and taking measures to enhance the body's ability to fight infection. Nutrition education, regular physical exercise, stress reduction, and elimination of recreational drug use are all important in promoting health.
- In recent years, the Department of Health and Human Services has recommended monitoring of $CD4^+$ lymphocytes and initiation of antiretroviral therapy and PCP prophylaxis for all persons who are HIV-positive. Prompt diagnosis and aggressive treatment of opportunistic infections and related conditions is indicated in advanced disease.
- AIDS clinical trials are research studies conducted to help find effective therapies to treat persons infected with HIV and have been very effective.
- Patient-centered case management is recommended for all HIV+ patients to improve patient care and coordinate resources.
- In contrast with modes of transmission of HIV in the United States, infection internationally is about 70% transmitted heterosexually. To decrease risk of infection, travelers to areas of high endemicity should be advised how to avoid infection.

Learning Activities and Application to Practice

In Class

- Discuss geographical, age, and racial variations in prevalence of HIV/AIDS using the statistics, graphs, and maps provided (see Table 16–1 and Figures 16–1, 16–2, and 16–3). What are some factors that might account for the variations?
- Invite a health care provider who works with HIV/AIDS clients to be a guest speaker. Encourage the speaker to discuss local statistics and characteristics of HIV-positive individuals and trends. Allow the speaker to share recent changes in treatment and anticipated changes. Are there any clinical trials being conducted in the area? What efforts are being conducted locally to encourage prevention of HIV?

In Clinical

- Practice Universal Precautions at all times. Encourage students to be alert to how other health care providers practice, or fail to practice, strict precautions. Have the students note these in a log or diary and share with other students.
- If possible, allow students to observe pre- and post-HIV counseling for at least one individual. Have them notice such factors as: What is the procedure for maintaining anonymity? What is the procedure for reporting positive findings? To whom is the

patient referred following a positive test result? If the client is HIV-negative, what recommendations does the counselor provide to encourage the client to remain HIV-negative?

REFERENCES

American College Health Association. (1990). *Safer Sex*. Baltimore, American College Health Association.

Burnett, C. B., Crawford, P. E., Duffy, J. R., et al. (1996). *Pocket Guide to Infection Prevention and Safe Practice*. St. Louis, Mosby-Year Book.

Casey, K. M. (1995). Pathophysiology of HIV-1, clinical course and treatment. In J. H. Flaskerud and P. J. Ungvarski (Eds.). *HIV/AIDS: A Guide to Nursing Care* (3rd ed.). Philadelphia, W. B. Saunders.

Centers for Disease Control and Prevention. (1995a). *HIV/AIDS Surveillance Report, 7* (2). Altanta, Centers for Disease Control and Prevention.

Centers for Disease Control and Prevention. (1995b). *Epidemiology & Prevention of Vaccine-Preventable Diseases*. Atlanta, Centers for Disease Control and Prevention.

Centers for Disease Control and Prevention. (1995c). USPHS/IDSA guidelines for the prevention of opportunistic infections in persons infected with human immunodeficiency virus: A summary. *Morbidity and Mortality Weekly Report, 44* (RR-8).

Centers for Disease Control and Prevention. (1995d). Case-control study of HIV seroconversion in health-care workers after percutaneous exposure to HIV-infected blood—France, United Kingdom and United States, January 1988–August 1994. *Morbidity and Mortality Weekly Report*, *44* (50).

Centers for Disease Control and Prevention. (1995e). U. S. Public Health Service recommendations for HIV counseling and voluntary testing for pregnant women. *Morbidity and Mortality Weekly Report, 44* (RR-7).

Centers for Disease Control and Prevention. (1994a). Summary of notifiable diseases, United States—1993. *Morbidity and Mortality Weekly Report*, *42* (53).

Centers for Disease Control and Prevention. (1994b). 1994 revised classification system for human immunodeficiency virus infection in children less than 13 years of age. *Morbidity and Mortality Weekly Report, 43* (RR-12).

Centers for Disease Control and Prevention. (1994c). Guidelines for preventing the transmission of *Mycobacterium tuberculosis* in health-care facilities, 1994. *Morbidity and Mortality Weekly Report, 43* (RR-13).

Centers for Disease Control. (1993). Standards for pediatric immunization practices. *Morbidity and Mortality Weekly Report 42* (RR-5).

Centers for Disease Control. (1992). 1993 revised classification system for HIV infection and expanded surveillance case definition for AIDS among adolescents and adults. *Morbidity and Mortality Weekly Report, 41* (RR-17).

Centers for Disease Control. (1990). The use of preventive therapy for tuberculosis infection in the United States. *Morbidity and Mortality Weekly Report, 39* (RR-8).

Centers for Disease Control. (1988). Update: Universal precautions for prevention of transmission of human immunodeficiency virus, hepatitis B virus and other bloodborne pathogens in health-care settings. *Morbidity and Mortality Weekly Report, 37* (24).

Dambro, M. R. (1996). *Griffith's 5-Minute Clinical Consult*. Baltimore, Williams & Wilkins.

Flaskerud, J. H. (1995). Overview of HIV disease and nursing. In J. H. Flaskerud and P. J. Ungvarski (Eds.). *HIV/AIDS: A Guide to Nursing Care* (3rd ed.). Philadelphia, W. B. Saunders.

Jong, E. C. (1995). The travel medical kit and emergency medical care abroad. In E. C. Jong and R. McMullen (Eds.). *The Travel & Tropical Medicine Manual* (2nd ed.). Philadelphia: W. B. Saunders.

Jong, E. C. and McMullen, R. (1995). Sexually transmitted disease and foreign travel. In E. C. Jong and R. McMullen (Eds.). *The Travel & Tropical Medicine Manual* (2nd ed.). Philadelphia: W. B. Saunders.

Kemp, C. and Stepp, L. (1995). Palliative care for patients with acquired immunodeficiency syndrome. *American Journal of Hospice & Palliative Care, 12* (6), 14–27.

Ungvarski, P. J. and Staats, J. A. (1995). Clinical manifestations of AIDS in adults. In J. H. Flaskerud and P. J. Ungvarski (Eds.). *HIV/AIDS: A Guide to Nursing Care* (3rd ed.). Philadelphia: W. B. Saunders.

U. S. Department of Health and Human Services. (1994). *Clinician's Handbook of Preventive Services*. Washington D. C., Government Printing Office. (Also marketed through the "GPO Sales Program and Federal Depository Libraries".)

U. S. Department of Health and Human Services. (1990). *Healthy People 2000: National Health Promotion and Disease Prevention Objectives*. Washington, D. C., Government Printing Office.

U. S. Department of Health and Human Services/Agency for Health Care Policy and Research. (1994). *Clinical Practice Guidelines: Evaluation and Management of Early HIV Infection* (Number 7). Rockville, MD.

U. S. Department of Health and Human Services/National Institute of Allergy and Infectious Diseases. (1989). *AIDS Clinical Trials: Talking it Over*. Bethesda, MD.

Wilson, M. E. (1995). Travel and HIV infection. In E. C. Jong and R. McMullen (Eds.). *The Travel & Tropical Medicine Manual* (2nd ed.). Philadelphia: W. B. Saunders.

17

Mental Health Care in Community-Based Nursing Practice

Case Study

Kay Morton is a Registered Nurse working in a public-sponsored primary care clinic for indigent and homeless people in a large southwestern city. The clinic is housed in a center that provides comprehensive care for the poor. The center provides two meals per day; counseling; and assistance with job training and employment, housing, child care, and a number of other services. In addition to administrative and support personnel, the center employees five social workers, two psychologists, two Registered Nurses, and a physician's assistant. Residents from an area medical school provide psychiatric and medical care, and other local physicians volunteer their services periodically. In addition to primary medical care, other related services offered at the center include drug and alcohol counseling and 12-step programs, psychological counseling, and psychiatric care.

Recently, Kay saw Jeannie Smith for follow-up psychiatric care. Jeannie is 22 years old and a participant in the center's intensive case management program. Jeannie has three children (ages 6, 5, and 2 years) and has been receiving public assistance for more than 6 years. During that time, her children have been in foster care on several occasions. She admits to using crack cocaine, marijuana, and a number of other street drugs in addition to alcohol. She was diagnosed with bipolar disorder 2 years ago and is currently on medication. Since beginning the program, Jeannie has been "clean," has passed a high school equivalency examination, is enrolled in a local community college, and works part time as a cashier. She and her children live in a subsidized apartment, and the center assists her with child care.

At the center, Jeannie was first seen by her case worker for her weekly visit. Following that, she went to the clinic. Kay admitted her and following routine clinic procedures, questioned her about compliance with her medication regimen, any observed side effects, and use of illicit drugs and asked if she had any other problems, questions, or concerns.

Jeannie replied that she had been taking her medications as prescribed and had noticed no side effects. Also, she has not been using any substances prohibited in the program. She reported that her children have been well, her job is "O.K.," and school is fairly difficult, but she is managing. Kay took Jeannie's vital signs and weighed her. The weight and vital signs were all consistent with previous readings. Following agency protocols and a physician's order, Kay collected a urine specimen from Jeannie to be sent for drug screening.

Following the interview with Kay, the psychiatric resident talked with Jeannie for about 20 minutes. To ensure that Jeannie's lithium levels were in therapeutic range, the physician asked Kay to obtain a sample of blood. Kay drew a small sample of blood from Jeannie's right arm, using careful sterile technique and attention to "universal precautions." She reviewed the purpose of the test with Jeannie and explained that the results would be back in a day or two. Jeannie verbalized understanding and left to keep her appointment with her psychologist.

"Mental health is a general term used to refer not only to the absence of mental disorders but also to the ability of an individual to negotiate the daily challenges and social interactions of life without experiencing cognitive, emotional or behavioral dysfunction. Mental health and mental disorders can be affected by numerous factors ranging from biologic and genetic vulnerabilities, acute or chronic physical dysfunction, to environmental conditions and stresses" (USDHHS, 1990, p. 208). Consider these statistics (U. S. Department of Health and Human Services [USDHHS], 1990; USDHHS, 1995):

- Mental disorders will affect an estimated 41 million Americans during some time in their lives
- About 7.5 million children suffer from mental and emotional disturbances (e.g., depression, autism, and attention deficit disorder)
- Schizophrenia affects about 1% of the adult population at any one time
- Depression and associated affective/mood disorders affect about 5% of the population of the United States at any one time
- Suicide, a potential outcome of mental illness and mental disorders, is the ninth leading cause of death in the United States
- Only about 17% of adults with serious mental health problems and only about 33% of children with problems receive services for them
- Mental disorders cost an estimated 75 *billion dollars* in 1992 (e.g., direct cost of health care, lost time from work)
- Persons hospitalized with major depression account for more bed days than any impairment except cardiovascular disorders
- Individuals with job-related stress and depression miss an average of 16 work days annually
- People with untreated mental illnesses consume almost twice as much medical care as the average individual

The use and abuse of illicit drugs and alcohol is strongly related to mental disorders and is both a cause and an effect of mental disorders. Use of drugs and alcohol is directly associated with violence, suicide, birth defects (including mental retardation), accidental injury, and long-term health problems (e.g., liver disease, heart disease, some forms of cancer, and acquired immunodeficiency syndrome [AIDS]). In the United States (USDHHS, 1990; USDHHS, 1996)

- Substance abuse is the cause of 120,000 deaths each year (100,000 attributed to alcohol and 20,000 attributed to drugs)
- Alcohol problems cost United States citizens 70 to 99 billion dollars per year
- Drug use costs 44 to 69 billion dollars per year
- Alcohol is implicated in nearly half of all deaths caused by motor vehicle crashes
- Between 24 and 40% of all general hospital patients are there because of complications related to alcoholism
- About 25% of adolescents are at very high risk of alcohol and other drug problems

- Alcohol use during pregnancy is the leading preventable cause of birth defects
- Alcohol and drug abuse may be both a cause and an effect of homelessness

Early identification, appropriate treatment, and rehabilitation can significantly reduce the duration and level of disability associated with mental disorders and decrease the possibly of relapse. Interventions to promote mental health and decrease mental disorders include focusing on decreasing stressors and/or increasing the capacity of the individual to cope with stress. Other interventions include the use of pharmacological agents and psychosocial interventions, such as strengthening interpersonal, psychological, and physical resources through counseling, support groups, and training.

Over the last 50 years, psychiatry and mental health services have changed dramatically. Until the mid-1900s, treatment of the mentally ill was largely carried out in long-term psychiatric hospitals. The development of psychotropic drugs in the 1950s led to dramatic breakthroughs in the treatment of mental illness and enabled thousands of patients to be treated on an outpatient basis (Richardson, 1993). The process of deinstitutionalization began in the early 1960s in response to legislation intended to move mental health care into the community. The Mental Retardation Facilities and Community Mental Health Centers Construction Act of 1964 (Public Law 88–164) was written to improve inpatient, outpatient, emergency, and day treatment, and consultation and education services for persons with mental disorders. As a result of these developments, between 1955 and 1980, the census of state and county mental hospitals declined from 559,000 to 138,000.

In 1955, 75% of patient care for mental illnesses took place in state hospitals. Today, 75% of patient care for mental disorders occurs in community-based settings (Sharfstein et al., 1995). Ambulatory, or outpatient, care for mental disorders can be provided in many settings and by a variety of professionals, paraprofessionals, and volunteers. Persons with mental problems may seek assistance from physicians and other professional clinicians (e.g., psychologists, counselors) in private practice, hospital outpatient departments, mental health centers or clinics, alcohol and drug units or outpatient clinics, emergency departments, family or social service agencies, crisis centers, volunteer services such as self-help programs (e.g., Alcoholics Anonymous, Narcotics Anonymous), and clergy or religious counselors (Narrow et al., 1993).

The number of visits that a patient needs varies greatly, depending on the mental health problem, diagnosis, or disorder. Therapeutic mental health services include individual, family, and group psy-

TABLE 17–1 **Use of Ambulatory Mental Health Services by Diagnosis**

Mental Disorder	Total Number of Persons (in millions)	Total Number of Visits/ Year (in millions)	Average Visits per Year per Patient (n)
Substance abuse	3.4	56.3	17
Schizophrenia	1.0	16.7	16
Bipolar affective disorder	1.1	16.0	15
Major depressive disorder	4.2	69.7	17
Dysthymia	3.5	65.9	19
Phobias	5.2	15.6	3
Panic disorder	1.1	21.2	19
OCD	1.5	30.4	21

Data from Narrow, W. E., Reiger, D. A., Rae, D. S., Manderscheid, R. W., and Locke, B. Z. (1993). Use of services by persons with mental and addictive disorders: Findings form the National Institute of Mental Health Epidemiologic Catchment Area Program. *Archives in General Psychiatry, 50,* 95–107.

TABLE 17–2 *Healthy People 2000*—Examples of Objectives for Issues in Psychosocial Health

Alcohol and Other Drugs

4.1—Reduce deaths caused by alcohol-related motor vehicle crashes to no more than 5.5 per 100,000 people (age-adjusted baseline: 9.8 per 100,000 in 1987)*

Special Population Targets

Alcohol-Related Motor Vehicle Crash Deaths (per 100,000)	*1987 Baseline (%)*	*2000 Target*
4.1a—Native American and Alaska Native men	40.4	35.0
4.1b—People 15–24 years of age	21.5	12.5

4.3—Reduce drug-related deaths to no more than 3 per 100,000 people (age-adjusted baseline: 3.8 per 100,000 in 1987)*

Special Population Targets

Drug-Related Deaths (per 100,000)	*1990 Baseline*	*2000 Target*
4.3a—Blacks	5.7	3.0
4.3b—Hispanics	4.3	3.0

4.6—Reduce the proportion of young people who have used alcohol, marijuana, and cocaine in the past month as follows:

Special Population Targets

Substance/Age	*1988 Baseline (%)*	*2000 Target (%)*
Alcohol/12–17 years of age	25.2	12.6
Alcohol/18–20 years of age	57.9	29.0
Marijuana/12–17 years of age	6.4	3.2
Marijuana/18–25 years of age	15.5	7.8
Cocaine/12–17 years of age	1.1	0.6
Cocaine/18–25 years of age	4.5	2.3

4.7—Reduce the proportion of high school seniors and college students engaging in recent occasions of heavy drinking of alcoholic beverages to no more than 28% of high school seniors and 32% of college students (baseline: 33% of high school seniors and 41.7% of college students in 1989)

4.13—Provide to children in all school districts and private schools primary and secondary educational programs on alcohol and other drugs, preferably as part of comprehensive school health education (baseline: 63% provided some instruction, 39% provided counseling, and 23% referred students for clinical assessments in 1987)

4.16—Increase to 50 the number of states that have enacted and enforce policies, beyond those in existence in 1989, to reduce access to alcoholic beverages by minors

4.18—Extend to 50 states legal blood alcohol concentration tolerance levels of 0.04% for motor vehicle drivers 21 years and older and 0.00% for those younger than 21 (baseline: 0 states in 1989)

4.19—Increase to at least 75% the proportion of primary care providers who screen for alcohol and other drug use problems and provide counseling and referral as needed (baseline: 19–63% of pediatricians, nurse practitioners, obstetricians/gynecologists, internists, and family physicians reported routinely provided services to patients in 1992)

TABLE 17–2 ***Healthy People 2000*—Examples of Objectives for Issues in Psychosocial Health** *Continued*

Mental Health and Mental Disorders

6.1—reduce suicides to no more than 10.5 per 100,000 people (age-adjusted baseline; 11.7 per 100,000 in 1987)*

Special Population Targets

Suicides (per 100,000)	*1987 Baseline*	*2000 Target*
6.1a—Youth 15–19 years of age	10.2	8.2
6.1b—Men 20–34 years of age	25.2	21.4
6.1c—White men age 65 years and older	46.7	39.2
6.1d—Native American and Alaska Native men in reservation states	20.1	17.0

6.3—Reduce to less than 17% the prevalence of mental disorders among children and adolescents (baseline: an estimated 20% among youth younger than 18 years in 1992)*

6.4—Reduce the prevalence of mental disorders (exclusive of substance abuse) among adults living in the community to less than 10.7% (baseline: 1-month point prevalence of 12.6% in 1984)

6.5—Reduce to less than 35% the proportion of people 18 years and older who experienced adverse health effects form stress within the past year (baseline: 42.6% in 1985)

6.6—Increase to at least 30% the proportion of people 18 years and older with severe, persistent mental disorders who use community support programs (baseline: 15% in 1986)

6.7—Increase to at least 54% the proportion of people with major depressive disorders who obtain treatment (baseline: 31% in 1982)

6.8—Increase to at least 20% the proportion of people 18 years and older who seek help in coping with personal and emotional problems (baseline: 11.1% in 1985)

6.11—Increase to at least 40% the proportion of work sites employing 50 or more people that provide programs to reduce employee stress (baseline: 26.6% in 1985)

6.13—Increase to at least 60% the proportion of primary care providers who routinely review with patients their cognitive, emotional, and behavioral functioning and resources available to deal with any problems that are identified (baseline: 7–40% of pediatricians, nurse practitioners, obstetricians/gynecologists, internists, and family physicians reported routinely providing services to patients in 1992)*

6.15—Reduce the prevalence of depressive (affective) disorders among adults living in the community to less than 4.3% (baseline; 1 month prevalence of 5.1% in 1984)*

Special Population Targets

Depressive Disorders	*1991 Baseline*	*2000 Target*
6.15a—Women	6.6	5.5

From U. S. Department of Health and Human Services. (1990). *Healthy People 2000: National Health Promotion and Disease Prevention Objectives.* Washington, D. C., Government Printing Office.

*From U. S. Department of Health and Human Services. (1996). *Healthy People 2000: Midcourse Review and 1995 Revisions:* Washington, D. C., Government Printing Office.

TABLE 17–3 **Diagnostic Criteria for Major Depressive Episode**

A. Five (or more) of the following symptoms have been present during the same 2-week period and represent a change from previous functioning; at least one of the symptoms is either (1) depressed mood or (2) loss of interest or pleasure.
Note: Do not include symptoms that are clearly due to a general medical condition, or mood-incongruent delusions or hallucinations.
   1. Depressed mood most of the day, nearly every day, as indicated by either subjective report (e.g., feels sad or empty) or observation made by others (e.g., appears tearful). **Note:** In children and adolescents, can be irritable mood.
   2. Markedly diminished interest or pleasure in all, or almost all, activities most of the day, nearly every day (as indicated by either subjective account or observation made by others).
   3. Significant weight loss when not dieting or weight gain (e.g., a change of more than 5% of body weight in a month), or decrease or increase in appetite nearly every day. **Note:** In children, consider failure to make expected weight gains.
   4. Insomnia or hypersomnia nearly every day.
   5. Psychomotor agitation or retardation nearly every day (observable by others, not merely subjective feelings of restlessness or being slowed down).
   6. Fatigue or loss of energy nearly every day.
   7. Feelings of worthlessness or excessive or inappropriate guilt (which may be delusional) nearly every day (not merely self-reproach or guilt about being sick).
   8. Diminished ability to think or concentrate, or indecisiveness, nearly every day (either by subjective account or as observed by others).
   9. Recurrent thoughts of death (not just fear of dying), recurrent suicidal ideation without a specific plan, or a suicide attempt or a specific plan for committing suicide.

B. The symptoms do not meet criteria for a mixed episode.

C. The symptoms cause clinically significant distress or impairment in social, occupational, or other important areas of functioning.

D. The symptoms are not due to the direct physiological effects of a substance (e.g., a drug of abuse, a medication) or a general medical condition (e.g., hypothyroidism).

E. The symptoms are not better accounted for by bereavement; i.e., after the loss of a loved one, the symptoms persist for longer than 2 months or are characterized by marked functional impairment, morbid preoccupation with worthlessness, suicidal ideation, psychotic symptoms, or psychomotor retardation.

chotherapy; hypnosis; psychodrama; expressive therapies (e.g., art therapy); milieu therapy; medications; electroconvulsive therapy; and psychosurgery (Sharfstein et al., 1995). Table 17–1 shows the number of persons with the most commonly diagnosed mental disorders and the approximate number of visits needed by each for professional and nonprofessional services.

Two priority areas of *Healthy People 2000* (USDHHS, 1990) address the related issues of mental health and problems associated with substance abuse. Mental Health and Mental Disorders (Priority Area #6) and Alcohol and Other Drugs (Priority Area #4) contain a number of objectives concerning mental health and related issues. Table 17–2 lists selected objectives from each of these priority areas.

This chapter discusses some of the most common mental disorders encountered by nurses in community-based practice. The correlating and contributing health problems and risks posed by the use of alcohol and illicit drugs also are described. Nursing roles and interventions are included throughout.

TABLE 17–4 **Diagnostic Criteria for Dysthymic Disorder**

A. Depressed mood for most of the day, for more days than not, as indicated either by subjective account or observation by others, for at least 2 years.
   Note: In children and adolescents, mood can be irritable and duration must be at least 1 year.
B. Presence, while depressed, of two (or more) of the following:
   1. Poor appetite or overeating
   2. Insomnia or hypersomnia
   3. Low energy or fatigue
   4. Low self-esteem
   5. Poor concentration or difficulty making decisions
   6. Feelings of hopelessness
C. During the 2-year period (1 year for children or adolescents) of the disturbance, the person has never been without the symptoms in Criteria A and B for more than 2 months at a time.
D. No major depressive episode has been present during the first 2 years of the disturbance (1 year for children and adolescents); i.e., the disturbance is not better accounted for by chronic major depressive disorder, or major depressive disorder, in partial remission.
   Note: There may have been a previous major depressive episode, provided there was a full remission (no significant signs or symptoms for 2 months) before development of the dysthymic disorder. In addition, after the initial 2 years (1 year in children or adolescents) of dysthymic disorder, there may be superimposed episodes of major depressive disorder, in which case both diagnoses may be given when the criteria are met for a major depressive episode.
E. There has never been a manic episode, a mixed episode, or a hypomanic episode, and criteria have never been met for cyclothymic disorder.
F. The disturbance does not occur exclusively during the course of a chronic psychotic disorder, such as schizophrenia or delusional disorder.
G. The symptoms are not due to the direct physiological effects of a substance (e.g., a drug of abuse, a medication) or a general medical condition (e.g., hypothyroidism).
H. The symptoms cause clinically significant distress or impairment in social, occupational, or other important areas of functioning.

Specify if:
   Early onset: if onset is before age 21 years
   Late onset: if onset is age 21 years or older
Specify (for most recent 2 years of dysthymic disorder):
   With Atypical Features

Mental Health and Mental Illness

Mental health is more than absence of mental illness. There are varying degrees of mental health, and there is not one characteristic that is indicative of good mental health, nor can lack of one characteristic indicate a mental illness. In general, mental health is determined by (1) how a person feels about himself or herself, (2) how a person feels about others, and (3) how a person meets the demands of everyday life (National Mental Health Association, 1996). Thus, *mental health* refers to the ability to adapt to distress by mobilizing internal and external resources to minimize tension. Mentally healthy individuals are independent, have high self-esteem, and are able to form meaningful interpersonal relationships (Antai-Otong, 1995).

In contrast, *mental illness* refers to maladaptive responses to distress and an inability to mobilize

TABLE 17–5 **Diagnostic Criteria for Manic Episode**

A. A distinct period of abnormally and persistently elevated, expansive, or irritable mood, lasting at least 1 week (or any duration if hospitalization is necessary).
B. During the period of mood disturbance, three (or more) of the following symptoms have persisted (four if the mood is only irritable) and have been present to a significant degree:
   1. Inflated self-esteem or grandiosity
   2. Decreased need for sleep (e.g., feels rested after only 3 hours of sleep)
   3. More talkative than usual or pressure to keep talking
   4. Flight of ideas or subjective experience that thoughts are racing
   5. Distractibility (i.e., attention too easily drawn to unimportant or irrelevant external stimuli)
   6. Increase in goal-directed activity (either socially, at work or school, or sexually) or psychomotor agitation
   7. Excessive involvement in pleasurable activities that have a high potential for painful consequences (e.g., engaging in unrestrained buying sprees, sexual indiscretions, or foolish business investments)
C. The symptoms do not meet criteria for a mixed episode.
D. The mood disturbance is sufficiently severe to cause marked impairment in occupational functioning or in usual social activities or relationships with others, or to necessitate hospitalization to prevent harm to self or others, or there are psychotic features.
E. The symptoms are not due to the direct physiological effects of a substance (e.g., a drug of abuse, a medication, or other treatment) or a general medical condition (e.g., hyperthyroidism).
   Note: Manic-like episodes that are clearly caused by somatic antidepressant treatment (e.g., medication, electroconvulsive therapy, light therapy) should not count toward a diagnosis of bipolar I disorder.

resources. The mentally ill person is often dependent, has low self-esteem, and has difficulty forming interpersonal relationships (Antai-Otong, 1995). In the *Diagnostic and Statistical Manual of Mental Disorders IV (DSM-IV)*, (American Psychiatric Association [APA], 1994) the APA has classified mental illnesses and outlined diagnostic criteria for some 300 mental disorders. Some of the most common disorders are discussed here. These include depression, anxiety disorders, attention deficit disorder, eating disorders, and substance abuse. In addition, suicide, a consequence of mental illness, is also described. Assessment and treatment of mental disorders concludes the chapter.

Depression

Depression affects about 15 million Americans each year. It is estimated about 25% of all women and 12% of all men will suffer at least one episode or occurrence of depression during their lifetime, and approximately 3 to 5% of teenagers experience clinical depression each year (National Institute of Mental Health [NIMH], 1994b). Most people (almost two thirds) with a depressive illness do not seek treatment, although most, even those with the most severe disorders, can be helped. Estimates of the cost of depression in the United States range from 30 to 44 billion dollars. In addition to direct costs, factors to be considered include the value of lost work days and impact on productivity (Greensberg et al., 1993).

The most prevalent types of depression are

- Major depression—manifested by a combination of symptoms (Table 17–3) that interfere with the ability to work, sleep, eat, and enjoy once-pleasurable activities
- Dysthymia—long-term (minimum of 2 years), chronic symptoms that do not disable but keep the individual from functioning or from feeling good (Table 17–4); some people with dysthymia also experience major depressive episodes
- Bipolar disorder (manic-depressive illness)—

produces cycles of depression and mania (Table 17–5)

RISK FACTORS AND SYMPTOMS

Nurses working in community-based settings should be aware of risk factors for developing depression and of symptoms that might indicate a depressive episode. They can then work to reduce risk factors and teach others to be aware of these symptoms. Health education should also include information on when and how to obtain treatment. Symptoms of depression and mania are included in Table 17–6. Risk factors for depression include (USDHHS/Office of Disease Prevention and Health Promotion [ODPHP], 1994)

- Prior episode(s) of depression
- Family history of depressive disorder
- Prior suicide attempt(s)
- Female gender
- Age of onset younger than 40 years
- Postpartum period
- Medical comorbidity
- Lack of social support
- Stressful life events
- Personal history of sexual abuse
- Current substance abuse

Women have significantly higher rates of depression than men. This may be because of several factors, including developmental roles, hormonal changes, and situational crises. Table 17–7 lists some of the factors that contribute to higher rates of depression in women.

The highest rates of depressive disorders are found among those 25 to 44 years of age, with rates apparently increasing among those born after 1945. This trend may be the result of psychosocial factors (e.g., single parenting, changing roles, stress). Married people and those in ongoing intimate relationships have a lower rate of clinical depression than those living alone. Overall, however, unhappily married people have the highest rates, whereas happily married men the lowest. About 32% of clinically depressed individuals have some form of substance abuse or dependence.

TABLE 17–6 **Symptoms of Depression and Mania**

Depression

- Persistent sad or "empty" mood
- Loss of interest or pleasure in ordinary activities, including sex
- Decreased energy, fatigue, being "slowed down"
- Sleep disturbance (insomnia, early-morning waking, or oversleeping)
- Eating disturbances (loss of appetite and weight loss, or overeating and weight gain)
- Difficulty concentrating, remembering, making decisions
- Feelings of hopelessness, pessimism
- Feelings of guilt, worthlessness, helplessness
- Thoughts of death or suicide; suicide attempts
- Irritability
- Excessive crying
- Chronic aches and pains that do not respond to treatment

Mania

- Excessively "high" mood
- Irritability
- Decreased need for sleep
- Increased energy
- Increased talking, moving, and sexual activity
- Racing thoughts
- Disturbed ability to make decisions
- Grandiose notions
- Being easily distracted

From National Institute of Mental Health. (1994). *Helpful Facts About Depressive Illnesses.* NIH Publication No. 94–3875. Rockville, MD, National Institute of Mental Health.

DEPRESSION IN CHILDREN AND ADOLESCENTS

According to the USDHHS/ODPHP (1994), approximately 1.8% of prepubertal children and 4.7% of adolescents have major depressive disorders. Risk factors for depression in children and adolescents include a history of verbal, physical, or sexual abuse; frequent separation from or loss

TABLE 17–7 **Risk Factors for Depression in Women**

Developmental Roles

- Adolescence—female high school students have higher rates of depression, anxiety disorders, eating disorders, and adjustment disorders than male students; contributing factors may include changes in roles and expectations and physical, intellectual, and hormonal changes
- Adulthood—multidemensional stresses (e.g., responsibilities at home and work, single parenthood, caring for children and aging parents); lack of an intimate, confiding relationship; and marital disputes increase depression

Reproductive Life Cycle

- Menstruation and premenstrual syndrome—depressed feelings, irritability, and other behavioral and emotional changes may occur; these symptoms usually begin after ovulation and worsen until menstruation begins; premenstrual syndrome is probably attributable to the variations in estrogen and other hormones
- Pregnancy—pregnancy (if desired) seldom contributes to depression; having an abortion does not *appear* to lead to a higher incidence of depression; women with infertility problems may be subject to extreme anxiety or sadness
- Postpartum depression—many women experience sadness ranging from transient "blues" to major depression to severe, incapacitating psychotic depression; many women who experience depressive illness after childbirth have had prior depressive episodes (though they may have not been diagnosed)
- Maternal depression—maternal depression may negatively affect a child's behavioral, psychological, and social development
- Menopause—in general, menopause is *not* associated with an increased risk of depression

Victimization

Women molested as children are more likely to have clinical depression at some time in their lives than those with no history of abuse; there may be a higher incidence of depression among women who were raped as adults and women who experience physical abuse and/or sexual harassment; this may be the result of fostering low self-esteem, helplessness, self-blame, and social isolation

Poverty

Low economic status contributes to isolation, uncertainty, frequent negative events, and poor access to resources

Depression in Later Adulthood

Depression in elderly women may be most often related to widowhood; this is usually temporary and often subsides within a year

Data from National Institute of Mental Health. (1994). *Helpful Facts About Depressive Illness.* NIH Publication No. 94–3875. Rockville, MD, National Institute of Mental Health.

of a loved one; family history of depression; incarceration; pregnancy; lower socioeconomic status; homosexuality; mental retardation; attention deficit disorder; hyperactivity; and chronic illness. Complications of depression in children and adolescents include poor school performance, poor peer relations, alcohol and drug abuse, promiscuity, teenage pregnancy, other psychiatric illnesses, and suicide (USDHHS/ODPHP, 1994).

Health care providers should recognize the symptoms of depression and refer for treatment as appropriate. Table 17–8 summarizes characteristics of depression that may be seen in all age groups.

TREATMENT

Treatment for depression includes pharmacological therapy, electroconvulsive therapy, psychotherapy, behavior therapy, or a combination of these. Antidepressant medication has been shown to treat depressive effectively and is the first-line treatment if (1) the depression is severe, (2) the person

TABLE 17–8 Characteristics of Depression Across the Life Span

Childhood

Infants and Preschoolers

Insidious onset
Apathy, fatigue, withdrawal
Poor appetite, weight loss
Agitation, sleeplessness
Rarely, spontaneous disclosure of feeling sad

Prepubertal Children

Possible disclosure of sadness, suicidal thoughts
Irritability, self-criticism, weepiness
Decreased initiative and responsiveness to stimulation, apathy
Fatigue, sleep disturbance
Enuresis, encopresis
Weight loss, anorexia
Somatic complaints
Poor school performance
Social withdrawal, increased aggressiveness

Adolescence

Feelings of sadness less frequent than in other age groups
Unhappy restlessness, boredom, irritability
Intense, labile affects
Low self-esteem, hopelessness, worthlessness
Associated anxiety
Feelings of loneliness and being unloved
Pessimism about the future
Loss of interest in friends and activities, apathy
Low frustration tolerance
Poor school performance
Argumentativeness
Increased conflict with peers
Acting-out behavior, e.g., running away, stealing, physical violence
Sexual activity
Substance abuse
Complaints of headaches, abdominal pain
Hypersomnia

Early and Middle Adulthood

Depressed mood
Anhedonia
Feelings of worthlessness, hopelessness, guilt
Reduced energy, fatigue
Sleep disturbance, especially early morning awakening and multiple nighttime awakenings
Decreased sexual interest and activity
Psychomotor retardation
Anxiety
Decreased appetite and weight loss or increased appetite and weight gain

Later Adulthood

Unlikely to complain of depressed mood or present with tearful affect
Feelings of helplessness
Pessimism about the future
Ruminating about problems
Critical and envious of others
Loss of self-esteem
Guilt feelings
Longer and more severe depressions than in middle adulthood
Perceived cognitive deficits
Somatic complaints
Constipation
Social withdrawal
Loss of motivation
Change of appetite

Core Symptoms Across Age Groups

Suicidal ideation
Diminished concentration
Sleep disturbance

From Tommasini, N. R. (1995). The client with a mood disorder (depression). In D. Antai-Otong (Ed.). *Psychiatric Nursing: Biological and Behavioral Concepts.* Philadelphia: W. B. Saunders, pp. 157–190.

has psychotic features, (3) the person is melancholic or has atypical symptoms, (4) the patient prefers medication, and/or (5) psychotherapy by a trained, competent psychotherapist is not available (Frank et al., 1993). Treatment for all mental disorders is addressed in greater detail later in this chapter.

Anxiety Disorders

Anxiety disorders are a group of mental illnesses characterized by feelings of severe anxiety, resulting symptoms, and efforts (sometime extreme) to avoid those symptoms. Anxiety disorders are the most common of all of the mental disorders, affecting as many as 9% of the general population at any time. Anxiety disorders may be attributed to genetic makeup, as well as life experiences of the individual. Some of the more commonly encountered anxiety disorders are generalized anxiety disorder (GAD), panic disorder (sometimes accompanied by agoraphobia), phobias, obsessive-compulsive disorder (OCD), and posttraumatic stress disorder (PTSD) (NIMH, 1995). These are discussed briefly here.

GENERALIZED ANXIETY DISORDER

Generalized anxiety disorder is characterized by chronic, unrealistic, and exaggerated worry and tension about one or more life circumstances lasting 6 months or longer without anything seeming to provoke it (Katon, 1994). Symptoms include trembling, twitching muscle tension, headaches, irritability, sweating or hot flashes, dyspnea, nausea, and feeling a "lump" in the throat. GAD is more common in women than in men, and a familial tendency often exists. Diagnostic criteria for GAD are presented in Table 17–9.

TABLE 17–9 **Diagnostic Criteria for Generalized Anxiety Disorder**

A. Excessive anxiety and worry (apprehensive expectation), occurring more days than not for at least 6 months, about a number of events or activities (such as work or school performance)
B. The person finds it difficult to control the worry
C. The anxiety and worry are associated with three (or more) of the following six symptoms (with at least some symptoms present for more days than not for the past 6 months); **note:** only one item is required in children
   1. Restlessness or feeling keyed up or on edge
   2. Being easily fatigued
   3. Difficulty concentrating or mind going blank
   4. Irritability
   5. Muscle tension
   6. Sleep disturbance (difficulty falling or staying asleep or restless unsatisfying sleep)
D. The focus of the anxiety and worry is not confined to features of an axis I disorder; e.g., the anxiety or worry is not about having a panic attack (as in panic disorder); being embarrassed in public (as in social phobia), being contaminated (as in OCD), being away from home or close relatives (as in separation anxiety disorder), gaining weight (as in anorexia nervosa), or having a serious illness (as in hypochondriasis), and the anxiety and worry do not occur exclusively during PTSD
E. The anxiety, worry, or physical symptoms cause clinically significant distress or impairment in social, occupational, or other important areas of functioning
F. The disturbance is not due to the direct physiological effects of a substance (e.g., a drug of abuse, a medication) or a general medical condition (e.g., hyperthyroidism) and does not occur exclusively during a mood disorder, a psychotic disorder, or a pervasive developmental disorder.

TABLE 17–10 Diagnostic Criteria for Panic Disorder with and Without Agoraphobia

Diagnostic Criteria for Panic Disorder without Agoraphobia

A. Both 1 and 2
   1. Recurrent unexpected panic attack
   2. At least one of the attacks has been followed by 1 month (or more) of one (or more) of the following:
      a. Persistent concern about having additional attacks
      b. Worry abut the implications of the attack or its consequences (e.g., losing control, having a heart attack, "going crazy")
      c. a significant change in behavior related to the attacks

B. Absence of agoraphobia

C. The panic attacks are not due to the direct physiological effects of a substance (e.g., a drug of abuse, a medication) or a general medical condition (e.g., hyperthyroidism)

D. The panic attacks are not better accounted for by another mental disorder, such as social phobia (e.g., occurring on exposure to feared social situations), specific phobia (e.g., on exposure to a specific phobic situation), OCD (e.g., on exposure to dirt in someone with an obsession about contamination), PTSD (e.g., in response to stimuli associated with a severe stressor), or separation anxiety disorder (e.g., in response to being away from home or close relatives)

Diagnostic Criteria for Panic Disorder with Agoraphobia

A. Both 1 and 2
   1. Recurrent unexpected panic attacks
   2. At least one of the attacks has been followed by 1 month (or more) of one (or more) of the following:
      a. Persistent concern about having additional attacks
      b. Worry about the implications of the attack or its consequences (e.g., losing control, having a heart attack, "going crazy")
      c. a significant change in behavior related to the attacks

B. The presence of agoraphobia

C. The panic attacks are not caused by the direct physiological effects of a substance (e.g., a drug of abuse, a medication) or a general medical condition (e.g., hyperthyroidism)

D. The panic attacks are not better accounted for by another mental disorder, such as social phobia (e.g., occurring on exposure to feared social situations), specific phobia (e.g., on exposure to a specific phobic situation), OCD (e.g, on exposure to dirt in someone with an obsession about contamination), PTSD (e.g., in response to stimuli associated with a severe stressor), or separation anxiety disorder (e.g., in response to being away from home or close relatives

Reprinted with permission from the *Diagnostic and Statistical Manual of Mental Disorders, Fourth Edition.* Copyright 1994 Amrican Psychiatric Association.

PANIC DISORDER

Panic disorder strikes at least 3 to 6 million Americans (1.6–2.9% of women and 0.4–1.7% of men) and can occur at any age but most often begins in young adulthood (average age, 17–30 years). Panic disorder typically develops in three stages, with patients potentially stopping at any stage or progressing through all three. Individuals often have their first attack or cluster of attacks after a variety of life stresses. The initial attack may occur suddenly and unexpectedly while the patient is performing everyday tasks. Typically, he or she experiences tachycardia; dyspnea; dizziness; chest pain; nausea; numbness or tingling of the hands and feet; trembling or shaking; sweating; choking; or a feeling that he or she is going to die, go crazy, or do something uncontrolled. This can be extremely frightening. A diagnosis of panic disorder is made when attacks occur with some degree of frequency or regularity.

During the second stage, the anxiety attacks become increasingly frequent and severe, and the individual develops anticipatory anxiety (fear of having a panic attack). During this phase, events and circumstances associated with the attack may be selectively avoided, leading to phobic behaviors (e.g., if a woman has an attack while driving, she may become anxious the next time she needs to drive, and she may begin to avoid driving and then refuse to drive altogether). In this phase, the patient's life may become progressively constricted.

As the avoidance behavior intensifies, the third stage may develop, in which the patient begins to withdraw further to avoid being in places or situations from which escape might be difficult or embarrassing or help unavailable in the event of a panic attack (e.g., church, elevators, movie theaters) (Katon, 1994). The fear of being in these situations or places can lead to agoraphobia (literally, fear of the marketplace or open places). Agoraphobics frequently progress to the point where they cannot leave their homes without experiencing anxiety. Agoraphobia is the most common phobia leading to the use of health services, particularly when accompanied by panic attacks. About one third of all people who experience panic attacks eventually develop agoraphobia.

Panic disorder is often accompanied by other conditions. If not treated, 60 to 90% of patients with panic disorder develop a major depression at some time in their lives (Katon, 1994). Alcoholism is also common. Cognitive-behavioral therapy and medication can help 70 to 90% of people with panic disorder. Table 17–10 contains diagnostic criteria for panic disorder with and without agoraphobia.

PHOBIAS

A phobia is an irrational fear of something (an object or situation), and as many as 10% of Americans are affected by phobias. Adults with phobias realize their fears are irrational, but facing the feared object or situation might bring on severe anxiety or a panic attack. Phobias may begin in childhood but usually first appear in adolescence or adulthood.

Social phobia is a persistent and intense fear of and compelling desire to avoid a situation that would expose the individual to a situation that might be humiliating and embarrassing. Its tendency is familial and may be accompanied by depression or alcoholism. Social phobia often begins in childhood or early adolescence. Individuals suffering from social phobia think that others are very competent in public but that they are not. Small mistakes are exaggerated. The most common social phobia is a fear of public speaking. Other examples include being unable to urinate in a public bathroom and not being able to answer questions in social situations. Most people with social phobias can be treated with cognitive-behavior therapy and medication.

Simple phobias (excluding panic attack or social phobia) involve a persistent fear of and compelling desire to avoid certain objects or situations. Common objects of phobias are spiders, snakes, dogs, cats, and situations such as flying, heights, and closed-in spaces. The person often recognizes that the fear is excessive or unreasonable but nonetheless avoids the situation or endures it with intense anxiety. Systematic desensitization and normal exposure are the most effective treatments for simple phobias. Medication produces minimal benefit (Katon, 1994).

OBSESSIVE-COMPULSIVE DISORDER

Obsessive-compulsive disorder is characterized by anxious thoughts and rituals that the individual has difficulty controlling. The person with OCD is overcome with the urge to engage in some ritual to avoid a persistent frightening thought, idea, image, or event—the *obsession. Compulsions* are the rituals or behaviors that are repeatedly performed to prevent, neutralize, or dispel the dreaded obsession. When the individual tries to resist the compulsion, anxiety increases. Common compulsions include hand-washing, counting, checking, or touching (Robinson, 1996).

Obsessive-compulsive disease is diagnosed only when the compulsive activities consume at least an hour a day and interfere with daily life. Most individuals recognize that what whey are doing is senseless but are unable to control the compulsion. About 2% of Americans are afflicted with OCD, which often appears in the teenage years or early adulthood. Depression or other anxiety disorders often accompany OCD. Clomipramine (Anafranil) and fluoxetine (Prozac) have been effective in treating OCD. Behavioral therapy may also help.

POSTTRAUMATIC STRESS DISORDER

Posttraumatic stress disorder is a debilitating condition that follows a terrifying event. Individuals with PTSD have recurring, persistent, frightening thoughts and memories of their ordeal. Traumatic incidents that trigger PTSD may have threatened that individual's life or the life of someone else. Incidents include "shell shock" or "battle fatigue" common to war veterans, violent attack (e.g., kidnapping, rape, mugging), serious accidents, or natural disasters (e.g., earthquake, tornado) or witnessing mass destruction or injury, such as after an airplane crash. Sometimes the individual is unable to recall an important aspect of the traumatic event (Katon, 1994).

People with PTSD repeatedly relive the trauma in the form of nightmares and/or disturbing recollections, flashbacks, or hallucinations during the day. As a result, they often have sleep disturbances, depression, and feelings of detachment or emotional numbness, and/or are easily startled. They may avoid places or situations that bring back memories (e.g., a woman raped in an elevator may refuse to ride in elevators), and anniversaries of the event are often very difficult. PTSD occurs at all ages and may be accompanied by depression, substance abuse, and/or anxiety. PTSD usually begins within 3 months of the trauma, and the course of the disorder varies. Some individuals recover within 6 months; the condition becomes chronic in others. Infrequently, the illness does not manifest until years after the traumatic event.

Posttraumatic stress disorder is treated with antidepressants and antianxiety medications and psychotherapy. Support from family and friends can be very beneficial.

Eating Disorders

Eating disorders are becoming increasingly prevalent in the United States. Indeed, the most common eating disorders, anorexia nervosa and bulimia nervosa, affect about 3 million U. S. residents. Currently, it is estimated that anorexia affects 1% of girls 12 to 18 years of age (Farley, 1994), and that as many as 2 to 8% of adolescent and college-aged women have some symptoms of bulimia (Decker and Freeman, 1996).

Eating disorders almost exclusively affect females; males account for only 5 to 10% of bulimia and anorexia cases. The vast majority of patients diagnosed with eating disorders are white. This, however, may be because of socioeconomic factors rather than race, as females in middle and upper socioeconomic groups are most frequently affected. Anorexia and bulimia are often triggered by developmental milestones (e.g., puberty, first sexual contact) or another crisis (e.g., death of a loved one, ridicule over weight, starting college).

BULIMIA NERVOSA

"The essential features of bulimia are binge eating and inappropriate compensatory methods to prevent weight gain" (APA, 1994, p. 545). A "binge" is defined as eating an "abnormal" amount of food at a "discrete period of time" (usually less than 2 hours) (APA, 1994). For example, a bulimic might eat an entire pie, half a cake, or a half gallon of ice cream at one sitting. Snacking throughout the day is not considered "bingeing."

To lose or maintain weight, the bulimic practices "purging," which usually involves self-induced vomiting caused by gagging, using an emetic, or simply mentally willing the action. Laxatives, diuretics, fasting, and excessive exercise may also be employed to control weight.

Bulimia typically begins in adolescence or during the early 20s and usually in conjunction with a diet. Members of certain professions that emphasize weight and/or appearance (e.g., dancers, flight attendants, athletes, actors, models) are at high risk (Decker and Freeman, 1996).

A number of health problems may result from bulimia. Electrolyte imbalance can result in fatigue, seizures, muscle cramps, arrhythmias, and decreased bone density. Vomiting can damage the esophagus, stomach, teeth, and gums.

ANOREXIA NERVOSA

The person suffering from anorexia nervosa becomes obsessed with a fear of fat and with losing weight. Anorexia nervosa often develops with a fairly gradual decrease in caloric intake. However, the decrease in caloric intake continues until the anorexic is consuming almost nothing. Anorexia usually begins in early adolescence (12–14 years is the most common age group) and may be limited to a single episode of dramatic weight loss within a few months followed by recovery, or the illness may last for many years.

As stated earlier, anorexia nervosa almost exclusively affects white adolescent girls. Other characteristics of girls who develop anorexia are that they are well-behaved and eager to please; are perfectionists; may have a poor self-image; are dependent on others' opinions, introverted, and insecure; are overly compliant and deferential to others' wishes; and are emotionally reserved (Decker and Freeman, 1996).

In response to the severely decreased caloric intake, the body tries to compensate by slowing down body processes. Menstruation ceases; blood pressure, pulse, and respiration rates slow; and thyroid activity diminishes. Electrolyte imbalance can become very severe. Other symptoms include mild anemia, joint swelling, and reduced muscle mass. Anorexia nervosa can be life threatening and has a mortality rate of 5 to 18%. In 1990, 70 deaths in the United States were attributed to anorexia.

TREATMENT

Treatment for eating disorders includes nutrition counseling, psychotherapy, and behavior modification and may take a year or more. Hospitalization may be required for patients with serious complications. Self-help groups and support groups can be very beneficial for both the patient and the family. Many bulimics appear to respond to antidepressants. Anorexia nervosa, however, does not appear as responsive to medication.

Nurses who frequently work with adolescent girls and young women in community settings such as schools and clinics should be aware of the risk factors, signs, and symptoms of anorexia and bulimia and be prepared to intervene. Tables 17–11 and 17–12 list the diagnostic criteria for bulimia and anorexia, respectively.

TABLE 17–11 **Diagnostic Criteria for Bulimia Nervosa**

A. Recurrent episodes of binge eating: An episode of binge eating is characterized by both of the following:
   1. Eating, in a discrete period of time (e.g., within any 2-hour period), an amount of food that is definitely larger than most people would eat during a similar period of time and under similar circumstances
   2. A sense of lack of control over eating during the episode (e.g., a feeling that one cannot stop eating or control what or how much one is eating)

B. Recurrent inappropriate compensatory behavior to prevent weight gain, such as self-induced vomiting; misuse of laxatives, diuretics, enemas, or other medications; fasting; or excessive exercise

C. The binge eating and inappropriate compensatory behaviors both occur, on average, at least twice a week for 3 months

D. Self-evaluation is unduly influenced by body shape and weight

E. The disturbance does not occur exclusively during episodes of anorexia nervosa

Specify type

Purging type: during the current episode of bulimia nervosa, the person has regularly engaged in self-induced vomiting or the misuse of laxatives, diuretics, or enemas

Nonpurging type: during the current episode of bulimia nervosa, the person has used other inappropriate compensatory behaviors, such as fasting or excessive exercise, but has not regularly engaged in self-induced vomiting or the misuse of laxatives, diuretics, or enemas

Attention Deficit Hyperactivity Disorder

One of the most common conditions encountered by nurses who work with children in community settings is Attention Deficit Disorder (ADD) or Attention Deficit Hyperactivity Disorder (ADHD). (Here the disorder is referred to as ADHD.) ADHD affects 3 to 5% of all children in the United States (about 2 million) (NIMH, 1994a). Behaviors that might indicate ADHD usually appear before age 7 years and are often accompanied by related problems, such as learning disability, anxiety, and depression. The three major characteristics of ADHD are inattention, hyperactivity, and impulsivity. Table 17–13 presents the diagnostic criteria for ADHD.

The cause of ADHD is not known, but it is important to note that it is *not* caused by minor head injuries, birth complications, food allergies, too much sugar, poor home life, poor schools, or too much television. Maternal substance use and abuse (e.g., alcohol, cigarettes, cocaine) *may* affect the brain of the developing baby and produce symptoms of ADHD later in life. This, however, accounts for only a small percentage of those affected (NIMH, 1994a).

Attention disorders run in families, as children

TABLE 17–12 **Diagnostic Criteria for Anorexia Nervosa**
. .

A. Refusal to maintain body weight at or above a minimally normal weight for age and height (e.g., weight loss leading to maintenance of body weight less than 85% of that expected; or failure to make expected weight gain during period of growth, leading to body weight less than 85% of that expected)
B. Intense fear of gaining weight or becoming fat, even though underweight
C. Disturbance in the way in which one's body weight or shape is experienced, undue influence of body weight or shape on self-evaluation, or denial of the seriousness of the current low body weight
D. In postmenarcheal females, amenorrhea, i.e., the absence of at least three consecutive menstrual cycles (a woman is considered to have amenorrhea if her periods occur only following hormone, e.g., estrogen, administration)
Specify type:
 Restricting type: during the current episode of anorexia nervosa, the person has not regularly engaged in binge eating or purging behavior (i.e., self-induced vomiting or the misuse of laxatives, diuretics, or enemas)
 Binge-eating/purging type: during the current episode of anorexia nervosa, the person has regularly engaged in binge eating or purging behavior (i.e., self-induced vomiting or the misuse of laxatives, diuretics, or enemas)

. .

Reprinted with permission from the *Diagnostic and Statistical Manual of Mental Disorders, Fourth Edition.* Copyright 1994 American Psychiatric Association.

diagnosed with ADHD usually have at least one close relative who also has ADHD, and at least one third of all fathers who had ADHD as children have children with symptoms. Additionally, in the majority of sets of identical twins in which one has the disorder, the other does also (NIMH, 1994a). Although symptoms and signs may be noticed by parents, it is often teachers who recognize the behaviors consistent with attention deficit disorders and suggest referral for assessment and treatment.

Experts caution that diagnosis of attention disorders should be made following a comprehensive physical, psychological, social, and behavioral evaluation and not based solely on anecdotal reports from parents. The evaluation should rule out other possible reasons for the behavior (e.g., emotional problems, poor vision or hearing, physical problems) and should include input from teachers, parents, and others who know the child well. Intelligence and achievement testing may also be performed to rule out or identify a learning disability.

Symptoms of ADHD are typically managed through a combination of behavior therapy, emotional counseling, and practical support. Use of medication is becoming increasingly commonplace in the management of ADHD. It is very important, however, that children with attention disorders and their families understand that medication does not "cure" the disorder; it just temporarily controls symptoms.

Curiously, stimulants are the medications that have been shown to be successful in treating attention disorders in both children and adults. The most commonly used medications are methylphenidate (Ritalin), dextroamphetamine (Dexedrine or Dextrostat), and pemoline (Cylert). About 90% of children with ADHD show improvement when taking one of these drugs. These medications are short acting (lasting 2–4 hours) and therefore may need to be taken several times each day. Recently, sustained-release preparations, which require fewer doses, have been made available for some of the medications.

Effective doses vary among children, and drug regimens for treatment of ADHD vary among physicians. Some physicians recommend keeping children on medication only during school and

TABLE 17–13 Diagnostic Criteria for Attention Deficit/Hyperactivity Disorder

A. Either (1) or (2):
 (1) Six (or more) of the following symptoms of *inattention* have persisted for at least 6 months to a degree that is maladaptive and inconsistent with developmental level

 Inattention
 a. Often fails to give close attention to details or makes careless mistakes in schoolwork, work, or other activities
 b. Often has difficulty sustaining attention in tasks or play activities
 c. Often does not seem to listen when spoken to directly
 d. Often does not follow through on instructions and fails to finish schoolwork, chores, or duties in the workplace (not due to oppositional behavior or failure to understand instructions)
 e. Often has difficulty organizing tasks and activities
 f. Often avoids, dislikes, or is reluctant to engage in tasks that require sustained mental effort (such as schoolwork or homework)
 g. Often loses things necessary for tasks or activities (e.g., toys, school assignments, pencils, books, or tools)
 h. Is often easily distracted by extraneous stimuli
 i. Is often forgetful in daily activities
 (2) Six (or more) of the following symptoms of *hyperactivity-impulsivity* have persisted for at least 6 months to a degree that is maladaptive and inconsistent with developmental level

 Hyperactivity
 a. Often fidgets with hands or feet or squirms in seat
 b. Often leaves seat in classroom or in other situations in which remaining seated is expected
 c. Often runs about or climbs excessively in situations in which it is inappropriate (in adolescents or adults, may be limited to subjective feelings of restlessness)
 d. Often has difficulty playing or engaging in leisure activities quietly
 e. Is often "on the go" or often acts as if "driven by a motor"
 f. Often talks excessively

 Impulsivity
 g. Often blurts out answers before quesitions have been completed
 h. Often has difficulty awaiting turn
 i. Often interrupts or intrudes on others (e.g., butts into conversations or games)
B. Some hyperactive-impulsive or inattentive symptoms that caused impairment were present before age 7 years
C. Some impairment from the symptoms is present in two or more settings (e.g., at school [or work] and at home)
D. There must be clear evidence of clinically significant impairment in social, academic, or occupational functioning
E. The symptoms do not occur exclusively during the course of a pervasive developmental disorder, schizophrenia, or other psychotic disorder and are not better accounted for by another mental disorder (e.g., mood disorder, anxiety disorder, dissociative disorder, or a personality disorder)

Code based on type:
 314.01—Attention-deficit/hyperactivity disorder, combined type: if both criteria A1 and A2 are met for the past 6 months
 314.00—Attention-deficit/hyperactivity disorder, predominantly inattentive type: if criterion A1 is met but criterion A2 is not met for the past 6 months
 314.01—Attention-deficity/hyperactivity disorder, predominantly hyperactive-impulsive type: if criterion A2 is met but criterion A1 is not met for the past 6 months

 Coding note: For individuals (especially adolescents and adults) who currently have symptoms that no longer meet full criteria, "in partial remission" should be specified

have the child stop taking the medication on weekends and during summer vacation. Others prescribe medication every day, assuming that this regimen is more beneficial in helping establish positive behavioral patterns and work habits.

Medications used to treat ADHD have some potential adverse effects. Appetite suppression is fairly common and may contribute to growth retardation. Periodic assessment of height and weight is therefore important. Sleeping difficulties are also possible. There is concern that long-term use of pemoline (Cylert) might affect the liver. Therefore, liver function must be assessed periodically in patients taking this medication.

Substance Abuse

Substance abuse refers to patterns of use of alcohol and/or other drugs that result in health conse-

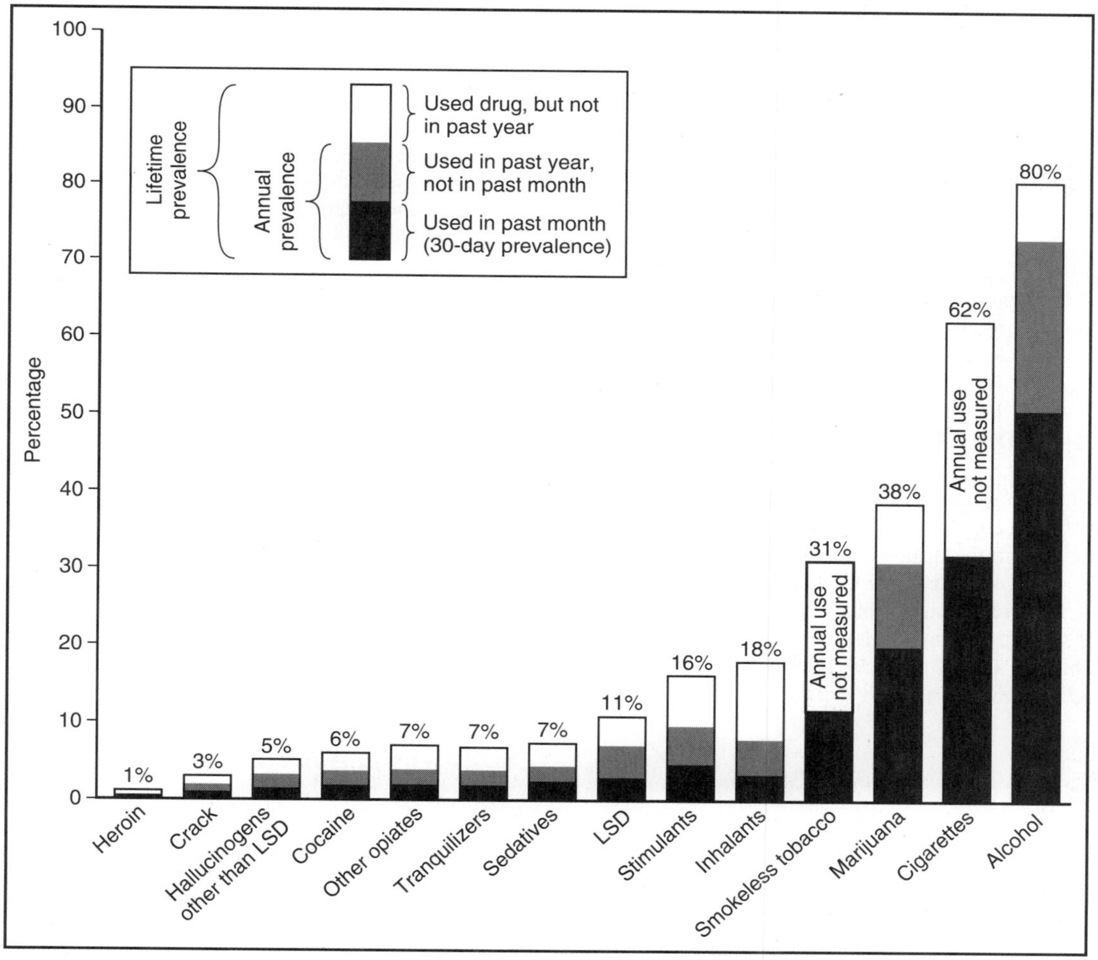

FIGURE 17–1 Prevalence and recency of use of various types of drugs for 12th graders, 1994. (Johnston, L. D., O'Malley, P. M., Bachman, J. G. [1993]. *National Survey Results on Drug Use from Monitoring the Future Study, 1975–1992.* Vol I. NIH Publ. No 93-3597. Washington, D. C., Government Printing Office.)

quences or impairment in social, psychological, and occupational functioning (Robert Wood Johnson Foundation, 1993). The toll caused by alcohol and other drugs on society is staggering. The economic costs of alcohol alone are massive. Alcohol and drug use is involved in several of the leading causes of morbidity and mortality in the United States, including accidental injury, suicide, homicide, liver disease, certain types of cancer, and AIDS. A number of legal and illegal substances used by many Americans, including alcohol, cigarettes, marijuana, heroin, and many others, are harmful. It is important to note that substance abuse often begins in adolescence. Figure 17–1 shows the frequency of use of alcohol, cigarettes, and illicit drugs among 12th graders.

ALCOHOL ABUSE

Alcoholism is the greatest drug problem in the United States today. Indeed, about 10% of the adult population has a chronic, heavy intake of alcohol and shows symptoms of alcoholism. Table 17–14 lists some facts about alcohol abuse.

ILLICIT DRUG USE

Illicit drugs used in the United States include opioids (e.g., heroin, morphine), cocaine (e.g., crack), amphetamines, hallucinogens (e.g., lysergic acid diethylamide [LSD], phencyclidine [PCP]), marijuana, inhalants (e.g., airplane model glue, spray paint, nail polish remover, gasoline). Table 17–15 lists a few relevant statistics on the use and abuse of illicit drugs.

RISK FACTORS FOR SUBSTANCE ABUSE

A number of risk factors have been identified that can contribute to the likelihood that an individual might abuse alcohol and/or other drugs. Table 17–16 lists these by developmental stage. Nurses who work in community settings such as clinics, physicians' offices, schools, and work sites should be knowledgeable about risk factors that contribute to substance abuse and when to intervene to reduce them, whenever possible.

TABLE 17–14 **Fast Facts About Alcohol Use and Abuse**

- Alcohol abuse costs U. S. residents almost $100 billion annually, the majority (71%) being in productivity losses associated with illness and death
- During the past decade, alcohol consumption in the United States has declined, most notably because of a decrease in consumption of distilled liquor; in contrast, beer consumption has remained stable, and wine consumption has increased slightly
- By eighth grade, almost 70% of adolescents state that they have tried alcohol at least once; the average age of first use is 14 years
- Abuse varies markedly based on cultural and ethnic groups; white, Native American, and Hispanic high school seniors reportedly drink the most (45–48% of boys drink heavily); by comparison, only 19% of Asian-Americans and 24% of black high school seniors drink heavily
- Alcohol consumption is highest between 18 and 34 years of age when about 62% of individuals report using alcohol during the last month
- Almost half of all fatal traffic accidents involve alcohol
- Drinking also contributes to a large percentage of deaths from falls, fires or burns, and drownings

Data from Robert Wood Johnson Foundation. (1993). *Substance Abuse: The Nation's Number One Health Problem.* Waltham, MA, Institute for Health Policy, Brandeis University.

SIGNS AND SYMPTOMS OF SUBSTANCE ABUSE

Nurses should also be aware of the signs and symptoms that might indicate use and/or abuse of alcohol and other drugs. To help nurses recognize these symptoms of substance use and withdrawal and identify appropriate treatment, Table 17–17 describes each. Tables 17–18 and 17–19 present the diagnostic criteria for substance dependence and substance abuse, respectively.

TABLE 17–15 **Fast Facts About the Use and Abuse of Illicit Drugs**

- Drug abuse costs U. S. residents about $67 billion annually; in contrast to alcohol abuse, much of the costs of illicit drug use are from costs related to crime, property destruction, and public attempts to control their use
- The use of illicit drugs has declined rather substantially; in the late 1970s, almost 40% of high school seniors reported using drugs compared with 14% in 1992; marijuana use among those 18–25 years of age peaked at 35% in 1979 and fell to 13% in 1991; likewise, cocaine use peaked in 1979 at 13% and dropped to 2% in 1991
- Males are more than three times as likely as females to be heavy drinkers and more than twice as likely to use marijuana weekly; males and females are equally likely to use cocaine
- At least half of all people arrested for major crimes (homicide, theft, assault) were using illicit drugs at the time of their arrest
- Deaths from illicit drugs are often from a combination of two or more illicit drugs or drugs combined with alcohol; heroin or cocaine is involved in two thirds of drug deaths; almost 40% of illicit drug deaths are among adults between 30 and 39 years (perhaps indicating chronic problems due to drug abuse); blacks are more than twice as likely to die from the direct effects of illicit drugs as whites
- More than 33% of new AIDS cases occur among injecting drug users or people having sexual contact with them
- Among convicted inmates, 84% of women reported they had used illicit drugs at some time, and 40% reported daily use; for those arrested for prostitution, 85% tested positive for illicit drugs, and 65% of women arrested for homicide tested positive for illicit drugs
- In contrast, men most likely to be under the influence were arrested for drug sale or possession (80%) or larceny or theft (65%)

Data from Robert Wood Johnson Foundation. (1993). *Substance Abuse: The Nation's Number One Health Problem.* Waltham, MA, Institute for Health Policy, Brandeis University.

TREATMENT FOR SUBSTANCE ABUSE

An estimated 18 million people who use alcohol and other drugs are in need of treatment, and less than one fourth will get it. Unlike health care for other conditions, most of the funding for drug and alcohol treatment facilities comes from federal block grants and state and local government funds. Private insurance, Medicaid, and other public insurance programs contribute less than a third of the total funding for treatment.

Substance abuse treatment is effective for many people, and most people need some kind of treatment to recover from substance abuse (Plumlee, 1995). The key to effective treatment is to match the client's needs with the intervention strategy most appropriate for him or her (Robert Wood Johnson Foundation, 1993).

The vast majority of clients in alcohol and/or drug treatment programs are outpatients. Alcohol and drug treatment services are provided by family practitioners, internists, psychiatrists, and other medical specialists and in emergency rooms.

Self-help groups are an important part of recovery for many. The most common models of treatment consist of education and participation in "12-step" groups (Plumlee, 1995).

Education

Intense and ongoing education about the disease of alcoholism or other drug addiction to break the abuser's denial may be helpful, including

- Initiation of the Twelve Steps of Alcoholics Anonymous (AA)
- Required reading of literature from AA or Narcotics Anonymous (NA) (as appropriate)
- Attendance at the meeting of AA or NA
- Skill building to maintain abstinence

Twelve-Step Groups

Participation in 12-step groups (e.g., NA and AA) gives social support and structure that assists in

TABLE 17–16 **Risk Factors for Alcohol and Other Drug Abuse by Stage of Life**

Childhood
- Fetal exposure to alcohol and other drugs (AOD)
- Parents who are substance abusers
- Physical, sexual, or psychological abuse
- Economic disadvantage
- Delinquency
- Mental health problems such as depression and suicidal ideation
- Disability

Adolescence
- AOD use by parents
- Low self-esteem
- Depression
- Psychological distress
- Poor relationship with parents
- Low sense of social responsibility
- Lack of religious commitment
- Low academic performance and motivation
- Peer use of AOD
- Participation in deviant, aggressive behavior

Young Adulthood
- Exposure to drug users in social and work environments
- Marital and work instability
- Unemployment
- Divorce
- Psychological or psychiatric difficulties

Middle Adulthood
- Bereavement, especially as a result of loss of spouse or significant other
- Adverse work conditions or unemployment
- Changes in health status or appearance
- Socioeconomic stressors
- Environmental changes or relocation
- Divorce, separation, or remarriage
- Difficulties with children or changes in child-rearing responsibilities

Older Adulthood
- Retirement or role status change
- Loss of loved ones
- Changes in health status and mobility
- Increased sensitivity to effects of alcohol and other drugs
- Housing relocations
- Affective changes (e.g., anxiety and depression)
- History of previous misuse or abuse of AOD
- Solitude or social contexts that foster use of AOD
- Negative self-concept

From U. S. Office of Substance Abuse Prevention. (1992). *Nurse Training Course: Alcohol and Other Drug Abuse Prevention.* Rockville, MD, National Training System, U. S. Public Health Service.

the recovery process. Nurses who are in a position to identify those in need of these services should be knowledgeable about these programs and ready to supply information and referral. To this end, Table 17–20 shows the Twelve Steps of AA. Further information can be obtained by contacting local programs or national offices (see Table 17–28).

Suicide

Suicide is the most serious potential outcome of mental disorders and is the ninth leading cause of death in the United States. Each year, more than 30,000 United States residents take their own lives (USDHHS, 1995). Depression, schizophrenia, panic disorder, and alcohol and other drug abuse have been implicated in both attempted and completed suicides (USDHHS, 1990). Table 17–21 lists some statistics regarding suicide of which the nurse in community-based practice should be aware.

One trend that is of particular concern is the steady increase in suicide among all youth 15 to 25 years of age since the 1950s. Suicide is now the third leading cause of death in that age group. In other age groups, suicide is also a significant

TABLE 17–17 **Signs of Intoxication, Indications of Withdrawal, and Treatment Modalities for Selected Psychoactive Substances**

Substance	Signs of Intoxication	Indications of Withdrawal	Treatment Modalities
Alcohol	Decreased alertness, impaired judgment, slurred speech, nausea, double vision, vertigo, staggering, unpredictable emotional changes, stupor, unconsciousness, increased reaction time	Anxiety, insomnia, tremors, delirium, convulsions	Detoxification, psychotherapy, group therapy, family therapy, self-help groups (AA, Al-Anon), pharmacological therapy, residential programs, referral for vocational rehabilitation and social services as needed
Sedatives, hypnotics, anxiolytics	Slurred speech, slow, shallow respiration, cold and clammy skin, nystagmus, weak and rapid pulse, drowsiness, blurred vision, unconsciousness, disorientation, depression, poor judgment, motor impairment	Anxiety, insomnia, tremors, delirium, convulsions (may occur up to 2 weeks after stopping use of anxiolytics)	Detoxification, psychotherapy, and group therapy (for underlying psychiatric disorders)
Opioids	Sedation, hypertension, respiratory depression, impaired intellectual function, constipation, pupillary constriction, watery eyes, increased pulse and blood pressure	Restlessness, irritability, tremors, loss of appetite, panic, chills, sweating, cramps, watery eyes, runny nose, nausea, vomiting, muscle spasms, impaired coordination, depressed reflexes, dilated pupils, yawning	Pharmacological therapy (methadone, opioid antagonists), therapeutic communities (Synanon, Odyssey House, Phoenix House), group therapy, assistance with social skills, vocational training and job placement, family therapy, self-help groups (NA, Chemical Dependency Anonymous), psychotherapy
Cocaine	Irritability; anxiety; slow, weak pulse; slow, shallow breathing; sweating; dilated pupils; increased blood pressure; insomnia; seizures; dysinhibition; impulsivity; compulsive actions; hypersexuality; hypervigilance; hyperactivity	*Early crash:* agitation, depression, anorexia, high level of craving, suicidal ideation *Middle crash:* fatigue, depression, no craving, insomnia *Late crash:* exhaustion, hypersomnolence, hyperphagia, no craving *Early withdrawal;* normal sleep and mood, low craving, low anxiety *Middle and late withdrawal:* anhedonia, anxiety anergy, high level of craving exacerbated by conditioned cues *Extinction:* normal hedonic response and mood, episodic craving triggered by conditioned cues	Hospitalization, self-help groups, contingency contracting (client agreement to urinary monitoring and acceptance of aversive contingencies for positive results), pharmacological therapy (tricyclic antidepressants)

Table continued on following page

Amphetamines	Sweating, dilated pupils, increased blood pressure, agitation, fever, irritability, headache, chills, insomnia, agitation, tremors, seizures, wakefulness, hyperactivity, confusion, paranoia	Fatigue, hunger, long period of sleep, disorientation, severe depression	No established treatment guidelines; may be similar to treatment for cocaine abuse
Hallucinogens	Dilated pupils, mood swings, elevated blood pressure, paranoia, bizarre behavior, nausea, and vomiting, tremors, panic, flushing, fever, sweating, agitation, aggression, nystagmus (with phencyclidine)	Slight irritability, restlessness, insomnia, reduced energy level, depression	Detoxification, psychotherapy (for underlying psychiatric disorders), group therapy, residential programs
Cannabis (marijuana, hashish)	Reddened eyes; increased pulse, respiration, and blood pressure; laughter; confusion; panic; drowsiness	Insomnia, hyperactivity, decreased appetite	Same as for hallucinogens, self-help groups
Inhalants	Giddiness, drowsiness, increased vital signs, headache, nausea, fainting, stupor, fatigue, slurred speech, disorientation, delirium	None reported	Psychosocial interventions, psychotherapy (for underlying psychiatric disorder), sociodrama, vocational rehabilitation, family therapy, social support services
Nicotine	Headache; loss of appetite; nausea; increased pulse, blood pressure, and muscle tone	Nervousness, increased appetite, sleep disturbances, anxiety, irritability	Aversive conditioning, desensitization, substitution, hypnotherapy, group therapy, relaxation training, supportive therapy, abrupt abstinence

Adapted from Clark, M. J. (1996). Substance abuse. In M. J. Clark (Ed.). *Nursing in the Community,* (2nd ed.). Stamford, CT; Appleton & Lange, pp. 807–837.

TABLE 17–18 Diagnotic Criteria for Substance Dependence

A maladaptive pattern of substance use, leading to clinically significant impairment or distress, as manifested by three (or more) of the following, occurring at any time in the same 12-month period:

1. Tolerance, as defined by either of the following:
   a. A need for markedly increased amounts of the substance to achieve intoxication or desired effect
   b. Markedly diminished effect with continued use of the same amount of the substance
2. Withdrawal, as manifested by either of the following:
   a. The characteristc withdrawal syndrome for the substance (refer to criteria A and B of the criteria sets for withdrawal from the specific substances)
   b. The same (or a closely related) substance is taken to relieve or avoid withdrawal symptoms
3. The substance is often taken in larger amounts or over a longer period than was intended
4. There is a persistent desire or unsuccessful effort to cut down or control substance use
5. A great deal of time is spent in activities necessary to obtain the substance (e.g., chain-smoking), or recover from its effects
6. Important social, occupational, or recreational activities are given up or reduced because of substance use
7. The substance use is continued despite knowledge of having a persistent or recurrent physical or psychological problem that is likely to have been caused or exacerbated by the substance (e.g., current cocaine use despite recognition of cocaine-induced depression, or continued drinking despite recognition that an ulcer was made worse by alcohol consumption)

Specifiy if

With physiological dependence: evidence of tolerance or withdrawal (i.e., either item 1 or 2 is present)
Without physiological dependence: no evidence of tolerance or withdrawal (i.e., neither item 1 nor 2 is present)

Reprinted with permission from the *Diagnostic and Statistical Manual of Mental Disorders, Fourth Edition.* Copyright 1994 American Psychiatric Association.

TABLE 17–19 Diagnostic Criteria for Substance Abuse

A. A maladaptive pattern of substance use leading to clinically significant impairment or distress, as manifested by one (or more) or the following, occurring within a 12-month period:
   1. Recurrent substance use resulting in a failure to fulfill major role obligations at work, school, or home (e.g., repeated absences or poor work performance related to substance use; substance-related absences, suspensions, or expulsions from school; neglect of children or household)
   2. Recurrent substance use in situations in which it is physically hazardous (e.g., driving an automobile or operating a machine when impaired by substance use)
   3. Recurrent substance-related legal problems (e.g., arrests for substance-related disorderly conduct)
   4. Continued substance use despite having persistent or recurrent social or interpersonal problems caused or exacerbated by the effects of the substance (e.g., arguments with spouse about consequences of intoxication, physical fights)

B. The symptoms have never met the criteria for substance dependence for this class of substance

Reprinted with permission from the *Diagnostic and Statistical Manual of Mental Disorders, Fourth Edition.* Copyright 1994 American Psychiatric Association.

TABLE 17–20 **The Twelve Steps of Alcoholics Anonymous**

1. Admitted we were powerless over alcohol—that our lives had become unmanageable
2. Came to believe that a Power greater than ourselves could restore us to sanity
3. Made a decision to turn our will and our lives over to the care of God *as we understood Him*
4. Made a searching and fearless moral inventory of ourselves
5. Admitted to God, to ourselves, and to another human being the exact nature of our wrongs
6. Were entirely ready to have God remove all these defects of character
7. Humbly asked Him to remove our shortcomings
8. Made a list of all persons we had harmed and became willing to make amends to them all
9. Made direct amends to such people wherever possible, except when to do so would injure them or others
10. Continued to take personal inventory and, when we were wrong, promptly admitted it
11. Sought through prayer and meditation to improve our conscious contact with God *as we understood Him,* praying only for knowledge of His will for us and the power to carry that out
12. Having had a spiritual awakening as the result of these steps, we tried to carry this message to alcoholics, and to practice these principles in all our affairs

The Twelve Steps are reprinted with permission of Alcoholics Anonymous World Services, Inc. Permission to reprint this material does not mean that AA has reviewed or approved the contents of this publication, nor that AA agrees with the views expressed herein. AA is a program of recovery from alcoholism—use of the Twelve Steps in connection with programs and activities which are patterned after AA, but which address other problems, does not imply otherwise.

cause of death. In 1990, 265 children 10 to 14 years of age and 4,750 people 15 to 24 years of age committed suicide. Table 17–22 shows the change in suicide rates for adolescents and young adults over the past four decades. As this table illustrates, rates have been rising alarmingly, particularly in males.

Risk factors for adolescent suicide include a strong family history of psychiatric disorders (e.g., depression or suicidal behavior), previous suicide attempts, serious medical illness, family violence, alcohol and other drug abuse, and accessibility to firearms (USDHHS/ODPHP, 1994). To combat the high rates of suicide among adolescents and young adults, the National Center for Injury Prevention and Control outlined general recommendations, which are listed in Table 17–23.

Identification of Mental Disorders

Whether the nurse is working in a physician's office, a clinic, home health, a school, occupational health, or another setting, recognition of signs and symptoms that might indicate a mental disorder is an important component of practice. For example, a student might come to the school nurse's office concerned about a "friend" who induces vomiting in the bathroom after lunch each day; an occupational health nurse might observe signs consistent with alcohol abuse in an employee; or a patient might visit a clinic for a routine visit but mention that for the last several weeks she has been unable to sleep, has lost several pounds, and is no longer interested in her normal activities. In each of these situations, the nurse should continue to assess for other signs and symptoms that might indicate a mental disorder and be prepared to intervene should concerns be supported.

Often, the assessment process includes direct questioning or observation. At other times, a standardized assessment tool or questionnaire might be employed. Tables 17–24 through 17–26 contain examples of instruments that are available to elicit information about symptoms of anxiety or depression or conditions such as alcohol abuse. However, whenever using these or other screening tools, the nurse should be prepared *in advance* to intervene based on assessment data. Very frequently, this involves referral to other health pro-

TABLE 17–21 **Suicide Facts**

Completed Suicides (United States, 1993)

- Suicide is the ninth leading cause of death in the United States, accounting for 1.4% of all deaths (in contrast, 33% of deaths are from heart disease, 23% are from cancer, and 6.6% are from cerebrovascular disease—the three leading causes)
- More men than women die by suicide
  - The gender ratio is more than 4:1
  - More than 72% of all suicides are committed by white men
  - Nearly 80% of all firearm suicides are committed by white men
- The highest suicide rates are for persons older than 65 years (rate 73.6/100,000)
- Suicide is the third leading cause of death among young people 15–24 years of age (following unintentional injuries and homicide); in this age group.
  - The rate was 13.2/100,000 in 1993 (up from 13.0 in 1992)
  - The total number of deaths in 1993 was 4,849
  - The gender ratio was 5.5:1.0 (men:women)

Risk Factors (Frequently Occur in Combination)

- Almost all people who kill themselves have a diagnosable mental or substance abuse disorder; the majority have more than one disorder
- Adverse life events in combination with other strong risk factors (mental or substance abuse disorders and impulsivity) may lead to suicide
- Familial factors in highly dysfunctional families can be associated with suicide
  - Family history of mental or substance abuse disorder
  - Family history of suicide
  - Family violence, including emotional, physical, or sexual abuse
- Prior suicide attempt
- Firearm in the home
- Incarceration
- Exposure to the suicidal behavior of others (e.g., family members, peers, and/or the media in news or fiction stories)

Attempted Suicides

- There are an estimated 8–25 attempted suicides to one completion; the ratio is higher in women and youth and lower in men and the elderly
- More women than men report a history of attempted suicide (gender ratio 2:1)
- The strongest risk factors for attempted suicide in youth are depression, alcohol or other drug use disorder, and aggressive or disruptive behaviors
- The majority of suicide attempts are expressions of extreme distress that need to be addressed and not just a harmless bid for attention

Prevention

- Because suicide is a highly complex behavior, preventive interventions must also be complex and intensive to have lasting effects
- Recognition of mental and substance abuse disorders and appropriate treatment are the most promising ways to prevent suicide in older persons
- Limiting young people's access to firearms and other forms of responsible firearm ownership, especially in conjunction with the prevention of mental and addictive disorders, may be beneficial for prevention of firearm suicides
- School-based, information-only prevention programs focusing on suicide may actually increase distress in the young people who are most vulnerable
- School and community prevention programs designed to address suicide as part of a broader focus on mental health (e.g., incorporating coping skills in response to stress, substance abuse, aggressive behaviors) are most likely to be successful

Adapted from National Institute of Mental Health. (1996). *Suicide Facts.* Rockville, MD, National Institute of Mental Health.

TABLE 17–22 **Suicide Rates* for Persons 15–24 Years of Age, by Age Group and Sex—United States, 1950, 1960, 1980, and 1990**

Age Group (Years)	Sex	Year				
		1950	*1960*	*1970*	*1980*	*1990*
15–19	Male	3.5	5.6	8.8	13.8	18.1
	Female	1.8	1.6	2.9	3.0	3.7
	Total	2.7	3.6	5.9	8.5	11.1
20–24	Male	9.3	11.5	19.2	26.8	25.7
	Female	3.3	2.9	5.6	5.5	4.1
	Total	6.2	7.1	12.2	16.1	15.1
15–24	Male	6.5	8.2	13.5	20.2	22.0
	Female	2.6	2.2	4.2	4.3	3.9
	Total	4.5	5.2	8.8	12.3	13.2

*Per 100,000 persons.

From Centers for Disease Control and Prevention. (1994). Programs for the prevention of suicide among adolescents and young adults, *Morbidity and Mortality Weekly Report, 43*(RR-6).

fessionals for further assessment, testing, counseling, and treatment. The nurse who suspects that a student has an eating disorder can talk with his or her parents and teachers, the school counselor and principal, and others to determine the best course of action to follow up on assessment findings and associated concerns. If a client describes signs and symptoms consistent with depression, the nurse should chart the reported information and explain to the patient's physician the comments that were voiced. When an employee is suspected of alcohol abuse, the occupational nurse should follow company policy on how, when, and under what circumstances the employee and his or her supervisor should be informed of the concerns. The employee should be given information on available treatment options and support groups.

Treatment of Mental Disorders

The goals of treatment for mental illness are to reduce symptoms, improve personal and social functioning, develop and strengthen coping skills, and promote behaviors to improve the individual's life. Basic approaches to the treatment of mental disorders include pharmacotherapy, psychotherapy, and/or behavior therapy (USDHHS/Public Health Service, 1994).

PSYCHOTHERAPEUTIC MEDICATIONS

Psychotherapeutic medications do not cure mental illness; rather, they act by controlling symptoms (NIMH, 1995b). As with medications for physical health problems, the appropriateness of psychotherapeutic medications and their prescribed regimen depends on the diagnosis, side effects, and patient response. Table 17–27 lists some of the most commonly used psychotherapeutic medications. Indications and adverse effects and nursing implications for the different types of medications are briefly discussed.

Antipsychotic medications are used to reduce symptoms of schizophrenia. Most antipsychotic medications are *neuroleptics*. Neuroleptics are quite effective but may produce a number of side effects. The most common side effects are drowsiness, tachycardia, orthostatic hypotension, weight gain, photosensitivity, and menstrual irregularities. Often, side effects diminish after a few weeks.

TABLE 17–23 Examples of Suicide Prevention Programs and General Recommendations on Prevention of Suicide Among Adolescents and Young Adults

Suicide Prevention Programs

- School gatekeeper training—school staff are taught to identify and refer students at risk for suicide
- Community gatekeeper training—community members (e.g., clergy, police, recreation staff) and clinical health care providers who see adolescent patients are trained to identify and refer persons who are at risk for suicide
- General suicide education—students are taught about suicide, including warning signs and how to seek help for themselves or others
- Screening programs—questionnaires or other screening instruments are used to identify high-risk adolescents and young adults and provide further assessment and treatment
- Peer support programs—peer relationships and competency in social skills among high-risk adolescents and young adults are encouraged
- Crisis centers and hotlines—trained volunteers and paid staff provide telephone counseling and other services for suicidal persons
- Restriction of access to lethal means—activities and programs that restrict access to handguns, drugs, and other common means of suicide are encouraged
- Intervention after a suicide—focus on friends and relatives of persons who have committed suicide to help prevent or contain suicide clusters and help adolescents and young adults cope effectively with feelings of loss that follow the sudden death or suicide of a peer

Suicide Prevention Recommendations

- Ensure that suicide prevention programs are linked as closely as possible with professional mental health resources in the community
- Avoid reliance on one prevention strategy—use of more than one of the types of programs detailed above is recommended
- Expand suicide prevention efforts for young adults
- Incorporate evaluation efforts into suicide prevention programs

From Centers for Disease Control and Prevention. (1994). Programs for the prevention of suicide among adolescents and young adults, *Morbidity and Mortality Weekly Report, 43*(RR-6), 3–8.

More serious adverse effects of neuroleptics include "extrapyramidal reactions" (movement disorders resulting from the effect of the drug on the extrapyramidal motor system) (Lehne and Scott, 1996). Acute dystonia (characterized by spasms or cramping of the muscles of the tongue, face, neck, or back), parkinsonism (including bradykinesia, masklike face, drooling, tremor, rigidity, shuffling gait), and akathisia (restlessness characterized by constant pacing and squirming) are extrapyramidal reactions sometimes seen early in treatment with antipsychotic drugs (Lehne and Scott, 1996; Pennebaker and Riley, 1995). These adverse effects tend to decrease with time or can be managed with other medications (e.g., antiparkinsonian agents).

The most serious extrapyramidal adverse effect of use of antipsychotic agents, however, is tardive dyskinesia. Tardive dyskinesia develops in 20 to 40% of patients during long-term therapy and produces involuntary movement of the tongue and face. Eating difficulty and weight loss may result. Tardive dyskinesia is permanent, although some symptoms decline after the dosage is reduced or the drug withdrawn (Lehne and Scott, 1996).

Clozapine (Clozaril) and risperidone (Risperdal) are termed "atypical neuroleptics." These are relatively new medications that have been shown to be more effective than traditional antipsychotic medications for some people with schizophrenia. These medications have less risk of extrapyramidal side effects, including tardive dyskinesia, than other antipsychotics. Other complications or adverse effects are possible, however. Clozapine,

TABLE 17–24 **Center for Epidemiologic Studies Depression Scale**

During the Past Week	Rarely or None of the Time (Less than 1 Day)	Some or a Little of the Time (1–2 Days)	Occasionally or a Moderate Amount of the Time (3–4 Days)	Most or All of the Time (5–7 Days)
1. I was bothered by things that don't usually bother me.	0	1	2	3
2. I did not feel like eating; my appetite was poor.	0	1	2	3
3. I felt that I could not shake off the blues even with the help of my family or friends.	0	1	2	3
4. I felt that I was just as good as other people.	3	2	1	0
5. I had trouble keeping my mind on what I was doing.	0	1	2	3
6. I felt depressed.	0	1	2	3
7. I felt everything I did was an effort.	0	1	2	3
8. I felt hopeful about the future.	3	2	1	0
9. I thought my life had been a failure.	0	1	2	3
10. I felt fearful.	0	1	2	3
11. My sleep was restless.	0	1	2	3
12. I was happy.	3	2	1	0
13. I talked less than usual.	0	1	2	3
14. I felt lonely.	0	1	2	3
15. People were unfriendly.	0	1	2	3
16. I enjoyed life.	3	2	1	0
17. I had crying spells.	0	1	2	3
18. I felt sad.	0	1	2	3
19. I felt that people disliked me.	0	1	2	3
20. I could not get "going."	0	1	2	3

Interpretation: A total score of 22 or higher is indicative of depression when this scale is used in primary care.

From Radloff, L. S. (1977). The CES-D scale: A self-report depression scale for research in the general population. *Applied Psychologic Measurement.* 1;385–401.

TABLE 17–25 **Social Readjustment Rating Scale***

Rank	Life Event	Mean Value	Rank	Life Event	Mean Value
1	Death of spouse	100	23	Son or daughter leaving home	29
2	Divorce	73	24	Trouble with in-laws	29
3	Marital separation	65	25	Outstanding personal achievement	28
4	Jail term	63	26	Wife begins or stops work	26
5	Death of close family member	63	27	Begin or end school	26
6	Personal injury or illness	53	28	Change in living conditions	25
7	Marriage	50	29	Change in personal habits	24
8	Fired at work	47	30	Trouble with boss	23
9	Marital reconciliation	45	31	Change in work hours or conditions	20
10	Retirement	45	32	Change in residence	20
11	Change in health of family member	44	33	Change in schools	20
12	Pregnancy	40	34	Change in recreation	19
13	Sex difficulties	39	35	Change in church activities	19
14	Gain of new family member	39	36	Change in social activities	18
15	Business readjustment	39	37	Mortgage or loan less than $10,000	17
16	Change in financial state	38	38	Change in sleeping habits	16
17	Death of close friend	37	39	Change in number of family get-to-gethers	15
18	Change to different line of work	36	40	Change in eating habits	15
19	Change in number of arguments with spouse	35	41	Vacation	13
20	Mortgage over $10,000	31	42	Christmas	12
21	Foreclosure on mortgage or loan	30	43	Minor violations of the law	11
22	Change in responsibilities at work	29			

Life Crisis Categories and LCU Scores*

No life crisis	0–149
Mild life crisis	150–199
Moderate life crisis	200–299
Major life crisis	300 or more

*The LCU score includes those life event items experienced during a 1-year period. Reprinted by permission of the publisher from Holmes, T. H., and Rahe, R. H. (1967). The Social Readjustment Rating Scale, *Journal of Psychosomatic Research, 11.* Copyright 1967 by Elsevier Science Inc.

the most commonly used atypical neuroleptic, is known to cause agranulocytosis in 1 to 2% of patients. Because this condition is potentially fatal, persons on Clozapine must have *weekly* white blood cell counts performed to assess for signs of agranulocytosis. Treatment is stopped if the white blood cell count is below 3,000 or the granulocyte count is under 1,500. Risperidone, the newest atypical neuroleptic, was introduced in 1994 and has fewer side effects and no reported cases of agranulocytosis (Lehne and Scott, 1996).

Antimanic Medications

Lithium is the most frequently used medication for treatment of bipolar disorders. Response to treatment with lithium varies somewhat between individual patients. In addition, the range between an effective dose and a toxic dose is small, so serum lithium levels must be monitored closely. It is recommended that levels be checked routinely at the beginning of treatment to determine the

TABLE 17–26 **The CAGE Questionnaire***

"Have you ever felt you ought to **C**ut down on drinking?"
"Have people **A**nnoyed you by criticizing your drinking?"
"Have you ever felt bad or **G**uilty about your drinking?"
"Have you ever had a drink first thing in the morning to steady your nerves or get rid of a hangover (**E**ye-opener)?"

*One "yes" response should raise suspicions of alcohol abuse. More than one "yes" response should be considered a strong indication that alcohol abuse exists.

From Ewing, J. A. (1984). Detecting alcoholism: The CAGE questionnaire. *Journal of the American Medical Association, 252*(14), 1905–1907. Copyright 1984, American Medical Assocation.

optimal maintenance dosage and every few months thereafter (NIMH, 1995b).

Side effects are often worse during the initial stage of lithium therapy and include drowsiness, weakness, nausea, vomiting, fatigue, hand tremors, increased thrust, and weight gain. Long-term lithium use may affect thyroid function; therefore, thyroid function tests should also be performed periodically.

Anticonvulsants

Occasionally, anticonvulsants are used to treat mania. The most common side effects of anticonvulsants include drowsiness, dizziness, confusion, visual disturbances, memory impairment, and nausea. Periodic blood tests are needed to monitor white blood cell counts and for anemia.

Antidepressants

Antidepressants are used most often for serious depression, but they can also be helpful for mild depression and anxiety. The choice of medications is usually based on the individual patient's symptoms. Most medications take 1 to 3 weeks before improvement is seen. If little or no change occurs in symptoms after 5 to 6 weeks, a different medication should be tried. Treatment is usually continued for a minimum of several months and may last up to a year or more.

Tricyclic antidepressants are commonly used for treatment of major depression. Side effects vary somewhat between medications and the reaction of the individual to the medication. Potential side effects include drowsiness, blurred vision, dry mouth, constipation, weight gain, orthostatic hypotension, dysuria, fatigue, and weakness. Often, side effects diminish or disappear during the course of treatment. Tricyclics may interfere with other medications and substances, including thyroid hormone, antihypertensives, oral contraceptives, sleeping medications, antipsychotic medications, diuretics, antihistamines, aspirin, vitamin C, alcohol, and tobacco.

An overdose of tricyclic antidepressant medications may produce tachycardia, dilated pupils, and flushed face. In extreme cases, overdose may cause agitation, which may progress to confusion, loss of consciousness, seizures, arrhythmias, cardiorespiratory collapse, and death (NIMH, 1995b).

Monoamine oxidase inhibitors (MAOIs) are more often used for "atypical" depression in which symptoms like anxiety, panic attacks, and phobias are present. MAOIs may cause a serious reaction with certain foods (e.g., aged cheeses, foods containing monosodium glutamate) and beverages (e.g., red wines) and medications (e.g., antihistamines, decongestants, local anesthetics, amphetamines, insulin, some narcotics, and antiparkinsonian medications). Reactions may produce hypertension, headache, nausea, vomiting, tachycardia, confusion, psychotic symptoms, seizures, stroke, and coma (NIMH, 1995b). Persons taking MAOIs should be given a list of restricted foods, beverages, and medications and encouraged to strictly comply with the restrictions.

Selective serotonin reuptake inhibitors (SSRIs) are the newest class of antidepressants available in the United States and have a more rapid onset of action than do other antidepressants. Improvement is usually seen in 1 to 3 weeks after initiation of therapy (Pennebaker and Riley, 1995). Gastrointestinal problems, headache, insomnia, anxiety, and agitation are the most common side effects of

TABLE 17–27 Psychotherapeutic Medications

Generic Name	Trade Name
Antipsychotic Medications	
Chlorpromazine	Thorazine
Chlorprothixene	Taractan
Clozapine	Clozaril
Fluphenazine	Permitil
	Prolixin
Haloperidol	Haldol
Loxapine	Loxitane
Mesoridazine	Serentil
Molindone	Moban
Perphenazine	Trilafon
Pimozide (for Tourette's syndrome)	Orap
Risperidone	
Thioridazine	
Thiothixene	Risperdal
Trifluoperazine	Mellaril
Triflupromazine	Navane
Antimanic Medications	Stelazine
	Vesprin
Carbamazepine	
Divalproex sodium	
Lithium carbonate	Tegretol
	Depakote
	Eskalith
	Lithane
	Lithobid
Lithium citrate	Cibalith-S
Antidepressant Medications	
Amitriptyline	Elavil
Amoxapine	Asendin
Bupropion	Wellbutrin
Desipramine	Norpramin
	Pertofrane
Doxepin	Adapin
	Sinequan
Clomipramine	Anafranil
Fluvoxamine (SSRI)	Luvox
Fluoxetine (SSRI)	Prozac
Imipramine	Tofranil

Generic Name	Trade Name
Antidepressant Medications *Continued*	
Isocarboxazid (MAOI)	Marplan (discontinued in 1994)
Maprotiline	Ludiomil
Nefazodone	Serzone
Nortriptyline	Aventyl
	Pamelor
Paroxetine (SSRI)	Paxil
Phenelzine (MAOI)	Nardil
Protriptyline	Vivactil
Sertraline (SSRI)	Zoloft
Tranylcypromine (MAOI)	Parnate
Trazodone	Desyrel
Trimipramine	Surmontil
Venlafaxine	Effexor
Antianxiety Medications (All of These Medications, Except Buspirone, Are Benzodiazepines)	
Alprazolam	Xanax
Buspirone	BuSpar
Chlordiazepoxide	Librax
	Libritabs
	Librium
Clorazepate	Tranxene
	Valium
Diazepam	Paxipam
Halazepam	Ativan
Lorazepam	Serax
Oxazepam	Centrax
Prazepam	
Stimulants (Given for Attention Deficit/ Hyperactivity Disorder)	
Dextroamphetamine	Dexedrine
Methylphenidate	Ritalin
Pemoline	Cylert

From National Institute of Health. (1995). *Medications.* NIH Publication No 95-3929. Rockville, MD, National Institute of Mental Health.

SSRIs. Ejaculatory delay in men and skin rashes, which may be severe, have also been noted (Lehne and Scott, 1996). In addition, SSRIs may decrease appetite.

Serious complications have resulted when SSRIs are used in conjunction with other medications. In particular, fluoxetine (Prozac) should not be combined with MAOIs and should only be used with caution with tricyclic antidepressants (Lehne and Scott, 1996). Finally, although apparently rare, suicidal thoughts and overtly violent behaviors have been traced to Prozac.

Antianxiety Medications

Benzodiazepines are medications used to treat most anxiety disorders. They have been shown to be safe and effective and have low addictive potential. The most commonly used benzodiazepines are alprazolam (Xanax), diazepam (Valium), clonazepam (Klonopin), and lorazepam (Ativan). Antianxiety medications usually act rapidly. Dosage varies greatly, depending on the symptoms and the individual's body chemistry. Common side effects include drowsiness, loss of coordination, fatigue, and mental slowing or confusion. Combination of benzodiazepines and alcohol can produce serious interactions and potentially life-threatening complications, and patients should be warned accordingly.

Stimulants

Stimulants are primarily used to treat symptoms of ADHD and narcolepsy. The most common side effects are decreased appetite and difficulty in falling asleep. Some children report gastrointestinal problems, headache, and depression. Growth retardation has been documented in some children, and careful, ongoing assessment of growth patterns is recommended while children are taking stimulants.

PSYCHOTHERAPY

"Psychotherapies rely primarily on structured conversation aimed at changing a patient's attitudes, feelings, beliefs, defenses, personality, and behavior. The therapist's procedures vary across schools of psychotherapy and with the nature of the patient's problem" (Sharfstein et al., 1995, p. 237). Psychotherapy is often used in conjunction with medication to treat many mental disorders. Various types of psychotherapy include (NIMH, 1994b)

- Individual or interpersonal therapy—focuses on the patient's current life and relationships within the family, social, and work environments
- Family therapy—involves discussions and problem-solving sessions with every member of a family—sometimes with the entire group, sometimes with individuals
- Couple therapy—used to develop the relationship and minimize problems through understanding how individual conflicts are expressed in the couple's interactions
- Group therapy—involves a small group of people with similar problems who, with the guidance of a therapist, discuss individual issues and help each other with problems
- Play therapy—a technique used for establishing communication and resolving problems with young children
- Cognitive therapy—works to identify and correct distorted thought patterns that can lead to troublesome feelings and behaviors; often combined with behavioral therapy

Short-term psychotherapy is often used when situational stresses (e.g., death in the family, divorce, physical illness) produce problems. In these cases, therapy may only last a few weeks or months, with the goal of helping the individual resolve the problem as quickly as possible. Long-term therapy may last for several months to several years and emphasize underlying problems that started in childhood (NIMH, 1994b).

BEHAVIORAL THERAPY

Behavioral therapy uses learning principles to change thought patterns and behaviors systematically. Behavior therapy is used to encourage the

TABLE 17–28 **Resources for Mental Health and Mental Disorders**

Mental Health/Mental Illness

Department of Health and Human Services
Public Health Service
National Institutes of Health

National Institute of Mental Health
5600 Fishers Lane
Room 7C-02
Rockville, MD 20857
(301) 443-4513

National Institute of Mental Health
Center for Mental Health Services
Office of Consumer, Family, and Public Information
National CMHS Clearinghouse
5600 Fishers Lane
Room 13-103
Rockville, MD 20857
(800) 789-CMHS (2647)

National Mental Health Assocation
1021 Prince Street
Alexandria, VA 22314-2971
(703) 684-7722
(800) 969-NMHA (6642)

American Psychiatric Association
1400 K Street, NW, Suite 1101
Washington, D. C. 20005
(202) 682-6000

American Psychological Association
750 First Street, NE
Washington, D. C. 20002-4242
(202) 336-5500

American Psychiatric Nurses' Association
1200 19th Street, NW, Suite 300
Washington, D. C. 20036
(202) 857-1133

National Association of Social Workers
750 First Street, NE, Suite 700
Washington, D. C. 20002-4241
(202) 408-8600
(800) 638-8799

Depression

National Institute of Mental Health
Depression Awareness, Recognition, and Treatment Program (D/ART)
5600 Fishers Lane
Room 10-85
Rockville, MD 20857
(301) 443-4140
(800) 421-4211

National Depressive and Manic Depressive Association
730 North Franklin Street
Suite 501
Chicago, IL 60610
(312) 642-0049

Depression and Related Affective Disorders Association
Meyer 3-181
600 North Wolfe Street
Baltimore, MD 21287-7381
(410) 955-4647

Suicide

National Adolescent Suicide Hotline
(800) 621-4000

Anxiety Disorders

Anxiety Disorders Association of America
6000 Executive Boulevard, Suite 513
Rockville, MD 20852
(301) 231-8368
(301) 231-9350

National Anxiety Foundation
3135 Custer Drive
Lexington, KY 40517-4001
(800) 755-1576

Panic Disorder Information Line
(800) 64-PANIC (72642)

Table continued on following page

TABLE 17–28 **Resources for Mental Health and Mental Disorders** *Continued*

Attention Deficit/Hyperactivity Disorder

Attention Deficit Information Network (ADIN)
475 Hillside Avenue
Needham, MA 02194
(617) 455-9895

Children and Adults with Attention Deficit Disorders (CHADD)
499 NW 70th Avenue, Suite 109
Plantation, FL 33317
(305) 587-3700

Federation of Families for Children's Mental Health
1021 Prince Street
Alexandria, VA 22314
(703) 684-7710

National Center for Learning Disabilities
99 Park Avenue, 6th Floor
New York, NY 10016
(212) 687-7211

National Information Center for Children and Youth with Disabilities
P. O. Box 1492
Washington, D. C. 20013
(800) 695-0285

Eating Disorders

American Anorexia/Bulimia Association, Inc.
418 E. 76th Street
New York, NY 10021
(212) 734-1114

Anorexia Nervosa and Related Eating Disorders, Inc.
P. O. Box 5102
Eugene, OR 97405
(503) 344-1144

National Anorexic Aid Society
1925 East Dublin-Granville Road
Columbus, OH 43229
(614) 436-1112

National Association of Anorexia Nervosa and Associated Disorders
P. O. Box 7
HIghland Park, IL 60035
(708) 831-3438

Alcohol and Drug Abuse

Public Health Service
Substance Abuse and Mental Health Services Administration
National Clearinghouse for Alcohol and Drug Information
P. O. Box 2345
Rockville, MD 200847-2345
(800) 729-6686

National Institutes of Health

National Institute on Alcohol Abuse and Alcoholism
5600 Fishers Lane
Rockville, MD 20857
(301) 443-3885

National Institute on Drug Abuse
5600 Fishers Lane
Rockville, MD 20857
(301) 443-6480

National Drug and Alcohol Treatment Hotline
(800) 662-HELP

Cocaine Hotline
(800) COCAINE (262-2463)

Alcoholics Anonymous World Services
475 Riverside Drive
Grand Central Station
New York, NY 10163
(212) 870-3400

Narcotics Anonymous
P. O. Box 9999
Van Nuys, CA 91409
(818) 780-3951

Al-Anon
Family Group Headquarters
Midtown Station
New York, NY 10018
(212) 302-7240

Miscellaneous

Gamblers Anonymous
(800) 472-0443

individual to learn specific skills to obtain rewards and satisfaction. Stress management, biofeedback, and relaxation training are examples of behavior therapy (NIMH, 1994b).

SUMMARY

As discussed throughout this chapter, mental disorders are very common and are most often identified and treated in community settings. Therefore, all nurses who work in the community should be knowledgeable about risk factors, as well as signs and symptoms that might indicate a mental disorder, and be prepared to intervene. This chapter has described some of the more common mental disorders, including assessment of risk factors and symptoms, overview of diagnostic criteria, and basic treatment regimens.

To assist nurses in gaining more information on any of the topics covered, Table 17–28 lists a number of resources. In addition to these resources, the nurse in community-based practice is strongly encouraged to develop a list of area individuals, groups, agencies, and organizations that provide services for persons with mental disorders and their families.

Brochures and teaching materials are available free of charge from many organizations listed, and a supply of appropriate materials can be made available for all who come in contact with the health care provider. For example, a school nurse can display brochures on eating disorders, depression in teenagers, and prevention of alcohol and drug abuse in adolescents in or near the school clinic. Likewise, a variety of educational materials describing threats to mental health and mental disorders should be easily available in work site settings and primary care clinics. These measures can help to demystify mental illness and assist those who need treatment to seek out care.

Key Points

- *Mental health* refers to the absence of mental disorders as well as the ability of an individual to negotiate the daily challenges and social interactions of life without experiencing cognitive, emotional, or behavioral dysfunction.
- Approximately 75% of patient care for mental disorders occurs in community-based settings. Providers include physicians, psychologists, counselors, clergy, and laypersons. Settings for care include outpatient departments, mental health centers and clinics, alcohol and drug units, emergency departments, family or social service agencies, crisis centers, and volunteer services (self-help programs).
- Depression affects about 15 million people in the United States each year. Nurses in community-based practice should be aware of risk factors and symptoms of depression and routinely assess those in high-risk groups. Treatment for depression includes pharmacological therapy, electroconvulsive therapy, behavior therapy, and/or psychotherapy.
- Anxiety disorders are the most common mental disorder, affecting up to 9% of the general population. The most common anxiety disorders are GAD (chronic, unrealistic, and exaggerated worry), panic disorder (sometimes accompanied by agoraphobia), phobias, OCD, and PTSD. Anxiety disorders are treated with antidepressants, antianxiety medications, behavior therapy, and psychotherapy.
- Eating disorders are becoming increasingly prevalent in the United States. Bulimia is characterized by binge eating and "purging" (self-induced vomiting, use of laxatives, diuretics, fasting, and excessive exercise). Individuals with anorexia nervosa are obsessed with a fear of fat and with losing weight. Anorexia and

bulimia usually develop during adolescence. Nurses who work with adolescents and young adults should be aware of the signs and symptoms of eating disorders and screen those considered to be "at risk." Treatment includes counseling, psychotherapy, and behavior modification.

- Attention deficit hyperactivity disorder affects 3 to 5% of all children and is characterized by inattention, hyperactivity, and impulsivity. A diagnosis of ADD or ADHD should be made following a comprehensive physical, psychological, social, and behavioral evaluation to rule out other possible reasons for the behavior. ADHD is usually managed through a combination of behavior therapy, emotional counseling, practical support, and medication.
- A number of legal and illegal substances used by Americans are potentially harmful. Alcoholism is the greatest drug problem in the United States today. Illicit drugs used include opioids (e.g, heroin, morphine), cocaine, amphetamines, hallucinogens, marijuana, and inhalants. Nurses in community-based settings should be aware of risk factors of substance abuse, signs of intoxication and withdrawal, and treatment of the most common psychoactive substances and refer accordingly.
- Suicide is the most serious potential outcome of mental disorders and is the ninth leading cause of death in the United States. Risk factors for suicide include a family history of psychiatric disorders, previous suicide attempts, serious medical illness, family violence, alcohol and other drug abuse, and accessibility to firearms.
- Treatment of mental disorders includes use of psychotherapeutic medications (e.g., antipsychotics, antimanics, anticonvulsant medications, antidepressants, antianxiety medications, and stimulants), psychotherapy, and behavior therapy.

Learning Activities and Application to Practice

In Class

- Invite a guest speaker from an area mental health center. Ask the speaker to share information on the most commonly encountered mental health problems and how they are managed. Include signs and symptoms that might indicate a mental disorder and how to refer a client for help. Conclude with strategies and interventions on how to promote mental health within the community.
- Divide students into groups of four to six and assign each group one of the commonly encountered mental health problems described in this chapter (e.g., depression, anxiety disorders, eating disorders, substance abuse). Encourage each group to discuss if they have encountered the problem in practice and if so describe how the problem was identified and treated. Have each group devise primary, secondary, and tertiary prevention strategies to address the mental health problem and share ideas with the class.
- Discuss the *Healthy People 2000* objectives related to "Alcohol and Other Drugs" and "Mental Health and Mental Disorders." Examine differences related to age, race/ethnic group, and gender (e.g., suicide is most common among white males; alcohol-related motor vehicle deaths for American Indians are 400% higher than for

the population as a whole). Identify factors that contribute to differences and outline strategies to address these factors.

- Discuss use of screening tools like those contained in the chapter for mental health problems such as depression or substance abuse. How and when might they be used most effectively?

In Clinical

- Assign students to identify, investigate, and visit area organizations and providers that care for persons with mental disorders or work to improve mental health. During the visit have the student learn what services are available, how services are accessed, what interventions are provided, and what the responsibilities of nurses are. Share findings with the clinical group.
- Have students identify the most common mental disorder encountered in the community-based setting to which they are assigned (e.g., if they are in elementary school—ADD; if in a high school—eating disorders or substance abuse; if working with women or elders—depression). Compile or develop materials that could be used for health education in that setting. Develop a forum to share the materials with other health professionals at the setting or with members of the group or "community" (e.g., a seminar for parents of children diagnosed with ADD/ADHD).

REFERENCES

American Psychiatric Association. (1994). Diagnostic and Statistical Manual of Mental Disorders (4th ed.). Washington, D. C., American Psychiatric Association.

Antai-Otong, D. (1995). Foundations of psychiatric nursing practice. In D. Antai-Otong (Ed.). *Psychiatric Nursing: Biological and Behavioral Concepts*. Philadelphia, W. B. Saunders, pp. 65–78.

Clark, M. J. (1996). Substance abuse. In M. J. Clark, *Nursing in the Community* (2nd ed.). Stamford, CT, Appleton & Lange, pp. 807–837.

Decker, W. A. and Freeman, M. (1996). The journey challenged by eating disorders. In V. B. Carson and E. N. Arnold (Eds.). *Mental Health Nursing: The Nurse-Patient Journey.* Philadelphia, W. B. Saunders, pp. 909–926.

Ewing, J. A. (1984). Detecting alcoholism: The CAGE questionnaire. *Journal of the American Medical Association, 252* (14), 1905–1907.

Farley, D. (1994). Eating disorders: When thinness becomes an obsession. *Current Issues in Women's Health, 2,* 33–37.

Frank, E., Karp, J. F., and Rush, A. J. (1993). Efficacy of treatments for major depression. *Psychopharmacology Bulletin, 29* (4), 457–475.

Greensberg, P. E., Stiglin, L. E., Finkelstein, S. N., and Berndt, E. R. (1993). The economic burden of depression in 1990. *Journal of Clinical Psychiatry, 54* (11), 405–418.

Holmes, T. H. and Rahe, R. H. (1967). The social readjustment rating scale. *Journal of Psychosomatic Research, 11,* 213–217.

Johnston, L. D., O'Malley, P. M., and Bachman, J. G. (1993). *National survey results on drug use from monitoring the future study, 1975–1992.* Vol I. NIH Pub. No 93–3597. Washington, D. C., Government Printing Office.

Katon, W. (1994). *Panic Disorder in the Medical Setting.* NIH Publication No 94–3482. Washington, D. C., National Institutes of Mental Health.

Lehne, R. A., and Scott, D. (1996). Psychopharmacology. In V. B. Carson and E. N. Arnold (Eds.). *Mental Health Nursing: The Nurse-Patient Journey.* Philadelphia, W. B. Saunders, pp. 523–570.

Narrow, W. E., Reiger, D. A., Rae, D. S., Manderscheid, R. W., and Locke, B. Z. (1993). Use of services by persons with mental and addictive disorders: Findings from the National Institute of Mental Health Epidemiologic Catchment Area Program. *Archives in General Psychiatry, 50*, 95–107.

National Institute of Mental Health. (1995a). *Anxiety Disorders.* NIH Publication No. 95–3879. Rockville, MD, National Institute of Mental Health.

National Institute of Mental Health. (1994a). *Attention Deficit Hyperactivity Disorder.* NIH Publication No. 94–3572. Rockville, MD, National Institute of Mental Health.

National Institute of Mental Health. (1994b). *Helpful Facts About Depressive Illnesses.* NIH Publication No. 94–3875. Rockville, MD, National Institute of Mental Health.

National Institute of Mental Health. (1995b). *Medications*. NIH Publication No. 95–3929. Rockville, MD, National Institute of Mental Health.

National Institute of Mental Health. (1996). *Suicide Facts*. Rockville, MD, National Institute of Mental Health.

National Mental Health Association. (1996). *Mental Health and You*. Alexandria, VA, National Mental Health Association.

Pennebaker, D. F. and Riley, J. (1995). Psychopharmacological therapy. In D. Antai-Otong (Ed.). *Psychiatric Nursing: Biological and Behavioral Concepts*. Philadelphia, W. B. Saunders, pp. 543–576.

Plumlee, A. A. (1995). The client with addictive behaviors. In D. Antai-Otong (Ed.). *Psychiatric Nursing: Biological and Behavioral Concepts*. Philadelphia, W. B. Saunders, pp. 357–386.

Radloff, L. S. (1977). The CES-D Scale: A self-report depression scale for research in the general population. *Applied Psychological Measurement, 1,* 385–401.

Richardson, M. (1993). Mental health services. In S. J. Williams and P. R. Torrens (Eds.). *Introduction to Health Services* (4th ed.). Albany, NY, Delmar Publishers.

Robert Wood Johnson Foundation. (1993). *Substance Abuse: The Nation's Number One Health Problem*. Waltham, MA, Institute for Health Policy, Brandeis University.

Robinson, L. (1996). The journey threatened by stress and anxiety disorders. In V. B. Carson and E. N. Arnold (Eds.). *Mental Health Nursing: The Nurse-Patient Journey*. Philadelphia, W. B. Saunders, 691–724.

Sharfstein, S. S., Stoline, A. M., and Koran, L. (1995). Mental health services. In A. R. Kovner (Ed.). *Jonas's Health Care Delivery in the United States* (5th ed.). New York, Springer Publishing Co.

Tommasini, N. R. (1995). The client with a mood disorder (depression). In D. Antai-Otong (Ed.). *Psychiatric Nursing: Biological and Behavioral Concepts*. Philadelphia, W. B. Saunders, pp. 157–190.

U. S. Department of Health and Human Services. (1990). *Healthy People 2000: National Health Promotion and Disease Prevention Objectives*. Washington, D. C., Government Printing Office.

U. S. Department of Health and Human Services. (1995). *Healthy People 2000: Midcourse Review and 1995 Revisions*. Washington, D. C., Government Printing Office.

U. S. Department of Health and Human Services/Public Health Service. (1994). *A Consumer's Guide to Mental Health Services*. NIH Publication No. 94–3585. Rockville, MD, Government Printing Office.

U. S. Department of Health and Human Services/Office of Disease Prevention and Health Promotion. (1994). *Clinician's Handbook of Preventive Services*. Washington, D. C., Government Printing Office.

Index

Note: Page numbers in *italics* refer to illustrations; page numbers followed by t refer to tables.